HEART DISEASE IN MEN

HEART DISEASE IN MEN

ALICE B. TODD
AND
MARGO H. MOSLEY
EDITORS

Nova Science Publishers, Inc.
New York

LIBRARY OF CONGRESS CATALOGING-IN-PUBLICATION DATA

Heart disease in men / Alice B. Todd and Margo H. Mosley (editors).
p. ; cm.
Includes index.
ISBN 978-1-60692-297-2 (hardcover)
1. Heart--Diseases. 2. Men--Diseases. I. Todd, Alice B. II. Mosley, Margo H.
[DNLM: 1. Heart Diseases. 2. Men's Health. WG 210 H4345 2009]
RC681.H367 2009
616.1'2--dc22

2008038154

Published by Nova Science Publishers, Inc. ✦ New York

CONTENTS

Preface		**vii**
Research and Review Studies		**1**
Chapter 1	Familial Primary Arrhythmias: Genes, Mechanisms and Treatment: Present Perspective *Z.A. Bhuiyan and A.A.M. Wilde*	**3**
Chapter 2	Syncope and Orthostatic Hypotension *Antonio Franco Folino*	**45**
Chapter 3	Using Multiple Images Post-stress to Enhance Diagnostic Accuracy of Myocardial Perfusion Imaging: The Clinical Importance of Determining Washin and Washout Indicates a Parabolic Function Between Coronary Perfusion (Blood Flow) and Cellular ("Uptake/Release") Function *Richard M. Fleming , Gordon M. Harrington and Riaz Baqir*	**75**
Chapter 4	Depression, Suicide Risk and Heart Disease in Men *Maurizio Pompili, Marco Innamorati, Ilaria Cuomo, Giovanni Manfredi, Roberto Tatarelli and David Lester*	**101**
Chapter 5	Magnetically Supported Percutaneous Coronary Interventions *Mark Patterson*	**125**
Chapter 6	Psychosocial Functioning in Adults with Congenital Heart Disease: The Same in Males as in Females? *Elisabeth H.M. van Rijen and Elisabeth M.W.J. Utens*	**145**
Chapter 7	The Use of Cardiovascular Biomarkers for the Assessment of Heart Disease in Men *David C. Gaze*	**167**
Chapter 8	Immune Responses to Heat Shock Proteins in Chronic Periodontitis and Coronary Heart Disease *A. Hasan, D. Sadoh and M. Foo*	**183**

Chapter 9	The Role of Drug Eluting Stents: Facts and Fiction 2008 *Marco Balducelli*	**201**
Chapter 10	Dose Individualization of Drugs Based on Body Composition *Michael Barras and Bruce Green*	**219**
Chapter 11	Diagnostic Clues of Etiological Investigations for Cardiomyopathy *Yasuharu Tokuda*	**243**
Chapter 12	The Role of Natriuretic Peptides in Investigation of Various Cardiovascular Diseases *K. Kotaška and R. Průša*	**259**
Chapter 13	Sex-Related Differences in Time to Surgical Revascularization and Postoperative Mortality *B. Sobolev, G. Fradet, L. Kuramoto and A. Levy*	**275**
Chapter 14	Cardiovascular Disease and Erectile Dysfunction The Evolving Role of Phosphodiesterase-5-Inhibitors *Ujjaini Khanderia and Randolph E. Regal*	**293**
Chapter 15	Congenital Heart Disease in Adults- Challenges and Management Issues *Rajesh Vijayvergiya and Puspendra Garg*	**317**
Chapter 16	Coronary Artery Surgery in Men: Risks and Outcomes *Justin D. Blasberg and Sandhya K. Balaram*	**333**
Chapter 17	Evaluation of Coronary Artery Disease by Exercise Echocardiography *Jesus Peteiro and Beatriz Bouzas*	**347**
Chapter 18	Changes in Research Focus with Time. The Oslo-Study of 1972/73 and Until Today *Lise Lund Håheim*	**365**
Chapter 19	Diabetic Nephropathy - A Ticking Cardiovascular Bomb *Ole Torffvit*	**381**
Index		**391**

PREFACE

Heart disease is an umbrella term for a number of different diseases affecting the heart. As of 2007, it is the leading cause of death in the United States,England, Canada and Wales, killing one person every 34 seconds in the United States alone.Heart disease is synonymous with cardiac disease but not with cardiovascular disease which is any disease of the heart or blood vessels. Among the many types of heart disease are, for example: Angina; Arrhythmia; Congenital heart disease; Coronary artery disease (CAD); Dilated cardiomyopathy; Heart attack (myocardial infarction); Heart failure; Hypertrophic cardiomyopathy; Mitral regurgitation; Mitral valve prolapse; and Pulmonary stenosis. This new book brings together important recent research on heart disease with a focus on men and heart disease.

As explained in Chapter 1, the Heart is a specialised organ that contracts synchronously, pumping blood to the body and to the lungs. The upper two chambers of the heart are called atria (right and left), the bottom two chambers are called ventricles (right and left). Right atrium receives deoxygenated blood from all parts of the body except for the lungs and transports them to right ventricle. The left atrium receives oxygenated blood from the lungs and transports them to the left ventricle and then to rest of the body. Cardiac excitation originates in the sinoatrial (SA) node and propagates through the atria into the atrial-ventricular (AV) node. The impulse then propagates through the Purkinje conduction system to the ventricles which then contract. The synchronized pumping action of the heart is caused by a flow of electricity through the heart that repeats itself in a cycle.

As explained in Chapter 2, syncope is a symptom, usually defined as a transient, sudden loss of consciousness and postural tone, ultimately caused by an insufficient cerebral perfusion with a critical reduction of the blood flow to the reticular activating system.

Syncope is commonly classified in 5 main forms: the neurally mediated syncope, the form characterized by the presence of an orthostatic hypotension, the episodes due to cardiac arrhythmias or structural cardiac diseases, and the vascular steal syndromes.

Each form is characterized by specific anatomical substrates and by particular pathophysiological mechanisms.

Neurally mediated syncope, is the most frequent cause of loss of consciousness. It is the result of an autonomic reflex that has as a final effect the reduction of sympathetic drive, the increase of vagal activity, and consequently bradycardia and hypotension. Also carotid sinus hypersensitivity can be one of the triggers for neurally mediated syncope.

Orthostatic hypotension is mainly caused by a primitive or secondary failure of the autonomic nervous system, unable to compensate the reduction of blood pressure during orthostatism.

Cardiac causes of syncope are principally represented by structural heart disease and arrhythmias. Both lead to syncope by a significant reduction of cardiac output.

Finally, vascular steal syndromes cause syncope when, due to a proximal obstruction of subclavian vein, the blood is deviated to the arm from the vertebral artery and the circle of Willis, inducing a cerebral hypoperfusion.

Other causes of loss of consciousness include neurologic or psychiatric disorders such as drop attacks, epilepsy, psychogenic syncope, and vertebrobasilar transient ischemic attack.

Even though most of the patients have a favorable prognosis, in some cases the limit dividing syncope from sudden death can be very narrow, particularly in patients with heart diseases. For this reason, the first diagnostic step should be oriented to an early detection of the cardiac causes of syncope. Subsequently, specific diagnostic pathways to identify other different forms of syncope are required. However, in spite of a complete assessment, in about the 20-25% of the patients the cause remains unknown.

The foremost aim of the treatment in the forms of syncope due to cardiac causes, is the reduction of mortality. In these cases an accurate screening of the patients is necessary to determine the indication to cardiac pacing or defibrillator implant.

In the other patients the aim of the treatment should be the reduction of recurrences and the improvement of the quality of life.

Myocardial perfusion imaging (MPI) has evolved over the last several decades with improvements in equipment and isotopes. Despite these advances, sensitivity and specificity of the methodology remains 65-90%. Numerous investigators have recommended changes in protocols and quantification of data to increase the diagnostic accuracy of this non-invasive physiologic test. Initial investigations have demonstrated differences in initial and delayed results post stress which have increased the ability to detect cardiomyopathies and vasospastic coronary artery disease. Chapter 3 explored MPI stress validity using early (5 minute) and delayed (60 minute) post stress imaging and findings noted on cardiac catheterization.

Methods: Records of forty-one individuals undergoing cardiac evaluation were studied for pharmacologic and exercise stress approaches with either Sestamibi or Myoview using standardized protocols. Twenty-two (54%) were diagnostically studied following MPI in the cardiac catheterization laboratory. Findings from the post stress images were used to determine washin/washout rates (WR) for total, anterior and inferior regions of myocardium and compared with findings from coronary angiography.

Results: Fifty four percent (22 of 41) of the subjects studied underwent coronary angiography. Reading of MPI dynamic images at 60 minutes post stress resulted in 9 false (FNs) negatives (41%) and 2 false (FPs) positives (9%) in the anterior myocardium. Visual reading of inferior ischemia from dynamic images lead to 9 FNs (41%) and 3 FPs (14%). Evaluation of WR from multiple images obtained at 5 and 60 minutes post stress demonstrated a significant correlation between total heart WR and the average percent diameter (%DS) stenosis ($r=0.45$, $p<0.05$) and between inferior WR and inferior %DS ($r=0.68$, $p<0.001$). There was no correlation between anterior WR and anterior %DS for individuals with washout. However, when myocardial infarction/injury (MII) was taken into account there was an improved correlation ($r=0.21$) between anterior WR and anterior %DS. When washin occurred (total, anterior or inferior) a critical stenosis was noted at or near the ostium of a major epicardial vessel supplying a "large" region of viable myocardium at risk. This study also showed a significant increase in the incidence of MII in inferior regions of the heart when compared with anterior regions. The relationship between heart to lung (H:L) ratio was negatively ($r=-0.38$, p=NS) correlated with the presence of anterior MII. The relationship between left ventricular ejection fraction (EF) and anterior washout (W. Ant) was significant ($r=0.46$, $p<0.002$).

Conclusions: Initial static (5 minute) and delayed dynamic (60 minutes) images demonstrate changes between initial and delayed imaging which cannot be accounted for on the basis of radioactive decay alone and which can be quantified as WR. Both washin and washout WR, clearly demonstrates that the uptake and release of Tc 99m compounds is an active process influenced by both myocardial ischemia and MII; although, primarily ischemia and as such can be used to not only more accurately detect ischemia compared with using the 60 minute image alone, but to also allow determination of %DS. An absence of WR is seen only with individuals who have no ischemia and no MII, viz. "normals" who were limited in this study, since the referral of such subjects did not occur in this setting. Total WR and Inferior WR were highly correlated with % DS seen on coronary angiography. These results confirm earlier findings that such information appeared to be diagnostically important in determining coronary intervention of viable myocardium supplied by severely stenotic arteries missed using only the single set of images obtained at 60 minutes post stress. Our findings confirm earlier work on WR and the degree of cardiomyopathy/CHF in individuals with reduced left ventricular ejection fractions (LVEF) resulting from anterior MII and ischemia. This study is the first to demonstrate that using multiple (static and dynamic) imaging post stress increases the diagnostic accuracy of detecting ischemia and resulted in important diagnostic decisions about patient care/treatment (e.g. Coronary artery stenting), which was not apparent using only the 60 minute image. On inquiry the American Heart Association could cite no prior information regarding the incidence of MII in different regions of the heart. This study demonstrated a significant difference in regional MII and the ability to confidently correlate %DS from the total and inferior WR, in addition to removing the effect of diaphragmatic attenuation noted with the 60 minute image only despite the use of Gadolinium for attenuation correction. Further work is needed to determine if WR obtained from multiple imaging at rest could increase the diagnostic information gleaned regarding the extent of myocardial damage (stunned, hibernating or infarcted) present and perhaps provide insight into why certain regions of the heart are more prone to MII. For example, does the architecture of the right coronary artery predispose it to flow limitations not seen in the other epicardial arteries, just as it makes it more difficult for the interventionalist to angioplasty or stent longer lesions without injury to the artery. Assessment of static images during intermediate times (between 5 and 60 minutes) and using multiple head static imaging may yield additional diagnostic information, the benefit of which can only be determined by looking at the results. Finally, these findings demonstrated a parabolic interactive model between coronary blood flow and cellular "uptake/release" of Technetium-99m tracers which more accurately detects coronary ischemia using a multiple post-stress imaging washin/washout model.

Depression strongly affects the quality of life of patients with heart diseases. Mood disorders in general, together with chronic medical conditions, result in a unique and additional impairment of patient functioning. Depression also increases the risk of morbidity and mortality related to cardiac disorders and may play an important role in the development of angina, hypertension, myocardial infarction, arrhythmias and sudden cardiac death. Lastly, depression may be linked with suicide. Studies on the link between heart disease and suicide risk are rare in the literature, but it appears that patients with coronary heart disease engage in more suicidal behavior independently of depression. A cross-sectional ecological study has reported that the use of calcium channel blockers (commonly prescribed in heart disease) could increase the risk of suicide. On the other hand, other researchers have found no increased risk of suicide associated with these drugs. Back in the 1960s, Farberow and colleagues studied 90 patients with cardiorespiratory illness: 45 patients who completed suicide and 45 nonsuicide controls. These authors found that the suicidal patients were more emotionally disturbed both before and while in the hospital. They were reported to be more hostile, anxious, agitated, apprehensive, depressed, and distressed over their illness than were the controls. These patients required more frequent hospitalization than the controls and had more difficult interpersonal relationships with the staff. They were called dependent–dissatisfied, a label already used by the authors for suicidal psychiatric patients to indicate the type of patient who was continually complaining, demanding, insisting, and controlling. These patients showed inflexibility and lack of adaptability, continually making demands on others regardless of their effect on them. They turned to hospital and staff for support, but consistently succeeded in alienating them with their insatiable demands for special attention. They seemed to need constantly repeated evidence of self-worth from outside sources in order to maintain their feelings of self-esteem. More recently, Pompili and colleagues explored suicidality and associated traits, such as hopelessness, in a sample of cardiac patients and controls. The authors found that patients with heart disease do not differ in these traits from control patients with other internal medicine disorders. Although their medical conditions were more serious than those of the control patients, this apparently had no impact on their hopelessness or suicidality. Men are generally at higher risk of suicide, but in this investigation, they were only slightly more hopeless than women. Implications regarding suicide risk and mood disorders in men are discussed in Chapter 4.

Magnetic navigation is the use of a magnetic field to actively re-orientate a magnetically-enabled wire or device. The field is directed by external magnets that are repositioned by a computer-controlled system. This young technology could lead to a significant evolution in the practice of coronary interventional procedures as it enhances or introduces 3 specific capabilities of exact tip orientation, computer-enhanced control and orientation of the magnetic field, and computer processing.

Chapter 5 will describe the system, review current evidence and progress and potential future advances of this technology.

As a result of dramatically improved survival rates for children with congenital heart disease, a new patient population of adults with congenital heart disease has emerged over the last decades, as Chapter 6 presents. Since very little was known about long-term psychosocial outcomes in these patients, several studies have been done into the psychosocial functioning of adults with congenital heart disease.

For most of these studies, the main question has been whether psychosocial functioning of adults with congenital heart disease was comparable to that of their healthy peers from the general population. Within the population of adults with congenital heart disease, the effects of cardiac diagnosis and operative variables on psychosocial functioning have frequently been described. However, the effects of *gender* on psychosocial outcome in these patients have rarely been studied.

In most studies, no comparisons were made between male respectively female patients with same-sex persons from the general population, nor has the role of gender been explored directly between male versus female patients with congenital heart disease. This can be considered remarkable, since gender-differences in psychosocial functioning have been found in the general population. Therefore it seems unwarranted to assume that the psychosocial functioning of males with congenital heart disease will be comparable to that of female patients.

As discussed in Chapter 7, cardiovascular disease (CVD) is the leading cause of death in the Western World. CVD is not a disease of old age: evidence from autopsy studies demonstrated the presence of atheroma in coronary arteries in children as young as seven years old. CVD does not occur in isolated succinct episodes but occurs as a continuous spectrum, from initiation of atheroma formation, destabilization, development of cardiac ischemia through to cellular necrosis and cardiac dysfunction. The symptomatic part of the disease spectrum is known as the acute coronary syndrome (ACS). ACS is due to the rupture or erosion of atheroma. This produces, depending on its size, surrounding vascular anatomy and the degree of collateral vessels present, a mismatch between oxygen supply and demand resulting in tissue ischemia. This may progress to cardiomyocyte necrosis, known as a myocardial infarction (MI). Post-MI survival results in remodelling of the myocardium and the development of cardiac failure. A number of blood-borne biomarkers are available which can aid in the diagnosis of all of disease stages: the risk assessment of developing CVD, assessing the risk of plaque rupture, diagnosis and prognosis of ACS and the subsequent assessment of myocardial dysfunction.

The most challenging stage with respect to biomarkers and one of current research focus is the detection of cardiac ischemia. A number of potential ischemia markers have been investigated. However, to date, only one, ischemia-modified albumin (IMA) has been clinically validated. The problem associated with developing an ischemia marker is that there is currently no reference standard for diagnosis. This is problematic when assessing the sensitivity and specificity of any candidate biomarker. Measurement of the cardiac structural proteins, the troponins is now recognised as the gold standard test for detection of myocardial necrosis. The sensitive nature of these tests has also revealed that myocardial necrosis is also found in a range of other clinical situations, including trauma, pulmonary embolism, renal failure, multiple organ failure or in cases of arduous physical exercise. This highlights the need to assess biomarker status in conjunction with the clinical picture at presentation. The natriuretic peptides, in particular the B-type and its N-terminal pro-hormone cleaved subunit are diagnostic and prognostic in both acute ACS and detecting post infarction myocardial dysfunction. The role of the B type natriuretic peptides in detection of cardiac failure, both acute and chronic, is well defined. Their role in ACS remains the subject of further studies.

Coronary heart disease (CHD) shares a number of features with chronic periodontitis (CP) including risk factors such as smoking and diabetes; an aetiopathogenesis implicating a number of microbial species, as well as chronic inflammation. However, the link between these two conditions remains unclear. The prevalence of CHD increases with age and is higher in males than females. CP is a chronic inflammatory condition which destroys the supporting tissues of teeth and also increases in prevalence with age. Immune responses against heat shock proteins (HSP) can be cross-reactive among bacterial and human antigens. There is evidence that microbial HSP65 and human HSP60 is involved in periodontal disease and CHD and may therefore provide a mechanistic link between CP and CHD. The aim of this study is to investigate immune responses to the human HSP60 and microbial HSP65 in patients with CP and CHD and relate these to the level of inflammation. The authors collected serum samples from 100 male subjects divided into 4 groups, each matched for age: (a) Healthy control group with minimal gingivitis, (b) CP, (c) CHD with gingivitis (d) CHD with CP. ELISA was used to determine the levels of serum anti-HSP and C-reactive protein (CRP) in the 4 groups. Peripheral blood mononuclear cells were also isolated from these 4 groups and stimulated with HSPs. Significant lymphoproliferation was seen in CHD with or without CP when stimulated with human HSP60. CRP and serum anti-human HSP60 IgG were elevated in the patients groups compared to the healthy control group, but not serum anti-microbial HSP 65 IgG,. In view of the potential confounding effects of smoking in CP and CHD, a group of current smokers (n=24) were also recruited to investigate whether smoking affects HSP immune responses.There was no significant difference in HSP-induced lymphoproliferation between smokers and non-smokers in any of the four groups. There was a significant correlation between CRP and lymphoproliferative responses to Human HSP60.

Chapter 8 shows that serum anti-human HSP60 IgG and serum CRP are raised in CHD with or without CP. In CHD with or without CP, serum CRP levels correlated significantly with human HSP60-induced lymphoproliferation, but not with anti-HSP antibody levels.

Since the introduction of drug eluting stents (DES), discussed in Chapter 9, in the treatment of coronary artery disease in 2002, many randomized clinical trials (RCTs) have been published. At the same time, as often is the case in medicine, utilization of these devices has grown far beyond the approved indications derived from RCTs (on-label). The DES employment in the "real world" scenario generated several registry studies intended to deem their actual safety and efficacy. Only a couple of years after the DES introduction in the market, reports arose about serious safety concerns. Cases of fatal late stent thrombosis began to appear in the literature and thorough revision of DES implant follow up were accomplished. Some researchers reported about an apparent excess in late mortality of patients who were treated with a DES more than 12 months before. As a result, many interventional cardiologists panicked and began to reduce consistently their utilization of DES. Like a wave in a sea storm generates and then is destroyed by the following calm, the same is happening for DES use in interventional cardiology. Stimulated by these alarming calls several other investigators began to report the results of wide national or regional registries that contradicted the previous catastrophic and hurried conclusions. Complete endothelization is often delayed and sometimes never totally accomplished after DES. This is due to the non selective action of drugs blocking cellular replication of endothelial cells, essential to the integrity of all biological processes and the prevention of clot formation and, probably, of polymers to which the drugs are attached and that are not biocompatible. Such intrinsic limitation of the DES is magnified in cases of difficult anatomic conditions (implant in small vessels, bifurcation stenosis, chronic total occlusions etc.) and probably also in particular unfavourable clinical substrates (diabetes, acute myocardial infarction), namely in all the so-called "off-label" indications. Paradoxically, it is particularly in these clinical and anatomic conditions that the potential of DES advantage over conventional treatment could display at the most. To solve these problems DES are changing in terms of different mechanical and biological solutions ultimately aimed at removing their weaknesses and sometimes even changing the philosophy of the device (as for the biodegradable stent approach). At the same time cardiologists are looking for a real comprehension of patients' peculiarities that must be the guide to find the most appropriate and tailored solutions as in most other fields in medicine.

The effect of body composition on the disposition of drugs is an important topic for clinicians due to the escalating prevalence of obesity. In the United States alone, approximately 25% of adults are obese (body mass index ≥30 kg/m^2) and 65% are either overweight or obese (body mass index ≥25 kg/m^2). This discernable growth in obesity is directly correlated with morbidity and mortality from cardiovascular disease. Nevertheless, only a limited number of studies have evaluated the impact of obesity-associated physiological changes on the time course of drug effect.

For many drugs, a dose approved for use in normal-weighted subjects is unlikely to result in the desired pharmacodynamic response if given to obese subjects. However, there are few guidelines that can aid the clinician to choose an optimal dose for the obese population. This knowledge deficit can be partly attributed to the exclusion of obese subjects from clinical trials, but also because there has not been a suitable body size descriptor to allow dose adjustment across a wide range of body compositions. The effect of body composition on drug disposition, drug response, and therefore patient outcomes is particularly pertinent in cardiovascular medicine where excessive drug exposure results in adverse drug events, and suboptimal drug exposure leads to clinical failure.

To help ensure drug exposure in the obese is similar to normal-weighted subjects, maintenance doses of drugs need to be chosen based upon some metric that is correlated with drug clearance. Adipose tissue has little metabolic activity and is therefore unlikely to contribute towards a drug's clearance (CL) while lean body weight (LBW) encapsulates 99% of the body's metabolic processes and is therefore intuitively more likely to be representative of a drug's CL. Dosing regimens adjusted by LBW rather than total body weight (TBW) are therefore more likely to result in comparable exposures across the spectrum of body compositions.

Recently, the hypothesis that drug CL is correlated with LBW rather than TBW has sparked interest in the development of novel individualized dose strategies in the field of cardiology. The benefits of dose individualization are well established in contemporary cardiovascular pharmacotherapy, and essential for drugs with a narrow therapeutic index; for example digoxin, warfarin and unfractionated heparin. Chapter 10 discusses concepts and evidence for drug dosing based upon LBW, principally in the obese population. The authors discuss historical methods to improve dosing across body compositions; recent advances and future directions with a focus on strategies significant to cardiovascular disease.

Cardiomyopathy is a disease of the myocardium that leads to impaired cardiac function and its common anatomical classifications include dilated, hypertrophic and restrictive cardiomyopathies. Many causes can precipitate a cardiomyopathy and the cause should be identified whenever possible since specific treatment, if available, can significantly improve the prognosis. In Chapter 11, the authors present the diagnostic clues and pitfalls for etiological investigations in patients with cardiomyopathy. The two major categories of the differential diagnosis are primary (idiopathic, familial and endomyocardial disease) and secondary myocardial involvement. Secondary causes include ischemic, valvular, hypertensive, infectious, inflammatory, metabolic, genetic, nutritional, toxic and peripartum cardiomyopathies. In this chapter, the authors focus on the non-cardiovascular causes of cardiomyopathy, i.e., etiologies other than ischemic, valvular, hypertensive, primary myocardial diseases, since physicians caring for patients with cardiomyopathy, mostly cardiologists, may find it difficult to determine these non-cardiovascular causes as part of the etiological diagnosis for cardiomyopathy. Since clinical examinations are simple and less expensive, but still can reveal many important clues for the crucial diagnosis, it is important to pay careful attention not only to laboratory, electrophysiological and imaging studies, but also to clinical examinations, such as history and physical examinations.

Chapter 12 discusses natriuretic peptides, which are well established serum biomarkers for acute and chronic heart failures. The prevalence of heart diseases increases markedly with age. Among all investigated neurohormones and natriuretic peptides, BNP and NT-proBNP are the best markers to rule out left ventricular dysfunction. The levels of BNP and NT-proBNP increase with the severity of the left ventricular impairment. Natriuretic peptides show good ability to discriminate patients with mild and severe left ventricular dysfunction. Brain natriuretic peptides are due to their higher sensitivity, specificity and negative predictive values well approved in diagnosis of severe and moderate left ventricular dysfunction. Various studies have pointed out the role of brain natriuretic peptides as markers of myocardial dysfunction. Natriuretic peptides play significant role as prognostic factors and long term clinical outcome predictors after acute myocardial infarction. Levels of natriuretic peptides A and B increase significantly in patiens with congenital and valvular heart diseases including transposition of great arteries and ventricular septal defect, thus, natriuretic peptides are clinicaly useful markers for monitoring various types of heart diseases of different etiology.

In Chapter 13, the authors compare the risk of postoperative in-hospital death between men and women undergoing coronary artery bypass grafting. Using data from a populationbased registry, they examine whether postoperative mortality during admission for the procedure differed between the sexes and whether any such differences were related to the time that patients waited for surgery, independent of other risk factors. The authors found a significant difference in the risk of death: 1.4% for men and 2.4% for women. Postoperative death was more likely among patients who were older, had higher operative risk, and had more coexisting medical conditions. After adjustment for clinical risk factors, the rate of postoperative mortality was similar for men and women in the highrisk group but differed for the lower risk groups. In terms of other aspects of care, we also found differences between the sexes in time to surgical revascularization, but only among those with lower operative risk. However, the time that patients waited for surgery after diagnostic catheterization did not influence the difference in the risk of postoperative death between men and women.

In Chapter 14, the authors review the association between ED and underlying CVD. The pharmacology, clinical efficacy and safety of the available phosphodiesterase -5 inhibitors (PDEIs) will be discussed. Clinical trials that have investigated the use of PDEIs in men with ED and concomitant cardiovascular conditions such as heart failure (HF), hypertension, pulmonary hypertension, diabetes mellitus, and coronary artery disease will be addressed.

As presented in Chapter 15, advances in diagnostic, percutaneous and surgical interventions in pediatric patients suffering from congenital heart disease (CHD) has resulted in increased number of adults with partial or totally corrected CHD. In developed countries, the burden of adult congenital heart disease (ACHD) constitute more of intervened patients, while in developing countries there is more number of un-intervened complicated ACHD patients. It has resulted into a significant number of ACHD populations world-wide. They present the challenging and complicated problems like atrial and ventricular arrhythmias, sudden cardiac death, infective endocarditis, congestive heart failure, right heart failure, pulmonary hypertension and Eisenmenger syndrome, hyperviscosity syndrome, and issues related with exercise and pregnancy. There are technical problems in management of CHD patients once they develop ventricular systolic dysfunction, pulmonary hypertension, atrial or ventricular tachy-arrhythmias and associated co-morbid illnesses. Post intervention patients have problems like graft infection, malfunction, valvular regurgitation and under-sizing in a growing child. There is also a need for heart and heart lung transplantation in few of the un-operable CHD patients during adulthood, which requires the technical expertise for surgery and intensive post-operative and follow-up management; which is available at limited centers in the world. To deal with these unusual problems of adult CHD patients, there is a need for multi-disciplinary, comprehensive approach involving pediatrician, cardiologist, electro-physiologist, pediatric cardiac surgeon, anesthesiologist, internist, psychiatrist and social worker. There is a need to setup adult CHD clinics with trained specialists, who can deal and coordinate different problems of this emerging sub-specialty of the cardiology. As the trained specialists are very limited, there is an urgent need for comprehensive training of health manpower in this field. There is also a need for development of cheap, easy and innovative therapies for management of these patients, so that poor patients can also be benefited.

Over the past fifteen years, gender studies in coronary artery bypass graft (CABG) surgery outcomes have focused on women, although the majority of patients diagnosed with coronary artery disease and those who undergo intervention are predominantly male. A marked increase in public interest in women's health accompanied by new scientific research has produced increasing evidence that women carry a higher operative mortality after CABG surgery. The fact that this data remains somewhat controversial emphasizes the complexity of the issue. It has become clear that differences in profiles between men and women contribute to variation in outcomes after CABG. Biologic differences play a role in etiology, progression, and treatment outcomes. Furthermore, some risk factors have been shown to be unique to each gender. Ultimately, determination of specific independent predictors for long-term mortality after CABG may be helpful in improving surgical results. The purpose of Chapter 16 is to summarize and analyze the current body of knowledge of male gender as an independent variable in coronary artery bypass surgery.

Stress echocardiography is an established tool for clinical decision making, with and average sensitivity of 80% and specificity of 86%. Among available stress techniques, exercise is safer and more physiologic, therefore represents the first choice for the patient able to exercise. Peak exercise imaging, although challenged in treadmill, has greater sensitivity than post-exercise imaging. Apical images are as good as those acquired during the post-exercise period. Some tips may increase the successfulness of peak treadmill exercise imaging, as explained in Chapter 17.

The role of new technology is promising for exercise echo. Doppler tissue and speckle imaging can assess myocardial velocities and deformation. Doppler tissue imaging increases the agreement and accuracy among novel readers, although it is not better than visual assessment performed by experienced observers. The role of speckle imaging is hopeful, as it can easily measure myocardial torsion, which has been found to be diminished under ischemic conditions. Finally, 3-dimensional echocardiography can also be used during exercise since a full volume of the entire myocardium can be acquired in only a few cardiac cycles.

Heart disease has been the focus for researchers for many years. The focus has changed and new factors are being investigated. This is illustrated following the Oslo-Study of

1972/73 until today. New knowledge was needed to curb the increasing incidence and mortality from heart disease in Norway. The Oslo-study was conducted on men only who were at higher risk than women at the time. Traditional risk factors as total serum cholesterol, triglycerides, serum glucose, blood pressure, BMI and smoking were at center of the investigation both for intervention and for long term follow-up analyses. Later focus has been on the vascular inflammation that is a central effect mechanism linked to arteriosclerosis looking into markers of endothelial function, C-reactive protein, antigens of oral bacteria, and environmental factors. With the general increase in BMI and hence Type 2 diabetes related factors on BMI increase as metabolic syndrome, physical activity at leisure, repeated weight reduction are receiving important attention. Continued research into the disease mechanism in heart disease has brought forward a lot of knowledge for primary and secondary heart disease prevention, as shown in Chapter 18.

Chapter 19 studies diabetic nephropathy, which with the early sign called microalbuminuria is associated with silent myocardial ischemia. It has a poor prognosis with more than seven times higher mortality than in diabetic patients without albuminuria. A multifactorial approach is necessary in order to reach full effect of treatment. With such the risk for cardiovascular disease and mortality may decrease by 50%.

RESEARCH AND REVIEW STUDIES

In: Heart Disease in Men
Editors: A.B. Todd and M.H. Mosley, pp. 3-44

ISBN: 978-1-60692-297-2

Chapter 1

Familial Primary Arrhythmias: Genes, Mechanisms and Treatment: Present Perspective

Z.A. Bhuiyan and A.A.M. Wilde

Department of Clinical Genetics and Cardiology, Academic Medical Centre, University of Amsterdam, The Netherlands

Abstract

The Heart is a specialised organ that contracts synchronously, pumping blood to the body and to the lungs. The upper two chambers of the heart are called atria (right and left), the bottom two chambers are called ventricles (right and left). Right atrium receives deoxygenated blood from all parts of the body except for the lungs and transports them to right ventricle. The left atrium receives oxygenated blood from the lungs and transports them to the left ventricle and then to rest of the body. Cardiac excitation originates in the sinoatrial (SA) node and propagates through the atria into the atrial-ventricular (AV) node. The impulse then propagates through the Purkinje conduction system to the ventricles which then contract. The synchronized pumping action of the heart is caused by a flow of electricity through the heart that repeats itself in a cycle.

Heart Muscle, Gap Junction, Desmosome and Ion Channel

Three layers of tissues, epicardium, myocardium and the endocardium form the outer to inner layers of the heart. Cardiac myocytes are the major functioning cells in the heart and are extensively coupled so that impulses propagate rapidly and uniformly.

Individual cardiomyocytes are separated from each other by a specialised boundary called the intercalated disc (ICD), where gap junction proteins, desmosomes and ion channels are located [1]. Gap junctions consist of tightly packed connexins which permit intercellular exchange of small molecules and excitatory current flow between neighbouring cells. Desmosomes alongwith adherens junctions are responsible for the mechanical attachments of individual cardiomyocytes. All these components of the intercalated disc are topologically segregated and serve distinct functions; disruption of one affects the function of others, predisposing the heart to arrhythmias [1-3].

Cardiac Action Potential

The cardiac action potential (AP) is generated by orchestrated interactions between various ion channels (figure 1). The standard model used to describe the cardiac action potential is the action potential of the ventricular myocyte. This action potential has 5 phases (numbered 0-4).

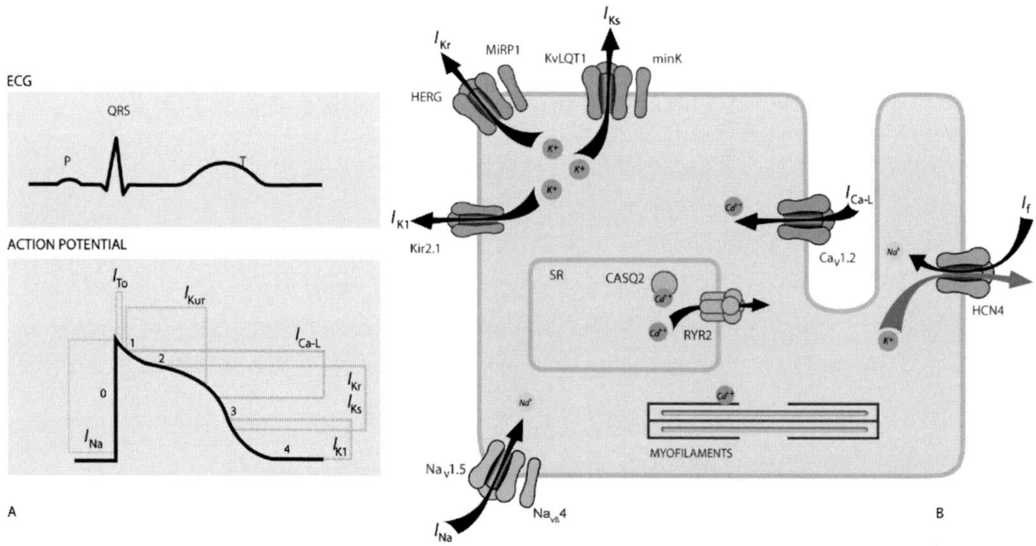

Figure 1. Ionic currents contributing to the ventricular action potential (A) and schematic representation of a cardiomyocyte displaying (only) those proteins involved in the pathogenesis of inherited arrhythmia syndromes (B). In panel A, the action potential is aligned with its approximate time of action during the ECG. In panel B, ankyrin-B, an adapter protein involved in the long QT syndrome type 4, is not depicted. (Reproduced with modification and permission from authors).[12]

Phase 4 (figure 1) is the resting membrane potential, and during this phase the cell is not being stimulated. Phase 4 corresponds with the diastole during which the heart is both electrically and mechanically quiescent and atria and ventricles are filled with blood. In this phase, atrial and ventricular myocytes have a stable, negative resting membrane potential of about -85 mV.

Phase 0 (figure 1) is the rapid depolarization phase, dominated by the sodium channel, which generates a large and fast inward current, I_{Na}, to depolarize the membrane. Upon activation, channels enter into an inactivated stage which is non-conducting and refractory. The ability of the cell to open the fast Na^+ channels during phase 0 is related to the membrane potential at the moment of excitation. If the membrane potential is at its baseline (about -85 mV), all the fast Na^+ channels are closed, and excitation will open them all, causing a large influx of Na^+ ions into the cell. If, however, the membrane potential is less negative, the cell may not be excitable, and conduction through the heart may be hampered, increasing the risk for arrhythmias. Phase 0 of the cardiac action potential is the trigger for the initiation of the contraction of the atria and ventricles [4].

Phase 1 (figure 1) is the early repolarisation phase. Repolarisation results from the rapid activation and inactivation of the outward, repolarising, transient K^+ current I_{to} against the background of a decrease in sodium channel permeability and an increase in calcium channel permeability [4]. This influx of calcium ions (Ca^{2+}) into the cell signals Ryanodine receptors (RyR2s) on the sarcoplasmic reticulum to release of Ca^{2+} into the cytosol. This Ca^{2+} induced release of Ca^{2+} leads to tropomyosin translocation and myofilament contraction.

A delicate balance between inward and outward currents results in the plateau phase of the repolarisation phases 2 and 3 (figure 1). The repolarization phase is mediated by the orchestrated activities of the delayed rectifier K^+ currents (I_{Kr} and I_{Ks}), the inward rectifier K^+ current (I_{K1}) along with a gradual decrease in net depolarizing currents. The resting membrane potential of the myocytes is maintained by the background I_{K1} (phase 4), which is linked to the next cycle of AP initiated by new influx of I_{Na}.

Summation of these action potentials can be detected on the body surface electrocardiogram (ECG) (figure 1). Atrial depolarization manifest on the ECG as P waves, while ventricular depolarization and repolarizations are seen as QRS and T waves, respectively (figure 1).

Arrhythmia Mechanism and Types

Abnormalities in impulse generation, during propagation, or the duration and configuration of individual cardiac action potentials form the basis of disorders of cardiac rhythm. Cardiac arrhythmias are responsible for an estimated one million cases of syncope and sudden cardiac death (SCD), only among Europeans and Americans each year [5]. Familial arrhythmias comprise a significant percentage in this population. Genetics and pathophysiology of the familial arrhythmias are quite complex and we have just begun to understand the intricate and complex processes behind the mechanism of arrhythmogenesis.

First reports linking genetic mutations to primary arrhythmias were published between 1995 and 1997 from the laboratory of Dr. Mark T. Keating and Dr. Pascal Guicheney [6-11]. Thereafter, during the last 13 years, we have observed potential discoveries linking mutations in cardiac ion channels, gap junction protein encoding genes with a wide variety of inherited arrhythmia syndromes [12]. Well coordinated crosstalks between the structural and electrical components of the heart are required for proper cardiac function [2,13]. Disruption in this communication could predispose the heart to arrhythmias with or without any structural defects in the heart [1,13].

Arrhythmias are classified into two main categories: bradycardia and tachycardia. Tachycardia is subclassified into supraventricular and ventricular tachycardia. In bradycardia, the heart rate is less than 60 beats per minute. A heart rate faster than 100 beats per minute is called tachycardia. Supraventricular arrhythmias originate from the atria. As named, ventricular arrhythmias originates from the ventricles. A fast uncoordinated heart rate is called fibrillation. Ventricular fibrillation (VF) is one of the most serious forms of all arrhythmias. General mechanisms of tachyarrhythmias include reentry, triggered activity (early after depolarizations, EAD; delayed after depolarizations, DAD), and abnormal automaticity [4].

Supraventricular Arrhythmia

A very common supraventricular arrhythmia is atrial fibrillation. A normal heart beats between 60 and 100 times a minute. During atrial fibrillation, the atria beat at 400 to 600 times per minute. In response to this, the ventricles usually beat irregularly with variable heart rate, depending on the conduction properties of the AV node. Atrial fibrillation is usually seen in patients with cardiovascular diseases, but could also be due to a genetic pathology. Once AF is developed, it is well possible that it might last lifetime.

Ventricular Arrhythmias

Tachyarrhythmias that originate in the ventricles are more debilitating than those that originate in the atria. In sustained ventricular tachycardia (VT), consecutive impulses arise from the ventricles at a heart rate of 100 beats or more per minute, which stops sometimes automatically without any intervention. But prolonged sustained VTs need to be intervened by drug treatment or electrical conversion. Prolonged sustained VTs might degenerate further into a totally disorganized electrical activity known as VF. VF also can many times present as the first manifestation of arrhythmia, which could be lethal in many occasions.

Cardiac Channelopathies

Ion channels are pore-forming protein complexes that provide controlled inward and outward ionic currents across the cell membranes, which is critical for cardiac contractility, rhythm generation and propagation. Channelopathies could be either congenital (often resulting from mutation/s in various genes) or acquired (resulting from autoimmune attack or drug effect on an ion channel). A large number of dysfunctions are caused by mutations in genes coding for cardiac ion channels. Long QT syndrome (LQTS), Short QT syndrome (SQTS), Sick sinus syndrome (SSS), Isolated Cardiac Conduction defect (ICCD), Brugada syndrome (BrS), Atrial Fibrillation (AF) and Catecholaminergic Polymorphic Ventricular Tachycardia (CPVT) are the presently known cardiac channelopathies.

Long QT syndrome (LQTS)

Congenital LQTS is an inherited disorder defined by prolongation of the QT interval. Patients with all forms of LQTS are predisposed to the ventricular tachyarrhythmia torsade de pointes (TdP) leading to recurrent syncope or sudden cardiac death. In many cases, syncope or sudden death could be the first and the only manifestation. LQTS affects an estimated 1 in 2,000 people world wide [14].

Table 1. Summary of genes and chromosomal loci (where genes are not known) for LQTS.

Disease name	Diseases causing gene (encoded protein)	Functional effect	Arrhythmia onset	Resting ECG	ECG at onset of arrhythmia	QT change with exercise	Response to β-blockers	Extracardiac features
LQT1	*KCNQ1* (K_vLQT1)	decreased I_{Ks}	emotinal or physical stress, swimming, diving	broad based T wave	tachycardia	relative increase	yes	no
LQT2	*KCNH2* (HERG)	decreased I_{Kr}	emotinal or physical stress, sudden loud noise	low-aplitude T wave with notching	with pause	some shortening	yes, less than LQT1 response	no
LQT3	*SCN5A* (α-subunit of sodium channel, Na_v1.5)	increased late sodium current	rest, sleep	long isoelectric ST segment	pause? bradycardia	adequate shortening	ns	no
LQT4	*Ank-B/ANK2* (ANK2)	disruption of localization and post-translational stability of Na^+/Ca^{2+} exchanger	ns	bradycardia, atrial arrhythmia	ns	ns	ns	no
LQT5	*KCNE1* (minK)	decreased I_{Ks}	ns	ns	ns	ns	yes	no
LQT6	*KCNE2* (miRP1)	decreased I_{Ks}	auditory/acoustic stimulus like alarm clock noise, door ringing bell	ns	ns	ns	ns	no
LQT7	KCNJ2 (*Kir2.1*)	decrased I_{K1}	exercise	large U-wave, extrasystoles	ns	ns	no	yes*

Table 1. Continued

Disease name	Diseases causing gene (encoded protein)	Functional effect	Arrhythmia onset	Resting ECG	ECG at onset of arrhythmia	QT change with exercise	Response to β-blockers	Extracardiac features
LQT8	*CACNA1C* (α-1 subunit of $I_{Ca\text{-}L}$)	increased L-type calcium current	ns	very long QT interval	ns	ns	ns	yes**
LQT9	*CAV3* (CAV3)	increased late sodium current	ns	ns	ns	ns	ns	ns
LQT10	*SCN4B* ($Na_{V\beta}4$)	increased late sodium current	ns	ns	ns	ns	ns	ns
LQT11	AKAP9	decreased I_{Ks}	ns	ns	ns	ns	ns	ns
LQT12	*SNTN1* (SNTN1)	Increased late sodium current				ns	ns	ns
JLNS	biallelic mutations in *KCNQ1* or *KCNE1*	loss of I_{Ks}	see LQT1	ns	ns	ns	yes	ns
LQT1 (recessive)	biallelic mutations in *KCNQ1*	near absence of I_{Ks}	see LQT1	ns	ns	ns	yes	ns

ns: not specified

*skeletal muscle periodic paralysis, cleft palate, low set ears, short stature.

** syndactyly, baldness at birth, small teeth, and occasionally cardiac structural malformations, autism, mental retardation, facial dysmorphic features.

The ECG hallmark of the LQTS is, as its name suggests, prolongation of the QT interval (corrected for heart rate i.e. QTc). Normal values of QTc are 440ms in males and 450 ms in females. In children age-dependent (and gender dependent) values are relevant. Values above 480ms in the absence of an identified cause are generally considered highly suspect for LQTS. The molecular basis of LQTS is heterogeneous and to date, mutations in at least 12 different genes have been reported in LQTS patients (table 1). Up to 70% of LQTS patients are reported to have a mutation in one of the 12 reported genes. Among the presently known 12 types of LQTS, the most common are LQT1, LQT2 and LQT3, caused by mutations in cardiac ion channel genes *KCNQ1*, *KCNH2* and *SCN5A*, respectively. Mutations in these three genes constitute more than 90% of genotyped patients [6-11,15]. Among the remaining nine genes implicated in LQTS, *ANK2*, *CAV3*, and *AKAP9* are regulatory/chaperone genes, *KCNE1*, *KCNE2*, *KCNJ2* and *SCN4B* are ancillary subunits of major ion channel genes and *CACNA1C* is the pore forming α-subunit of the cardiac L-type calcium channel gene (table 1). Mutations in these genes, combined, comprise the remaining 10% of the presently genotyped LQTS.

Among all reported mutations in LQT1 to LQT3, missense mutations are most common (72%), followed by frameshift mutations (10%), in-frame deletions, and nonsense and splice-site mutations (5% to 7% each) [15]. Around 8% of the LQTS patients carry mutations in two LQTS causing genes and had longer QTc and also 3.5 fold more risk of cardiac arrest [16]. Early after depolarization (EAD) is considered as the initiating arrhythmogenic mechanism in LQTS [4].

LQT1: Mutations in the *KCNQ1* gene cause the commonest form of LQTS referred to as LQT1, comprising around 50% of the total genotyped LQT patients. KvLQT1 (coded by *KCNQ1*) along with its β-subunit minK (coded by *KCNE1*) co-assemble to form the cardiac K^+ channel (figure 1), which is responsible for the slowly activating delayed rectifier outward K^+ current (I_{Ks}). In this form of the disease, syncope or sudden death is triggered by adrenergic drives e.g. emotional stress, physical exertion, diving, swimming [17]. Schwartz et al. (2001) reported that LQT1 patients experienced the majority of their events (62%) during exercise and only 3% during rest/sleep [18]. Swimming is a typical trigger for cardiac events in these patients. Mutation/s (mostly missense) in *KCNQ1* cause loss-of-function of the mutant allele but this non-functional allele still could exert a dominant negative effect on the normal/wild type allele, which is the pathologic basis of autosomal dominant LQT1 (figure 2). Truncating mutations in the *KCNQ1* are also non-functional and are not able (mostly) to exert dominant negative effect on the normal allele and hence the mono-allelic truncating *KCNQ1* mutation carriers usually lack any significant phenotypes, neither on ECG nor clinically.

Pathogenic mutations in the *KCNQ1* could be located all over the coding exons (including their intronic junctions). Among all the mutations, patients with mutations at the transmembrane domains are at higher risk of LQTS-related cardiac events and have greater sensitivity to sympathetic stimulation [19-20]. Homozygous or compound heterozygous mutations in the *KCNQ1* gene are rare, but when present, cause the recessive type of the disease, Jervell and Lange-Nielsen syndrome (JLNS). Clinical phenotype in JLNS patients are severer (also longer QTc) than the dominant LQT1, and the cardiac manifestations appear more frequently during the early childhood [21]. Patients with JLNS suffer additionally from

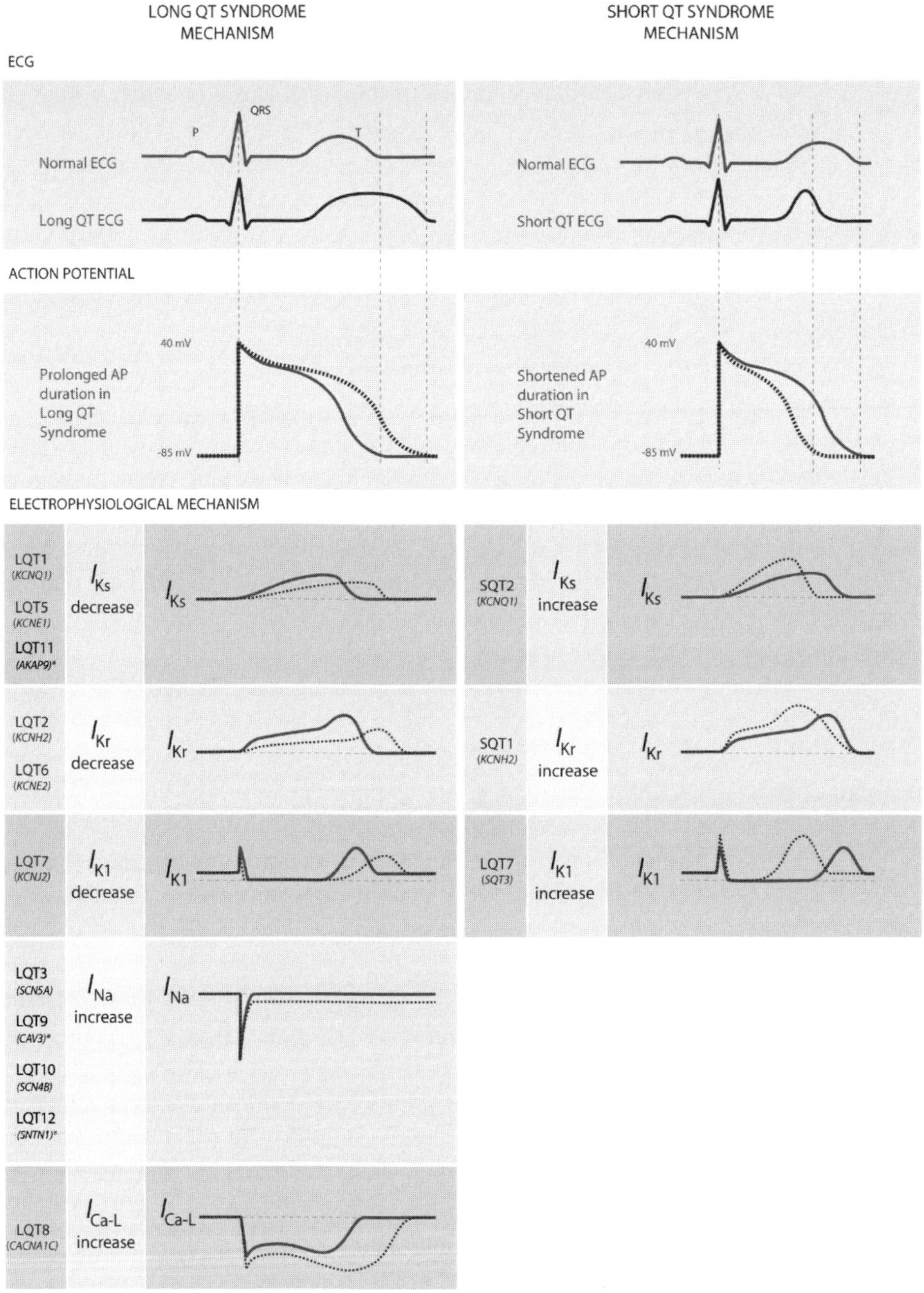

Figure 2. Pathophysiologic mechanisms of ion channel mutations in long QT syndrome (LQTS) and short QT syndrome (SQTS). (A) Schematic ECG representation. The red dotted line represents QT interval prolongation (left panel) and shortening (right panel) as can be observed in the LQTS and SQTS, respectively. (B) The ventricular action potential (AP). The red dotted line represents prolongation (left) and shortening (right) of action potential duration (APD) as can be observed in the LQTS and SQTS, respectively. *denotes the genes whose mutation/s indirectly causes the mentioned LQTS. (Reproduced with modification and permission from the authors).[12]

bilateral sensorineural deafness. JLNS causing homozygous *KCNQ1* mutations are predominantly truncating (except several missense mutations), leading to complete loss/absence of the functional K_vLQT1 protein and I_{Ks} channel. This $I_{Ks,}$ is also present in the inner ear and is required to maintain normal hearing. Total absence of I_{Ks} function in the inner ear leads to deafness in these patients. In some cases, homozygous/compound heterozygous *KCNQ1* mutation carriers could still have some residual I_{Ks} functions left, these patients suffer only from arrhythmias but not from deafness. We have shown in several patients from Saudi Arabia that residual amount of I_{Ks} (as little as 10%), could still maintain normal hearing in homozygous *KCNQ1* mutation carrier patients, but not the normal cardiac electrical function [22].

LQT2: LQT2 is equally prevalent as LQT1, accounting for 35-40% of genotyped LQT patients . Mutations in the *KCNH2* gene are responsible for the LQT2 form of LQTS. *KCNH2* encodes for the HERG protein, and mutations could cause reduction in the rapid component of the delayed rectifier repolarizing current (I_{Kr}). This reduction of the I_{Kr} contributes to lengthening of the QT interval (figures 1 and 2). Molecular mechanisms that account for reduced I_{Kr} current in these patients are disruption of I_{Kr} channel synthesis, membrane trafficking, gating, or permeation, and degradation of mutant mRNA by the nonsense-mediated mRNA decay (NMD) pathway [23-24]. 29% of the syncopal attacks in LQT2 occur during rest/sleep and only 13% of the syncopal attacks were reported during exercise [18]. Sudden startling noises e.g. alarm clock noise, telephone ringing often trigger syncopal events in these patients [18, 25]. Patients with mutations in the pore region of the *KCNH2* gene are at markedly increased risk for arrhythmia-related cardiac events compared with patients with nonpore mutations [26]. In neonates, 2:1 Atrioventricular block (AVB) is preferentially associated with *KCNH2* mutations [27]. Complete AV block complicated by LQTS were also found in 17% of adult patients with a mutation in the *KCNH2* gene [28]. Homozygous mutations in *KCNH2* are rare and when present, patients suffer from a severe form of LQTS, with 2:1 AV block and severe ventricular arrhythmias, well before and immediately after birth [24,29-31]. Homozygous nonsense *KCNH2* mutation carriers could have arrhythmia as early as during the intrauterine stages of life [24,29].

LQT-3: LQT3 accounts for $\leq$10% of genotyped LQTS patients. LQT3 is caused by gain of function mutations that disrupt fast inactivation of the α-subunit ($Na_v1.5$) of the voltage-gated sodium channels encoded by *SCN5A* (figure 1 and 2). Normally, wild-type (WT) Na^+ channels open in response to membrane depolarization, then enter into an inactivation state that prevents reopening during sustained depolarization [32]. LQT-3 causing mutations in *SCN5A* exert their deleterious effects by disrupting the inactivation process either by reducing the rate of channel inactivation or by increasing the likelihood of recovery from inactivation [32-33]. As a result, the inward sodium current persists abnormally during the plateau phase of the cardiac action potential (figure 2). This persistent entry of positive electrical currents prolong the duration of the action potential.

LQT3 patients experience the majority of their events (39%) during during sleep/rest [18], and about 13% of the events were reported to occur during exercise [18]. Genotype and phenotype relationship in *SCN5A* mutations is intricate and complex. In several instances single *SCN5A* mutation were shown to exert two or even three distinct phenotypes of arrhythmias in the same family [34-36]. Male patients with a mutation at the LQT3 locus could develop symptoms much earlier than the female patients [37]. Homozygous *SCN5A* mutations have been described in Long-QT syndrome with functional 2:1 AV block [38].

LQT-4: LQT-4 represents the first non-channel form of LQTS. A mutation in *ANK2*, a member of a family of versatile membrane adapters, leads to intracellular calcium overload which contributes to the LQT4 syndrome (table 1). In addition to QT prolongation, this syndrome is associated with sinus bradycardia and paroxysmal atrial fibrillation [39-40].

ANK2 is required for the localization and post-translational stability of Na^+/Ca^{2+} exchanger in cardiomyocytes [41]. Pathogenic effect of the ANK2 mutations could be moderate to severe and the clinical expressions depend on the severity of the mutation. All mutations (<10) till date described are missense mutations.

LQT-5: The MinK protein is a cardiac K^+ channel accessory subunit encoded by the *KCNE1* gene. Mutations in *KCNE1* are associated with the LQT5 form of LQTS (figure 1 and 2) [42-43]. *KCNE1* mutations reduce I_{Ks} and also exert dominant-negative effect on the wild type normal allele, which causes delayed cardiac repolarization (figures 1 and 2), leading to an increased risk of arrhythmia in the heterozygous carriers [9]. To date, <20 LQT5-related *KCNE1* mutations (all missense) have been reported, but this number and the incidence of mutations are very small compared with the principal LQTS mutations (LQT1-3). Heterozygous *KCNE1* mutation carriers were observed to have milder LQTS phenotypes in a study from Japan [44]. Homozygous *KCNE1* mutation carriers suffer from JLNS [45-46].

LQT-6: *KCNE2* gene encodes MinK-related peptide 1 (MiRP1), a β-subunit of the cardiac potassium channel I_{Kr} (figures 1 and 2). Mutations in *KCNE2* cause defects in the rapidly activating component of the delayed rectifier potassium current (I_{Kr}), responsible for the LQT6 [47]. Reported mutations in *KCNE2* gene till date are <15, all are missense. Auditory/acoustic stimulus like alarm clock noise, door ringing bell etc. could provoke syncopal attacks in *KCNE2* mutation carriers similar to *KCNH2* mutation carriers [48].

LQT-7: This syndrome is also known as Andersen-Tawil syndrome (ATS). ATS is a rare disorder, manifested by occasional syncope and cardiac arrest. ECG features include mild QT interval prolongation, abnormal U waves, frequent ventricular ectopy, bidirectional ventricular tachycardia (VT) and polymorphic VT. This syndrome also exhibits extracardiac features which include skeletal muscle periodic paralysis and developmental problems, such as cleft palate, low set ears, short stature, and developmental features in the limbs [49]. Majority of clinically diagnosed ATS patients are reported to have a mutation in *KCNJ2* [49]. *KCNJ2* encodes a pore-forming subunit of inwardly rectifying potassium channels (I_{K1}), which maintains normal resting membrane potentials (figures 1 and 2) [50-51]. To date, ≥35 heterozygous *KCNJ2* mutations are reported in ATS, and ATS causing mutations in *KCNJ2* showed loss-of-function and dominant negative suppression effects [52]. The clinical severity of ventricular arrhythmias are usually milder in ATS than in other types of LQTS [49]; however, there are reports of aborted sudden death in unrelated ATS patients [53-54].

LQT-8: Also known as Timothy syndrome (TS), combines severe QT prolongation with syndactyly, baldness at birth, and small teeth in 100% of cases and less penetrant cardiac structural malformations, autism, mental retardation, and facial dysmorphic features [55].

There are two subtypes: TS1 and TS2. Mutations in the α-1 subunit of the L-type calcium current (I_{Ca-L}) encoding gene *CACNA1C* lead to LQT-8 (both subtypes). To date 13 cases of TS1 were reported and all occurred due to a single de novo missense G406R mutation in the exon 8A of *CACNA1C* gene [55]. All TS1 individuals have syndactyly (webbing of fingers and toes) [56]. Comparatively severer variant, TS2, arises due to mutations in exon 8. None of the two reported TS2 patients had syndactyly. TS1 and TS2 mutations in *CACNA1C* lead to a gain of function defect, augmenting the depolarising Ca^{2+} current during the plateau phase of the action potential (figures 1 and 2), thereby prolongs the action potential duration (figure 1 and 2).

LQT-9 and LQT-10: Fairly recent genes associated with LQTS are *CAV3,* which encodes Caveolin-3, and *SCN4B,* which encodes $Na_{V\beta}4$, an auxiliary β-subunit of the cardiac sodium channel.

Mutations in *CAV3* and *SCN4B* produce gain of function in late I_{Na}, causing an LQT3-like phenotype [57-59] (figures 1 and 2). They are named as LQT-9 (associated with *CAV3* mutation) and LQT-10 (associated with *SCN4B* mutation).

LQT-11: In the heart, sympathetic nervous system (SNS) regulation of cardiac action potential duration (APD) is mediated by β-adrenergic receptor (β-AR) activation, which requires assembly of AKAP9 (Yotiao) with the α-subunit (KvLQT1) of the I_{Ks} channel. Mutation in *AKAP9* causes LQT-11 [60] (figure 2). To date only one mutation (S1570L) has been reported in *AKAP9* with a detection rate of 2% [60]. Mutation in *AKAP9* negatively affects the interaction between KvLQT1 and AKAP9 (Yotiao) and prolongs the action potential duration.

LQT-12: The most recent gene reported to cause LQTS is α-1-Syntrophin (*SNTN1*). SNTN-1 mutation causes gain of function of the cardiac sodium channel $Na_v1.5$, pathophysiologic basis of LQT-12 [61] (figure 2).

Acquired LQTS

Acquired LQTS is caused by factors and substances that decreases potassium flux and impair the ability of the myocardium to repolarize. Well-recognized conditions that negatively influence the "repolarization reserve" are female gender, hypokalemia, and drugs that inhibit cardiac potassium channels [62]. A number of commonly prescribed drugs could preferentially bind and block the HERG channel (encoded by *KCNH2*) due to its unique structure and increases predisposition to drug-induced arrhythmia [63-64]. Mutations or polymorphisms in HERG may facilitate this binding [65].

Certain variants of MiRP1 (encoded by KCNE2) also contribute to a significant fraction of cases of drug-induced LQTS [66]. One example is T8A-MiRP1 is a common SNP in the MiRP1, reported in about 1.6% of healthy individuals [47]. Individuals harbouring this SNP had a normal electrocardiogram at rest but developed a very long QT interval on Bactrim [trimethoprim/sulfamethoxazole (TMP/SMX)] therapy due to the fact that the channels formed with T8A-MiRP1 are inhibited by SMX [66].

S1103Y and L1825P in SCN5A have also been associated with acquired LQT3 [67-69]. Drugs affecting the intracellular calcium overload also could cause acquired variant LQTS in otherwise normal individuals. Procainamide and Quinidine induces LQTS and torsades de pointes in otherwise normal individuals who carried a SNP E1813K in the ANK2 [70]. These drugs suppress the ANK2 function in individuals harbouring the SNP E1813K and prolong the QT interval inducing intracellular calcium load. Autoimmune mediated LQTS has also been described in a patient with IgG containing anti-HERG antibodies [71].

Electrocardiographic (ECG) Features in the Three Common Forms of Long QT Syndrome

Typical ST-T-wave patterns are present in the majority of genotyped LQTS patients and can be used to identify LQT1, LQT2, and possibly LQT3 genotypes [72-73].

The LQT1 form of the long-QT syndrome is associated with a broad T wave without shortening of the QT interval at exercise (figure 3A). LQT2 is associated with low-amplitude, often bifid, T waves (figure 3B). LQT3 is associated with a long isoelectric segment and a narrow-based, tall T wave (figure 3C). Pause dependence of TdP onset in congenital LQTS is genotype specific, being predominant in LQT2 but almost absent in LQT1 [74]. Although patterns may suggest a specific genotype of the long-QT syndrome, exceptions have been described.

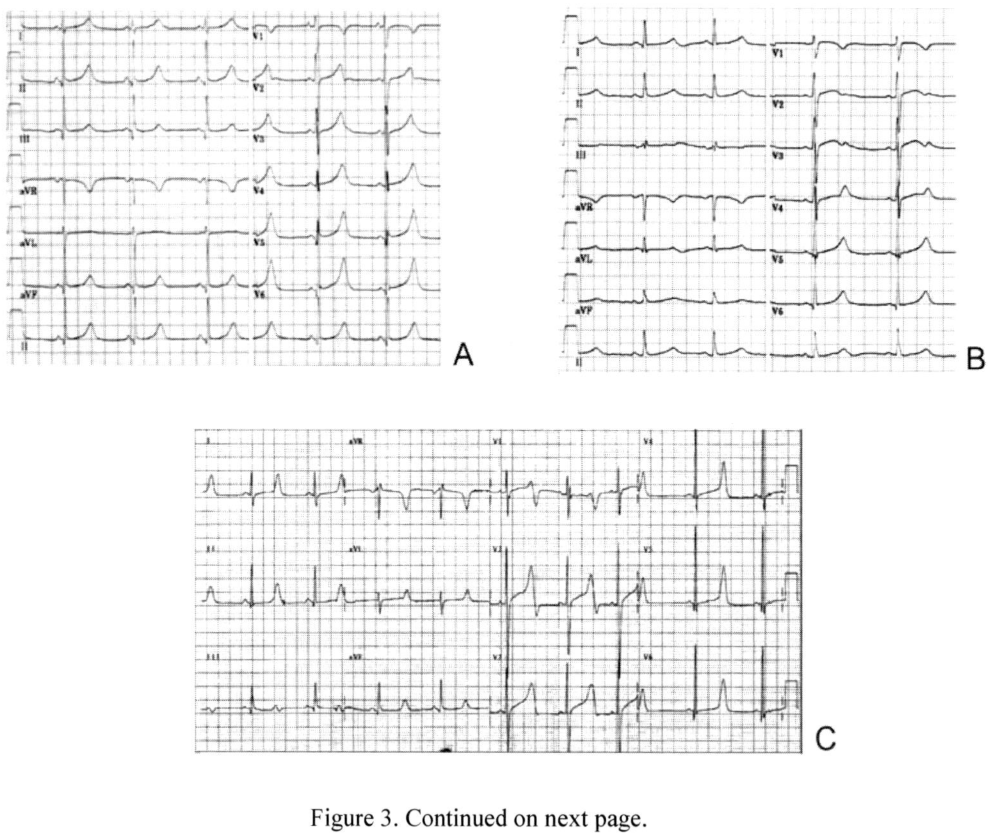

Figure 3. Continued on next page.

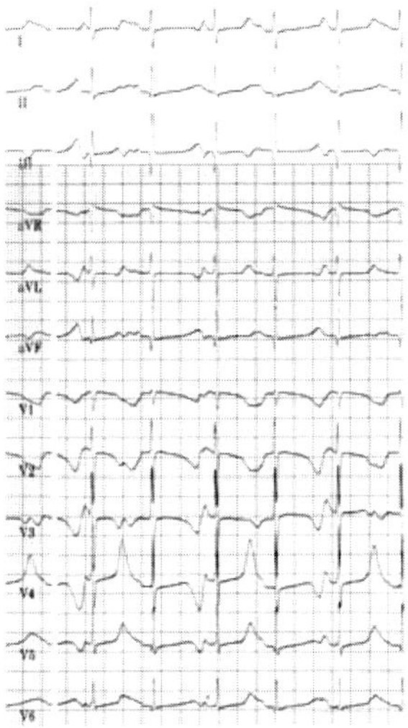

D

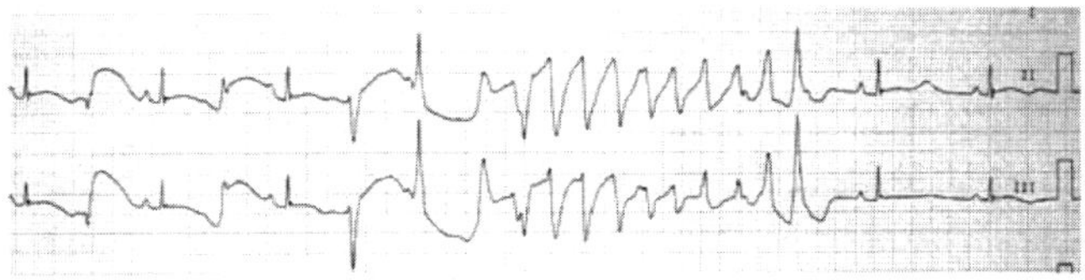

E

Figure 3. ECG recordings from patients with LQT1, LQT2 and LQT3 and LQT8. **A)** 12 lead ECG of a 18 year old male with a *KCNQ1* mutation. The QT interval is prolonged (QTc= ± 500ms). The ST segment has a broad base and relatively large amplitude. Conduction interval is normal (standard calibration). **B)** 12 lead ECG of a 14 year old girl with a *KCNH2* mutation. The QT interval is prolonged (QTc, ±520ms). The ST segment is notched in lead V3 and has relatively low amplitude in the extremity leads. Conduction interval is normal (standard calibration). **C)** 12 lead ECG of a 12 year old boy with a *SCN5A* mutation. The QT interval is prolonged (QTc. ± 600 ms). The ST segment has a long (almost) isoelectric segment with a large, sharp and narrow T wave. Conduction interval is normal (standard calibration). **D)** 12 lead ECG of a 2 year old boy with a *CACNA1C* mutation. The QT interval is very prolonged (620 ms; QTc= 911 ms) with upright T wave. The ST segment shows T wave alternans which are most evident in leads V3-V5. **E)** Two lead ECG (lead II and III) from a 14 year old girl with *KCNH2* mutation. In the middle part of ECG a TdP episode is seen that lasts a few seconds and terminates spontaneously. Prior to the TdP episode, ventricular extrasystoles disturb a regular sinus rhythm. Note the prolonged QTc particularly after the arrhythmia.

Mutation list and their carrier patients are still inadequate in number to perform such genotype specific ECG analysis in LQT4-LQT12 patients.

Genotype-Phenotype

Clinical expression of LQTS is not uniform, variation in penetrance and expression are influenced by age, gender, genotype, environmental factors, therapy, and possibly by not yet identified modifier genes. The genotype-phenotype correlation in heterozygous carriers has been investigated in detail in the LQT1, LQT2 and LQT3 syndrome patients, as these 3 forms constitute more than 90% of genotyped LQTS patients [15]. During childhood, the risk of cardiac events is significantly higher in LQT1 males than in LQT1 females, whereas no significant gender-related differences were seen in the risk of cardiac events among LQT2 and LQT3 carriers. During adulthood (also after age 40) LQT2 and LQT1 patients had a significantly higher risk of cardiac events in females than respective males [75-77]. In general, lethality of cardiac events seems to be predominant in LQT3 patients than in LQT1 and LQT2 patients [78]. Women with LQTS have a reduced risk for cardiac events during pregnancy, but an increased risk during the 9-month postpartum period, especially among women with the LQT2 genotype [79]. The QTc is an independent predictor of risk among patients with a mutation at the LQT1 locus and those with a mutation at the LQT2 locus but not among those with a mutation at the LQT3 locus [37].

Intrauterine Death, Sudden Deaths in Infants, Children and Adults: Role of Mutations in Ion Channel Genes

Recurrent third-trimester fetal loss was reported in heterozygous R1623Q SCN5A mutation carriers in a single report [80]. But, Intrauterine death has been reported several times due to homozygous *KCNH2* mutations [24,29]. Sudden cardiac death (SCD) in children could often be caused by a mutation in the cardiac ion channel gene [81-83]. In a report, >50% of the children with an unexplained SCD was shown to have a mutation in one of the known cardiac ion channel genes [84]. Though, mutations in *SCN5A* seem to be predominant in SIDS [85-86], mutations in *KCNQ1* were also reported. New additions to this list are mutations in *KCNH2*, *KCNE2* and *CAV3*, *SCN4B* and *SCN3B* [87a,b]. In 12% of the Sudden Arrhythmic Death Syndrome between 16-64 yrs of age were found to have LQTS [88].

Diagnosis

Most common clinical features of LQTS patients are palpitations, presyncope, syncope and sudden death. These clinical features also could be seen in patients with other arrhythmia syndromes e.g. catecholaminergic polymorphic ventricular tachycardia and secondary arrhythmia syndromes (due to various cardiomyopathies).

A proper history taking relevant to the disease is required, which in many occasions lead to the specific subtype of LQTS. This history taking includes the proband him/herself and also of any family members with similar history. History also should be focused on precipitating factor/s which provoked the symptoms e.g. swimming, alarm noise, door ringing bell etc.

Physical examinations and Echocardiography (or MRI/CT) are required to exclude the presence of any structural abnormality in index patients with LQTS. An ECG exhibiting prolonged QTc at rest in a structurally normal heart is the sine qua non to the diagnosis. To rule out the acquired cases of LQTS (occurs in 5 to 20% of cases) patients should be screened for serum electrolytes (K^+, Ca^{2+}, Mg^{2+}), hypothyroidism and other eliciting factors. Patients should be inquired about the use of drugs that can prolong the QT interval, which includes several antiarrhythmic drugs (www.torsades.org).

A great percentage (30-40%) of individuals with LQT1 has a non-diagnostic QTc at rest, and concealed LQT1, therefore unmasking LQT1 is clinically important as LQT1 represents one of the two most common subtypes of LQTS [89]. Exercise or epinephrine QT stress test could sometime (not always) help in differentiating between a rare but functionally irrelevant "mutation" in *KCNQ1* versus a pathogenic, LQT1-causing mutation [89-91]. Sotalol also could help in unmasking the concealed LQT [92].

Similarly, identification of occult LQT2 patients remains an unresolved problem. Shimizu et al [93] demonstrated that epinephrine bolus (but not steady state epinephrine) increased Tpe in LQT2 patients. Erythromycin was also found prolong the Tpe in LQT2 patients and could be used in unmasking the disease [94].

Single Nucleotide Polymorphism (SNP), Ethnicity and LQTS Predisposition

The term Single nucleotide polymorphism (SNP) refers to single nucleotide DNA sequence variations within the genome, and which seems to exert no pathogenic effect. SNPs are present all over the genome (exons, introns, gene regulatory regions) and can change the amino acid codon (non-synonymous changes) and can also be silent (synonymous changes). Some SNPs are found in equal frequency in all populations and some of them can be seen prevalently in specific ethnic/regional populations. For a nucleotide variation to be considered an SNP, generally accepted criteria are that this variant should be present in at least 1% of the population (Human Genome data base, NCBI). SNPs are usually considered harmless, but there are SNPs which can enhance the risk of a disease in specific populations. For example, S1103Y is a common SNP in SCN5A, about 13.2% of African Americans carry the Y1103 allele. Heterozygous carriers for this genotype seem to be associated with increased risk for arrhythmia in adults with 8-fold increased risk of arrhythmias without marked channel dysfunction in vitro [95]. Infants with African-Americans origin with 2 copies of the common synonymous SNP S1103Y in SCN5A are predisposed to 24-fold increased risk for SIDS [67, 95-96]. Similarly, R1193Q comprises 12% of the alleles in Han Chinese compared to <0.2% in other populations, considerably increasing the risk for LQTs (and some times Brugada Syndrome) in the Han Chinese population [97]. L1622I codon in ANK2 is conserved across species, and about 4% of the Africans share this allele [98]. Effect of this SNP on arrhythmia susceptibility in the African populations remain to be studied.

Clinical Management of LQTS

Cessation of all drugs known to prolong the QT interval and the correction of electrolyte imbalances and/or precipitating metabolic conditions should be the primary focus while treating LQTS patients. Because syncope or death in the LQTS is often adrenergically mediated, restriction of patients' participation in athletic activities is generally recommended [17]. It is not known whether this restriction should be extended to patients with forms of the disease in which adrenergic stressors are not prominent [17]. Silent mutation carriers should be counselled about the characteristics of the disorder and also need to be properly informed about the risk of mutation transmission to offspring, also mentioning the fact that that offspring of a silent mutation carrier could express the disease phenotype when carried the mutation unlike his/her silent mutation carrier parent.

The mainstay of therapy for the long-QT syndrome is and has been β-blockade. Long-acting preparations such as nadolol and metoprolol are usually used, and the efficacy of β - blockade is assessed by blunting of the exercise heart rate (e.g., by >20%) [17-18]. The percentages of patients who were free of recurrence with β-blocker therapy was reported to be higher and the death rate was lower among LQT1 patients (81% and 4%, respectively) than the LQT2 (59% and 4%, respectively) and LQT3 (50% and 17%, respectively) patients. Furthermore β-blockade can be used as a prophylactic treatment in silent mutation carriers to reduce SCD. Since, women with LQTS (especially LQT2) have an increased risk during the 9-month postpartum period, β-blockers should be prescribed to reduce any cardiac events during this high-risk period [79]. An implantable cardioverter–defibrillators (ICDs) can be considered for patients with recurrent syncope despite β-blocker therapy or in patients with high risk for cardiac arrest (e.g. symptomatic LQT2 and LQT3 with a documented QTc prolongation). β-blockers have limited efficacy in JLNS in which and early therapy with implanted cardioverter/defibrillators were recommended. [21]. Another effective anti-adrenergic therapy is ablation of the left stellate ganglion. This therapy has been shown to be effective alike β-blockers, particularly in LQT1 patients [18,99]. LCSD should be considered in patients with recurrent syncope despite beta-blockade and in patients who experience arrhythmia storms with an implanted defibrillator [99]. Sodium-channel blockers such as mexiletine and flecainide may normalize the QTc interval in patients with the LQT3 subtype, but they may also increase the risk of sudden death in patients with overlapping Brugada syndrome; their role as primary therapy in LQT3 thus remains uncertain. In vitro analysis was performed to check the efficacy of mexiletine showed some mutations are responsive to mexiletine and some are not [100]. Low-dose flecainide was reported as a promising therapeutic agent for LQTS patients with DeltaKPQ mutation carriers in the SCN5A [101]. These findings should be carefully addressed in the clinical setting in patient care. LCSD should also be considered in all forms of LQTS patients with recurrent syncope despite β-blockade and in patients who experience arrhythmia storms with an implanted defibrillator [99]. Pacing has limited value in the treatment of LQTs but might be used to allow full dose β-blocker therapy or in young infants to postpone ICD implantation. A pause-dependent arrhythmias (LQT2) may be prevented by pacing and pacing protocols that favor relatively fast heart rates can prove useful in patients as they may prevent electrical storm [102]. Several compounds (Nicorandil, NS3623) act as potassium channel openers and correct the QTc interval, are still in the experimental stage [103-104]. Though, they seem to work as potassium channel activator, further functional and clinical research studies are required before they could be brought to the clinic.

Short QT Syndrome

The short QT syndrome (SQTS) has been recognized recently as a new entity characterized by ion channel mutations, leading to sudden cardiac death due to VF associated with short refractory periods.

The short QT syndrome has been characterized by major and minor cardiac events, or symptoms. The major events include syncope, ventricular fibrillation and sudden cardiac death. The minor events include palpitations, light headedness/ dizziness, and paroxysmal atrial fibrillation. Sudden cardiac death could be frequent first symptom and first clinical presentation. Most patients have a significant family history of sudden cardiac death of relatives with a variable age distribution, ranging from 3 months to 70 years of age. The mean age of SQTS diagnosis is 30 years [105]. It has been suggested that sudden infant death syndrome may in some cases be attributed to SQTS [106].

Table 2. Summary of genes and chromosomal loci (where genes are not known) for SQTS, BrS, CCD, SSS, CPVT and FAF.

Disease name	Disease causing gene (encoded protein)	Functional effect of disease causing mutation	ECG
SQT-1	*KCNH2* (HERG)	increased I_{Kr}	short QT interval of typically less than 300 ms with tall peaked, narrow symmetrical T waves.
SQT-2	*KCNQ1* (K_vLQT1)	increased I_{Ks}	
SQT-3	*KCNJ2* (Kir2.1)	increased I_{K1}	
BrS-1	*SCN5A* (α-subunit of sodium channel $Na_v1.5$)	reduced surface $Na_v1.5$	ST-segment elevation in the right precordial leads (V1-V3), with or without the presence of incomplete or complete right bundle branch block
BrS-2	*GPD1-L* (glycerol-3-phosphate dehydrogenase 1 like)		
BrS-3	*CACNA1C* (α-1 subunit of I_{Ca-L})		
BrS-4	*CACNB2b* (β-2b subunit of I_{Ca-L})		
BrS-5	*SCN1B* (β-1 subunit of sodium channel)		
CCD-1	unknown (19q13.2-q13.3)	unknown	cardiac conduction defect at all cardiac levels.
CCD-2	*SCN5A* (α-subunit of sodium channel $Na_v1.5$)	reduced surface $Na_v1.5$	
CCD-3	unknown (chr 16q23-q24)	unknown	

Table 2. Continued

Disease name	Disease causing gene (encoded protein)	Functional effect of disease causing mutation	ECG
SSS-1	*HCN4* (Hyperpolarization activated cyclic nucleotide gated channel-4)	unknown	sinus bradycardia, sinus arrest, and/or sinoatrial block. Episodes of atrial tachycardias coexisting with sinus bradycardia.
SSS-2	*SCN5A* (α-subunit of sodium channel $Na_v1.5$)	reduced surface $Na_v1.5$	cardiac conduction defect
CPVT-1	*RyR2* (RyR2)	premature cytosolic release of Ca^{2+}	ventricular premature complexes, later in bigeminy, followed by bidirectional or polymorphic ventricular tachycardia
CPVT-2	*CASQ2* (CASQ2)	premature cytosolic release of Ca^{2+}	same
CPVT3	gene unknown (chr 7p14-21)	unknown	same
FAF1	gene unknown (chr 10q22-q24)	unknown	atrial fibrillation, no specific features
FAF-2	gene unknown (chr 6q14-q16)	unknown	atrial fibrillation, no specific features
FAF -3	*KCNQ1* (I_{Ks})	unknown	atrial fibrillation, no specific features
FAF -4	*KCNE2* (miRP1)	unknown	atrial fibrillation, no specific features
FAF -5	*GJA5* (Connexin 40)	unknown	atrial fibrillation, no specific features
FAF -6	*KCNA5* (I_{Kur})	unknown	atrial fibrillation, no specific features
FAF -7	gene unknown (chr 5p15)	unknown	prolonged SA P-wave

SQT: Short QT syndrome; BrS: Brugada syndrome; CCD: Cardiac Conduction Disease; SSS: Sick Sinus Syndrome; CPVT: Catecholaminergic Polymorphic Ventricular Tachycardia; FAF: Familial Atrial Fibrillation

ECG is characterized by a short QT interval of typically less than 300 ms with tall peaked, narrow symmetrical T waves. Short refractory periods lead to a propensity to develop atrial or ventricular fibrillation at electrophysiology study. SQTS is a genetically heterogeneous disease characterized by at least three different gene mutations of potassium channels involved in cardiac repolarization. Three forms of SQTS have been diagnosed due to mutations in three different genes (table 2), which are as follows:

SQT-1: A mutation in *KCNH2* which causes gain of function (contrary to loss of function mutations) is responsible for SQT-1 (figures 1 and 2). To date, only one missense mutation in *KCNH2*(N588K) have been described in SQT-1, that lead to gain of function and shortening of the action potential duration [107-108].

SQT-2: Mutation in the *KCNQ1* gene could also result in accelerated activation kinetics consistent with a gain of function in the outward current and is considered the pathophysiology of short QT syndrome (SQT-2) (figures 1 and 2) [109-110].

SQT-3: *KCNJ2* encodes the pore-forming subunit of inwardly rectifying potassium channel (I_{K1}). Mutation in this gene which causes gain of function of the I_{K1} channel, and the generated current do not decrease to the extent of normal potassium channels, shortens the action potential (figures 1 and 2). ECG shows unique features of asymmetric tall T waves with a rapid descending portion [111]. The QT-interval in the described patients are in the 320 ms range. The clinical syndrome is extremely heterogeneous with variation in symptoms and risk of sudden cardiac death within an individual genotype. At this point in time, it is difficult to link genotypes with definite phenotypic expression [112].

Given the high incidence of sudden cardiac death in SQTS, an ICD is recommended unless there is an absolute contraindication to implantation. Pharmacologic therapy is a potential alternative to ICDs in patients in whom ICD implant is not feasible. Hydroquinidine so far has been as the only agent to revert short QT interval to normal [113-114].

Brugada Syndrome

Brugada syndrome (BrS) is a leading cause of death due to ventricular arrhythmias among young men in Southeast Asia, and also responsible for a considerable numbers of sudden cardiac deaths worldwide. Among patients presenting with the syndrome, 20-50% are reported with a family history of sudden cardiac death.

Heterozygous mutations in the cardiac Na^+ channel SCN5A cause approximately 20% of the cases of BrS. Heterozygous mutations in the α-1 (*CACNA1C*) and the β-2b subunits (*CACNB2*) of the cardiac L-type calcium channel genes (figure 1 and table 2) were recently reported in BrS patients (8%) in combination with short QT interval [115]. Mutation in *GPD1-L* and *SCN1B* gene has also been implicated in BrS comprising <2 % of BrS patients [116-117]. All these BrS causing mutations, either by trafficking deficiency or abrogation in the electrical property, or affecting its binding to the adaptor molecule ankyrin-G prevents accumulation of *SCN5A* encoded $Na_v1.5$ at cell surface sites in ventricular cardiomyocytes [116,119], which results in premature closing of the sodium channel or less available channels during phase 1 of the action potential (figure 1). This loss or deficient sodium channel function manifests the BrS specific ECG in these patients (figure 4). Sodium channel blockers, cocaine, antidepressants and antihistamines are also known to facilitate the Brugada-type ECG by reducing the inward sodium current [120-121]. Actually, sodium channel blockers are clinically in use to unmask BrS in those cases in which there is a strong suspicion of the disease but no electrocardiographic proof. Reentry is considered the dominant mechanism in Brugada syndrome based on conduction slowing, easy VT/VF induction during electrophysiological study and the polymorphic nature of the arrhythmias [122].

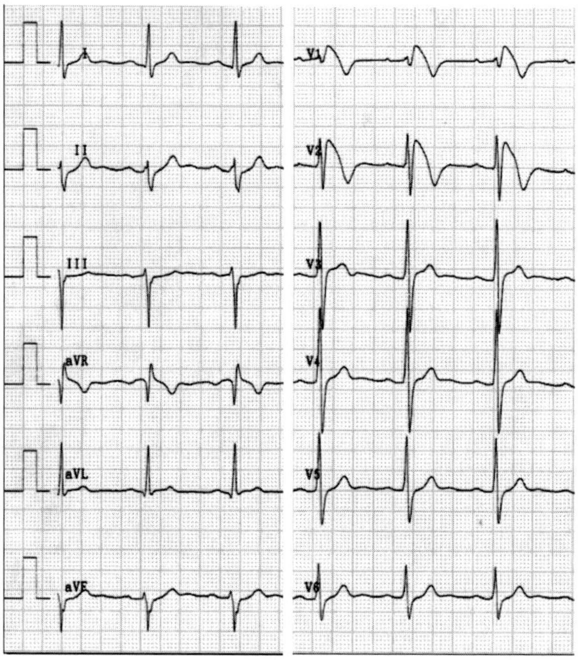

Figure 4. 12 lead ECG of a 38-yr old resuscitated male with BrS. The electrocardiographic hallmark of the disease is clearly present i.e. the coved type ECG (marked ST-elevation) in the right precordial leads, conduction intervals are prolonged (PR 210 ms, QRS 120 ms) and the electrical axis is leftward. This ECG is indicative for a SCN5A mutation and that is indeed what this patient had.

The main ECG findings in BrS are ST-segment elevation in the right precordial leads (V1-V3), with or without the presence of incomplete or complete right bundle branch block (figure 4). Occasionally, like in a French family with BrS, ST segment elevation and prominent J wave were observed in the inferior and also in right precordial leads. But, some family members showed classic ECG pattern of ST segment elevation in the right precordial and not in the inferior leads [123]. Among the two major types of ST segment elevations in BrS, coved-type morphology is required for the diagnosis, while the saddle-back type is an intermediate form that requires confirmation using pharmacological challenge (conversion into coved-type) or genetic analysis [122]. A large majority of BrS patients goes undetected without a mutation. ECG characteristics indicative for SCN5A mutations are longer conduction intervals and higher ST amplitude [124].

In the largest population of children affected by BrS described to date, fever represented the most important precipitating factor for arrhythmic events [125]. Patients with a spontaneously appearing Brugada ECG have a high risk for sudden arrhythmic death secondary to ventricular tachycardia/fibrillation [120-121]. In the adult population, the risk of arrhythmic events is higher in previously symptomatic patients [120].

Controversy exists in the management of asymptomatic patients with the classic ECG pattern. Therapeutic intervention with antipyretics or termination of the culprit medication (e.g. antidepressants and antihistamines) is warranted and carrier family members should be informed that some medications and disease states (fever) might increase their risk of arrhythmias.[121] In patients with previous symptoms (most likely) related to the occurrence of ventricular arrhythmias, there is general agreement that they should be protected with an implantable defibrillator. Longer follow-up in well-controlled clinical trials will be needed to better understand how to manage asymptomatic patients.

Cardiac Conduction Defect or Lev-Lenègre Syndrome

Progressive cardiac conduction defect (PCCD) is a frequent disease commonly attributed to degeneration and fibrosis of the His bundle and its branches. Cardiac conduction disease (CCD) is mostly encountered as a consequence of cardiac injury (caused by ischaemia or surgery), as the major cardiac manifestation of neuromuscular diseases, or in association with congenital cardiac abnormalities. However, isolated cardiac conduction disease (ICCD), with a progressive nature in some instances (also known as Lenegre and Lev disease) has also been described.

Three distinct genetic forms have been distinguished in families displaying an autosomal dominant inheritance (table 2). One form involves mutations in *SCN5A*. Mutations in *SCN5A* cause (progressive) cardiac conduction defect, also called hereditary Len`egre disease, characterized by an age-related alteration in the conduction of the cardiac impulse through the His-Purkinje system, ultimately leading to a pacemaker implantation but no ST-segment elevation [126]. An intriguing overlap exists between Lenegre disease and BrS: decreased availability of the sodium channel accounts for both clinical entities [127-128]. Linkage to chromosome 19q13.2–q13.3 and chromosome 16q23–24 has respectively been identified in two kindreds with the disorder (table 2). The causative gene at each of these locus is yet to be identified.

Patients with CCD or Lev-Lenègre disease are usually treated with conventional pacemaker therapy. Dual chamber pacing (DDD pace makers) or VVI PM's are mostly used in patients without or with atrial fibrillation.

Sick Sinus Syndrome

Sick sinus syndrome (SSS) encompasses a broad array of disturbances involving sinus node dysfunction. Common clinical manifestations are syncope, presyncope, dizziness, and fatigue. ECG typically manifests sinus bradycardia, sinus arrest, and/or sinoatrial block. Episodes of atrial tachycardias coexisting with sinus bradycardia ('tachycardia-bradycardia syndrome') are also common in this disorder. SSS occurs most often in the elderly associated with underlying heart disease or previous cardiac surgery, but can also occur in the fetus, infant, or child without heart disease or other contributing factors, in which case it is considered to be a congenital disorder [129]. In a significant portion of patients, however, this disease appears in the absence of an identifiable cardiac abnormality or other associated conditions. Compound heterozygous mutations in *SCN5A* gene have been described in five individuals between 2 years to 9 years with SSS [129] (table 2). Schulze-Bahr et al. (2003) first reported a frameshift mutation (1631delC) in the pace-maker gene *HCN4*, in a 66 yr old woman of idiopathic sick sinus syndrome [130] (table 2). One year later, Ueda et al. (2004) reported a missense D553N mutation in a 43-year-old woman who experienced first syncope at her 20 yrs followed by recurrent syncope at 34 yrs [131]. Co-segregation of D553N with the phenotype being found in her family in two other affected individuals. These sporadic two cases were followed by two reports where the authors reported missense mutations (S672R and G480R) in the critical regions of *HCN4* gene segregating in a large family with sinus bradycardia [132-133]. The heart rate varied from 43 to 60 beats per minute in persons with the mutated gene in both families. Sporadic *HCN4* mutation carriers reported by Schulze-Bahr et al. (2003) and Ueda et al. (2004) had complex array of rhythm disturbances [130-131], which seems in contrast with the bradycardia as the only clinical abnormality in the familial patients described by Nof et al. (2007) and Milanesi et al. (2006) [132-133]. Additionally, sinus node dysfunction were also observed in combination with other cardiac arrhythmias, including LQTS, BrS, idiopathic ventricular fibrillation, PCCD and CPVT [134-135].

Regarding therapy of SSS, pacemaker therapy may be appropriate in some cases, drug suppression of arrhythmias in others, and both strategies may be required in many individuals.

Anticoagulation is critical for treatment of many individuals with SND, particularly those with paroxysmal or persistent atrial fibrillation. In general, pacemaker therapy is indicated and has proven to be highly effective in patients with SND when bradyarrhythmia has been demonstrated to account for symptoms [136].

Catecholaminergic Polymorphic Ventricular Tachycardia (CPVT)

Catecholaminergic Polymorphic Ventricular Tachycardia (CPVT) is an arrhythmogenic disorder of the heart characterized by a reproducible form of polymorphic ventricular tachycardia, inducible by physical activity, stress or catecholamine infusion, which can deteriorate into ventricular fibrillation. Patients present with recurrent syncope, seizures or sudden death following physical activity or emotional stress. CPVT can be inherited as an autosomal dominant or recessive trait. ECG parameters, including the QTc interval are generally normal or borderline prolonged, however sinus bradycardia is frequently observed. The hall mark of the disease comprises ventricular arrhythmias of varying morphology that do not exist under resting conditions but appear only upon physical exercise, excitement or catecholamine administration (figure 5). These arrhythmias are first seen as ventricular premature complexes, later in bigeminy, followed by bidirectional or polymorphic ventricular tachycardia eventually leading to ventricular fibrillation. Clinical penetrance in this disease ranges from 25 to 100%, with an average of 70 to 80%. Syncope appears to be the first symptom in more than half of the patients. When untreated, the mortality to CPVT is high, reaching 30-50% by the age of 30 years.

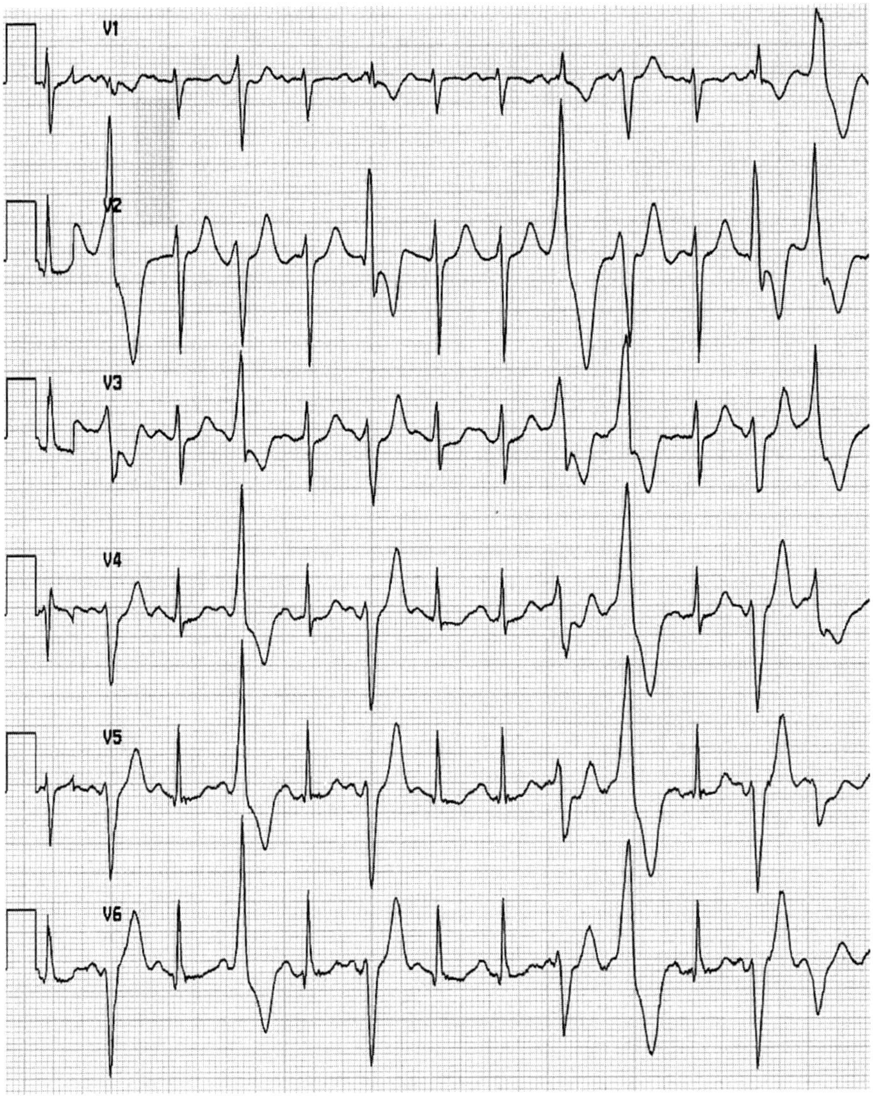

Figure 5. 6 lead (precordial leads, usual calibration) ECG of an individual harbouring a CPVT1 causing mutation in *RyR2* gene, recorded during exercise stress test. The ECG shows a sinus tachycardia interrupted by isolated polymorphic extrasystoles and polymorphic extrasystoles in doublets.

The gene locus corresponding for autosomal dominantly inherited CPVT[1] was initially mapped to chromosome 1q42-43, with eventual identification of missense mutations in the RyR2 gene in 50-60% of the patients (figure 1 and table 2) [137-141]. In a recent report 2% of SIDS cases have been linked to CPVT causing mutations in RyR2 [142]. Mutations in RyR2 are mostly missense mutations (only few are deletion of an amino acid), mutations are clustered in the N-terminal, Central and C-terminal domains of RyR2 (our observation; [143]). We have for the first time reported an inframe deletion of a complete exon of RyR2 gene caused by replication error due to Alu-repeat slippage [135]. Patients in two families with this deletion suffered from CPVT, combined with additional features of dilated cardiomyopathy (DCM), progressive AV-block, sino-atrial node (SAN) dysfunction, atrial fibrillation (AF) and atrial standstill (ASS) [135]. Second variant of CPVT [2] is caused by homozygous or compound heterozygous null mutation in the *CASQ2* gene [144-146]. Recently, we have reported a third variant of CPVT (3) with recessive mode of inheritance. Pathogenic locus for CPVT[3] has been mapped to chromosome 7p14-p22, for which the gene still remain to be discovered [147). Clinical symptoms of CPVT [3] appeared early in childhood (7-12 years) and in three of the four cases, the first appearance of symptoms turned into a fatal outcome [147].

The cardiac ryanodine receptor (RyR2) and CASQ2 governs the release of Ca^{2+} from the sarcoplasmic reticulum, which initiates muscle contraction (figure 1). Mutations in these genes lead to premature release of calcium from the intracellular stores, thereby causes increased cytosolic Ca^{2+} concentration and which causes arrhythmia. Delayed after depolarizations (DAD) is considered the dominant mechanism for arrhythmogenesis in CPVT [148].

β-blockers without sympathomimetic activity are clinically effective in reducing syncope in CPVT patients, but implantation of an automatic internal defibrillator is occasionally needed in these patients. Patients whose symptoms are not adequately controlled by means of β- blockade or ICD, LCSD could be considered an effective alternative treatment for catecholaminergic polymorphic ventricular tachycardia [149].

Atrial Fibrillation

Atrial fibrillation is a rhythm disorder characterized by chaotic electrical activity of cardiac atria and is the most common type of sustained cardiac arrhythmias. AF is a leading cause of cardiovascular morbidity, and stroke. Most cases of AF are seen in association with other cardiac or systemic conditions, but, 10% to 30% of patients were reported to have lone AF [150]. Though, our basic understanding about the ionic and molecular mechanisms of AF is still at the initial stage, increased inward rectifier K^+ current and altered Ca^{2+} handling are presently thought to be the pathophysiologic basis of AF [151]. Gain of function mutations in *KCNQ1, KCNE2, KCNE3* and *KCNE5* has been reported in AF [152-155] (table 2). Loss of function mutation (E375X) in *KCNA5* gene has also been reported in a family with lone AF [156] (table 2).

Mutations in cardiac gap-junction protein connexin 40 (*GJA5*) have been found in 25% of patients of idiopathic atrial fibrillation [157]. Among the total 4-reported *GJA5* mutations, three are somatic, one is a germline mutation. The cardiac gap-junction protein connexin 40 (*GJA5*) is expressed selectively in atrial myocytes and mediates the coordinated electrical activation of the atria. A recent report suggests that mutations in *SCN5A* may predispose patients with or without underlying heart disease to AF accounting for 6% of the AF cases [158]. AF can also present in 2% of patients with genetically proven LQTS, BrS, SQTS and CPVT [135, 159-161]. Darbar et al. (2008) recently reported a novel AF locus on chromosome 5p15, where the causative gene remains to be identified [162] (table 2). Mutations in *SCN1B* and *SCN2B* have also been recently reported in AF [163] (table 2).

Overlap Syndromes

LQTS causing SCN5A mutations are associated with gain-of-function defect of the encoding Na^+ channel, while BrS and ICCD causing mutations are typically associated with loss-of-function defects. Hence, two opposite functional pathophysiology are responsible for LQTS and BrS.

There are several reports of where LQTS and BrS were observed in patients due to single identical mutation in the SCN5A gene. An insertion of an aspartic acid residue (1795insD) in the C-terminus of SCN5A can result in BrS, LQTS and ICCD features in the same patients [34, 164]. Also conduction at all cardiac levels is hampered in these patients. The deletion of a lysine (K1500) was found to be associated with BrS, LQTS, and ICCD [165]. A French study in several families with BrS or ICCD identified a missense mutation G1406R pathogenic to both phenotypes [35]. E1784K mutation in SCN5A was recently described in a family with LQT3, BrS and SND [36]. How can a single mutation cause both phenotypes in the same patient (and also in mice) with the opposite effect on the channel function? Electrophysiology analysis, *invitro* and also with 1795insD transgenic mice provided an answer. Drastic reduction of peak sodium current (causing BrS phenotype), delayed time course of fast inactivation and small persistent sodium current pathogenic to LQT3 were observed in heterologous expression system and also in mice [164,166].

V1516D mutation in ANK2 was reported both in LQTS and BrS patients [70]. Very recently Darbar et al. (2008, Circulation) elaborated that BrS and/or LQT3 causing mutations could also cause lone AF [158]. AV block, DCM, Right ventricular fibrosis and conduction delay, sinus node dysfunction) were also observed with mutations in LQT/Brugada causing SCN5A gene [134, 167-168]. Mutations in the *CAV3* gene were originally described in the autosomal-dominant limb-girdle muscular dystrophies, rippling muscle disease, idiopathic hyper-CK-emia [169-170]. Mutation in this gene also recently has been described in LQTS patients. Despite no phenotype overlap, diverse diseases are observed due to mutations in the same gene. This could be due to the fact that functional aberration due to mutation/s in CAV3, an adapter molecule for ion channel, could be mild to severe depending on the location of the mutation and could also be the fact that pathological consequences of certain mutations are organ specific.

We have also recently observed expanded clinical phenotypes (sinoatrial node and atrioventricular node dysfunction, atrial fibrillation, atrial standstill, and dilated cardiomyopathy) in patients harbouring an inframe deletion of amino-terminal 35-amino acids in the RyR2 [135]. All the reported RyR2 missense mutation carriers contrarily suffer from CPVT only phenotype [137-141].

Variability in clinical penetrance and sometimes with additional phenotypes due to identical cardiac ion channel mutations is likely to be modified, synergized (or attenuated) by environmental factors, gender and individual genetic back up. This individual variation in disease susceptibility could be due to SNPs located inside the pathogenic gene or could be located in a place far from the primary disease locus, and which might directly or indirectly be involved in the functional circuit of the pathogenetic gene. K897T is an otherwise harmless, frequently observed SNP in the *KCNH2* gene, which was described to unmask the subclinical LQT2 phenotype in a patient who carried both A1116V mutation and the K897T SNP in the *KCNH2* gene [171]. 3-other family members who harboured the A1116V mutation (but not K897T) were devoid of any clinical symptoms [171].Though, in this study conclusion was drawn from the findings of a single symptomatic carrier, the approach of this study was quite novel. We recommend to perform similar study with more patients. Severity in clinical phenotype and longer QT intervals were also reported in patients who co-harboured a common SNP D85N in minK (encoded by *KCNE1*) along with the pathogenic LQT1 causing mutation in *KCNQ1* gene [16]. A block of 6-SNPs in the promoter region of SCN5A modulates the phenotypes in Brugada patients, being prevalent among the South Asians, and was shown to be associated with cardiac conduction disease prevalence/preponderance among South Asians [172]. Another intragenic SNP H558R in SCN5A encoded $Na_v1.5$ was also described as a modulator in BrS patients, where R558 carriers had attenuated BrS phenotype [173]. Similar extensive studies (including replication studies) with both intragenic and extragenic SNP markers are required, which might answer about the interindividual variability, also ethnic variability in disease vulnerability and progression.

Future Directions

During the last decade, we have seen growing list of genes and mutations linked to pathophysiology of arrhythmias of genetic origin. But, we still lack genetic pathobiological evidences for a large number of patients with inherited arrhythmias or sporadic arrhythmias with a suspected genetic origin. Efforts are at full speed to identify new genes, germline mutations and also in characterizing the mutations into pathophysiology of various congenital arrhythmias. Somatic mutations though common in various oncological disorders, were also recently reported in cardiac gap-junction protein connexin 40 (*GJA5*) in AF patients [157]. Somatic mutations are present only in the affected tissues or organs and are not transmitted to the offsprings unlike the germline mutations. Perhaps, due to limitations in access, somatic mutations have not been seriously looked for in most cardiac ion channel or desmosomal genes, which might add to the list of genes and mutations. In our study, including others in this field [137-141], we could see that yield in RyR2 mutation in familial CPVT cases is >80%, but this rate drops to ~50% in sporadic cases, though their CPVT diagnosis were clinically confirmed by experienced cardiologists in this field. Mutations confined to the diseased tissues (somatic mutations) might be checked for RyR2 in mutation negative CPVT cases. A pilot screening could be initiated with the archival cardiac tissues.

Gene copy-number variations (CNV) can influence disease phenotypes, which were also reported in various familial diseases [174]. Role of CNVs in cardiac arrhythmia pathogenesis also might shed new light in arrhythmia pathology.

We see an intriguing observation about HERG autoantibody mediated LQT2 [71]. Studies are also awaited about the role of autoantibody mediated various cardiac channelopathies.

Studies also lack about the modulators (some say modifier) which perhaps play a pivotal role in disease pathogenesis, manifestation and progression. Disease penetration among mutation carriers vary, sometimes even within the family members. What makes them susceptible despite having both the same mutation, why one develops fibrillation earlier than other, even why some one does not develop it at all even within the family? Complex interaction of various factors (SNPs, environment), perhaps play a role in the interindividual variation of disease expression. As we have previously mentioned, we see only few studies elucidating the modifier effect of an otherwise silent/innocuous SNPs (within the causative gene and or in the genes in the functional network) in exaggerating/ameliorating the clinical presentation of arrhythmias [16,171,175]. β-adrenergic blockade is the first line of treatment in patients with arrhythmias. Modifier/modulatory effect of common SNPs of the adrenergic signalling pathway genes on the clinical severity, therapy outcomes, both in cardiac channelopathies and desmopathies remain to be extensively studied. We also miss twin studies conducted in this field, which would have shed more light into this topic of gene environment interaction in familial arrhythmia cases due to a known mutation.

Extensive studies are required not only characterizing each ion channel function, their signalling pathways with identification of important signalling molecules are also crucial. This would lead to the identification of novel surrogate clinical/bio markers in disease diagnosis and progression and novel therapeutic intervention. Very few studies are focusing on the gene and mutation specific clinical management. Current treatments for arrhythmias are also limited mainly to β-blockers and in therapy resistant cases by expensive devices such as implantable defibrillators and pacemakers. Novel therapeutic approaches including biological interference treatment modalities may be developed.

Functional Role of Nonsense Mediated Decay (NMD) in Arrhythmogenesis

We [23-24] have shown for the first time the role of nonsense-mediated decay (NMD] into the pathogenesis of LQT2 arrhythmias. NMD removes aberrant mRNAs with premature termination codons from eukaryotic cells [176]. In our study, we have found that heterozygous Q1070X KCNH2 mutation carriers have virtually no LQT2 phenotypes, on the other hand homozygous carriers suffered from intrauterine fatal arrhythmias, severest phenotype observed among the reported in homozygous KCNH2 mutation carriers [24,29-31]. In vitro functional assay with the HERG Q1070X mutant showed normal cellular localisation and electrical properties. We have eventually discovered that the mutant Q1070X mRNAs are susceptible to NMD degradation, which leaves nearly negligible amount of mRNA to make any functional HERG protein. This finding also explains why heterozygous carriers have no phenotype as the mutant allele is unable to translate to protein and confer its dominant negative effect on WT HERG for functional aberration. Haploinsufficiency of HERG did not cause LQT2 phenotypes in our studied patients [24]. From the published report, we see that not all non-sense or frameshift *KCNH2* mutation carriers are without any phenotypes [23,177]. This could possibly due to the fact that, not all non-sense or frameshift KCNH2 mutations are equally susceptible to NMD degradation, which needs to be investigated. Interindividual variation in NMD might also be evident in some cases which remain to be investigated [178].

Emerging Role of microRNA in Arrhythmia Pathogenicity

We have mentioned in the beginning of this chapter that an extensive crosstalk between mechanical and electrical junctions is required for proper, coordinated heart function. Several recent reports add a new component, microRNA (miRNA), in this crosstalk, orchestrated function of which are also essential to prevent the heart from generating arrhythmias. miRNAs are endogenous ~22-nucleotide non-coding RNAs that regulate gene expression at the post-transcriptional level by annealing to inexactly complementary sequences in the 3'-untranslated regions of target mRNAs of protein-coding genes [179]. MiRNAs negatively regulate gene expression by promoting mRNA degradation and inhibiting mRNA translation. MiR-133 was found to repress *KCNH2* expression and prolonged the QT interval in diabetic hearts of experimental animals [179]. An elevated level of miR-1 was observed in patients with coronary artery disease, which has been reproduced in the mouse heart model of myocardial infarction [180]. This increased miR-1 reduced the expression of Cx43 and Kir2.1, which in return caused slowed electrical conduction and prolongation of repolarization potential and predisposed the heart to arrhythmias [180].

Given the emerging role of miRNAs in arrhythmogenesis, more research is needed especially in the context of their role into the pathogenetic mechanism of arrhythmias. Modulation of expression of cardiac miRNAs might be a potential a future therapeutic strategies, but more studies are required before bringing it to clinic. Their route of delivery is also required to be studied. This might help in developing a novel therapeutic strategy. Studies are also required in the context of expression of various ion-channel genes, miRNAs due to various stimuli. A global understanding from various dimensions is required to understand the pathobiology of arrhythmias, which has the potential to lead to a gene, individual specific, effective clinical management of arrhythmias.

References

[1] Kucera JP, Rohr S, Rudy Y. Localization of sodium channels in intercalated disks modulates cardiac conduction. *Circ Res*. 2002 ;91:1176-82.

[2a] Oxford EM, Musa H, Maass K, Coombs W, Taffet SM, Delmar M. Connexin43 remodeling caused by inhibition of plakophilin-2 expression in cardiac cells. *Circ Res*. 2007;101:703-11.

[2b] Oxford EM, Everitt M, Coombs W, Fox PR, Kraus M, Gelzer AR, Saffitz J, Taffet SM, Moïse NS, Delmar M. Molecular composition of the intercalated disc in a spontaneous canine animal model of arrhythmogenic right ventricular dysplasia/cardiomyopathy. *Heart Rhythm*. 2007 ;4: 1196-205.

[3] Rohr S. Molecular Crosstalk Between Mechanical and Electrical Junctions at the Intercalated Disc. *Circulation Research*. 2007;101: 637-639

[4] Zipes DP, Jalife J. *Cardiac Electrophysiology*: From Cell to Bedside. 2004, 4th edition, W. B. Saunders Co, Philadelphia, USA.

[5] Priori SG, Aliot E, Blømstrom-Lundqvist C, Bossaert L, Breithardt G, Brugada P, Camm JA, Cappato R, Cobbe SM, Di MC, Maron BJ, McKenna WJ, Pedersen AK, Ravens U, Schwartz PJ, Trusz-Gluza M, Vardas P, Wellens HJ, Zipes DP. *Task Force on Sudden Cardiac Death*, European Society of Cardiology. Europace. 2002;4: 3-18.

[6] Wang Q, Shen J, Splawski I, Atkinson D, Li Z, Robinson JL, Moss AJ, Towbin JA, Keating MT. SCN5A mutations associated with an inherited cardiac arrhythmia, long QT syndrome. *Cell*. 1995;80:805-11.

[7] Curran ME, Splawski I, Timothy KW, Vincent GM, Green ED, Keating MT. A molecular basis for cardiac arrhythmia: HERG mutations cause long QT syndrome. *Cell.* 1995;80:795-803.

[8] Wang Q, Curran ME, Splawski I, Burn TC, Millholland JM, VanRaay TJ, Shen J, Timothy KW, Vincent GM, de Jager T, Schwartz PJ, Towbin JA, Moss AJ, Atkinson DL, Landes GM, Connors TD, Keating MT. Positional cloning of a novel potassium channel gene: KVLQT1 mutations cause cardiac arrhythmias. *Nat Genet.* 1996 ;12: 17-23.

[9] Splawski I, Tristani-Firouzi M, Lehmann MH, Sanguinetti MC, Keating MT. Mutations in the hminK gene cause long QT syndrome and suppress IKs function. *Nat Genet.* 1997;17:338-40

[10] Sanguinetti MC, Jiang C, Curran ME, Keating MT. A mechanistic link between an inherited and an acquired cardiac arrhythmia: HERG encodes the IKr potassium channel. *Cell.* 1995; 81: 299-307.

[11] Neyroud N, Tesson F, Denjoy I, Leibovici M, Donger C, Barhanin J, Fauré S, Gary F, Coumel P, Petit C, Schwartz K, Guicheney P. A novel mutation in the potassium channel gene KVLQT1 causes the Jervell and Lange-Nielsen cardioauditory syndrome. *Nat Genet.* 1997;15:186-9.

[12] Wilde AA, Bezzina CR. Genetics of cardiac arrhythmias. *Heart* 2005; 91:1352-8. Review.

[13] Saffitz JE. Adhesion molecules: why they are important to the electrophysiologist. *J Cardiovasc Electrophysiol.* 2006;17: 225-9.

[14] Crotti L, Stramba-Badiale M, Pedrazzini M. Prevalence of the Long QT Syndrome. *Circulation* 2005; 112 (suppl. II): "abstr" 3097.

[15] Splawski I, Shen J, Timothy KW, Lehmann MH, Priori S, Robinson JL, Moss AJ, Schwartz PJ, Towbin JA, Vincent GM, Keating MT. Spectrum of mutations in long-QT syndrome genes. KVLQT1, HERG, SCN5A, KCNE1, and KCNE2. *Circulation.* 2000; 102: 1178-85.

[16] Westenskow P, Splawski I, Timothy KW, Keating MT, Sanguinetti MC. Compound mutations: a common cause of severe long-QT syndrome. *Circulation.* 2004;109:1834-41.

[17] Roden DM. Clinical practice. Long-QT syndrome. *N Engl J Med.* 2008;358:169-76. Review.

[18] Schwartz PJ, Priori SG, Spazzolini C, Moss AJ, Vincent GM, Napolitano C, Denjoy I, Guicheney P, Breithardt G, Keating MT, Towbin JA, Beggs AH, Brink P, Wilde AA, Toivonen L, Zareba W, Robinson JL, Timothy KW, Corfield V, Wattanasirichaigoon D, Corbett C, Haverkamp W, Schulze-Bahr E, Lehmann MH, Schwartz K, Coumel P, Bloise R. Genotype-phenotype correlation in the long-QT syndrome: gene-specific triggers for life-threatening arrhythmias. *Circulation.* 2001;103:89-95.

[19] Shimizu W, Horie M, Ohno S, Takenaka K, Yamaguchi M, Shimizu M, Washizuka T, Aizawa Y, Nakamura K, Ohe T, Aiba T, Miyamoto Y, Yoshimasa Y, Towbin JA, Priori SG, Kamakura S. Mutation site-specific differences in arrhythmic risk and sensitivity to sympathetic stimulation in the LQT1 form of congenital long QT syndrome: multicenter study in Japan. *J Am Coll Cardiol.* 2004;44:117-25.

[20] Moss AJ, Shimizu W, Wilde AA, Towbin JA, Zareba W, Robinson JL, Qi M, Vincent GM, Ackerman MJ, Kaufman ES, Hofman N, Seth R, Kamakura S, Miyamoto Y,

Goldenberg I, Andrews ML, McNitt S. Clinical aspects of type-1 long-QT syndrome by location, coding type, and biophysical function of mutations involving the KCNQ1 gene. *Circulation*. 2007;115: 2481-9.

[21] Schwartz PJ, Spazzolini C, Crotti L, Bathen J, Amlie JP, Timothy K, Shkolnikova M, Berul CI, Bitner-Glindzicz M, Toivonen L, Horie M, Schulze-Bahr E, Denjoy I. The Jervell and Lange-Nielsen syndrome: natural history, molecular basis, and clinical outcome. *Circulation*. 2006;113: 783-90.

[22] Bhuiyan ZA, Momenah TS, Kupershmidt S, Potet F, Alders M, Mannens MMAM, Wilde AAM. A homozygous intronic mutation leading to incomplete skipping of exon-2 in KCNQ1 rescues hearing in Jervell and Lange-Nielsen syndrome. *Heart Rhythm. May Supplement* 2008; 5: 5, PO2-54

[23] Gong Q, Zhang L, Vincent GM, Horne BD, Zhou Z. Nonsense mutations in hERG cause a decrease in mutant mRNA transcripts by nonsense-mediated mRNA decay in human long-QT syndrome. *Circulation*. 2007;116:17-24.

[24] Bhuiyan ZA, Momenah TS, Gong Q, Amin AS, Ghamdi SA, Carvalho JS, Homfray T, Mannens MM, Zhou Z, Wilde AA. Recurrent intrauterine fetal loss due to near absence of HERG: clinical and functional characterization of a homozygous nonsense HERG Q1070X mutation. *Heart Rhythm*. 2008;5: 553-61.

[25] Wilde AA, Jongbloed RJ, Doevendans PA, Düren DR, Hauer RN, van Langen IM, van Tintelen JP, Smeets HJ, Meyer H, Geelen JL. Auditory stimuli as a trigger for arrhythmic events differentiate HERG-related (LQTS2) patients from KVLQT1-related patients (LQTS1). *J Am Coll Cardiol*. 1999;33: 327-32.

[26] Moss AJ, Zareba W, Kaufman ES, Gartman E, Peterson DR, Benhorin J, Towbin JA, Keating MT, Priori SG, Schwartz PJ, Vincent GM, Robinson JL, Andrews ML, Feng C, Hall WJ, Medina A, Zhang L, Wang Z. Increased risk of arrhythmic events in long-QT syndrome with mutations in the pore region of the human ether-a-go-go-related gene potassium channel. *Circulation*. 2002;105: 794-9.

[27] Lupoglazoff JM, Denjoy I, Villain E, Fressart V, Simon F, Bozio A, Berthet M, Benammar N, Hainque B, Guicheney P. Long QT syndrome in neonates: conduction disorders associated with HERG mutations and sinus bradycardia with KCNQ1 mutations. *J Am Coll Cardiol*. 2004;43: 826-30.

[28] Chevalier P, Bellocq C, Millat G, Piqueras E, Potet F, Schott JJ, Baró I, Lemarec H, Barhanin J, Rousson R, Rodriguez-Lafrasse C. Torsades de pointes complicating atrioventricular block: evidence for a genetic predisposition. *Heart Rhythm*. 2007;4:170-4.

[29] Hoorntje T, Alders M, van Tintelen P, van der Lip K, Sreeram N, van der Wal A, Mannens M, Wilde A. Homozygous premature truncation of the HERG protein : the human HERG knockout. *Circulation*. 1999;100:1264-7

[30] Piippo K, Laitinen P, Swan H, Toivonen L, Viitasalo M, Pasternack M, Paavonen K, Chapman H, Wann KT, Hirvelä E, Sajantila A, Kontula K. Homozygosity for a HERG potassium channel mutation causes a severe form of long QT syndrome: identification of an apparent founder mutation in the Finns. *J Am Coll Cardiol*. 2000; 35:1919-25

[31] Johnson WH Jr, Yang P, Yang T, Lau YR, Mostella BA, Wolff DJ, Roden DM, Benson DW. Clinical, genetic, and biophysical characterization of a homozygous HERG mutation causing severe neonatal long QT syndrome. *Pediatr Res*. 2003;53: 744-8.

[32] Catterall WA. From ionic currents to molecular mechanisms: the structure and function of voltage-gated sodium channels. *Neuron* 2000; 26:13–25.

[33] Clancy CE, Kass RS. Theoretical investigation of the neuronal Na+ channel SCN1A: abnormal gating and epilepsy. *Biophys J.* 2004;86: 2606-14.

[34] Bezzina C, Veldkamp MW, van Den Berg MP, Postma AV, Rook MB, Viersma JW, van Langen IM, Tan-Sindhunata G, Bink-Boelkens MT, van Der Hout AH, Mannens MM, Wilde AA. A single Na(+) channel mutation causing both long-QT and Brugada syndromes. *Circ Res.* 1999;85:1206-13.

[35] Kyndt F, Probst V, Potet F, Demolombe S, Chevallier JC, Baro I, Moisan JP, Boisseau P, Schott JJ, Escande D, Le Marec H. Novel SCN5A mutation leading either to isolated cardiac conduction defect or Brugada syndrome in a large French family. *Circulation.* 2001;104: 3081-6.

[36] Makita N, Behr E, Shimizu W, Horie M, Sunami A, Crotti L, Schulze-Bahr E, Fukuhara S, Mochizuki N, Makiyama T, Itoh H, Christiansen M, McKeown P, Miyamoto K, Kamakura S, Tsutsui H, Schwartz PJ, George AL, Roden DM. The E1784K mutation in SCN5A is associated with mixed clinical phenotype of type 3 long QT syndrome. *J Clin Invest.* 2008;118: 2219-2229.

[37] Priori SG, Schwartz PJ, Napolitano C, Bloise R, Ronchetti E, Grillo M, Vicentini A, Spazzolini C, Nastoli J, Bottelli G, Folli R, Cappelletti D. Risk stratification in the long-QT syndrome. *N Engl J Med.* 2003; 348:1866-74.

[38] Lupoglazoff JM, Cheav T, Baroudi G, Berthet M, Denjoy I, Cauchemez B, Extramiana F, Chahine M, Guicheney P. Homozygous SCN5A mutation in long-QT syndrome with functional two-to-one atrioventricular block. *Circ Res.* 2001;89:E16-21.

[39] Schott JJ, Charpentier F, Peltier S, Foley P, Drouin E, Bouhour JB, Donnelly P, Vergnaud G, Bachner L, Moisan JP, Marec HL, Pascal O. Mapping of a gene for long QT syndrome to chromosome 4q25-27. *Am J Hum Genet.* 1995; 57:1114-22.

[40] Mohler PJ, Schott JJ, Gramolini AO, et al. Ankyrin-B mutation causes type 4 long-QT cardiac arrhythmia and sudden cardiac death. *Nature* 2003; 421: 634-639.

[41] Cunha SR, Bhasin N, Mohler PJ. Targeting and stability of Na/Ca exchanger 1 in cardiomyocytes requires direct interaction with the membrane adaptor ankyrin-B. *J Biol Chem.* 2007 ; 282:4875-83.

[42] Barhanin J, Lesage F, Guillemare E, Fink M, Lazdunski M, Romey G. K(V)LQT1 and IsK (minK) proteins associate to form the I(Ks) cardiac potassium current. *Nature.* 1996;384: 78-80.

[43] Sanguinetti MC, Curran ME, Zou A, Shen J, Spector PS, Atkinson DL, Keating MT. Coassembly of K(V)LQT1 and minK (IsK) proteins to form cardiac I(Ks) potassium channel. *Nature.* 1996; 384: 80-3.

[44] Ohno S, Zankov DP, Yoshida H, Tsuji K, Makiyama T, Itoh H, Akao M, Hancox JC, Kita T, Horie M. N- and C-terminal KCNE1 mutations cause distinct phenotypes of long QT syndrome. *Heart Rhythm.* 2007;4:332-40.

[45] Schulze-Bahr, E., Wang, Q., Wedekind, H., Haverkamp, W., Chen, Q., Sun, Y., Rubie, C., Hordt, M., Towbin, J. A., Borggrefe, M., Assmann, G., Qu, X., Somberg, J. C., Breithardt, G., Oberti, C., Funke, H., 1997. KCNE1 mutations cause Jervell and Lange-Nielsen syndrome. (Letter) *Nat. Genet.* 17: 267-268. 1997.

[46] Duggal, P., Vesely, M. R., Wattanasirichaigoon, D., Villafane, J., Kaushik, V., Beggs, A. H., 1998. Mutation of the gene for IKs associated with both Jervell and Lange-Nielsen and Romano-Ward forms of long-QT syndrome. *Circulation*. 97: 142-146.

[47] Abbott GW, Sesti F, Splawski I, Buck ME, Lehmann MH, Timothy KW, Keating MT, Goldstein SA. MiRP1 forms IKr potassium channels with HERG and is associated with cardiac arrhythmia. *Cell*. 1999; 97: 175-87.

[48] Gordon E, Panaghie G, Deng L, Bee KJ, Roepke TK, Krogh-Madsen T, Christini DJ, Ostrer H, Basson CT, Chung W, Abbott GW. A KCNE2 mutation in a patient with cardiac arrhythmia induced by auditory stimuli and serum electrolyte imbalance. *Cardiovasc Res*. 2008; 77: 98-106.

[49] Plaster NM, Tawil R, Tristani-Firouzi M, Canún S, Bendahhou S, Tsunoda A, Donaldson MR, Iannaccone ST, Brunt E, Barohn R, Clark J, Deymeer F, George AL Jr, Fish FA, Hahn A, Nitu A, Ozdemir C, Serdaroglu P, Subramony SH, Wolfe G, Fu YH, Ptácek LJ. Mutations in Kir2.1 cause the developmental and episodic electrical phenotypes of Andersen's syndrome. *Cell*. 2001;105:511-9.

[50] Kubo Y, Baldwin TJ, Jan YN, Jan LY. Primary structure and functional expression of a mouse inward rectifier potassium channel. *Nature*. 1993;362:127-33.

[51] Raab-Graham KF, Radeke CM, Vandenberg CA. Molecular cloning and expression of a human heart inward rectifier potassium channel. *Neuroreport*. 1994 ;5: 2501-5.

[52] Tristani-Firouzi M, Jensen JL, Donaldson MR, Sansone V, Meola G, Hahn A, Bendahhou S, Kwiecinski H, Fidzianska A, Plaster N, Fu YH, Ptacek LJ, Tawil R. Functional and clinical characterization of KCNJ2 mutations associated with LQT7 (Andersen syndrome). *J Clin Invest*. 2002;110: 381-8.

[53] Hosaka Y, Hanawa H, Washizuka T, Chinushi M, Yamashita F, Yoshida T, Komura S, Watanabe H, Aizawa Y. Function, subcellular localization and assembly of a novel mutation of KCNJ2 in Andersen's syndrome. *J Mol Cell Cardiol*. 2003;35:409-15.

[54] Kobori A, Sarai N, Shimizu W, Nakamura Y, Murakami Y, Makiyama T, Ohno S, Takenaka K, Ninomiya T, Fujiwara Y, Matsuoka S, Takano M, Noma A, Kita T, Horie M. Additional gene variants reduce effectiveness of beta-blockers in the LQT1 form of long QT syndrome. *J Cardiovasc Electrophysiol*. 2004;15:190-9.

[55] Splawski I, Timothy KW, Sharpe LM, Decher N, Kumar P, Bloise R, Napolitano C, Schwartz PJ, Joseph RM, Condouris K, Tager-Flusberg H, Priori SG, Sanguinetti MC, Keating MT. Ca(V)1.2 calcium channel dysfunction causes a multisystem disorder including arrhythmia and autism. Cell. 2004;119:19-31.

[56] Marks ML, Whisler SL, Clericuzio C, Keating M. A new form of long QT syndrome associated with syndactyly. *J Am Coll Cardiol*. 1995;25:59-64. Review.

[57] Vatta M, Ackerman MJ, Ye B, Makielski JC, Ughanze EE, Taylor EW, Tester DJ, Balijepalli RC, Foell JD, Li Z, Kamp TJ, Towbin JA. Mutant caveolin-3 induces persistent late sodium current and is associated with long-QT syndrome. *Circulation*. 2006;114: 2104-12.

[58] Cronk LB, Ye B, Kaku T, Tester DJ, Vatta M, Makielski JC, Ackerman MJ. Novel mechanism for sudden infant death syndrome: persistent late sodium current secondary to mutations in caveolin-3. *Heart Rhythm*. 2007 ;4:161-6.

[59] Medeiros-Domingo A, Kaku T, Tester DJ, Iturralde-Torres P, Itty A, Ye B, Valdivia C, Ueda K, Canizales-Quinteros S, Tusié-Luna MT, Makielski JC, Ackerman MJ.

SCN4B-encoded sodium channel beta4 subunit in congenital long-QT syndrome. *Circulation*. 2007;116:134-42.

[60] Chen L, Marquardt ML, Tester DJ, Sampson KJ, Ackerman MJ, Kass RS. Mutation of an A-kinase-anchoring protein causes long-QT syndrome. *Proc Natl Acad Sci U S A*. 2007;104:20990-5.

[61] Wu G, Ai T, Kim JJ, Mohapatra B, Xi Y, Li Z, Abbasi S, Purevjav E, Samani K, Ackerman MJ, Qi M, Moss AM, Shimizu W, Towbin JA, Cheng J, Vatta M. Alpha-1-Syntrophin Mutation and the Long QT Syndrome: a disease of sodium channel disruption. *Circulation: Arrhythmia and Electrophysiology*. 2008

[62] Roden DM. Mechanisms and management of proarrhythmia. Am J Cardiol. 1998;82:49I-57I. Review.

[63] Mitcheson JS, Chen J, Lin M, Culberson C, Sanguinetti MC. A structural basis for drug-induced long QT syndrome. *Proc Natl Acad Sci U S A*. 2000; 97:12329-33.

[64] Kannankeril PJ, Roden DM. Drug-induced long QT and torsade de pointes: recent advances. *Curr Opin Cardiol*. 2007;22:39-43. Review.

[65] Liu J, Zhang M, Jiang M, Tseng GN. Structural and functional role of the extracellular s5-p linker in the HERG potassium channel. *J Gen Physiol*. 2002;120:723-37.

[66] Sesti F, Abbott GW, Wei J, Murray KT, Saksena S, Schwartz PJ, Priori SG, Roden DM, George AL Jr, Goldstein SA. A common polymorphism associated with antibiotic-induced cardiac arrhythmia. *Proc Natl Acad Sci U S A*. 2000;97:10613-8.

[67] Splawski I, Timothy KW, Tateyama M, Clancy CE, Malhotra A, Beggs AH, Cappuccio FP, Sagnella GA, Kass RS, and Keating MT. Variant of SCN5A sodium channel implicated in risk of cardiac arrhythmia. *Science* 2002; 297: 1333–1336.

[68] Makita N, Horie M, Nakamura T, Ai T, Sasaki K, Yokoi H, Sakurai M, Sakuma I, Otani H, Sawa H, Kitabatake A. Drug-induced long-QT syndrome associated with a subclinical SCN5A mutation. *Circulation*. 2002;106:1269-74.

[69] Liu K, Yang T, Viswanathan PC, Roden DM. New mechanism contributing to drug-induced arrhythmia: rescue of a misprocessed LQT3 mutant. *Circulation*. 2005;112:3239-46.

[70] Mohler PJ, Le Scouarnec S, Denjoy I, Lowe JS, Guicheney P, Caron L, Driskell IM, Schott JJ, Norris K, Leenhardt A, Kim RB, Escande D, Roden DM. Defining the cellular phenotype of "ankyrin-B syndrome" variants: human ANK2 variants associated with clinical phenotypes display a spectrum of activities in cardiomyocytes. *Circulation*. 2007;115:432-41.

[71] Nakamura K, Katayama Y, Kusano KF, Haraoka K, Tani Y, Nagase S, Morita H, Miura D, Fujimoto Y, Furukawa T, Ueda K, Aizawa Y, Kimura A, Kurachi Y, Ohe T. Anti-KCNH2 antibody-induced long QT syndrome: novel acquired form of long QT syndrome. *J Am Coll Cardiol*. 2007; 50: 1808-9.

[72] Moss AJ, Zareba W, Benhorin J, Locati EH, Hall WJ, Robinson JL, Schwartz PJ, Towbin JA, Vincent GM, Lehmann MH. ECG T-wave patterns in genetically distinct forms of the hereditary long QT syndrome. *Circulation*. 1995;92:2929-34.

[73] Zhang L, Timothy KW, Vincent GM, Lehmann MH, Fox J, Giuli LC, Shen J, Splawski I, Priori SG, Compton SJ, Yanowitz F, Benhorin J, Moss AJ, Schwartz PJ, Robinson JL, Wang Q, Zareba W, Keating MT, Towbin JA, Napolitano C, Medina A. Spectrum of ST-T-wave patterns and repolarization parameters in congenital long-QT syndrome: ECG findings identify genotypes. *Circulation*. 2000;102: 2849-55.

[74] Tan HL, Bardai A, Shimizu W, Moss AJ, Schulze-Bahr E, Noda T, Wilde AA. Genotype-specific onset of arrhythmias in congenital long-QT syndrome: possible therapy implications. *Circulation*. 2006;114: 2096-103.

[75] Locati EH, Zareba W, Moss AJ, Schwartz PJ, Vincent GM, Lehmann MH, Towbin JA, Priori SG, Napolitano C, Robinson JL, Andrews M, Timothy K, Hall WJ. Age- and sex-related differences in clinical manifestations in patients with congenital long-QT syndrome: findings from the International LQTS Registry. *Circulation*. 1998;97:2237-44.

[76] Zareba W, Moss AJ, Schwartz PJ, Vincent GM, Robinson JL, Priori SG, Benhorin J, Locati EH, Towbin JA, Keating MT, Lehmann MH, Hall WJ. Influence of genotype on the clinical course of the long-QT syndrome. International Long-QT Syndrome Registry Research Group. *N Engl J Med*. 1998;339: 960-5.

[77] Goldenberg I, Moss AJ, Bradley J, Polonsky S, Peterson DR, McNitt S, Zareba W, Andrews ML, Robinson JL, Ackerman MJ, Benhorin J, Kaufman ES, Locati EH, Napolitano C, Priori SG, Qi M, Schwartz PJ, Towbin JA, Vincent GM, Zhang L. Long-QT syndrome after age 40. *Circulation*. 2008;117: 2192-201.

[78] Zareba W, Moss AJ, Locati EH, Lehmann MH, Peterson DR, Hall WJ, Schwartz PJ, Vincent GM, Priori SG, Benhorin J, Towbin JA, Robinson JL, Andrews ML, Napolitano C, Timothy K, Zhang L, Medina A; International Long QT Syndrome Registry. Modulating effects of age and gender on the clinical course of long QT syndrome by genotype. *J Am Coll Cardiol*. 2003;42:103-9.

[79] Seth R, Moss AJ, McNitt S, Zareba W, Andrews ML, Qi M, Robinson JL, Goldenberg I, Ackerman MJ, Benhorin J, Kaufman ES, Locati EH, Napolitano C, Priori SG, Schwartz PJ, Towbin JA, Vincent GM, Zhang L. Long QT syndrome and pregnancy. J Am Coll Cardiol. 2007; 49:1092-8.

[80] Miller TE, Estrella E, Myerburg RJ, Garcia de Viera J, Moreno N, Rusconi P, Ahearn ME, Baumbach L, Kurlansky P, Wolff G, Bishopric NH. Recurrent third-trimester fetal loss and maternal mosaicism for long-QT syndrome. *Circulation*. 2004;109:3029-34.

[81a] Schwartz PJ, Priori SG, Dumaine R, Napolitano C, Antzelevitch C, Stramba-Badiale M, Richard TA, Berti MR, Bloise R.A molecular link between the sudden infant death syndrome and the long-QT syndrome. *N Engl J Med*. 2000;343: 262-7.

[81b] Schwartz PJ, Priori SG, Bloise R, Napolitano C, Ronchetti E, Piccinini A, Goj C, Breithardt G, Schulze-Bahr E, Wedekind H, Nastoli J. Molecular diagnosis in a child with sudden infant death syndrome. *Lancet*. 2001;358:1342-3.

[82] Christiansen M, Tønder N, Larsen LA, Andersen PS, Simonsen H, Oyen N, Kanters JK, Jacobsen JR, Fosdal I, Wettrell G, Kjeldsen K. Mutations in the HERG K+-ion channel: a novel link between long QT syndrome and sudden infant death syndrome. *Am J Cardiol*. 2005; 95: 433-4. (SIDS)

[83] Tester DJ, Ackerman MJ. Postmortem long QT syndrome genetic testing for sudden unexplained death in the young. *J Am Coll Cardiol*. 2007;49:240-6.

[84] Hofman N, Tan HL, Clur SA, Alders M, van Langen IM, Wilde AA. Contribution of inherited heart disease to sudden cardiac death in childhood. *Pediatrics*. 2007;120:e967-73.

[85] Wedekind H, Smits JP, Schulze-Bahr E, Arnold R, Veldkamp MW, Bajanowski T, Borggrefe M, Brinkmann B, Warnecke I, Funke H, Bhuiyan ZA, Wilde AA, Breithardt

G, Haverkamp W. De novo mutation in the SCN5A gene associated with early onset of sudden infant death. *Circulation*. 2001;104:1158-64.

[86] Wang DW, Desai RR, Crotti L, Arnestad M, Insolia R, Pedrazzini M, Ferrandi C, Vege A, Rognum T, Schwartz PJ, George AL Jr. Cardiac sodium channel dysfunction in sudden infant death syndrome. *Circulation*. 2007;115:368-76.

[87a] Van Norstrand DW, Valdivia CR, Tester DJ, Ueda K, London B, Makielski JC, Ackerman MJ. Molecular and functional characterization of novel glycerol-3-phosphate dehydrogenase 1 like gene (GPD1-L) mutations in sudden infant death syndrome. *Circulation*. 2007;116:2253-9.

[87b] Van Norstrand D, Pundi KN, Tester DJ, Medeiros-Domingo A, Valdivia CR, Makielski JC, Ackerman MJ. Identification of cardiac sodium channel beta subunit mutations in sudden infant death syndrome. *Heart Rhythm* 2008; 5: 5 May Supplement 2008 AB45-1

[88] Behr E, Wood DA, Wright M, Syrris P, Sheppard MN, Casey A, Davies MJ, McKenna W; Sudden Arrhythmic Death Syndrome Steering Group. Cardiological assessment of first-degree relatives in sudden arrhythmic death syndrome. *Lancet*. 2003;362:1457-9.

[89] Takenaka K, Ai T, Shimizu W, Kobori A, Ninomiya T, Otani H, Kubota T, Takaki H, Kamakura S, Horie M. Exercise stress test amplifies genotype-phenotype correlation in the LQT1 and LQT2 forms of the long-QT syndrome. *Circulation*. 2003;107: 838-44.

[90] Magnano AR, Talathoti N, Hallur R, Bloomfield DM, Garan H. Sympathomimetic infusion and cardiac repolarization: the normative effects of epinephrine and isoproterenol in healthy subjects. J Cardiovasc *Electrophysiol*. 2006;17: 983-9.

[91] Ackerman MJ. Unmasking concealed long QT syndrome. *Heart Rhythm*. 2008 ;5:8-10.

[92] Kääb S, Hinterseer M, Näbauer M, Steinbeck G. Sotalol testing unmasks altered repolarization in patients with suspected acquired long-QT-syndrome--a case-control pilot study using i.v. sotalol. *Eur Heart J*. 2003;24:649-57.

[93] Shimizu W, Noda T, Takaki H, Kurita T, Nagaya N, Satomi K, Suyama K, Aihara N, Kamakura S, Sunagawa K, Echigo S, Nakamura K, Ohe T, Towbin JA, Napolitano C, Priori SG. Epinephrine unmasks latent mutation carriers with LQT1 form of congenital long-QT syndrome. *J Am Coll Cardiol*. 2003;41:633-42.

[94] Jeyaraj D, Abernethy DP, Natarajan RN, Dettmer MM, Dikshteyn M, Meredith DM, Patel K, Allareddy RR, Lewis SA, Kaufman ES. I(Kr) channel blockade to unmask occult congenital long QT syndrome. *Heart Rhythm*. 2008;5:2-7.

[95] Plant LD, Bowers PN, Liu Q, Morgan T, Zhang T, State MW, Chen W, Kittles RA, Goldstein SA. A common cardiac sodium channel variant associated with sudden infant death in African Americans, SCN5A S1103Y. *J Clin Invest*. 2006;116:430-5.

[96] Van Norstrand DW, Tester DJ, Ackerman MJ. Overrepresentation of the proarrhythmic, sudden death predisposing sodium channel polymorphism S1103Y in a population-based cohort of African-American sudden infant death syndrome. *Heart Rhythm*. 2008;5:712-5.

[97] Hwang HW, Chen JJ, Lin YJ, Shieh RC, Lee MT, Hung SI, Wu JY, Chen YT, Niu DM, Hwang BT. R1193Q of SCN5A, a Brugada and long QT mutation, is a common polymorphism in Han Chinese. *J Med Genet*. 2005 ;42:e7;

[98] Mohler PJ, Healy JA, Xue H, Puca AA, Kline CF, Allingham RR, Kranias EG, Rockman HA, Bennett V. Ankyrin-B syndrome: enhanced cardiac function balanced by risk of cardiac death and premature senescence. *PLoS ONE*. 2007;2:e1051

[99] Schwartz PJ, Priori SG, Cerrone M, Spazzolini C, Odero A, Napolitano C, Bloise R, De Ferrari GM, Klersy C, Moss AJ, Zareba W, Robinson JL, Hall WJ, Brink PA, Toivonen L, Epstein AE, Li C, Hu D. Left cardiac sympathetic denervation in the management of high-risk patients affected by the long-QT syndrome. *Circulation.* 2004;109:1826-33.

[100] Ruan Y, Liu N, Bloise R, Napolitano C, Priori SG. Gating properties of SCN5A mutations and the response to mexiletine in long-QT syndrome type 3 patients. *Circulation.* 2007;116:1137-44.

[101] Moss AJ, Windle JR, Hall WJ, Zareba W, Robinson JL, McNitt S, Severski P, Rosero S, Daubert JP, Qi M, Cieciorka M, Manalan AS. Safety and efficacy of flecainide in subjects with Long QT-3 syndrome (DeltaKPQ mutation): a randomized, double-blind, placebo-controlled clinical trial. Ann Noninvasive *Electrocardiol.* 2005;10 (4 Suppl):59-66.

[102] Viskin S. Cardiac pacing in the long QT syndrome: review of available data and practical recommendations. *J Cardiovasc Electrophysiol.* 2000;11:593-600.

[103] Shimizu W, Antzelevitch C. Effects of a K(+) channel opener to reduce transmural dispersion of repolarization and prevent torsade de pointes in LQT1, LQT2, and LQT3 models of the long-QT syndrome. *Circulation.* 2000;102:706-12.

[104] Diness TG, Yeh YH, Qi XY, Chartier D, Tsuji Y, Hansen RS, Olesen SP, Grunnet M, Nattel S. Antiarrhythmic properties of a rapid delayed-rectifier current activator in rabbit models of acquired long QT syndrome. *Cardiovasc Res.* 2008;79:61-9.

[105] Giustetto C, Di Monte F, Wolpert C, Borggrefe M, Schimpf R, Sbragia P, Leone G, Maury P, Anttonen O, Haissaguerre M, Gaita F. Short QT syndrome: clinical findings and diagnostic-therapeutic implications. *Eur Heart J.* 2006;27:2440-7.

[106] Morphet JA.The short QT syndrome and sudden infant death syndrome. Can J Cardiol. 2007;23:105. Brugada R, Hong K, Dumaine R, Cordeiro J, Gaita F, Borggrefe M, Menendez TM, Brugada J, Pollevick GD, Wolpert C, Burashnikov E, Matsuo K, Wu YS, Guerchicoff A, Bianchi F, Giustetto C, Schimpf R, Brugada P, Antzelevitch C.Sudden death associated with short-QT syndrome linked to mutations in HERG. *Circulation.* 2004;109:30-5.

[107] Brugada R, Hong K, Dumaine R, Cordeiro J, Gaita F, Borggrefe M, Menendez TM, Brugada J, Pollevick GD, Wolpert C, Burashnikov E, Matsuo K, Wu YS, Guerchicoff A, Bianchi F, Giustetto C, Schimpf R, Brugada P, Antzelevitch C. Sudden death associated with short-QT syndrome linked to mutations in HERG. *Circulation.* 2004;109:30-5.

[108] Cordeiro JM, Brugada R, Wu YS, Hong K, Dumaine R. Modulation of I(Kr) inactivation by mutation N588K in KCNH2: a link to arrhythmogenesis in short QT syndrome. *Cardiovasc Res.* 2005;67:498-509.

[109] Bellocq C, van Ginneken AC, Bezzina CR, Alders M, Escande D, Mannens MM, Baró I, Wilde AA. Mutation in the KCNQ1 gene leading to the short QT-interval syndrome. *Circulation.* 2004;109: 2394-7.

[110] Hong K, Piper DR, Diaz-Valdecantos A, Brugada J, Oliva A, Burashnikov E, Santos-de-Soto J, Grueso-Montero J, Diaz-Enfante E, Brugada P, Sachse F, Sanguinetti MC, Brugada R. De novo KCNQ1 mutation responsible for atrial fibrillation and short QT syndrome in utero. *Cardiovasc Res.* 2005;68:433-40.

[111] Priori SG, Pandit SV, Rivolta I, Berenfeld O, Ronchetti E, Dhamoon A, Napolitano C, Anumonwo J, di Barletta MR, Gudapakkam S, Bosi G, Stramba-Badiale M, Jalife J. A novel form of short QT syndrome (SQT3) is caused by a mutation in the KCNJ2 gene. *Circ Res*. 2005;96:800-7.

[112] Borggrefe M, Wolpert C, Antzelevitch C, Veltmann C, Giustetto C, Gaita F, Schimpf R. Short QT syndrome. Genotype-phenotype correlations. *J Electrocardiol*. 2005;38(4 Suppl):75-80. Review.

[113] Gaita F, Giustetto C, Bianchi F, Schimpf R, Haissaguerre M, Calò L, Brugada R, Antzelevitch C, Borggrefe M, Wolpert C. Short QT syndrome: pharmacological treatment. *J Am Coll Cardiol*. 2004;43:1494-9.

[114] McPate MJ, Duncan RS, Witchel HJ, Hancox JC. Disopyramide is an effective inhibitor of mutant HERG K+ channels involved in variant 1 short QT syndrome. *J Mol Cell Cardiol*. 2006;41:563-6.

[115] Antzelevitch C, Pollevick GD, Cordeiro JM, Casis O, Sanguinetti MC, Aizawa Y, Guerchicoff A, Pfeiffer R, Oliva A, Wollnik B, Gelber P, Bonaros EP Jr, Burashnikov E, Wu Y, Sargent JD, Schickel S, Oberheiden R, Bhatia A, Hsu LF, Haïssaguerre M, Schimpf R, Borggrefe M, Wolpert C. Loss-of-function mutations in the cardiac calcium channel underlie a new clinical entity characterized by ST-segment elevation, short QT intervals, and sudden cardiac death. *Circulation*. 2007;115:442-9.

[116] London B, Michalec M, Mehdi H, Zhu X, Kerchner L, Sanyal S, Viswanathan PC, Pfahnl AE, Shang LL, Madhusudanan M, Baty CJ, Lagana S, Aleong R, Gutmann R, Ackerman MJ, McNamara DM, Weiss R, Dudley SC Jr. Mutation in glycerol-3-phosphate dehydrogenase 1 like gene (GPD1-L) decreases cardiac Na+ current and causes inherited arrhythmias. *Circulation*. 2007;116:2260-8.

[117] Van Norstrand DW, Valdivia CR, Tester DJ, Ueda K, London B, Makielski JC, Ackerman MJ. Molecular and functional characterization of novel glycerol-3-phosphate dehydrogenase 1 like gene (GPD1-L) mutations in sudden infant death syndrome. *Circulation*. 2007;116: 2253-9.

[118] Watanabe H, Koopmann TT, Le Scouarnec S, Yang T, Ingram CR, Schott JJ, Demolombe S, Probst V, Anselme F, Escande D, Wiesfeld AC, Pfeufer A, Kääb S, Wichmann HE, Hasdemir C, Aizawa Y, Wilde AA, Roden DM, Bezzina CR. Sodium channel beta1 subunit mutations associated with Brugada syndrome and cardiac conduction disease in humans. *J Clin Invest*. 2008;118:2260-2268.

[119] Mohler PJ, Splawski I, Napolitano C, Bottelli G, Sharpe L, Timothy K, Priori SG, Keating MT, Bennett V. A cardiac arrhythmia syndrome caused by loss of ankyrin-B function. *Proc Natl Acad Sci U S A*. 2004;101: 9137-42.

[120] Antzelevitch C, Brugada P, Borggrefe M, Brugada J, Brugada R, Corrado D, Gussak I, LeMarec H, Nademanee K, Perez Riera AR, Shimizu W, Schulze-Bahr E, Tan H, Wilde A. Brugada syndrome: report of the second consensus conference. *Heart Rhythm*. 2005 Apr;2(4):429-40.

[121] Junttila MJ, Gonzalez M, Lizotte E, Benito B, Vernooy K, Sarkozy A, Huikuri HV, Brugada P, Brugada J, Brugada R. Induced Brugada-type electrocardiogram, a sign for imminent malignant arrhythmias. *Circulation*. 2008;117:1890-3.

[122] Meregalli PG, Wilde AA, Tan HL. Pathophysiological mechanisms of Brugada syndrome: depolarization disorder, repolarization disorder, or more? *Cardiovasc. Res*. 2005; 67: 367-78

[123] Potet F, Mabo P, Le Coq G, Probst V, Schott JJ, Airaud F, Guihard G, Daubert JC, Escande D, Le Marec H. Novel brugada SCN5A mutation leading to ST segment elevation in the inferior or the right precordial leads. *J Cardiovasc Electrophysiol.* 2003;14:200-3.

[124] Smits JP, Eckardt L, Probst V, Bezzina CR, Schott JJ, Remme CA, Haverkamp W, Breithardt G, Escande D, Schulze-Bahr E, LeMarec H, Wilde AA. Genotype-phenotype relationship in Brugada syndrome: electrocardiographic features differentiate SCN5A-related patients from non-SCN5A-related patients. *J Am Coll Cardiol.* 2002;40:350-6.

[125] Probst V, Denjoy I, Meregalli PG, Amirault JC, Sacher F, Mansourati J, Babuty D, Villain E, Victor J, Schott JJ, Lupoglazoff JM, Mabo P, Veltmann C, Jesel L, Chevalier P, Clur SA, Haissaguerre M, Wolpert C, Le Marec H, Wilde AA. Clinical aspects and prognosis of Brugada syndrome in children. *Circulation.* 2007;115:2042-8.

[126] Schott JJ, Alshinawi C, Kyndt F, Probst V, Hoorntje TM, Hulsbeek M, Wilde AA, Escande D, Mannens MM, Le Marec H. Cardiac conduction defects associate with mutations in SCN5A. *Nat Genet.* 1999;23:20-1.

[127] Probst V, Kyndt F, Potet F, Trochu JN, Mialet G, Demolombe S, Schott JJ, Baró I, Escande D, Le Marec H. Haploinsufficiency in combination with aging causes SCN5A-linked hereditary Lenègre disease. *J Am Coll Cardiol.* 2003;41:643-52.

[128] Probst V, Allouis M, Sacher F, Pattier S, Babuty D, Mabo P, Mansourati J, Victor J, Nguyen JM, Schott JJ, Boisseau P, Escande D, Le Marec H. Progressive cardiac conduction defect is the prevailing phenotype in carriers of a Brugada syndrome SCN5A mutation. *J Cardiovasc Electrophysiol.* 2006;17:270-5.

[129] Benson DW, Wang DW, Dyment M, Knilans TK, Fish FA, Strieper MJ, Rhodes TH, George AL Jr. Congenital sick sinus syndrome caused by recessive mutations in the cardiac sodium channel gene (SCN5A). *J Clin Invest.* 2003;112:1019-28.

[130] Schulze-Bahr E, Neu A, Friederich P, Kaupp UB, Breithardt G, Pongs O, Isbrandt D. Pacemaker channel dysfunction in a patient with sinus node disease. *J Clin Invest.* 2003;111:1537-45.

[131] Ueda K, Nakamura K, Hayashi T, Inagaki N, Takahashi M, Arimura T, Morita H, Higashiuesato Y, Hirano Y, Yasunami M, Takishita S, Yamashina A, Ohe T, Sunamori M, Hiraoka M, Kimura A. Functional characterization of a trafficking-defective HCN4 mutation, D553N, associated with cardiac arrhythmia. *J Biol Chem.* 2004;279:27194-8.

[132] Nof E, Luria D, Brass D, Marek D, Lahat H, Reznik-Wolf H, Pras E, Dascal N, Eldar M, Glikson M. Point mutation in the HCN4 cardiac ion channel pore affecting synthesis, trafficking, and functional expression is associated with familial asymptomatic sinus bradycardia. *Circulation.* 2007;116: 463-70.

[133] Milanesi R, Baruscotti M, Gnecchi-Ruscone T, DiFrancesco D. Familial sinus bradycardia associated with a mutation in the cardiac pacemaker channel. *N Engl J Med.* 2006;354:151-7.

[134] Smits JP, Koopmann TT, Wilders R, Veldkamp MW, Opthof T, Bhuiyan ZA, Mannens MM, Balser JR, Tan HL, Bezzina CR, Wilde AA. A mutation in the human cardiac sodium channel (E161K) contributes to sick sinus syndrome, conduction disease and Brugada syndrome in two families. *J Mol Cell Cardiol.* 2005;38: 969-81.

[135] Bhuiyan ZA, van den Berg MP, van Tintelen JP, Bink-Boelkens MT, Wiesfeld AC, Alders M, Postma AV, van Langen I, Mannens MM, Wilde AA. Expanding spectrum

of human RYR2-related disease: new electrocardiographic, structural, and genetic features. *Circulation.* 2007;116:1569-76.

[136] Benditt DG, Sakaguchi S, Lurie KG, Lu F. Cardiovascular Medicine, Third Edition. 2007. Springer London.

[137] Laitinen PJ, Brown KM, Piippo K, Swan H, Devaney JM, Brahmbhatt B, Donarum EA, Marino M, Tiso N, Viitasalo M, Toivonen L, Stephan DA, Kontula K. Mutations of the cardiac ryanodine receptor (RYR2) gene in familial polymorphic ventricular tachycardia. *Circulation.* 2001;103: 485-90.

[138] Tiso N, Stephan DA, Nava A, Bagattin A, Devaney JM, Stanchi F, Larderet G, Brahmbhatt B, Brown K, Bauce B, Muriago M, Basso C, Thiene G, Danieli GA, Rampazzo A. Identification of mutations in the cardiac ryanodine receptor gene in families affected with arrhythmogenic right ventricular cardiomyopathy type 2 (ARVD2). *Hum Mol Genet.* 2001;10:189-94.

[139] Priori SG, Napolitano C, Tiso N, Memmi M, Vignati G, Bloise R, Sorrentino V, Danieli GA. Mutations in the cardiac ryanodine receptor gene (hRyR2) underlie catecholaminergic polymorphic ventricular tachycardia. *Circulation.* 2001;103:196-200.

[140] Bauce B, Rampazzo A, Basso C, Bagattin A, Daliento L, Tiso N, Turrini P, Thiene G, Danieli GA, Nava A. Screening for ryanodine receptor type 2 mutations in families with effort-induced polymorphic ventricular arrhythmias and sudden death: early diagnosis of asymptomatic carriers. *J Am Coll Cardiol.* 2002;40: 341-9.

[141] Postma AV, Denjoy I, Kamblock J, Alders M, Lupoglazoff JM, Vaksmann G, Dubosq-Bidot L, Sebillon P, Mannens MM, Guicheney P, Wilde AA. Catecholaminergic polymorphic ventricular tachycardia: RYR2 mutations, bradycardia, and follow up of the patients. *J Med Genet.* 2005;42:863-70.

[142] Tester DJ, Dura M, Carturan E, Reiken S, Wronska A, Marks AR, Ackerman MJ. A mechanism for sudden infant death syndrome (SIDS): stress-induced leak via ryanodine receptors. *Heart Rhythm.* 2007;4:733-9.

[143] Bagattin A, Veronese C, Bauce B, Wuyts W, Settimo L, Nava A, Rampazzo A, Danieli GA. Denaturing HPLC-based approach for detecting RYR2 mutations involved in malignant arrhythmias. *Clin Chem.* 2004; 50:1148-55.

[144] Lahat H, Pras E, Olender T, Avidan N, Ben-Asher E, Man O, Levy-Nissenbaum E, Khoury A, Lorber A, Goldman B, Lancet D, Eldar M. A missense mutation in a highly conserved region of CASQ2 is associated with autosomal recessive catecholamine-induced polymorphic ventricular tachycardia in Bedouin families from Israel. *Am. J. Hum. Genet.* 2001;69:1378-1384.

[145] Postma AV, Denjoy I, Hoorntje TM, Lupoglazoff JM, Da Costa A, Sebillon P, Mannens MM, Wilde AA, Guicheney P. Absence of calsequestrin 2 causes severe forms of catecholaminergic polymorphic ventricular tachycardia. *Circ Res* 2002 ; 91: e21-6.

[146] Song L, Alcalai R, Arad M, Wolf CM, Toka O, Conner DA, Berul CI, Eldar M, Seidman CE, Seidman JG. Calsequestrin 2 (CASQ2) mutations increase expression of calreticulin and ryanodine receptors, causing catecholaminergic polymorphic ventricular tachycardia. *J Clin Invest.* 2007;117:1814-23.

[147] Bhuiyan ZA, Hamdan MA, Shamsi ET, Postma AV, Mannens MM, Wilde AA, Al-Gazali L. A novel early onset lethal form of catecholaminergic polymorphic ventricular

tachycardia maps to chromosome 7p14-p22. *J Cardiovasc Electrophysiol.* 2007; 18:1060-6.

[148] Lehnart SE, Terrenoire C, Reiken S, Wehrens XH, Song LS, Tillman EJ, Mancarella S, Coromilas J, Lederer WJ, Kass RS, Marks AR. Stabilization of cardiac ryanodine receptor prevents intracellular calcium leak and arrhythmias. *Proc Natl Acad Sci U S A.* 2006;103:7906-10.

[149] Wilde AA, Bhuiyan ZA, Crotti L, Facchini M, De Ferrari GM, Paul T, Ferrandi C, Koolbergen DR, Odero A, Schwartz PJ. Left cardiac sympathetic denervation for catecholaminergic polymorphic ventricular tachycardia. *N Engl J Med.* 2008;358:2024-9.

[150] Darbar D. Genetics of atrial fibrillation: rare mutations, common polymorphisms, and clinical relevance. *Heart Rhythm.* 2008;5:483-6.

[151] Workman AJ, Kane KA, Andrew C. Rankin AC. Cellular bases for human atrial fibrillation. *Heart Rhythm* 2008;5: S1–S6

[152] Chen YH, Xu SJ, Bendahhou S, Wang XL, Wang Y, Xu WY, Jin HW, Sun H, Su XY, Zhuang QN, Yang YQ, Li YB, Liu Y, Xu HJ, Li XF, Ma N, Mou CP, Chen Z, Barhanin J, Huang W. KCNQ1 gain-of-function mutation in familial atrial fibrillation. *Science.* 2003;299:251-4.

[153] Yang Y, Xia M, Jin Q, Bendahhou S, Shi J, Chen Y, Liang B, Lin J, Liu Y, Liu B, Zhou Q, Zhang D, Wang R, Ma N, Su X, Niu K, Pei Y, Xu W, Chen Z, Wan H, Cui J, Barhanin J, Chen Y. Identification of a KCNE2 gain-of-function mutation in patients with familial atrial fibrillation. *Am J Hum Genet.* 2004;75:899-905.

[154] Ravn LS, Aizawa Y, Pollevick GD, Hofman-Bang J, Cordeiro JM, Dixen U, Jensen G, Wu Y, Burashnikov E, Haunso S, Guerchicoff A, Hu D, Svendsen JH, Christiansen M, Antzelevitch C. Gain of function in IKs secondary to a mutation in KCNE5 associated with atrial fibrillation. *Heart Rhythm.* 2008;5:427-35.

[155] Lundby A, Ravn LS, Svendsen JH, Hauns S, Olesen SP, Schmitt N. KCNE3 mutation V17M identified in a patient with lone atrial fibrillation. *Cell Physiol Biochem.* 2008;21:47-54.

[156] Olson TM, Alekseev AE, Liu XK, Park S, Zingman LV, Bienengraeber M, Sattiraju S, Ballew JD, Jahangir A, Terzic A. Kv1.5 channelopathy due to KCNA5 loss-of-function mutation causes human atrial fibrillation. *Hum Mol Genet.* 2006;15:2185-91.

[157] Gollob MH, Jones DL, Krahn AD, Danis L, Gong XQ, Shao Q, Liu X, Veinot JP, Tang AS, Stewart AF, Tesson F, Klein GJ, Yee R, Skanes AC, Guiraudon GM, Ebihara L, Bai D. Somatic mutations in the connexin 40 gene (GJA5) in atrial fibrillation. *N Engl J Med* 2006;354:2677-2688

[158] Darbar D, Kannankeril PJ, Donahue BS, Kucera G, Stubblefield T, Haines JL, George AL Jr, Roden DM. Cardiac sodium channel (SCN5A) variants associated with atrial fibrillation. *Circulation.* 2008;117:1927-35.

[159] Poglajen G, Fister M, Radovancevic B, Vrtovec B. Short QT interval and atrial fibrillation in patients without structural heart disease. *J Am Coll Cardiol.* 2006;47:1905-7.

[160] Johnson JN, Tester DJ, Perry J, Salisbury BA, Reed CR, Ackerman MJ. Prevalence of early-onset atrial fibrillation in congenital long QT syndrome. *Heart Rhythm.* 2008;5:704-9.

[161] Kusano KF, Taniyama M, Nakamura K, Miura D, Banba K, Nagase S, Morita H, Nishii N, Watanabe A, Tada T, Murakami M, Miyaji K, Hiramatsu S, Nakagawa K, Tanaka M, Miura A, Kimura H, Fuke S, Sumita W, Sakuragi S, Urakawa S, Iwasaki J, Ohe T. Atrial fibrillation in patients with Brugada syndrome relationships of gene mutation, electrophysiology, and clinical backgrounds. *J Am Coll Cardiol.* 2008;51:1169-75.

[162] Darbar D, Hardy A, Haines JL, Roden DM. Prolonged signal-averaged P-wave duration as an intermediate phenotype for familial atrial fibrillation. *J Am Coll Cardiol.* 2008;51:1083-9.

[163] Watanabe H, Darbar D, Ingram CR, Jiramongkolchai K, Chopra SS, Kucera G, Stubblefield T, Wang J, Roden DM. Loss of Function Mutations of Sodium Channel Beta-1 and Beta-2 Subunits Associated with Atrial Fibrillation and ST-segment Elevation. *Circulation.* 116: II_54. Abstract 356.

[164] Remme CA, Verkerk AO, Nuyens D, van Ginneken AC, van Brunschot S, Belterman CN, Wilders R, van Roon MA, Tan HL, Wilde AA, Carmeliet P, de Bakker JM, Veldkamp MW, Bezzina CR. Overlap syndrome of cardiac sodium channel disease in mice carrying the equivalent mutation of human SCN5A-1795insD. *Circulation.* 2006;114:2584-94.

[165] Grant AO, Carboni MP, Neplioueva V, Starmer CF, Memmi M, Napolitano C, Priori S. Long QT syndrome, Brugada syndrome, and conduction system disease are linked to a single sodium channel mutation. J Clin Invest. 2002;110:1201-9

[166] Veldkamp MW, Viswanathan PC, Bezzina C, Baartscheer A, Wilde AA, Balser JR. Two distinct congenital arrhythmias evoked by a multidysfunctional Na(+) channel. *Circ Res.* 2000;86:E91-7.

[167] McNair WP, Ku L, Taylor MR, Fain PR, Dao D, Wolfel E, Mestroni L; Familial Cardiomyopathy Registry Research Group. SCN5A mutation associated with dilated cardiomyopathy, conduction disorder, and arrhythmia. *Circulation.* 2004;110:2163-7.

[168] Coronel R, Casini S, Koopmann TT, Wilms-Schopman FJ, Verkerk AO, de Groot JR, Bhuiyan Z, Bezzina CR, Veldkamp MW, Linnenbank AC, van der Wal AC, Tan HL, Brugada P, Wilde AA, de Bakker JM. Right ventricular fibrosis and conduction delay in a patient with clinical signs of Brugada syndrome: a combined electrophysiological, genetic, histopathologic, and computational study. *Circulation.* 2005;112: 2769-77

[169] Minetti C, Sotgia F, Bruno C, Scartezzini P, Broda P, Bado M, Masetti E, Mazzocco M, Egeo A, Donati MA, Volonte D, Galbiati F, Cordone G, Bricarelli FD, Lisanti MP, Zara F. Mutations in the caveolin-3 gene cause autosomal dominant limb-girdle muscular dystrophy. *Nat Genet.* 1998 Apr;18(4):365-8.

[170] Carbone I, Bruno C, Sotgia F, Bado M, Broda P, Masetti E, Panella A, Zara F, Bricarelli FD, Cordone G, Lisanti MP, Minetti C. Mutation in the CAV3 gene causes partial caveolin-3 deficiency and hyperCKemia. *Neurology.* 2000;54:1373-6.

[171] Crotti L, Lundquist AL, Insolia R, Pedrazzini M, Ferrandi C, De Ferrari GM, Vicentini A, Yang P, Roden DM, George AL Jr, Schwartz PJ. KCNH2-K897T is a genetic modifier of latent congenital long-QT syndrome. *Circulation.* 2005;112:1251-8.

[172] Bezzina CR, Shimizu W, Yang P, Koopmann TT, Tanck MW, Miyamoto Y, Kamakura S, Roden DM, Wilde AA. Common sodium channel promoter haplotype in asian subjects underlies variability in cardiac conduction. *Circulation.* 2006;113:338-44.

[173] Junttila J, Lizotte E, Dube MP, Hong K, Benito B, DeZutter M, Sarkozy A, Huikuri HV, Vatta M, Towbin J, Brugada P, Brugada J, Brugada R. *Heart Rhythm. Supplement* 2008; 5, 5. P01-81

[174] McCarroll SA, Altshuler DM. Copy-number variation and association studies of human disease. *Nat Genet.* 2007;39 (7 Suppl):S37-42. Review.

[175] Schwartz PJ, Vanoli E, Crotti L, Spazzolini C, Ferrandi C, Goosen A, Hedley P, Heradien M, Bacchini S, Turco A, La Rovere MT, Bartoli A, George AL Jr, Brink PA. Neural control of heart rate is an arrhythmia risk modifier in long QT syndrome. *J Am Coll Cardiol.* 2008; 51: 920-9.

[176] Nagy E, Maquat LE. A rule for termination-codon position within intron-containing genes: when nonsense affects RNA abundance. *Trends Biochem Sci.* 1998;23:198-9.

[177] Choe CU, Schulze-Bahr E, Neu A, Xu J, Zhu ZI, Sauter K, Bahring R, Priori S, Guicheney P, Monnig G, Neapolitano C, Heidemann J, Clancy CE, Pongs O, Isbrandt D. C-terminal HERG (LQT2) mutations disrupt IKr channel regulation through 14-3-3epsilon. *Hum Mol Genet.* 2006; 15: 2888-902.

[178] Resta N, Susca FC, Di Giacomo MC, Stella A, Bukvic N, Bagnulo R, Simone C, Guanti G. A homozygous frameshift mutation in the ESCO2 gene: evidence of intertissue and interindividual variation in Nmd efficiency. *J Cell Physiol.* 2006;209: 67-73.

[179] Xiao J, Luo X, Lin H, Zhang Y, Lu Y, Wang N, Zhang Y, Yang B, Wang Z. MicroRNA miR-133 represses HERG K+ channel expression contributing to QT prolongation in diabetic hearts. *J Biol Chem.* 2007;282:12363-7.

[180] Yang B, Lin H, Xiao J, Lu Y, Luo X, Li B, Zhang Y, Xu C, Bai Y, Wang H, Chen G, Wang Z. The muscle-specific microRNA miR-1 regulates cardiac arrhythmogenic potential by targeting GJA1 and KCNJ2. *Nat Med.* 2007;13:486-91.

In: Heart Disease in Men
Editors: A.B. Todd and M.H. Mosley, pp. 45-73
ISBN: 978-1-60692-297-2

Chapter 2

Syncope and Orthostatic Hypotension

Antonio Franco Folino
Department of Cardiology, University of Padua, Italy

Abstract

Syncope is a symptom, usually defined as a transient, sudden loss of consciousness and postural tone, ultimately caused by an insufficient cerebral perfusion with a critical reduction of the blood flow to the reticular activating system.

Syncope is commonly classified in 5 main forms: the neurally mediated syncope, the form characterized by the presence of an orthostatic hypotension, the episodes due to cardiac arrhythmias or structural cardiac diseases, and the vascular steal syndromes.

Each form is characterized by specific anatomical substrates and by particular pathophysiological mechanisms.

Neurally mediated syncope, is the most frequent cause of loss of consciousness. It is the result of an autonomic reflex that has as a final effect the reduction of sympathetic drive, the increase of vagal activity, and consequently bradycardia and hypotension. Also carotid sinus hypersensitivity can be one of the triggers for neurally mediated syncope.

Orthostatic hypotension is mainly caused by a primitive or secondary failure of the autonomic nervous system, unable to compensate the reduction of blood pressure during orthostatism.

Cardiac causes of syncope are principally represented by structural heart disease and arrhythmias. Both lead to syncope by a significant reduction of cardiac output.

Finally, vascular steal syndromes cause syncope when, due to a proximal obstruction of subclavian vein, the blood is deviated to the arm from the vertebral artery and the circle of Willis, inducing a cerebral hypoperfusion.

Other causes of loss of consciousness include neurologic or psychiatric disorders such as drop attacks, epilepsy, psychogenic syncope, and vertebrobasilar transient ischemic attack.

Even though most of the patients have a favorable prognosis, in some cases the limit dividing syncope from sudden death can be very narrow, particularly in patients with heart diseases. For this reason, the first diagnostic step should be oriented to an early detection of the cardiac causes of syncope. Subsequently, specific diagnostic pathways to identify other different forms of syncope are required. However, in spite of a complete assessment, in about the 20-25% of the patients the cause remains unknown.

The foremost aim of the treatment in the forms of syncope due to cardiac causes, is the reduction of mortality. In these cases an accurate screening of the patients is necessary to determine the indication to cardiac pacing or defibrillator implant.

In the other patients the aim of the treatment should be the reduction of recurrences and the improvement of the quality of life.

Definition and Classification

Syncope is a symptom, usually defined as a transient, sudden loss of consciousness and postural tone, ultimately caused by an insufficient cerebral perfusion with a critical reduction of the blood flow to the reticular activating system.

A sudden lack of cerebral perfusion lasting 6-8 seconds, as well as a 20% reduction of oxygen supply to the brain, seem to be sufficient to cause a loss of consciousness.

Syncope has a large impact on the general population. In the long-term follow-up of the Framingham study, it occurred in 3% of men and in 3.5% of women, and 10.5% of the population experienced at least one episode of syncope during a mean follow-up of 17 years[1-2]. The prevalence of syncope increases with age, occurring in 0.7% of subjects 35 to 44 years old and in 5.6% of those older than 74 years. Syncope accounts for 3-5% of emergency room visits and 1-3% of hospital admissions [3].

However, we have to consider that very often syncope remains an isolated episode, not reported to a physician.

Annual mortality in patients with syncope strictly depends on the underlying cause. It is comprised between 18 and 33% in subjects with heart diseases, and between 0-12% in subjects with other causes of syncope. In the subjects with syncope of unknown origin mortality is around 6%[2].

The episodes of loss of consciousness have a relevant economical and social impact on the patients and on community. It is an event that often induces significant changes on the lifestyle of the patient, altering the course of his daily activities, causing anxiety and depression, until changes of work activity.

Table 1. Classification of syncope

1. Neurally mediated syncope
    a. Vasovagal syncope
    b. Carotid sinus syncope
    c. Situational syncope
        i. Micturition
        ii. Swallow
        iii. Cough
    d. Trigeminal and glossopharyngeal neuralgia
2. Orthostatic hypotension
    a. Non-neurogenic
    b. Neurogenic primitive
    c. Neurogenic secondary
3. Cardiac arrhythmias
4. Structural heart diseases
5. Vascular steal syndromes

The most recent classification of syncope considers 5 main forms, on the basis of its pathophysiology: neurally mediated form, syncope in patients with orthostatic hypotension, syncope due to cardiac arrhythmias or structural cardiac diseases, and syncope in vascular steal syndromes[4]. Other causes of real or apparent loss of consciousness principally include neurologic or psychiatric disorders such as drop attacks, epilepsy, falls, psychogenic syncope, and carotid or vertebro-basilar transient ischemic attack. (Table 1)

Neurally mediated syncope is the most frequent cause of syncope. It is the result of an autonomic reflex, that has as a final effect the reduction of sympathetic drive, the increase of vagal activity, and consequently bradycardia and hypotension[5].

Vasovagal syncope is the most common form of neurally mediated syncope, and is usually easily identified on the basis of its clinical presentation. It is induced by different stimuli, such as emotions, pain, prolonged orthostatism, invasive medical procedures.

Carotid sinus syndrome is a form of neurally mediated syncope. It represents a frequent cause of loss of consciousness in elderly, but its pathophysiology is still debated.

This category also includes situational syncope that occurs, reproducibly, during a specific activity, such as micturition, coughing or swallowing, and episodes due to trigeminal or glossopharyngeal nerves disease.

Orthostatic hypotension is mainly caused by a primitive or secondary failure of the autonomic nervous system, unable to compensate the reduction of blood pressure during orthostatism [6].

Cardiac causes of syncope are principally represented by structural heart disease and arrhythmias. Both lead to syncope by a significant reduction of cardiac output.

Finally, vascular steal syndromes cause syncope when, due to a proximal obstruction of subclavian vein, the blood is deviated to the arm from the vertebral artery and the circle of Willis, inducing a cerebral hypoperfusion.

Other causes of loss of consciousness include epilepsy, vertebro-basilar transient ischemic attack, hypoglycaemia, hypoxia and hypocapnia.

We have also to consider as a very different entity, from a pathogenetic point of view, the episodes of loss of postural tone in absence of alterations of consciousness, as in cataplexy, falls, drop attack, psychogenic syncope, and carotid transient ischemic attack.

Pathophysiological Mechanisms

Neurally Mediated Syncope

The episodes of neurally mediated syncope are triggered by a stimulation of peripheral receptors, sensitive to chemical or mechanical signals, widespread in different organs. The afferent signals via vagal and sympathetic fibers reach autonomic centers of brainstem, where they are modulated by neurohumoral agents, such as endorphins, serotonin, nitric oxide, vasopressin, or by signals from cortex, limbic system and hypothalamus. These upper centers are particularly activated in the case of emotion or fear, and are able by itself to induce a syncope. Probably derived from the most ancestral part of our nervous system they could be the result of a specific evolution of the brain, as proposed in some neuroevolutionary theories [7].

Efferent signals originate from the brainstem and cause a vasodilatation, mainly due to a reduction of sympathetic activity, and bradycardia, mediated by the vagus nerve. This represents the "peripheral arch" of the reflex, and is associated with a "central arch that induces a paradoxical, cerebral vasoconstriction. (Figure 1)

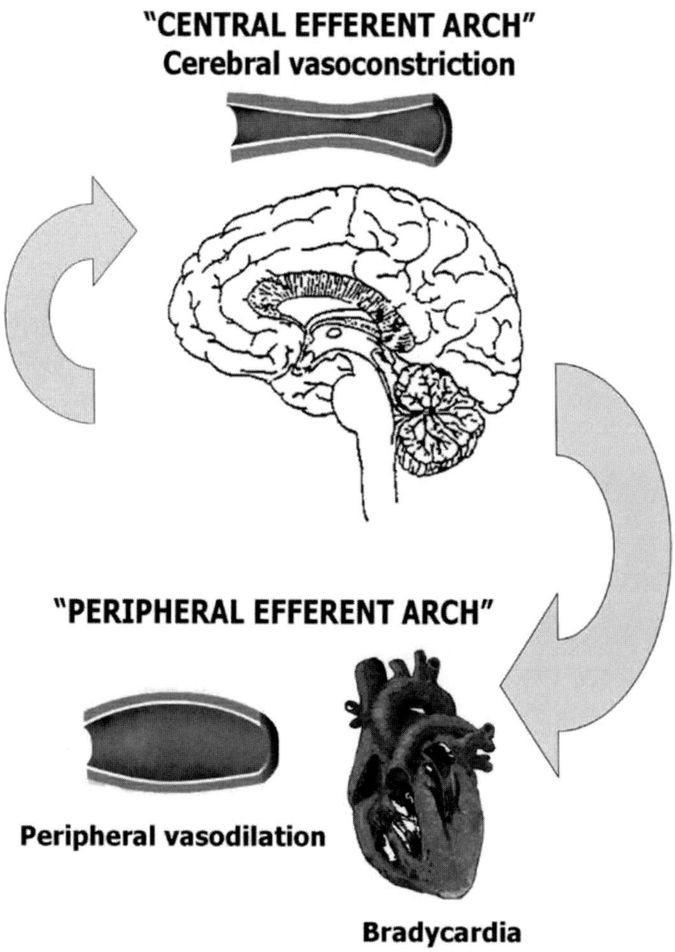

Figure 1. Efferent arches of vagal reflex. The efferent signals originating from brainstem follow two main pathways: the central arch, directed to the brain, induces local vasoconstriction; the peripheral arch, directed to heart and peripheral circulation induces bradycardia and vasodilation.

Among well characterized structures contributing to the induction of typical episodes of syncope, as for example in carotid sinus hypersensitivity or in post-micturition syncope, in most of vasovagal episodes a determinant role seems to be played by ventricular mechanoreceptors [8-9]. The activation of such structures is considered the most important final cause leading to the loss of consciousness, similarly to what happens in spontaneous episodes of syncope, during prolonged orthostatism [5,10-11]. In these conditions, an increased inotropic stimulus, induced by baroreflex activation, with a reduced left ventricular volume, due to a decrease of venous return, was supposed to activate the ventricular mechanoreceptors thereby eliciting, via vagal C fibers, a reflex bradycardia and hypotension, as a form of Bezold-Jarisch reflex. Several reports provided significant results supporting the so called "ventricular theory", even if a relevant cortical modulation as well as hypothalamic influences and neurohumoral agents resulted to be implicated [12-13]. Nevertheless, some studies excluded the presence of an increased ventricular contractility before syncope [14-15]. Therefore, also other alternative mechanisms should be considered.

More recently, also a reduction of atrial contribute to ventricular filling has been proposed as an additional mechanism in the pathogenesis of vasovagal syncope[15].

In the last years, very debated was the underlying mechanisms involved in carotid sinus syncope. Initially believed to be simply related to an hypersensitivity of carotid sinus receptors, it revealed a more articulated pathogenesis.

Carotid sinus receptors, autonomic centre of the brainstem, and the efferent limb of the reflex have all been incriminated. Recently, attention was addressed to two main hypotheses: an altered autonomic activity in the brainstem [16], and a chronic denervation of sternocleidomastoid muscle [17]. Spontaneous syncope generally occurs during accentuate neck movements or for an external pressure exerted on the neck.

Orthostatic Hypotension

Orthostatic hypotension is defined as a 20mmHg drop in systolic blood pressure or a 10mmHg drop in diastolic blood pressure within 3 minutes of standing or head-up tilt [18-19]. However, its presentation can be very different, appearing as a gradual progressive decline in blood pressure, over a more prolonged period of time, also resulting in symptoms, or in a less pronounced decrease of blood pressure but associated with significant symptoms. It can be also asymptomatic, in spite of a relevant decrease of blood pressure, depending on other factors as the operating range and efficiency of cerebral autoregulation.

The more frequent symptoms reported are blurred vision, lightheadedness, dizziness, palpitations and syncope.

During orthostatism 500-800ml of blood moves to lower extremities and splanchnic circulation, with a consequent reduction of venous return, cardiac output and arterial pressure. To compensate this situation, baroreceptors trigger a reflex increase of sympathetic activity, inducing an increase of peripheral vascular resistances, heart rate and contractility, finally restoring blood pressure.

This physiological mechanisms can be inefficient for alterations that occur at different levels, associated or not with autonomic disorders.

First of all, an absolute or relative decrease of plasma volume can preclude the maintenance of stable blood pressure in presence of a effective autonomic reflex. This occur during a significant hemorrhage or during chronic treatment with hypotensive drugs, particularly in elderly people. Some drugs cause a real volume depletion such as diuretics, or result in vasodilation, as calcium channel blockers, alpha-adrenergic or ß-blockers. Other drugs induce hypotension by central or peripheral effects. (Table 2)

Critical situations facilitating occurrence of symptomatic hypotension are meals consumption, when a substantial amount of plasma is confined in the gastrointestinal tract, or dehydration.

Orthostatic hypotension can be also caused by primitive or secondary disorders of autonomic nervous system. (Table 3)

The first include pure autonomic failure, reported in 1920s by Bradbury and Eggleston [20], where orthostatic hypotension is present without symptoms or signs of central neurodegeneration. In these subjects a reduced supine plasma level of norepinephrine is usually present and their clinical presentation is characterized by impotence and loss of libido, alterations of sudomotor function, urinary retention, incontinence and disturbed bowel. It usually involve elderly patients between 50 and 70 years and is more frequent in males [21].

Table 2. Pharmacological treatment that can cause orthostatic hypotension

- ✓ Alpha and beta blockers
- ✓ Other antihypertensives drugs
    - o Calcium channel blockers
    - o Diuretics
    - o Angiotensine converting enzyme inhibitors
- ✓ Bromocriptine
- ✓ Insulin
- ✓ MAO inhibitors
- ✓ Narcotics/sedatives
- ✓ Nitrates
- ✓ Phenothiazines
- ✓ Sildenafil
- ✓ Tricyclic antidepressants

Table 3. Autonomic disorders associated with orthostatic hypotension

- ✓ Primary autonomic disorders
    - o Pure autonomic failure
    - o Multiple-system atrophy (Shy-Drager syndrome)
    - o Parkinson's disease

- ✓ Secondary autonomic disorders
    - o Diabetes
    - o Amyloidosis
    - o Renal Failure
    - o Multiple myeloma
    - o Autoimmune diseases
    - o Familial dysautonomia
    - o Alcoholic polyneuropathy
    - o Paraneoplastic syndrome
    - o Cerebral cancer
    - o Syringomyelia
    - o Dopamine beta-hydroxylase deficiency
    - o Guillain-Barré syndrome

Another, more severe, primitive dysautonomia is multiple system atrophy (Shy-Drager syndrome)[22], which includes a combination of autonomic failure and progressive central neurodegeneration, has been divided into parkinsonian, cerebellar, and mixed forms.

The first is characterized by a more pronounced rigidity then tremor as present in Parkinson's disease, and with a loss of facial expression and limb akinesia. The cerebellar form is distinguished by a gait disturbance and truncal ataxia, speech disturbances and mild intention tremor of the extremities[23]. The patients with mixed forms present a combination of the symptoms reported in the parkinsonian and cerebellar forms.

Multiple system atrophy is a progressive disease that usually begins with mild autonomic symptoms. Orthostatic hypotension is associated with urinary and rectal incontinence, loss of sweating, followed by orthostatic hypotension, dysarthria, instability in ambulation, iris atrophy, tremulousness and muscular stiffness. Patients with multiple system atrophy generally have intact cardiac sympathetic innervation and a large decrease in blood pressure in response to ganglion blockade with trimethaphan [24], suggesting the presence of a preganglionic lesion responsible for this disease.

Finally, autonomic failure can occur in a small percentages of patients with Parkinson's disease. In these subjects a small or normal decrease in blood pressure in response to trimethaphan is present as well as a marked decreased or absent cardiac spillovers of norepinephrine, L-dopa, and dihydroxyphenylglycol, which provides neurochemical confirmation of a loss of sympathetic terminal innervation in the heart.

However, most chronic autonomic failure occurs as a secondary consequence of disease processes such as diabetes, amyloidosis, renal failure, multiple myeloma, autoimmune diseases, or due to toxic agents as alcohol.

In comparison with vasovagal syncope, where the decrease of blood pressure is often rapid, in the episodes due to dysautonomia it is more slow and progressive, and often occur with little warning [25], only when the patients reach very low values of blood pressure. Furthermore, another distinguishing characteristic is that in dysautonomic syncope a significant decrease of heart rate is not always present [26], whereas in patients with pure autonomic failure or multiple system atrophy a severe chronotropic incompetence, defined as a non adequate increase of heart rate during orthostatism (at least 10% more then baseline heart rate), can be observed [27].

A typical clinical feature of the subjects with autonomic failure is the simultaneous presence of orthostatic hypotension and supine hypertension. This situation, sometimes revealed during ambulatory blood pressure monitoring in hypertensive patients, represents a very difficult challenge in the treatment of both conditions[26].

Loss of consciousness due to dysautonomia tend to be more common in the morning after arising from sleep and are worsened by any condition that enhances peripheral venous pooling (eg, heat or alcohol).

Orthostatic Intolerance

The postural orthostatic tachycardia syndrome (POTS), also knows as chronic orthostatic intolerance is characterized by an exaggerated heart rate increase during orthostatism (>30bpm or heart rate >120bpm) associated with lightheadedness, dizziness, palpitations, fatigue, nausea and rarely syncope [28-29]. These symptoms generally disappear when the subjects lie in supine position and can be present with different severity, ranging from mild and rare, not interfering with a normal life, to serious and precocious, requiring wheelchair. This syndrome can occur after stressful situations as infections, sepsis, surgery or trauma

[29,30-31], with a high prevalence in female subjects (5:1)[32]. Orthostatic intolerance, which generally occurs in younger patients, rarely features rapid orthostatic hypotension, but delayed orthostatic hypotension can occur.

The etiology of this syndrome is still unclear, However, several hypothesis have been proposed. One of the first postulated theory considers that a central role is played by an impaired innervation of the vein or their response to sympathetic stimulation [33-34]. This induces a gravity dependent venous pooling in the lower extremities [35] and in the splanchnic area [36], with a consequent reduced venous return to the heart and a baroreflex mediated increase of heart rate. Other studies demonstrated a hypersensitivity to a noradrenalin infusion [37], as well as alterations of α and ß-receptors sensitivity, high plasma norepinephrine concentrations [38] and a baroreceptors dysfunction [39].

The occurrence of POTS in subjects after having suffered for a febrile illness suggested that in some cases an immune mediated pathogenesis could be present [32].

More recently, an alteration of kidneys innervation has been proposed, causing a reduction in erythropoietin levels. In fact, its administration demonstrated a clinical improvement in patients with POTS [40].

Finally, a genetic basis has been suggested by the identification of a defective gene coding for a norepinephrine transporter substance that induces an excessive increase of serum norepinephrine levels [41-42].

Two main primitive forms of this syndrome were proposed. The more frequent, the dysautonomic form, is characterized by a mild peripheral autonomic neuropathy causing an impaired increase of peripheral vascular resistances during orthostatism, resulting in a reflex tachycardia.

The second form, the hyperadrenergic, is probably related to an hypersensitivity of ß-adrenergic receptors. In these patients serum catecholamine levels are usually high and extreme tremulousness, migraine and anxiety are often present. It is still unclear whether this supersensitivity is primary or secondary to a denervation. However, the recent proposed genetic theories, showed as decrease of norepinephrine transporter substance, could impair the clearance of norepinephrine form the synaptic space and therefore induce an excessive sympathetic activation.

In patients with autonomic disorders, such as diabetes, amiloidosi, Sjogren's syndrome, pure autonomic failure or multiple systems atrophy, characterized by a peripheral autonomic denervation, a secondary form of POTS can be present.

Cardiac Syncope

Syncope can be caused by different heart diseases, representing the second more frequent cause of loss of consciousness. (Table 4) Schematically, we can divide the cardiac cause of syncope in two groups: those due to cardiac arrhythmias or to structural heart diseases. Either finally lead to syncope by a critical reduction of cardiac output.

Several brady or tachyarrhythmias can cause syncope. Among the first, sinus node dysfunction and atrioventricular conduction defects can induce a critical decrease of ventricular rate.

The tachyarrhythmias more frequently involved in syncope are those of ventricular origin, such as ventricular tachycardia and fibrillation. They can be due to different underlying heart diseases, for example coronary artery disease, long QT syndrome, arrhythmogenic right ventricular cardiomyopathy and Brugada syndrome. Supraventricular tachyarrhythmias more rarely cause syncope, usually only if an elevated ventricular rate is reached, as during atrial fibrillation or flutter, particularly in patients with Wolf-Parkinson-White syndrome, where accessory pathway can sustain a fast atrioventricular conduction.

Table 4. Causes of cardiac syncope

- ✓ Cardiac arrhythmias
  - o Sinus node dysfunction
  - o Supraventricular and ventricular tachyarrhythmias
  - o Atrioventricular conduction system disease
  - o Inherited syndromes (e.g. long QT syndrome, Brugada syndrome)
- ✓ Structural cardiac disease
  - o Valvular diseases (aortic stenosis)
  - o Acute myocardial infarction or ischemia
  - o Obstructive cardiomyopathy
  - o Atrial myxoma
  - o Acute aortic dissection
  - o Pericardial disease/tamponade
  - o Pulmonary embolus/pulmonary hypertension

Iatrogenic brady or tachyarrhythmias can also be induced by several drugs, particularly those exerting a direct effect on conduction system and inducing changes of the refractory periods of myocardial cells.

Structural cardiac disease, potentially causing syncope are cardiac valvular diseases, more frequently aortic stenosis, extensive myocardial infarction and obstructive cardiomyopathy, particularly the hypertrophic form. Also atrial myxoma as well as acute aortic dissection, pericardial tamponade and pulmonary embolism, can induce a dramatic reduction of cardiac output and syncope.

Vascular Steal Syndromes

This uncommon cause of syncope represents less than 0.1% of the episodes. Typically, subjects with a proximal occlusion of subclavian artery, with vigorous movements of the homolateral arm, induce an inversion of blood flow in the correspondent vertebral artery, distal to the occlusion, with an impairment of cerebral perfusion.

Exercise Related Syncope

In some occasions syncope occurs in athletes and untrained subjects while practicing physical exercise [43-45]. There are three critical situations in which it more frequently happens: during the effort, immediately after exercise is stopped and apart from exercise. In these three circumstances syncope is induced throughout very different and specific mechanisms, with relevant prognostic implications.

In the first case, we have to suspect that syncope is due to a tachyarrhythmias [46]. Particularly, effort induced ventricular tachycardia can be due to a not recognized heart diseases, such as right ventricular cardiomyopathy, or other forms of primitive or secondary cardiomyopathy. In some cases ventricular tachycardia or fibrillation can occur in subjects with anatomical anomalies of coronary arteries origin or course. Therefore, in these cases an accurate cardiological examination in is necessary.

In the second case, a neurally mediated syncope or an orthostatic hypotension are the more frequent causes. If during effort the subject stops suddenly exercise, the contribute of muscular contraction to blood flow circulation is abruptly missing. This contributes to a reduction of blood pressure, facilitated by an exercise related vasodilatation, triggering a vagal reflex throughout a reduction of venous return and vagal C-fibers stimulation, similarly to what happen during tilt induced syncope.

Finally, to explain the episodes of syncope that appear apart from exercise, particularly in endurance athletes, we have to consider that these subjects have some arrangements of circulation homeostasis such as an attenuation of baroreflex control of heart rate [47] and peripheral vascular resistances [48], increase of venous and arterials capacitance, dehydration, changes of some mechanical properties of myocardium causing a greater effective left ventricular diastolic chamber compliance and distensibility, and a steeper slope of Starling curve [49]. These modification can be advantageous for athletes performance but in some cases, particularly during hypovolaemia [50], became critical factors for the induction of neurally mediated syncope. These changes can also cause false positive response to Tilt Test in trained athletes. However, we have to consider that in this population false negative responses are very rare, therefore, a negative test requires an accurate diagnostic work-up to exclude the presence of other cardiological or neurological diseases.

Cerebral Autoregulation of Blood Flow

Whatever the specific mechanism involved, all the pathophysiological processes leading to syncope have a common final mechanism causing the loss of consciousness: the cerebral hypoperfusion [51]. Cerebral circulation cannot be considered as a static system, that passively undergo the modification of perfusion related to variation of cardiac output. In fact, cerebral circulation is maintained constant over a wide range of variation of perfusion pressure, by means of different integrated mechanisms based on the maintenance of a constant intracranial volume through the modulation of arterial and venous bed and the processes of production and absorption of the cerebrospinal fluid.

Therefore, within the high and low autoregulatory limit of blood pressure, usually ranging from about 60 to 140mmHg, cerebral blood flow remains constant. (Figure 2).

Cerebral autoregulation is organized by three different control pathways: myogenic, metabolic, and neurogenic [52-53]. The first is based on the intrinsic ability of smooth muscular cells of the arterioles to induce a vasoconstriction in response to a direct increase of cerebral blood pressure [54]. By means of the second, modifications of arteriolar resistance are induced by changes in local or systemic metabolism [52], with the secretion of vasoactive substances. A relevant influence is also played by CO_2 concentration [55]. Its increase induces a vasodilatation, whereas hypocapnia causes a vasoconstriction [56-57]. Therefore, an increase of CO_2 may enhance cerebral blood flow improving orthostatic tolerance [58], but its reduction, caused for example by hyperventilation, could represent a critical contributory factor in the decrease of cerebral perfusion during orthostatism [59]. Finally, the neurogenic mechanism is based on the presence of a rich innervation of cerebral vessels both by parasympathetic and sympathetic nerves [60]. The latter, believed to be the more important, causes a vasoconstriction that induce a shift of the autoregulation curve towards higher limits, hence protecting brain from high systemic blood pressure.

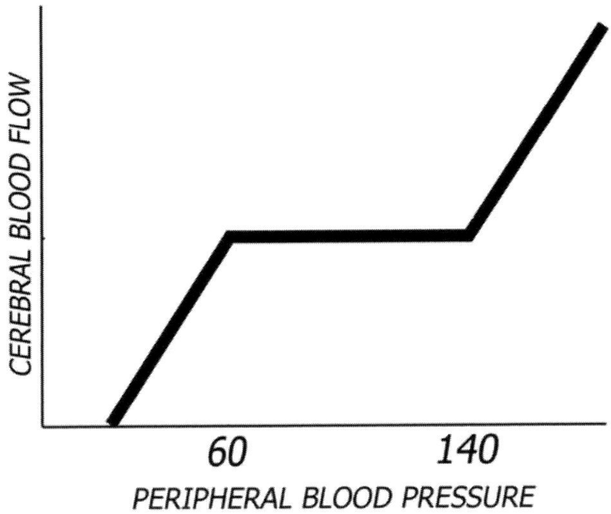

Figure 2. Schematic representation of the pressure/perfusion curve of cerebral autoregulation. When the systemic blood pressure fluctuates among 60-140 mmHg, a relatively constant value of cerebral blood flow is maintained. If blood pressure increases above the upper limit of cerebral autoregulation, cerebral perfusion increases proportionally. If blood pressure decreases below the lower limit of cerebral autoregulation, cerebral blood flow decrease proportionally.

Besides these three main mechanisms of cerebral autoregulation, there is a fourth important factor that in the last years has been shown to play a relevant role in the modulation of cerebrovascular resistance: the endothelial function. It intervenes influencing all the previous mechanisms mainly through the release of different mediators inducing relaxation or constriction of the vascular smooth muscle cells [61].

Arrhythmias and structural heart diseases induce syncope by a reduction of cardiac output. In these cases, cerebral autoregulation acts to compensate the consequent decrease of perfusion pressure by a reactive vasodilation. However, when the lower limit of autoregulation is reached the mechanisms cannot compensate the further fall of cerebral blood flow and syncope occurs.

More complex seems to be the role of cerebral autoregulation in neurally mediated and orthostatic syncope.

Cerebral Autoregulation and Syncope

Involvement of Cerebral Autoregulation in the Pathogenesis of Neurally Mediated Syncope

Neurally mediated syncope is the result of a composite reflex mechanism, formed by afferent signals that are integrated in the brainstem and modulated by different factors [62]. The working mechanism activated in a specific episode can differ in each patient, and probably also in the same patient in different episodes. Nevertheless, the final consequence is a compound of bradycardia and hypotension that represents the "efferent peripheral arch" of the reflex, that exerts its effects on systemic vasculature and on the heart [63]. (Figure 1)

Following the introduction of non-invasive techniques for the study of cerebral circulation, in particular transcranial Doppler, providing a real-time evaluation of cerebral blood flow, the interest was shifted to the modifications of cerebral perfusion during syncope and the efficiency of cerebral autoregulation, in the attempt to establish if the cerebral hypoperfusion is simply the passive results of the peripheral bradycardia and hypotension or if an active participation of cerebral autoregulation is present, as the expression of a concrete "efferent central arch" of the reflex.

Different studies demonstrated the presence of an active, paradoxical, cerebral vasoconstriction just before syncope, instead of the normal reduction of cerebrovascular resistance in response of a decrease of blood pressure, representing an important overwhelming factor leading to cerebral hypoperfusion, and therefore to loss of consciousness [64-68]. In some cases this effect was ascribed as the consequence of the hypocapnia due to the hyperventilation occurring before syncope, and not to an altered cerebral autoregulation. However, a paradoxical cerebral vasoconstriction was also demonstrated without a concomitant hyperventilation or hypoventilation and in absence of significant modifications of CO_2.

It was showed as in some patients the reduction of cerebral blood flow occurs consistently in advance in respect to the reflex hypotension-bradycardia [69], clearly excluding the possibility that cerebral hypoperfusion is dependent from a peripheral decrease of blood pressure, and confirming the presence of an independent mechanism involved in the pathogenesis of this form of syncope [70].

These mechanism could also explain the rare forms of syncope defined as "cerebral syncope" [71], occurring in absence of significant modification of blood pressure and heart rate. These episodes can be the extreme presentation of a pure "central" reflex directed to cerebral vessels, inducing an isolated cerebral vasoconstriction and a consequent loss of consciousness.

Cerebral Circulation in Orthostatic Hypotension and Chronic Orthostatic Intolerance

It was evidenced as in patients with orthostatic hypotension due to autonomic failure a widening of the autoregulation limits of the flow-pressure curve is present, probably reflecting a shift to higher values for the right limit to compensate the presence of a supine hypertension, and a shift towards lower values of the left limit to preserve cerebral perfusion during orthostatism when hypotension appears [72-73]. In subjects affected by multiple systemic atrophy an insufficient cerebral circulation, passively following the modifications of blood pressure toward higher or lower values, was also showed [74].

In orthostatic intolerance the appearance of symptoms can be associated with an increase of cerebral vascular resistance and cerebral hypoperfusion [75-76]. Occasionally was observed as cerebrovascular arteriolar vasoconstriction was primarily associated with hypocapnia due to hyperventilation [77].

In patients with orthostatic intolerance, peculiar, intermittent fluctuation of the cerebral blood flow velocity during tilt test was showed. These fluctuations were present before the development of hypotension, and earlier than in patients with vasovagal syncope [78]. This fact could reflect a specific abnormality of sympathetic innervation of cerebral vessels or an abnormal efferent sympathetic drive modulating cerebrovascular resistances.

Cerebral Autoregulation in Carotid Hypersensitivity

The role of an altered cerebral autoregulation in patients with carotid sinus hypersensitivity is controversial. In some cases a transient increase of cerebrovascular resistances preceding the critical reduction was showed [79]. In others, higher cerebral vascular resistances were evidenced [80].

Considering that autonomic control of cerebral vascular resistances is tonically active, we could suppose that in these patients adrenergic output is normally increased, and also moderate changes of arterial pressure are able to induce a selective further increase of sympathetic activity. This could be the result of a specific cerebrovascular disease or the cerebral involvement of a generalized atherosclerotic degeneration, or else related to the "central hypersensitivity" proposed in the genesis of carotid sinus syndrome [81].

Diagnostic Pathways

Syncope is a symptom that can be the expression of very different pathological conditions involving diverse organs and apparatus, and requiring specific diagnostic competencies. For this reason, the diagnostic approach often requires multidisciplinary competencies and must follows some simply but fundamental principles. First of all we have to reach a rapid diagnosis of the diseases where syncope represents a possible signal for life threatening condition: cardiac and cerebrovascular diseases.

Afterward, a specific, reasoned pathway should be followed, to avoid useless and expensive examination or prolong hospitalization.

The whole diagnostic pathway could be arranged in different steps where the information reached in the first sequence of tests can reach the diagnosis or guide the choice for the following procedures. (Table 5)

Table 5. Diagnosis of syncope

- ✓ **FIRST PHASE**
  - History
  - Physical examination
  - Electrocardiogram
  - Carotid sinus massage (>40 yrs)

- ✓ **SECOND PHASE**
  - Neurological disease suspected
    - Neurological examination
    - Carotid/vertebral artery echo-Doppler
    - EEG
    - TAC
    - MRI
  - Cardiac disease suspected
    - Echocardiogram
    - Exercise stress test
    - ECG monitoring (24-hour, 7-14 days)
    - High resolution ECG (signal averaging)
  - Neurally mediated syncope suspected (atypical symptoms)
    - Upright Tilt Test

- ✓ **THIRD PHASE**
  - Upright Tilt Test negative patients
    - Echocardiogram
    - Exercise stress test
    - ECG monitoring (24-hour, 7-14 days)
    - High resolution ECG (signal averaging)
  - Heart disease still possible
    - Implantable loop recorder (14 months)
    - trans-oesophageal electrophysiological study
    - Electrophysiological study
    - Coronary angiography
  - Patients with negative cardiological evaluation and symptoms typical for neurally mediated syncope
    - Upright Tilt Test

First Diagnostic Phase

The first diagnostic phase is essential to orient diagnosis, but very often also provide the final diagnosis.

History

An accurate history is the first determinant approach to the patients with syncope. It can provide a diagnosis in a very high number of cases [82], revealing the presence of known cardiac metabolic or neurological diseases, familial forms of cardiomyopathies or cases of sudden death, as well the occurrence of previous syncopal episodes. Moreover, the assumption of drugs potentially implicated in the episode of loss of consciousness should be considered.

Then, specific information on the characteristics of the episode must be collected. It is very important to consider the circumstances preceding the episode. Crowd, warm sites, stressful situations, prolonged standing or sitting often precede vasovagal syncope, sometimes occurring also during or after meal.

Neck movements or compressions are characteristic triggers for carotid sinus syncope.

Syncope occurring during physical exercise should address the diagnosis towards cardiac causes, whereas episodes occurring after exercise are sometime present as form of vasovagal syncope, particularly in endurance athletes. Typical situation for neurally mediated syncope are micturition, particularly during nighttimes, as well as defecation cough or swallow.

Indicative are also the characteristic of episodes onset. Palpitation is a non specific symptom. However, it could indicate that an arrhythmias is responsible for the syncope. Blurred vision is a very frequent symptom reported just before syncope. Its early onset is due to the effect of the intraocular pressure that facilitate the tendency of the retina's arteries to collapse in presence of a reduced systemic pressure. Therefore, it can be present in any case of syncope starting with a decrease of blood pressure.

On the contrary, nausea and sweating are specific symptoms, indicative of an incoming vasovagal syncope.

If convulsion are reported, it is very important to establish the precise moment of onset. In fact, this sign can be due either to a cerebral hypoperfusion and to a desynchronization of electrical cerebral activity. However, in the first case convulsions will be delayed and follow the loss of consciousness, whereas in case of epilepsy they will start early at the beginning of the episode.

Other signs indicative of a neurological origin of the episode are bilateral pupil dilatation and tongue bite. In contrast, urinary or fecal incontinency, often attribute to the presence of a epileptic crisis, are sometimes present also in case of other causes of syncope, when a marked and prolonged decrease of cerebral blood flow is present.

Occasionally, particularly in elderly people, we have to consider the presence of a retrograde amnesia after syncope, that can bring to deny the occurrence of prodromic symptoms. Also for this reason, the information that can be collected from witnesses are very important and can provide crucial indications.

Finally, also signs and symptoms characterizing the recovery of consciousness can be useful to address diagnosis. Patients with vasovagal symptoms usually have a rapid recovery, sometimes reporting nausea and vomiting, whereas those with epilepsy refer for muscular pain, disorientation or headache, with a slow resolution.

Physical Examination

In the contest of the first approach to the patient with loss of consciousness, we have also to include an accurate physical examination, mainly addressed to the identification of cardiac and neurological diseases. Moreover, a precise measurement of blood pressure, in supine and standing position, must be obtained. A reduction of 20 or more mmHg of systolic blood pressure or a reduction of 10 or more mmHg of diastolic pressure, in presence or not of symptoms, are indicative of orthostatic hypotension.

Electrocardiogram

Electrocardiogram represents a simple, not expansive, useful tool in the baseline diagnostic for syncope, suggesting the presence of structural heart disease, tachy or bradyarrhythmias, atrioventricular accessory pathways, long QT or Brugada syndromes.

Carotid Sinus Massage

In subjects older then 40 years, it is very important to perform a carotid sinus massage. This easy manoeuvre can provide a diagnosis of carotid sinus hypersensitivity.

It should be performed both in supine position and in orthostatism, for 5-10 seconds on right and left carotid, after an adequate interval. The test can be considered positive if a pause lasting 3 or more seconds, or a decrease of 50 or more mmHg of systolic blood pressure is induced.

In case of prolonged asystole, to reveal the presence of a concomitant, independent vasodepressor component, the manoeuvre can be repeated after atropine infusion.

Neurological side effects occur with an incidence of 1/5000 cases. Therefore, an accurate auscultation of both carotids, to detect murmurs due to atherosclerotic disease, should be performed.

This first diagnostic step can provide a final diagnosis in more than 50-55% of cases. For the other patients a diagnostic suspect should be done and the choice of further diagnostic tests guided on the basis of the information obtained.

Second Diagnostic Phase

The second step in the diagnosis of syncope will aim to define a suspect with more specific diagnostic tests.

If a neurological cause is supposed, the patient should be addressed to a neurologist for a specific physical examination and to establish the instrumental tests required to achieve the diagnosis.

In the case a heart disease is suspected, subsequent tests must be selected on the basis of the information collected in the first diagnostic phase. Echocardiogram can provide useful information on anatomical structures and on heart function, even though, rarely we can find the decisive elements in case of normal physical examination and ECG.

If the patients experienced a syncope during physical effort, exercise stress test is mandatory. The finding of an inducible myocardial ischemia is rarely present in patients with syncope. However, the test can be useful to reveal exercise induced arrhythmias or abnormality of blood pressure changes during effort and recovery.

When an arrhythmias is suspected to be the cause of syncope one of the more frequent test utilized is 24-hour Holter monitoring. However, in spite of its wide use, very rarely it can provide determinant information. Its diagnostic yield is considered to be about 2% [83]. The reasons for this limited utility is that it is extremely difficult to document a spontaneous episode of syncope, and that the arrhythmias eventually revealed can infrequently considered indicative if the patient is asymptomatic. Probably, we have to consider that the patients in which this test can be more useful are those older, with suspected bradyarrhythmias, where marked bradycardia, high degree AV block or asystole can be more frequently revealed.

In the last years other systems for external ECG monitoring lasting 7-15 days became available. These devices can identify arrhythmias and store the pertinent ECG, or store the entire recording for a post-processing analysis for arrhythmias; the opportunity for the patients to store the ECG during symptoms is also present. In some cases ECG can also be send to the hospital by phone, for a rapid analysis by the referring cardiologist.

High resolution ECG is a specific examination that reveals the presence of late potentials in the terminal portion of QRS complex, not recognizable with standard ECG. The instrument analyse conventional ECG signals by an amplification and filtering process, making visible potentials with an amplitude of μvolts. Subsequently, by an averaging procedure, the mean QRS complex is reconstructed on the basis of the only signal regularly present, permitting the elimination of electrical interferences that can impair a so delicate and precise analysis. From a clinical point of view, this test, evidencing delayed potential, reflecting the presence of myocardial areas with slow conduction, reveals essentially the presence of an arrhythmogenic anatomical substrate. This test was initially utilized in patients with myocardial infarction prone to develop ventricular tachycardia or fibrillation. Later, it was also applied in the diagnosis of patients with arrhythmogenic right ventricular cardiomyopathy.

If history is clearly typical for a neurally mediated syncope, and in absence of other abnormalities detected during the first diagnostic step, no more investigations are needed. However, in presence of syncopal episodes not always occurring with typical characteristics, Upright Tilt Test, can be useful in the diagnosis of vasovagal syncope. Different protocols were proposed for this test since its first use in the '80s [84]. Actually, it is performed by means of a tilting table with footboard, keeping the patients with an inclination of 60-70 degree for an interval of 20 minutes. If this first phase is negative, a sublingual nitrate is administered (spray 300-400μg) and the test continued for additional 15 minutes. The test is considered positive if syncope occurs or if presyncopal symptoms appear with a significant reduction of heart rate and/or blood pressure. Positive tests are usually classified in 3 main forms: mixed, when heart rate and blood pressure fall; vasodepressive, when blood pressure falls and heart rate decreases <10% of peak rate; cardioinhibitory without asystole, when heart rate decreases below 40bpm for more then 10, but without asystole lasting more then 3 seconds; cardioinhibitory with asystole, when asystole lasting more then 3 seconds occurs.

On the basis of patients selection and protocol utilized, the test is positive in about 55-70% of the subjects [85], consequently, the diagnostic yield of the test is ranging from 11 to 87% [86-87].

Different mechanisms have been proposed to explain tilt induced syncope, and test itself represented an important experimental condition to explore the modification of autonomic activity and circulation leading to the loss of consciousness. One of the more recognized mechanisms considers syncope as the result of a sequence of events involving different peripheral receptors, neural afferent and efferent pathways and central nucleus. First of all, passive orthostatism provokes a shift of circulating blood in subdiafragmatic venous system, with a filtration of aproteic fluid in interstitial space. These modifications of blood distribution cause a reduction of venous return, cardiac output and, consequently of blood pressure. This reduction induces a baroreflex activation of sympathetic activity resulting in a splancnic, renal and cutaneous vasoconstriction, and an increase of cardiac contractility and heart rate. In this situation we have a relatively empty heart vigorously contracting at an elevated heart rate. This induces a stimulation of ventricular mechanoreceptors, situated in the myocardial wall that sending afferent signal to the nucleus tractu solitario in the brainstem, induces a final vagal discharge, causing peripheral vasodilation and marked reduction of heart rate.

It is possible that this mechanism is involved also in the genesis of spontaneous episodes of neurally mediated syncope. However, we have to consider that either during Tilt Test and spontaneous episode the mechanism involved can vary also in the same subject.

In this diagnostic phase, Tilt Test should also be considered in patients with abnormalities revealed during cardiological evaluation, but with typical symptoms for a neurally mediated episode. These subjects represent the real challenge in the identification of the causes of syncope and risk stratification. In fact, the presence of positive cardiological elements requires a compete assessment to identify the underlying mechanism possibly responsible for syncope. On the other hand, if Tilt Test results positive, considering the possible presence of a cardiac life-threatening conditions, we cannot exclude that it represent a false positive or a positive response in a latent predisposition to develop neurally mediated reactions. Therefore, this patients, also in presence of a diagnostic Tilt Test have to be regularly followed and the implantation of a loop recorder should be considered.

Similarly, in patients suffering for episodes of loss of consciousness, in some occasions with characteristics suggesting a vasovagal origin and sometimes a neurological disease, even in presence of a positive Tilt Test, an exhaustive neurological investigation is mandatory.

Third Diagnostic Phase

At the end of the second diagnostic phase the origin of syncope can be determined in a high number of subjects.

However, in the case a definite diagnosis is not done and we suspect cardiac life-threatening conditions, some invasive examination should be carried out.

In the last years, an implantable ECG recorded was successfully utilized in the diagnosis of unexplained syncope. It comprises a light (17 gr) and small recorder, with a life of about 14 months, that is implanted subcutaneously on the upper part of the thorax (1st-4th rib). By means of two electrodes, placed on its surface, it records a closed loop ECG of about 42 minutes. Its is capable for automatic arrhythmias identification and storage for events such asystole, bradycardia or tachycardia. Moreover, the patient can activate a manual ECG storage by mean of a remote control, in case of symptoms or when recovers from syncope. The device will store permanently the last 42 minutes of ECG.

The stored ECG can be subsequently discharged by means of a programmer by telemetry, visualized and printed.

The use of this device provide the final diagnosis in a very high percentage of patients (65-88%) and highlighted some important epidemiological and pathophysiological aspects of syncope [83,88-90].

If some elements suggest the possible presence of atrioventricular re-entry arrhythmias, as in the case of nodal or atrioventricular accessory pathways, a trans-oesophageal electrophysiological study can provide the final diagnosis.

However, to obtain a complete evaluation of the electrophysiological properties of the specialized conduction system and myocardium, an invasive electrophysiological study is necessary, and in patients with structural heart disease, where bradyarrhythmias or tachyarrhythmias are suspected, it provides determinant elements in a high percentage of cases [91].

In patients with suspected congenital or acquired coronary artery diseases, where the non-invasive investigations failed to provide a definite diagnosis, a coronary angiography can be considered.

We have to consider that myocardial ischemia can induce a syncope throughout different mechanisms: by the induction of brady or tachyarrhythmias, but also by a direct reduction of cardiac contractility and therefore, cardiac output.

Following a complete evaluation in a relatively high number of patients, about 20-25%, a definite diagnosis cannot be achieved. However, we might suppose, on the basis of the incidence of the different causes of syncope and for the good prognosis of patients with unexplained syncope, that most of this patients have neurally mediated episodes, and some other patients have occasional, brady or tachyarrhythmias, not related with relevant forms of heart disease. In a very limited number of cases life-threatening conditions could be implicated.

Therapeutical Options

Syncope is a symptom presents in different diseases and conditions. Therefore, a specific treatment should be addressed following the final diagnosis, particularly in cardiological, neurological and psychiatric disorders, to improve quality of life and reduce mortality.

The hospitalization of patients referring for syncope should be considered in subjects with suspected or known significant neurological or heart diseases, presenting with significant ECG abnormalities, such as brady or tachyarrhythmias, or when syncope occurred during exercise. In some cases a family history of sudden death could be an additional information supporting the decision to hospitalize.

While the therapy of most of the causes of syncope are well standardized, the management of patients with neurally mediated syncope, particularly those suffering for vasovagal episodes, is still debated.

Neurally Mediated Syncope

Episodes of syncope ascribed to the presence of a carotid sinus hypersensitivity are in some cases considered an indication for permanent pacemaker implantation, particularly when bradycardia is documented [92].

In case of situational syncope the therapy is primarily addressed to avoid the trigger event, such as cough in cough syncope. However, sometimes is difficult to prevent episodes of micturition or defecation syncope. In these cases, suggest to the patient some strategies to decrease the chances of syncope could be useful. For example, decrease of liquid intake in the evening and a slower change of posture, with an intermediate sitting when getting out of the bed, to prevent micturition syncope. Increase of liquid intake and use of stool softeners in case of defecation syncope.

Trigeminal and glossopharyngeal neuralgia that sometimes triggers episodes of syncope should be accurately investigated to determine its precise etiology. The most frequent forms are idiopathic. However, in some cases an inflammatory or neoplastic origin should be considered.

Much more complex and articulated are the therapeutical options in case of vasovagal syncope. In this case, considering the low risk profile of the patients, the primary goal should be to reduce the symptomatic recurrences. The patient should be reassured, explaining the nature of this condition. The adoption of preventive measures can drastically improve symptoms. First of all, an increased intake of liquid and salt, inducing an enhancement of blood volume has been showed to reduce the episodes of syncope and improve orthostatic tolerance [93-94]. To avoid predisposing situations or triggering events, such as prolonged standing or sitting, crowded and hot environments, heavy meals, rapid changes of posture, is also essential to prevent episodes.

In some patients chronic therapies can facilitate syncope, particularly antihypertensive treatment by vasodilators. Therefore, a reduction or a discontinuation of these drugs should be considered.

Moreover, it is important to teach the patients to promptly recognize premonitory symptoms. Tilt Test can provide an opportunity to discuss with the patients the symptoms perceived just before faint. When recognized, the patient can begin some countermaneuvers such as supine position, legs crossing, isometric arm effort [95].

Many drugs have been used in the treatment of vasovagal syncope, with very different characteristics, mainly reflecting the uncertainty of the underlying mechanisms involved in this form of syncope: ß-blockers, theophylline, fludrocortisone, dysopiramide, etilefrine, scopolamine, clonidine, midodrine, paroxetine. However, no treatment showed and confirmed, in randomized and controlled trials, its efficacy in preventing vasovagal syncope [96-105].

Considering the cardioinhibitory component of the vasovagal reaction, since '80s different trials evaluated the efficacy of cardiac pacing in preventing this form of syncope, in some cases with positive results [106 110]. This studies included patients with frequent episodes, with a documented, important cardioinhibitory component. Particular algorithms of pacing (step rate, rate-drop response) were adopted. This mode of pacing induces a sequential atrioventricular stimulation with a relatively high rate (80-100ppm), for a limited time, when the spontaneous rhythm descend below a programmed basic rate (45-50bpm). The preservation of a physiological sequence of activation and the high rate stimulation intend to compensate not only the reduction of sinus rhythm, but also the decrease of blood pressure.

However, considering the absence of controlled, randomized, double blind studies, and the relevant placebo effect represented by a pacemaker implantation, the real efficacy of a permanent stimulation was rather dubious.

More recently, to discriminate this probable placebo effect, a randomized, perspective, controlled trial was conducted in two group of patients with activated (DDD) or inactivated (ODO) dual chamber pacing [111]. Results showed a comparable number of recurrences in the two groups, thus confirming as the invasive procedure can by itself to improve the clinical outcome of patients with vasovagal syncope.

Nevertheless, after a comprehensive evaluation of the results coming from all the different studies, we can conclude that DDD pacing can reduce the risk of syncope in selected patients with recurrent, refractory, highly-symptomatic, cardioinhibitory vasovagal syncope.

Orthostatic Hypotension

The first step in the treatment of orthostatic hypotension is the management of the underlying cause. Antihypertensive treatments, particularly vasodilators, or absolute blood volume depletion are reversible causes that should be corrected.

As a primary approach, the patients should be instructed to increase fluid and salt intake and to schedule a regular physical activity. Recumbent or seated exercise may be preferable to avoid orthostatic hypotension induced by intramuscular vasodilation. Moreover, hot environments should be avoided, as well rapid changes of posture, for example with an adequate period of sitting before getting out of the bed, accompanied by movements of the legs and dorsiflexion of the feet. Also large meals, eating foods that are rich in carbohydrates, and alcohol consumption should be avoided. In addition, several physical countermaneuvers such as legs crossing, stooping, squatting, and tensing the muscles of the leg or abdomen, can help to maintain an adequate blood pressure.

The use of compressive stockings, can be useful to minimize venous pooling, exerting a pressure sufficient to induce an adequate compression on the legs, and reasonably comfortable for the patient to encourage their use. Better results are obtained when the compression is extended to the waist, since a relevant quote of the peripheral pooling is confined in the splanchnic circulation.

The elevation of bed head's of about 10-20 degrees is useful to reduce the risk of a sudden hypotension when arising in the morning. Moreover, it can reduce supine hypertension.

Increasing periods of passive standing, know also as "Tilt Training", seems to be useful to improve tolerance to orthostatism.

Different drugs have been used in the treatment of orthostatic hypotension. The mineral corticoid fludrocortisone may be used in some patients to expand intravascular volume [112-114]. Moreover, it seems to increase the sensitivity of blood vessels to norepinephrine. However, side effects of this drug, such as hypokalemia or hypomagnesaemia, headache and supine hypertension, should be considered.

Midodrine, by stimulation of α-adrenergic receptors, induces an arteriolar and venous vasoconstriction, can be useful in some cases of orthostatic hypotension [115-117]. It is characterized by a short half-life, requiring to be administered 3-4 times per day. Also midodrine can cause supine hypertension.

Other α-adrenoreceptor agonists which act directly on α, β1, and β2 receptors and release norepinephrine from the postganglionic sympathetic neurons are ephedrine and pseudoephedrine [118].

Also Clonidine, an α_2 adrenoreceptor agonist, is sometimes useful in orthostatic hypotension, particularly in patients with autonomic failure and supine hypertension. The efficacy of this drug is due to its peripheral effect, especially in veins, raising blood pressure by a stimulation of α_2 receptors, classically hypersensitive in subjects with autonomic failure, for the chronic and progressive decrease of sympathetic activity.

Some studies showed as Fluoxetine, a serotonin reuptake inhibitor, may be useful in the treatment of orthostatic hypotension [119], influencing the regulation of blood pressure mediated by central nervous system.

Erythropoietin has been used to treat autonomic failure associated with decreased red cell mass or anaemia [120-122]. Even though, the aim of the treatment is generally considered the increase of haematocrit level, its effect on the improvement of orthostatic hypotension seems to be independent of red cell raise, but induced by a direct effect on peripheral vasculature.

More recently, two drugs showed positive effects on orthostatic hypotension.

The use of a vasopressin analogue, the desmopressin acetate, has been shown to supplement volume expansion and reduce nocturnal diuresis in multiple system atrophy patients [123].

In double blind, cross over, placebo controlled trials, administration of droxidopa, a synthetic amino acid, that is decarboxylated to norepinephrine by the enzyme L-aromatic amino acid decarboxylase, showed to increase standing blood pressure, ameliorate symptoms and improve standing ability in patients with neurogenic orthostatic hypotension due to degenerative autonomic disorders[124-126].

As a final consideration, we have to remember that all these treatment are palliative for symptoms, not curative, and have to be selected on the basis of the specific conditions of each patient considered.

References

[1] Savage DD, Corwin L, McGee DL, et al: Epidemiologic features of isolated syncope: the Framingham study. *Stroke*. 1985;16:626-629.

[2] Soteriades ES, Evans JC, Larson MG, et al: Incidence and prognosis of syncope. *N Engl J Med* 2002;347:878-885.

[3] Silverstein MD, Singer DE, Mulley A, et al: Patients with syncope admitted to medical intensive care units. *JAMA* 1982;248:1185-1189.

[4] Brignole M, Alboni P, Benditt DG, et al: Guidelines on management (diagnosis and treatment) of syncope – Update 2004. The task force on syncope, *European Society of Cardiology*. *Europace* 2004;6:467-537.

[5] Abboud FM: Neurocardiogenic syncope. *N Engl J Med* 1993;328:1117-1120.

[6] The consensus committee of American autonomic society and the American academy of neurology: Consensus statement on the definition of orthostatic hypotension, pure autonomic failure, and multiple system atrophy. *Neurology* 1996;46:1470.

[7] Brancha HS, Brancha AS, Williams AE, et al: The human fear-circuitry and fear-induced fainting in healthy individuals. The paleolithic-threat hypothesis. *Clin Auton res* 2005;15:238-241.

[8] Thoren P: Characteristic of left ventricular receptors with non-medullated vagal afferents. *Circ Res* 1977;40:415-421.

[9] Abboud FM: Ventricular syncope. Is the heart a sensory organ? *New Engl J Med* 1989;320:390-392.
[10] Rea R, Thames MD: Neural control mechanisms and vasovagal syncope. *J Cardiovasc Electrophysiol* 1993;4:587-595.
[11] Kosinski D, Grubb B, Temesy-Armos P: Pathophysiological aspects of neurocardiogenic syncope: current concepts and new perspectives. *Pacing Clin Electrophysiol* 1995;18:716-724.
[12] Shalev Y, Gal R, Tchou PJ, et al: Echocardiographic demonstration of decreased left ventricular dimensions and vigorous myocardial contraction during syncope induced by Head-up tilt test. *J Am Coll Cardiol* 1991;18:746-751.
[13] Nwosu EA, Rahco PS, Hanson P, et al: Hemodynamic and volumetric response of the normal left ventricle to upright tilt testing. *Am Heart J* 1994:128:106-113.
[14] Liu JE, Hahn RT, Stein KM, et al: Left ventricular geometry and function preceding neurally mediated syncope. *Circulation* 2000;101:777-783.
[15] Folino AF, Russo G, Buja G, et al: Contribution of decreased atrial function in the pathogenesis of neurally mediated syncope. *Am J Cardiol* 2006;97:1017-1024.
[16] O'Mahony D: Pathophysiology of carotid sinus hypersensitivity in elderly patients. *Lancet* 1995;346:950-952.
[17] Tea SH, Mansourati J, L'Heveder G, et al: New insight into the pathophysiology of carotid sinus syndrome. *Circulation* 1996;93:1411-1416.
[18] The definition of orthostatic hypotension, pure autonomic failure, and multiple system atrophy. *J Auton Nerv Syst* 1996;58:123-4.
[19] Gilman S, Low P, Quinn N, Albanese A, Ben-Shlomo Y, Fowler C, et al. Consensus statement on the diagnosis of multiple system atrophy. American Autonomic Society and American Academy of Neurology. *Clin Auton Res* 1998;8:359-362.
[20] Bradbury S, Eggleston C. Postural hypotension. A report of three cases. *Am Heart J.* 1925;1:73-86.
[21] Low PA, Bannister R. Multiple system atrophy and pure autonomic failure. In: Low P, ed. *Clinical Autonomic Disorders.* Philadelphia, Pa: Lippincott-Raven; 1997:555–575.
[22] Shy GM, Drager GA. A neurologic syndrome associated with orthostatic hypotension. *Arch Neural* 1960;3:511–527.
[23] Grubb BP. Neurocardiogenic syncope and related disorders of orthostatic intolerance. *Circulation* 2005;111;2997-3006.
[24] Shannon JR, Jordan J, Diedrich A, Pohar B, Black BK, Robertson D, Biaggioni I. Sympathetically mediated hypertension in autonomic failure. *Circulation* 2000;101:2710-5.
[25] Grubb BP, Kosinski D. Orthostatic hypotension: causes, classification and treatment. *Pacing Clin Electrophysiol.* 2003;26:892–901.
[26] Mathias C, Bannister R. Clinical features and evaluation of the primary chronic autonomic failure syndromes. In: Mathias C, Bannister R, eds. Autonomic Failure: A Textbook of Clinical Disorders of the Autonomic Nervous System. 45th ed. Oxford, UK: Oxford University Press; 1999:307–320.
[27] Schatz IT. Pure autonomic failure. In: Robertson D, Low RA, Polinsky RJ, eds. *Primer on the Autonomic Nervous System.* San Diego, Calif: Academic Press; 1996:239 –242.
[28] Low PA, Schondorf R, Rummans TA. Why do patients have orthostatic symptoms in POTS? *Clin Auton Res* 2001;11:223–4.

[29] Grubb BP, Kosinski DJ, Boehm K, et al. The postural orthostatic tachycardia syndrome: a neurocardiogenic variant identified during head-up tilt table testing. *Pacing Clin Electrophysiol* 1997;20:2205–12.

[30] Steward JM, Gewitz MH, Weldon A, et al. Orthostatic intolerance in adolescent chronic fatigue syndrome. *Pediatrics* 1999;103:116-121.

[31] Kanjwal Y, Kosinski D, Grubb BP. The postural orthostatic tachycardia syndrome: definitions, diagnosis, and management. *Pacing Clin Electrophysiol* 2003;26:1747–57.

[32] Schondorf R, Low P. Idiopathic postural tachycardia syndromes. In: Low P, (ed.), *Clinical Autonomic Disorders*. Boston MA: Little Brown and Company, 1993;641-652.

[33] Low PA, Caskey PE, Tuck RR, et al. Quantitative sudomotor axon reflex test in normal and neuropathic subjects. *Ann Neurol* 1983;14:573–80.

[34] Schondorf R, Low PA. Idiopathic postural orthostatic tachycardia syndrome: an attenuated form of acute pandysautonomia? *Neurology* 1993;43:132–7.

[35] Streeten DHP, Anderson GH Jr, Richardson R, et al. Abnormal orthostatic changes in blood pressure and heart rate in subjects with intact sympathetic nervous system function: Evidence for excessive venous pooling. *J Lab Clin Med* 1988;111:326-335.

[36] Hoeldtke RD, Davis KM. The orthostatic tachycardia syndrome: Evaluation of autonomic function and treatment with octreotide and ergot alkaloids. *J Clinic Endocrinol Metab* 1991;73:132-139.

[37] Street DHP, Pathogenesis of hyperadrenergic orthostatic hypotension: Evidence of disordered venous innervation exclusively in the lower limbs. *J Clinic Invest* 1990;86:1582-1588.

[38] Frohlich ED, Dustan HP, Tarazi RC. Hyperdynamic beta-adrenergic circulatory state. An overview. *Arch Intern Med* 1970;126:1068–9.

[39] Muenter Swift N, Charkoudian N, Dotson RM, et al. Baroreflex control of muscle sympathetic nerve activity in postural orthostatic tachycardia syndrome. *Am J Physiol Heart Circ Physiol* 2005;289:H1226–33.

[40] Hoeldtke RD, Streeten DHP. Treatment of orthostatic hypotension with erythropoietin. *N Eng J Med* 1993;329:611-615.

[41] Stober G, Nothen MM, Porzgen P, et al. Systematic search for variation in the human norepinephrine transporter gene: identification of five naturally occurring missense mutations and study of association with major psychiatric disorders. *Am J Med Genet* 1996;67:523–32.

[42] Shannon JR, Flattem NL, Jordan J, Jacob G, Black B, Biaggioni I, Blackely RD, Robertson D. Orthostatic intolerance and tachycardia associated with norepinephrine-transporter deficiency. *N Engl J Med* 2000;342:541-549.

[43] Kosinski DJ. Syncope in the athlete. In: Grubb BP, Olshansky B, eds. *Syncope: mechanisms and management.* Armonk: Futura Publishing, 1998:317-335.

[44] O'Connor F, Oriscello R, Levine BD. Exercise related syncope in the young athlete: reassurance, restriction or referral? *Am Fam Physician* 1999;60:2001-2008.

[45] Brignole M, Puggioni E. Exercise-related syncope: are athletes different from sedentary subjects? *Eur Heart J* 2003;23:1080-1082.

[46] Mounsey JP, Ferguson JD. The assessment and management of arrhythmias and syncope in the athlete. *Clin Sports Med* 2003;22:67-79.

[47] Smith ML, Graitzer HM, Hudson DL, Raven PB. Baroreflex function in endurance- and static exercise-trained men. *J Appl Physiol* 1988;64:585-591.

[48] Mack GW, Shi X, Nose H, Tripathi A, Nadel ER. Diminished baroreflex control of forearm vascular resistance in physically fit humans. *J Appl Physiol* 1987;63: 105-110.
[49] Levine BD, Lane LD, Buckey JC, Friedman DB, Blomqvist CG. Left ventricular pressure-volume and Frank-Starling relations in endurance athletes. *Circulation* 1991;84:1016-1023.
[50] Morikawa T, Sagawa S, Torii R, Endo Y, Yamazaki F, Shiraki K. Hypovolemic intolerance to lower body negative pressure in female runners. *Med Sci Sports Exerc* 2001;33:2058-2064.
[51] Jorgensen LG, Perko M, Perko G, et al. Middle cerebral artery velocity during head-up tilt induced hypovolemic shock in humans. *Clin Physiol.* 1993;13:323–336.
[52] Paulson OB, Strandgaard S, Edvinsson L. Cerebral autoregulation. *Cerebrovasc Brain Metab Rev* 1990;2:161–192.
[53] Aaslid R, Lindegaard KF, Sorteberg W, et al. Cerebral autoregulation dynamics in humans. *Stroke* 1989;20:45–52.
[54] Folkow B: Description of the myogenic hypothesis. *Circ Res* 1964;15:279–287.
[55] Ursino M, Lodi CA. Interaction among autoregulation, CO2 reactivity, and intracranial pressure: a mathematical model. *Am J Physiol Heart Circ Physiol* 1998;274: H1715–H1728.
[56] Shapiro W, Wasserman AJ, Baker JP, et al. Cerebrovascular response to acute hypocapnic and eucapnic hypoxia in normal man. *J Clin Invest* 1970;49: 2362–2368.
[57] Poulin MJ, Liang PJ, Robbins PA. Dynamics of the cerebral blood flow response to step changes in end-tidal PCO2 and PO2 in humans. *J Appl Physiol* 1996;81: 1084–1095.
[58] Novak V, Spies JM, Novak P, et al. Hypocapnia and cerebral hypoperfusion in orthostatic intolerance. *Stroke* 1998;29:1876–1881.
[59] Harms MP, Colier WN, Wieling W, et al. Orthostatic tolerance, cerebral oxygenation, and blood velocity in humans with sympathetic failure. *Stroke* 2000;31:1608–1614.
[60] Goadsby PJ, Edvinsson L. Neurovascular control of the cerebral circulation, in Edvinsson L, Krause DN (eds): *Cerebral blood flow and metabolism*. Philadelphia, PA, Lippincott Williams & Wilkins, 2002, pp 172-188.
[61] Andresen J, Shafi NI, Bryan RM. Endothelial influences on cerebrovascular tone. J Appl Physiol 2006;100:318-327.
[62] Mosqueda-Garcia R, Furlan R, Tank J, et al. The Elusive Pathophysiology of Neurally Mediated Syncope. *Circulation* 2000;102;2898-2906.
[63] Folino AF. Cerebral autoregulation in neurally mediated syncope: victim or executioner? *Heart* 2006;92:724-726.
[64] Grubb BP, Gerard G, Roush K, et al. Cerebral vasoconstriction during head-upright tilt-induced vasovagal syncope. A paradoxic and unexpected response. *Circulation* 1991;84:1157-1164.
[65] Krishnamurthy S, Wang X, Bhakta D, et al. Dynamic cardiorespiratory interaction during head-up tilt-mediated presyncope. *Am J Physiol Heart Circ Physiol* 2004;287:H2510–H2517.
[66] Carey BJ, Manktelow BN, Panerai RB, et al. Cerebral autoregulatory response to head-up tilt in normal subjects and patients with recurrent vasovagal syncope. *Circulation* 2001;104:898-902.

[67] Claydon VE, Hainsworth R. Cerebral autoregulation during orthostatic stress in healthy controls and in patients with posturally related syncope. *Clin Auton Res* 2003;13:321–329.

[68] Lagi A, Cencetti S, Corsoni V, et al. Cerebral vasoconstriction in vasovagal syncope: any link with symptoms? A transcranial Doppler study. *Circulation* 2001;104:2694-2698.

[69] Dan D, Hoag JB, Ellenbogen KA, et al. Cerebral blood flow velocity declines before arterial pressure in patients with orthostatic vasovagal presyncope. *J Am Coll Cardiol* 2002;39:1039-1045.

[70] Bondar RL, Kassam MS, Stein F, et al. Simultaneous cerebrovascular and cardiovascular response during presyncope. *Stroke* 1995;26:1794-1800.

[71] Grubb BP, Samoil D, Kosinski D, et al. Cerebral syncope: loss of consciousness associated with cerebral vasoconstriction in the absence of systemic hypotension. *Pacing Clin Electrophysiol* 1998;21:652-658.

[72] Depresseux JC, Rousseau JJ, Franck G. The autoregulation of cerebral blood flow, the cerebrovascular reactivity and their interaction in the Shy-Drager syndrome. *Eur Neurol* 1979;18:295-301.

[73] Brooks DJ, Redmond S, Mathias CJ, et al. The effect of orthostatic hypotension on cerebral blood flow and middle cerebral artery velocity in autonomic failure, with observations on the action of ephedrine. *J Neurol Neurosurg Psychiatry* 1989;52:962-966.

[74] Lagi A, Bacalli S, Cencetti S, et al. Cerebral autoregulation in orthostatic hypotension: a transcranial Doppler study. *Stroke* 1994;25:1771-1775.

[75] Schondorf R, Benoit J, Stein R. Cerebral autoregulation in orthostatic intolerance. *Ann NY Acad Sci* 2001;940:514-526.

[76] Hermosillo AG, Jordan JL, Vallejo M, et al. Cerebrovascular blood flow during the near syncopal phase of head-up tilt test: a comparative study in different types of neurally mediated syncope. *Europace* 2006;8:199-203.

[77] Novak V, Spies JM, Novak P, et al. Hypocapnia and cerebral hypoperfusion in orthostatic intolerance. *Stroke* 1998;29:1876–1881.

[78] Hermosillo AG, Jauregui-Renaud K, Kostine A, et al. Comparative study of cerebral blood flow between postural tachycardia and neurocardiogenic syncope, during head-up tilt test. *Europace* 2002;4:369-374.

[79] Leftheriotis G, Dupuis JM, Victor J. Cerebral hemodynamics in carotid sinus syndrome and atrioventricular block. *Am J Cardiol* 2000;86:504-508.

[80] Parry SW, Steen N, Baptist M, et al. Cerebral autoregulation is impaired in cardioinhibitory carotid sinus syndrome. *Heart* 2006;92:792–797.

[81] O'Mahony D. Pathophysiology of carotid sinus hypersensitivity in elderly patients. *Lancet* 1995;346:950-952.

[82] Kapoor WN. Diagnostic evaluation of syncope. *Am J Med.* 1991;90:91-106.

[83] Krahn AD, Klein GJ, Yee R. Recurrent syncope. Experience with an implantable loop recorder. *Cardiol Clin* 1997;15:313-326.

[84] Kenny RA, Ingram A, Bayliss J, Sutton R. Head-up tilt: a useful test for investigating unexplained syncope. *Lancet* 1986;1:1352-1355.

[85] Folino AF, Buja G, Martini B, Bassan L, Nava A. Upright tilt test: correlation between results and patient clinical features. *Pacing Clin Electrophysiol.* 1996;19:1582-1587.

[86] Kapoor WN. Evaluation and outcome of patients with syncope. *Medicine (Baltimore).* 1990;69:160-175.

[87] Kapoor WN. Evaluation and management of the patient with syncope. *JAMA.* 1992;268:2553-2560.

[88] Moya A, Brignole M, Menozzi C, et al. International Study on Syncope of Uncertain Etiology (ISSUE) Investigators. Mechanism of syncope in patients with isolated syncope and in patients with tilt-positive syncope. *Circulation.* 2001;104:1261-1267.

[89] Brignole M, Sutton R, Menozzi C, et al. International Study on Syncope of Uncertain Etiology 2 (ISSUE 2) Group. Early application of an implantable loop recorder allows effective specific therapy in patients with recurrent suspected neurally mediated syncope. *Eur Heart J* 2006;27:1085-1092.

[90] Krahn AD, Klein GJ, Norris C, Yee R. The etiology of syncope in patients with negative tilt table and electrophysiological testing. *Circulation* 1995; 92:1819-1824.

[91] Linzer M, Yang EH, Estes NA3rd, Wang P, Vorperian VR, Kapoor WN. Diagnosing syncope. Part 1: Value of history, physical examination, and electrocardiography. Clinical Efficacy Assessment Project of the American College of Physicians. *Ann Intern Med* 1997;126:989-996.

[92] Epstein AE, Dimarco JP, Ellenbogen KA, et al. ACC/AHA/HRS 2008 Guidelines for Device-Based Therapy of Cardiac Rhythm Abnormalities: Executive Summary A Report of the American College of Cardiology/American Heart Association Task Force on Practice Guidelines (Writing Committee to Revise the ACC/AHA/NASPE 2002 Guideline Update for Implantation of Cardiac Pacemakers and Antiarrhythmia Devices) Developed in Collaboration With the American Association for Thoracic Surgery and Society of Thoracic Surgeons. *J Am Coll Cardiol* 2008;51:2085-2105.

[93] Shroeder C, Bush VE, Norcliffe LJ, et al. Water drinking acutely improves orthostatic tolerance in healthy subjects. *Circulation* 2002;106:2806-2811.

[94] Lu CC, Diedrich A, Tung CS, Paranjape SY, Harris PA, Byrne DW, Jordan J, Robertson D. Water ingestion as prophylaxis against syncope. *Circulation* 2003;25:2660-2665.

[95] Brignole M, Croci F, Menozzi C, et al. Isometric arm counter-pressure maneuvers to abort impending vasovagal syncope. *J Am Coll Cardiol* 2002;40:20532059.

[96] Mahanonda N, Bhuripanyo K, Kangkagate C et al. Randomized double-blind, placebo-controlled trial of oral atenolol in patients with unexplained syncope and positive upright tilt table test results. *Am Heart J* 1995;130: 1250-1253.

[97] Jhamb DK, Singh B, Sharda B et al. Comparative study of the efficacy of metoprolol and verapamil in patients with syncope and positive head-up tilt test response. *Am Heart J* 1996; 132: 608-611.

[98] Ward CR, Gray JC, Gilroy JJ, Kenny RA. Midodrine: a role in the management of neurocardiogenic syncope. Heart 1998;79:45-49.

[99] Milstein S, Buetikofer J, Dunnigan A, Benditt DO, Gornick C, Reyes WJ. Usefulness of disopyramide for prevention of upright tilt-induced hypotension-bradycardia. *Am J Cardiol* 1990; 65: 1339-1344.

[100] Kelly PA, Mann DE, Adler SW, Fuenzalida CE, Reiter MJ. Low dose disopyramide often fails to prevent neurogenic syncope during head-up tilt testing. *PACE* 1994;17:573-576.

[101] Moya A. Permanyer-Miralda G, Sagrista-Sauleda J et al. Limitations of head-up tilt test for evaluating the efficacy of therapeutic interventions in patients with vasovagal syncope: results of a controlled study of etilefrine versus placebo. *J Am Coll Cardiol* 1995;25:65-69.

[102] Tarata TS, Wasmund SL, Smith ML, et al. Serotonin Reuptake Inhibitor (Paxil) Does Not Prevent the Vasovagal Reaction Associated With Carotid Sinus Massage and/or Lower Body Negative Pressure in Healthy Volunteers. *Circulation* 2002;106:1500-1504.

[103] Madrid A, Ortega 1, Rebollo GJ et al. Lack of efficacy of atenolol for the prevention of neurally-mediated syncope in highly symptomatic population: a prospective double-bind, randomized and placebo-controlled study. *J Am Coll Cardiol* 2001;37:554-557.

[104] Di Gerolamo E, Di brio C, Sabatini O, Leonzio L, Barbone C, Barsotti A. Effects of paroxetine hydrochloride, a selective serotonin reuptake inhibitor, on refractory vasovagal syncope: a randomized, double-bind, placebo-controlled study. *J Am Coll Cardiol* 1999;33:1227-1230.

[105] Salim MA, Di Sessa TG. Effectiveness of Fludrocortisone and Salt in Preventing Syncope Recurrence in Children A Double-Blind, Placebo-Controlled, Randomized Trial. *J Am Coll Cardiol* 2005;45:484-488.

[106] Fitzpatrick A, Theodorakis G, Ahmed R, Williams T, Sutton R. Dual chamber pacing aborts vasovagal syncope induced by head-up 60 degree tilt. *PACE* 1991;14:13-19.

[107] Sra J, Jazayeri MR, Avitali B et al. Comparison of cardiac pacing with drug therapy in the treatment of neurocardiogenic (vasovagal) syncope with bradycardia or asystole. *N Engl J Med* 1993; 328: 1085-1090.

[108] Benditt DG, Petersen M, Lune KG, Grubb BL, Sutton R. Cardiac pacing for prevention of recurrent vasovagal syncope. *Ann Int Med* 1995;122:204-209.

[109] Benditt DG, Sutton R, Gammage M et al. Rate-Drop Response Investigators Group. Rate-drop response cardiac pacing for vasovagal syncope. *J lntervent Cardiac Electrophys* 1999;3:27-33.

[110] Connolly SJ, Sheldon R, Roberts RS, Gent M. Vasovagal pacemaker study investigators. The North American vasovagal pacemaker study (VPS): A randomized trial of permanent cardiac pacing for the prevention of vasovagal syncope. *J Am Coll Cardiol* 1999;33:16-20.

[111] Connolly SJ, Sheldon R, Thorpe KE, et al. VPS II Investigators. Pacemaker therapy for prevention of syncope in patients with recurrent severe vasovagal syncope: Second Vasovagal Pacemaker Study (VPS II): a randomized trial. *JAMA* 2003;289:2224-2229.

[112] Lipsitz LA. Orthostatic hypotension in the elderly. *N Engl J Med* 1989;321:952-957.

[113] van Lieshout JJ, ten Harkel AD, Wieling W. Fludrocortisone and sleeping in the head-up position limit the postural decrease in cardiac output in autonomic failure. *Clin Auton Res* 2000;10:35-42.

[114] Chobanian AV, Volicer L, Tifft CP, Gavras H, Liang CS, Faxon D. Mineralocorticoid-induced hypertension in patients with orthostatic hypotension. *N Engl J Med* 1979;301:68-73.

[115] McTavish D, Goa KL. Midodrine: a review of it's pharmacological properties and therapeutic use in orthostatic hypotension and secondary hypotensive disorders. *Drugs* 1989;38:757-777.

[116] Low PA, Gilden JL, Freeman R, Sheng KN, McElligott MA. Efficacy of midodrine vs placebo in neurogenic orthostatic hypotension: a randomized, double-blind multicenter study. *JAMA* 1997;277:1046-1051.

[117] Wright RA, Kaufmann HC, Perera R, et al. A double-blind, dose-response study of midodrine in neurogenic orthostatic hypotension. *Neurology* 1998;51:120-124.

[118] Jordan J, Shannon JR, Biaggioni I, Norman R, Black BK, Robertson D. Contrasting actions of pressor agents in severe autonomic failure. *Am J Med* 1998;105:116-124.

[119] Grubb BP, Samoil D, Kosinski D, et al. Fluoxetine hydrochloride for the treatment of severe refractory orthostatic hypotension. *Am J Med* 1994;97:366-368.

[120] Hoeldtke RD, Streeten DH. Treatment of orthostatic hypotension with erythropoietin. *N Engl J Med* 1993;329:611-615.

[121] Perera R, Isola L, Kaufmann H. Effect of recombinant erythropoietin on anemia and orthostatic hypotension in primary autonomic failure. *Clin Auton Res* 1995;5:211-213.

[122] Biaggioni I, Robertson D, Krantz S, Jones M, Haile V. The anemia of primary autonomic failure and its reversal with recombinant erythropoietin. *Ann Intern Med* 1994;121:181-186.

[123] Sakakibara R, Matsuda S, Uchiyama T, Yoshiyama M, Yamanishi T, Hattori T. The effect of intranasal desmopressin on nocturnal waking in urination in multiple system atrophy patients with nocturnal polyuria. *Clin Auton Res* 2003;13:106-108.

[124] Kaufmann H, Saadia D, Voustianiouk A, Goldstein DS, Holmes C, Yahr MD, Nardin R, Freeman R. Norepinephrine precursor therapy in neurogenic orthostatic hypotension. *Circulation* 2003 ;108:724-728.

[125] Gibbons CH, Vernino SA, Kaufmann H, Freeman R. L-DOPS therapy for refractory orthostatic hypotension in autoimmune autonomic neuropathy. *Neurology* 2005;65:1104-1106.

[126] Goldstein DS, Holmes C, Kaufmann H, Freeman R. Clinical pharmacokinetics of the norepinephrine precursor L-threo-DOPS in primary chronic autonomic failure. *Clin Auton Res* 2004;14:363-368.

In: Heart Disease in Men
Editors: A.B. Todd and M.H. Mosley, pp. 75-100
ISBN: 978-1-60692-297-2

Chapter 3

USING MULTIPLE IMAGES POST-STRESS TO ENHANCE DIAGNOSTIC ACCURACY OF MYOCARDIAL PERFUSION IMAGING: THE CLINICAL IMPORTANCE OF DETERMINING WASHIN AND WASHOUT INDICATES A PARABOLIC FUNCTION BETWEEN CORONARY PERFUSION (BLOOD FLOW) AND CELLULAR ("UPTAKE/RELEASE") FUNCTION

***Richard M. Fleming*[1,a], *Gordon M. Harrington*[2,b] *and Riaz Baqir*[1,c]**

[1]Division of Cardiology, Veterans Affairs Hospital, Des Moines, IA
[2]University of Northern Iowa, Cedar Falls, IA 50614-0505

Abstract

Background: Myocardial perfusion imaging (MPI) has evolved over the last several decades with improvements in equipment and isotopes. Despite these advances, sensitivity and specificity of the methodology remains 65-90%. Numerous investigators have recommended changes in protocols and quantification of data to increase the diagnostic accuracy of this non-invasive physiologic test. Initial investigations have demonstrated differences in initial and delayed results post stress which have increased the ability to detect cardiomyopathies and vasospastic coronary artery disease. This study explored MPI stress validity using early (5 minute) and delayed (60 minute) post stress imaging and findings noted on cardiac catheterization.

[a] E-mail address: rmfmd7@hotmail.com. Corresponding Author: R. M. Fleming, M.D., VA Central Iowa Health Care System, Department of Internal Medicine, Division of Cardiology, 3600 30th Street, Des Moines, Iowa 50310
[b] E-mail address: gordon.harrington@uni.edu
[c] E-mail address: riazbaqirmd@aol.com

Methods: Records of forty-one individuals undergoing cardiac evaluation were studied for pharmacologic and exercise stress approaches with either Sestamibi or Myoview using standardized protocols. Twenty-two (54%) were diagnostically studied following MPI in the cardiac catheterization laboratory. Findings from the post stress images were used to determine washin/washout rates (WR) for total, anterior and inferior regions of myocardium and compared with findings from coronary angiography.

Results: Fifty-four percent (22 of 41) of the subjects studied underwent coronary angiography. Reading of MPI dynamic images at 60 minutes post stress resulted in 9 false (FNs) negatives (41%) and 2 false (FPs) positives (9%) in the anterior myocardium. Visual reading of inferior ischemia from dynamic images lead to 9 FNs (41%) and 3 FPs (14%). Evaluation of WR from multiple images obtained at 5 and 60 minutes post stress demonstrated a significant correlation between total heart WR and the average percent diameter (%DS) stenosis ($r=0.45$, $p<0.05$) and between inferior WR and inferior %DS ($r=0.68$, $p<0.001$). There was no correlation between anterior WR and anterior %DS for individuals with washout. However, when myocardial infarction/injury (MII) was taken into account there was an improved correlation ($r=0.21$) between anterior WR and anterior %DS. When washin occurred (total, anterior or inferior) a critical stenosis was noted at or near the ostium of a major epicardial vessel supplying a "large" region of viable myocardium at risk. This study also showed a significant increase in the incidence of MII in inferior regions of the heart when compared with anterior regions. The relationship between heart to lung (H:L) ratio was negatively ($r=-0.38$, p=NS) correlated with the presence of anterior MII. The relationship between left ventricular ejection fraction (EF) and anterior washout (W. Ant) was significant ($r=0.46$, $p<0.002$).

Conclusions: Initial static (5 minute) and delayed dynamic (60 minutes) images demonstrate changes between initial and delayed imaging which cannot be accounted for on the basis of radioactive decay alone and which can be quantified as WR. Both washin and washout WR, clearly demonstrates that the uptake and release of Tc 99m compounds is an active process influenced by both myocardial ischemia and MII; although, primarily ischemia and as such can be used to not only more accurately detect ischemia compared with using the 60 minute image alone, but to also allow determination of %DS. An absence of WR is seen only with individuals who have no ischemia and no MII, viz. "normals" who were limited in this study, since the referral of such subjects did not occur in this setting. Total WR and Inferior WR were highly correlated with % DS seen on coronary angiography. These results confirm earlier findings that such information appeared to be diagnostically important in determining coronary intervention of viable myocardium supplied by severely stenotic arteries missed using only the single set of images obtained at 60 minutes post stress. Our findings confirm earlier work on WR and the degree of cardiomyopathy/CHF in individuals with reduced left ventricular ejection fractions (LVEF) resulting from anterior MII and ischemia. This study is the first to demonstrate that using multiple (static and dynamic) imaging post stress increases the diagnostic accuracy of detecting ischemia and resulted in important diagnostic decisions about patient care/treatment (e.g. Coronary artery stenting), which was not apparent using only the 60 minute image. On inquiry the American Heart Association could cite no prior information regarding the incidence of MII in different regions of the heart. This study demonstrated a significant difference in regional MII and the ability to confidently correlate %DS from the total and inferior WR, in addition to removing the effect of diaphragmatic attenuation noted with the 60 minute image only despite the use of Gadolinium for attenuation correction. Further work is needed to determine if WR obtained from multiple imaging at rest could increase the diagnostic information gleaned regarding the extent of myocardial damage (stunned, hibernating or infarcted) present and perhaps provide insight into why certain regions of the heart are more prone to MII. For example, does the architecture of the right coronary artery predispose it to flow limitations not seen in the other epicardial arteries, just as it makes it more difficult for the interventionalist to angioplasty or stent longer lesions without injury to the artery. Assessment of static images during intermediate times (between 5 and 60 minutes) and using multiple head static imaging may yield additional diagnostic information, the benefit of which can only be determined by looking at the results. Finally, these findings demonstrated a parabolic interactive model between coronary blood flow and cellular "uptake/release" of Technetium-99m tracers which more accurately detects coronary ischemia using a multiple post-stress imaging washin/washout model.

Key words: myocardial washout, myocardial washin, washout rate (WR), multiple imaging, MPI, myocardial ischemia, myocardial infarction/injury (MII), data validity, MPI accuracy.

Background

While diagnostic testing and decision making in the treatment of atherosclerotic coronary artery disease (ASCAD/CAD) tends to revolve around evidence of anatomic (cardiac catheterization[1], coronary computed tomography, intravascular ultrasound[2,3], et cetera) disease, it has been well established that this inflammatory[4-6] process may smolder for years and that up to 85% of all myocardial infarctions occur with < 30% diameter narrowing. It is; therefore, important for us to look for new ways to uncover this smoldering inflammatory disease process when intervention may be more beneficial to the patient and potentially less costly to the patient and society at a time when health care costs are a major issue.

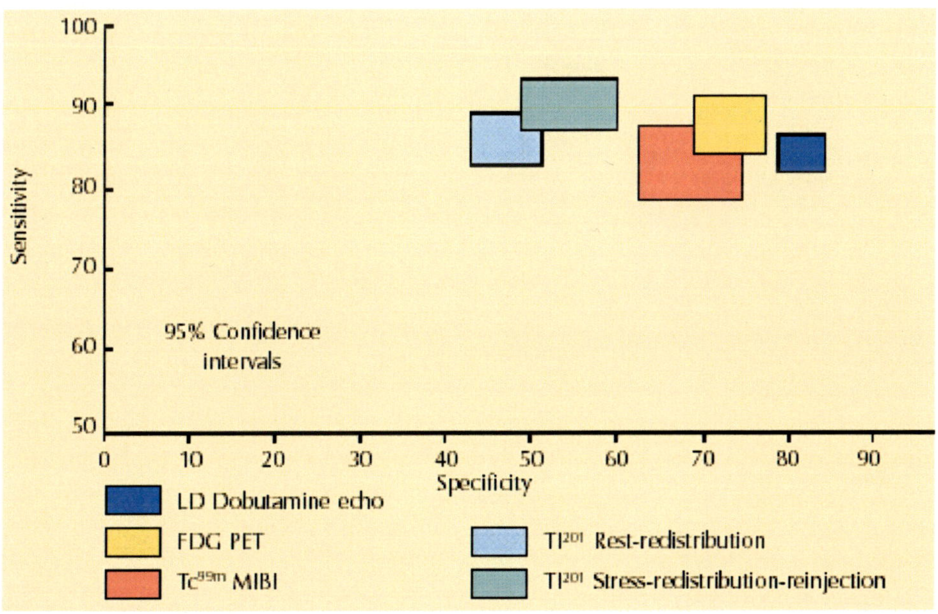

Figure 1. Sensitivity and Specificity of current approach. The 95% confidence intervals (CI) are shown for five different non-invasive diagnostic imaging approaches. The ability of MIBI to detect disease (sensitivity) using standard imaging approaches is less than 90%. The ability of MIBI to exclude disease (specificity) is less than 80% using standard approaches.

When teenagers learn to buy their first automobile, they learn an important lesson. Not every car that looks good runs well. This same lesson applies to the diagnosis and treatment of ASCAD. The lesson is to determine how well the car runs, or in this case, how well the heart runs. Hence the importance of physiologic testing; ie. testing to see how well the heart runs. Prior to nuclear imaging of the heart, now called myocardial perfusion[7,8] imaging (MPI), patients ran on a treadmill (exercise stress testing/EST) under the belief that this would precipitate chest pain (angina) and perhaps electrocardiographic and hemodynamic changes which would indicate problems with coronary blood flow. Until recently, it was believed that this was purely the result of narrowing within the lumen of the artery. It has since been demonstrated that angina is the result of regional blood flow[9,10] differences; hence, the importance of quantifying such areas of the heart by analyzing regions of interest (ROI). These differences in regional blood flow work through mechanisms as of yet not completely understood. The ability to precipitate these differences in regional blood flow can be accomplished via the utilization of MPI and pharmacologic or exercise stress testing. While nuclear tracers (isotopes) have improved over the years, many misconceptions[11-17] have plagued the field limiting the accuracy of MPI with sensitivities and specificities of 65-90% in most published investigations[18] as shown in figure 1.

During our initial[19,20] efforts to better understand the underlying inflammatory component of CAD via MPI, static and dynamic imaging revealed differences in the qualitative appearances of images seen following pharmacologic stressing of individuals. Furthermore, comparisons of initial static (5 minutes) and then dynamic (60 minutes) images demonstrated different results indicating that the technetium isotope Sestamibi does not simply "stick" to the myocardium as was once thought. Other investigators have noted similar differences between initial static and subsequent dynamic imaging of the heart[21-25] allowing for enhanced detection of congestive heart failure[22,26-29], cardiomyopathies[30,31], Prinzmetal 's angina[32,33] and underlying coronary artery disease[22,27,34-45] including evidence of washin[42,43] indicative of critical lesions not detected by conventional MPI. In the same way that thrombolysis in myocardial infarction (TIMI) flow is used to look for changes (sometimes subtle, sometimes not) in coronary blood flow in the cath lab, static and dynamic imaging following pharmacologic or EST allows us a more advanced look at the physiologic (imaging) function of the heart, in the same way that modern computers built into today's cars allow the detection of functional problems within the car before the trained (certified) mechanic can detect it.

Given these recent investigations into improving the detection of ischemia by quantifying isotope counts on multiple (sequential) images following pharmacologic and exercise stress, we set out to determine the validity of MPI readings at a US government facility based upon readings provided by a boarded nuclear medicine physician and results obtained by Boarded General Invasive Cardiologists in the cardiac catheterization laboratory. Static and dynamic ROIs were then analyzed to quantify changes in isotope counts at 5 and 60 minutes post stress. Assessment of the effect of both isotope decay (10% reduction over a 55 minute period of time) for technetium 99m compounds and the actual changes in isotope count (washin/washout rate; WR) were then compared with percent diameter stenosis (%DS) obtained by cardiac catheterization. The results of WR were then compared to %DS and the severity of myocardial infarction/injury (MII) to determine if we could (1) improve our detection of CAD by using WR and (2) to subsequently improve patient care and management as a result. We additionally set out to verify the relationship between heart to lung (H:L) ratios with both left ventricular ejection fraction and MII.

Methods

Forty-one subjects were studied at a Veterans Hospital following informed consent procedures for diagnostic studies. Patients were all referred by primary care providers to determine the extent of coronary artery disease. Participants signed informed consent (IC) for the stressor component of the study. IC is not required at the institution for injection or imaging of a nuclear isotope. All subjects were de-identified in accordance with Veterans Administration (VA) Manual 3, Part I, Chapter 9, Section 9A(4). Results of these diagnostic studies were obtained under the Freedom of Information Act (FOIA).

Myocardial Perfusion Imaging (MPI) Protocols

Patients were brought to the nuclear cardiology department in the fasting state with an intravenous catheter inserted into either the right or left antebrachium. Patients underwent pharmacologic stress (adenosine or dobutamine) or EST per standard VA protocols.

Adenosine Stress: Those receiving adenosine were given 140 mcg/kg/min for a total of 4 minutes with approximately 30 mCi of isotope (Sestamibi or Myoview) given at the completion of the second minute of adenosine infusion followed by a saline flush to assure delivery of the isotope into the venous system. Hemodynamic and electrocardiographic data were collected at baseline, at 2 and 4 minutes infusion, in addition to 1, 3 and 5 minutes post adenosine infusion. Patients then underwent static image acquisition 5 minutes after peak pharmacologic stress with the patient placed in a supine position and the camera positioned directly above the center of their sternum in the anterior position, immediately above the patient. Image acquisition required 2 minutes. Fifty-five minutes later (60 minutes post isotope infusion) multiple static step and shoot (dynamic) images were obtained as noted below.

Dobutamine Stress: Those receiving dobutamine[46-50] pharmacologic stress did so as already described in the literature. Hemodynamic and blood pressure monitoring occurred at 1 minute 30 seconds into each phase of the pharmacologic stress and during recovery until hemodynamically and clinically stable. The injection of the isotope was given at peak dobutamine infusion followed by 2 minutes of continued infusion of dobutamine at the peak rate. Patients then underwent static image acquisition 5 minutes after peak pharmacologic stress as described above. Fifty-five minutes later (60 minutes post isotope infusion) multiple static step and shoot (dynamic) images were obtained as noted below.

Exercise Stress (EST): Those following exercise stress imaging[17,49] were injected with the isotope after obtaining 85% maximum predicted heart rate (MPHR) and exercised for an additional two minutes per protocol as previously described in the literature. Hemodynamic and blood pressure monitoring occurred at 1 minute 30 seconds into each phase of the exercise stress and during recovery until hemodynamically and clinically stable. Patients static and dynamic images were then obtained as previously discussed.

Single Photon Emission Computed Tomography (SPECT) Cameras

Thirty-seven of the 41 studies were completed using a Philips Forte Dual Head SPECT camera using general all (GAP) purpose collimators with the heads positioned at 90 degrees per manufacturers specifications. A 15% window was used with a 64 by 64 matrix. A static image was acquired 5 minutes after isotope infusion as described previously[19,20]. At 60 minutes post-stress, a second image was taken with 32 views acquired using standard step and shoot approach with 25 seconds per view beginning in right anterior oblique (RAO) and terminating in the left posterior oblique (LPO) position. Jet stream software was used per manufacturer's instructions to quantitatively measure regions of interest (ROIs). Dynamic images were reconstructed using a Butterworth filter and standard back projection with reconstruction of short, horizontal and long axis views as previously described[17].

Four of the 41 studies were completed using a Picker Axis Dual Head SPECT camera using a low energy general all (LEGAR-PAR) purpose collimator with parallel hole positioning. The heads were positioned at 102 degrees per manufacturer specifications. Dynamic images were reconstructed using a Butterworth filter and standard back projection with reconstruction of short, horizontal and long axis views as described above. A 15% window was used with a 64 by 64 matrix with 34 views obtained over 30 seconds per view. Image acquisition began in the RAO position and terminated in the LPO position. Picker camera software was used for ROI measurements.

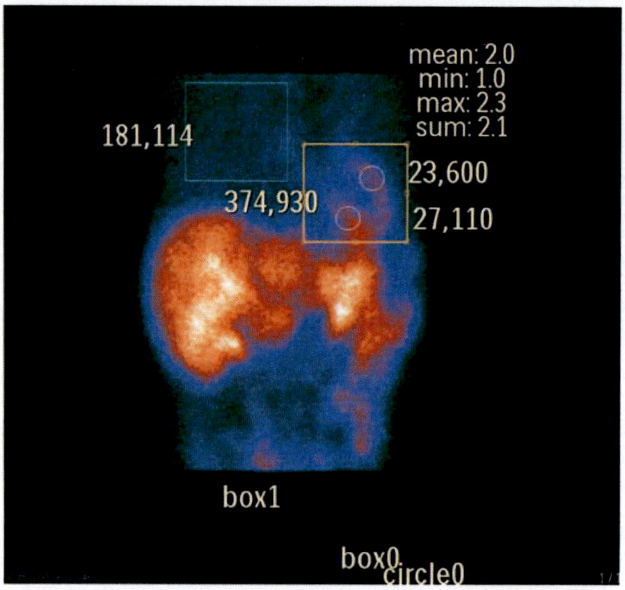

Figure 2. Static image taken at 5 minutes post stress with regions of interest defined and quantified. Static imaging at 5 minutes with regions of interest (ROI) showing total heart count of 374,930, total lung count of 181,114 with a calculated heart to lung (H:L) ratio of 2.0. The anterior ROI shows 23,600 count and the inferior ROI shows 27,110.

Washin and Washout Data (WR) Using Multiple Static and Dynamic Images

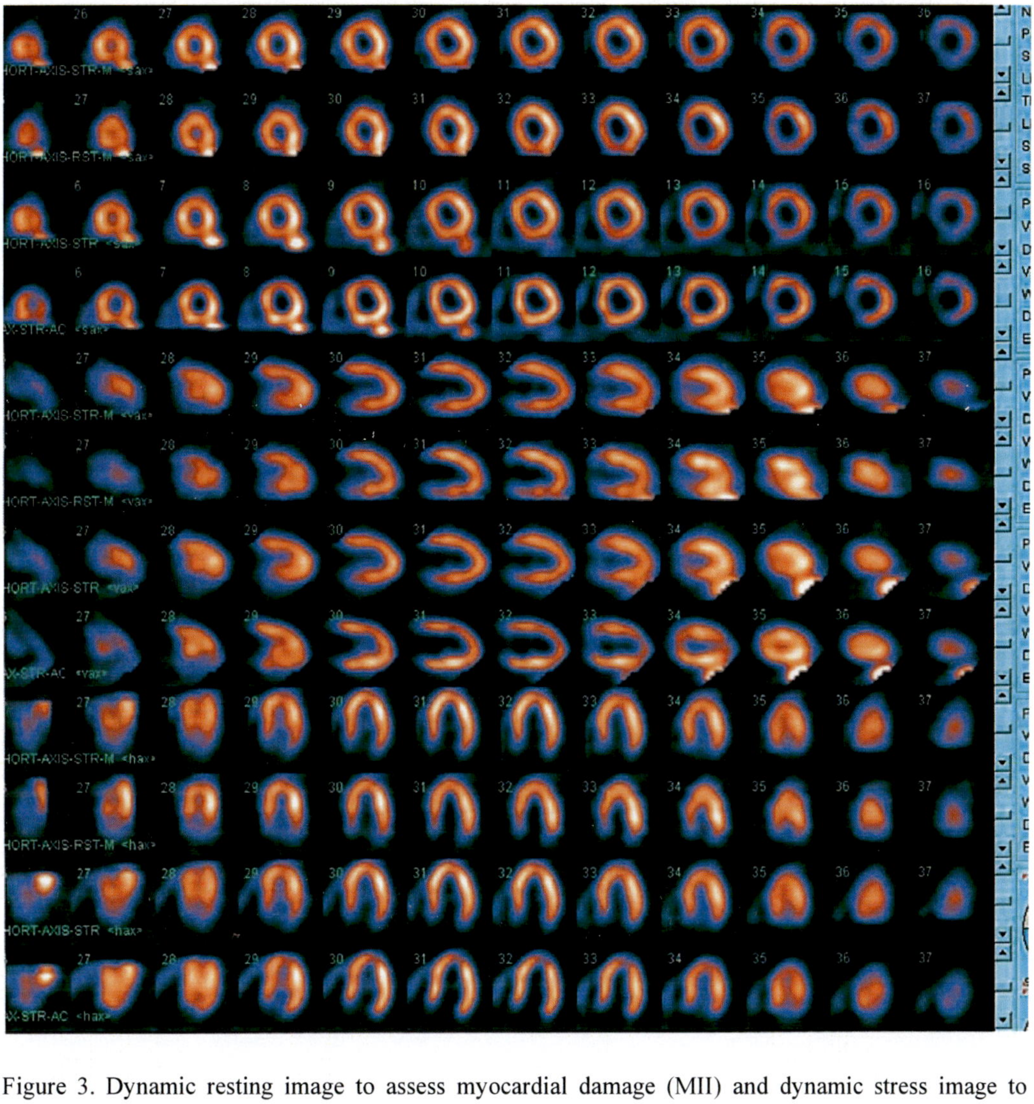

Figure 3. Dynamic resting image to assess myocardial damage (MII) and dynamic stress image to assess ischemia with and without attenuation (AC) correction. The same patient shown in figures 2, 3, 5 and 6 is displayed using coronal short axis (top 4 rows), vertical long axis (rows 5-8) and the horizontal (rows 9-12) long axis rows. Rows 1-2, 5-6, and 9-10 show images using non-attenuation corrected images. Rows 3-4, 7-8, and 11-12 show the same regions using AC. Rows 2,4,6,8,10 and 12 show resting images providing information regarding myocardial (MII) infarction/injury (infarction, stunned or hibernating) while rows 1,3,5,7,9 and 11 reveal the same regions of myocardium following pharmacologic stress; in this case adenosine. These images were interpreted as "normal" showing no evidence of infarction or ischemia.

The initial static image (figure 2) was analyzed for ROIs as noted above. Total heart, total lung, anterior and inferior myocardial assessment of isotope count activity were measured and recorded. From this, H:L ratios were calculated. Following the acquisition of the static image, dynamic imaging was obtained 55 minutes later. The dynamic images were reconstructed as previously described and shown in figure 3. From these dynamic images, an identical static image was chosen and matched to the initial static image (figure 4). Regions of interest were drawn using the same approach shown in figure 2. The ROIs from the final images (e.g. Figures 2 and 4) were used to calculate WRs for total heart (W.TH), anterior (W.Ant) and inferior (W. Inf) regions of the heart for each patient using the calculations shown below.

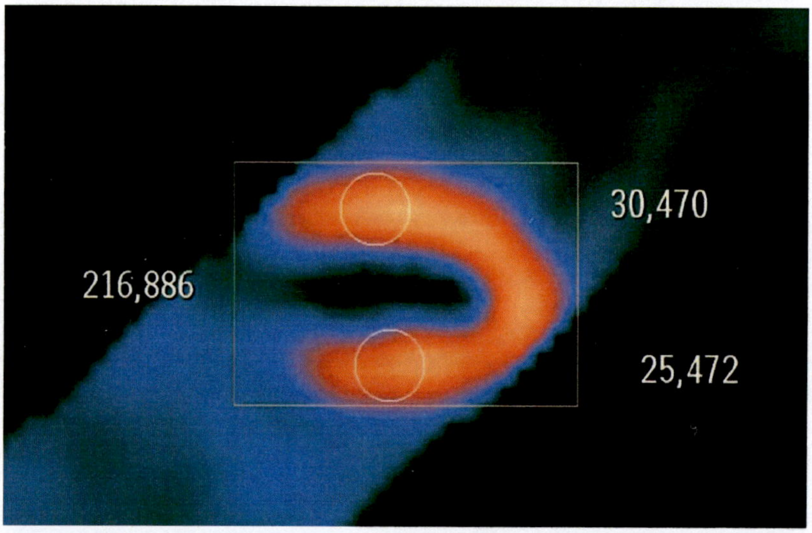

Figure 4. Regions of interest for assessment of washin/washout (WR) at 60 minutes. Reconstruction of the same myocardial region noted in figure 2, this time taken from the dynamic image result obtained at 60 minutes post stress, showing a total heart count of 216,886. The anterior ROI shows an increase in count activity (washin) of 30,470 compared with the activity of 23,600 (Figure 2) obtained at 5 minutes. The inferior ROI shows a count of 25,472 compared with the count activity of 27,110 (Figure 2) obtained 5 minutes post stress.

Visual Interpretation of Myocardial Perfusion Imaging (MPI)

A Board Certified Nuclear Medicine physician independently interpreted images using standard and AC images (figure 3) in all but four of the participants. These four studies were performed on the Picker camera which does not have AC capability, while the Philips camera was undergoing scheduled maintenance. The AC images obtained using the Philips camera used Gadolinium as a source with accompanying camera software. The reporting of ischemia by this hospital physician became the final reporting of patient results in accordance with hospital policy. Infarction was not reported by this physician other than to note if the resting and stress dynamic images matched or not. Myocardial infarction/injury (MII) was reported by a Boarded Nuclear Cardiologist who assigned a value of zero ("0") to regions without limitations in isotope uptake, one ("1") to regions with reduced but still present (partial thickness) isotope uptake and two ("2") if no isotope (full thickness) was observed in the region.

Washin & Washout Rate (WR) Calculations

The radioactive decay of Tc99m over a 55 minute period of time would result in 90% of the original isotope remaining if all of the isotope originally taken up by the myocardium was not released; but, simply retained and decayed over time. The WRs were calculated from both the attenuation and non-attenuated images. The static images were without AC.

W. TH (Total Heart Washin/Washout Rates) WR (%) =

(eq 1).

$$= \frac{\text{ROI counts (total heart) at 5 minutes - ROI counts (total heart) at 60 minutes}}{\text{ROI counts (total heart) at 5 minutes}} \times 100 - 10$$

W. Ant (Anterior Heart Washin/Washout Rates) WR(%) =

(eq 2).

$$= \frac{\text{ROI counts (anterior) at 5 minutes -ROI counts (anterior) at 60 minutes}}{\text{ROI counts (anterior) at 5 minutes}} \times 100 - 10$$

W. Inf (Inferior Heart Washin/Washout Rates) WR(%) =

(eq 3).

$$= \frac{\text{ROI counts (inferior) at 5 minutes -ROI counts (inferior) at 60 minutes}}{\text{ROI counts (inferior) at 5 minutes}} \times 100 - 10$$

Coronary Angiography[51,52].

Twenty-two of the subjects were brought to the cardiac catheterization laboratory for diagnostic evaluation of coronary lumen disease (percent diameter stenosis, %DS) in the fasting state. Patients were prepped in the usual manner after signing IC per hospital protocol. Coronary angiography was performed using Seldinger and Judkins techniques with arterial access obtained from either the right or left femoral artery. Subjects were subsequently injected with contrast using either Ultravist 370 for non-renally impaired individuals or Visipaque 320 for those with questions regarding renal function. A single head Philips Flat Detector (FD) 20 was used at 15 frames per second (fps) and an 8 inch field. Images were recorded digitally and reviewed by two Board Certified Invasive Cardiologists and matched to the specific regions of myocardium supplied (anterior, inferior). An example of injected left coronary arteries are shown in figures 5 and 6, taken immediately prior to and after placement of three stents as described.

Statistical Analysis. Quantification of isotope counts was made using the specific nuclear computer software provided by the camera companies. These quantified counts were recorded with calculations of WR as noted above. Chi-square analysis of comparison of disease present by cath and MPI were noted. Correlation coefficients, confidence intervals and p-value (significance levels) were determined between %DS and WRs using product-moment correlation. Statistical analysis and graphics were developed using R-2.6.0 and GGobi software.

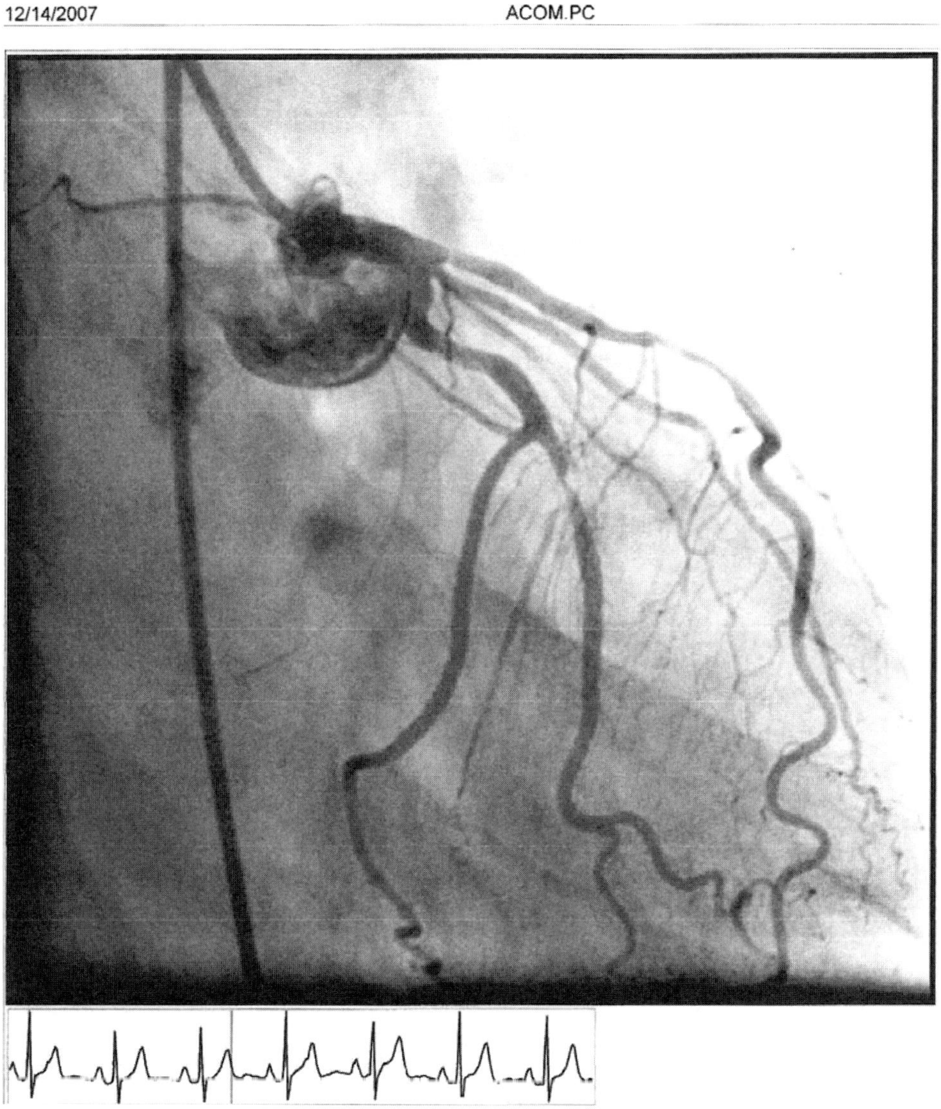

Figure 5. Critically diseased left anterior descending and circumflex arteries matching Washin/Washout (WR) data, prior to stenting.Cardiac catheterization revealed a "normal left main (LM) and right coronary artery (RCA). The left anterior descending (LAD) had an 80% DS ostial (beginning) lesion in addition to a 75% "long segmental" proximal lesion. The first diagonal had a 60 %DS lesion at the ostium. The proximal left circumflex (LCx) had a 40% DS proximal and an 80 %DS ostial lesion of the first obtuse marginal (OM1) was noted.

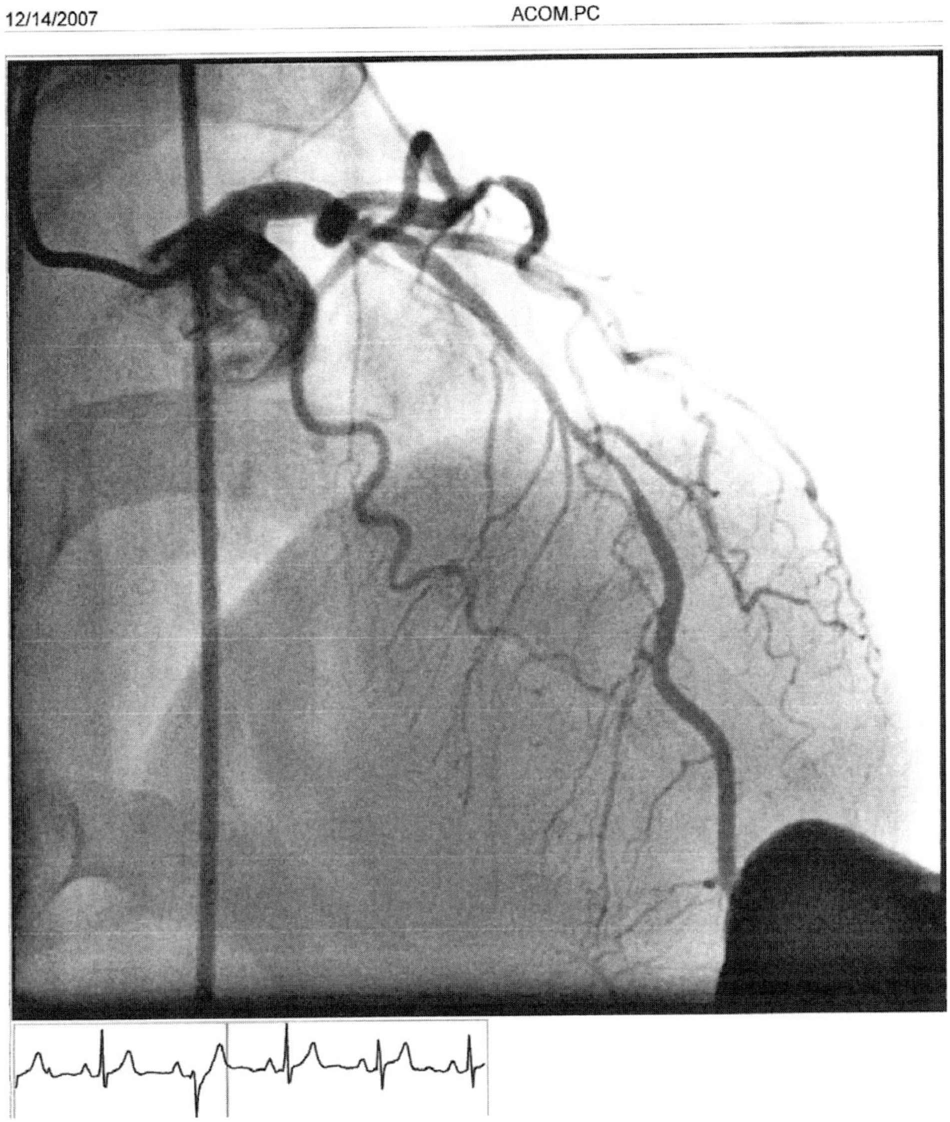

Figure 6. Critically diseased left anterior descending and circumflex arteries matching washin/washout (WR) data, after stenting. Cardiac catheterization of same arteries show in figure 5 following insertion of a cypher RX drug eluting 3.5 x 8 mm stent for the 80 %DS ostial lesion of the LAD, a cypher RX drug eluting 3.0 x 33 mm stent for the 75% DS proximal LAD lesion and a Cypher RX drug eluting 3.0 x 13 mm stent for the 80% DS ostial lesion of OM1.

Results

General: There were no statistical differences (p=NS) in any of the measured outcomes based upon the form of stress used or isotope selected.

Prevalence of MII: Multiple studies and papers have looked at the association with specific problems relative to the region of MII (e.g. aneurysms, first degree atrial-ventricular block, right ventricular versus left ventricular infarction), yet there appears to be no information[53] regarding the prevalence of myocardial infarction/injury (MII) in specific regions of myocardium. Of the 22 individuals who underwent cardiac catheterization, half of them (50%) had no evidence of MII anteriorly, while only two (9%) had no evidence of MII inferiorly. Of the 50% who did have MII anteriorly, more than half of these (6 of 11) had level one (less than full thickness) MII and less than one-quarter (23%) had evidence of full thickness MII. In contrast, almost three-quarters (73%) had evidence of full thickness MII inferiorly. As shown in Table 1, the same results held true for all individuals in the study independent of whether they had undergone cardiac catheterization or not.

Table 1. Incidence of myocardial infarction/injury (MII) as noted on resting images for both patients taken to cardiac catheterization and those who underwent MPI.

Group	0	1	2
Anterior (cath) n=22	n=11 (50%)	n=6 (27%)	n=5 (23%)
Inferior (cath) n=22	n=2 (9%)	n=4 (18%)	n=16 (73%)
Anterior (all) n=41	n=21 (51%)	n=12 (29%)	n=8 (20%)
Inferior (all) n=41	n=6 (15%)	n=9 (22%)	n=26 (63%)

0 = no evidence of myocardial injury, 1 = reduction in isotope activity, 2 = absence of isotope activity.

Visual Interpretation by MPI of the Presence of Ischemia: Interpretation of MPI post stress images taken at 60 minutes alone, without the information present during the initial 5 minute static images, were compared with cardiac catheterization data using both 50% DS and 70% DS as the cutoff for "significant" CAD. When the MPI report interpretation (which used only the 60 minute post-stress image) was reviewed and compared with the coronary angiogram, 12 of 18 (67% sensitivity) individuals with 50 %DS stenotic lesions present angiographically were reported as having ischemia on the MPI. Note that this approach did not require that the artery deemed to have significant disease match the myocardial region reported as ischemic. Only 1 of the 4 without disease on cardiac catheterization was deemed to be free of disease by MPI interpretation. When the same question was asked using 70% DS as the cutoff for CAD, interpretation of the 60 minute dynamic image yielded detection of disease in only 8 of the 15 cases (53% sensitivity) and reported only 1 of the 7 individuals as being free of significant disease.

In an effort to further look at the validity of MPI readings, we investigated the incidence of false negative (FN) and false positive (FP) results looking specifically at regions of myocardium and matching the results with the arteries which supplied those regions as confirmed by coronary angiography. When the findings of anterior disease were defined as 50 %DS, 9 of the 22 (41%) anterior studies were interpreted as being free (FN) of disease while 2 of the 22 (9%) were interpreted as having (FP) disease present on MPI but absent on angiography. The means that the overall interpretation of anterior disease using the 60 minute MPI image only was correct in 11 of 22 (50%) cases. The findings were similar when inferior disease was analyzed, where 9 of the 22 cases (41%) were determined to be free (FN) of disease, while 3 of the 22 (14%) were reported has having (FP) disease present on the 60 minute MPI image while being absent on coronary angiography. A total of 55% of the individuals studies were mis-diagnosed based upon the reading of the 60 minute dynamic image only without the information available from the 5 minute static image which allowed for the calculation of WR. When looked at in this same manner, using 70 %DS as the cutoff for CAD, 12 of the 22 individuals (55 %) were told that they did not have disease in an area where they actually did and needed treatment. Of these, 5 (42%) had disease anteriorly, 4 (33%) had inferior disease and 3 (25%) had disease in both the anterior and inferior regions. Of these individuals (as noted below and in Table 4), all had WRs more than twice the Tc99m decay, indicating ischemia in the arterial region with angiographically documented disease.

Washin/Washout (WR) Detection of Ischemia by Artery: The results obtained from AC and non-attenuation corrected dynamic images at 60 minutes did not change outcomes. For simplicity sake and since the 5 minute static images were derived without attenuation correction, further results discussed below will focus on standard (non-attenuated) images only and subsequent WRs. In an effort to determine the reliability of technician assessment of count activity and subsequently WR, four of the cases were reviewed by two technicians on separate occasions. They were asked to draw regions of interest (ROIs) for total heart, total lung, anterior and inferior regions on the 5 minute static image and total heart, anterior and inferior ROIs on the 60 minute dynamic image. As shown in table 2, the greatest inter-technologist reliability was seen with total heart (W.TH) washout or washin. Table 3 shows the correlations for all 41 subjects, comparing total heart washin/washout (W.TH), anterior washin/washout (W.Ant), inferior washin/washout (W.Inf), anteriorly (Ant Sten) %DS, inferiorly (Inf Sten) %DS and the average (Avg Sten) %DS.

Table 2. Comparison of Washin/Washout assessment between nuclear technologists.

ID	W.TH T1	W.TH T2	W.Ant T1	W.Ant T2	W.Inf T1	W.Inf T2
R	-10	-46	-6	16	6	19
S	-30	-13	-26	-44	0	-15
T	-34	-58	-55	-100	-17	-65
U	-16	0	15	0	21	4

W.TH = total washin/washout rate, W. Ant = anterior washin/washout rate, W. Inf = inferior washin/washout rate, T1 = Nuclear medicine tech # 1, T2= Nuclear medicine tech #2.

Table 3. Correlations of static and dynamic imaging Washin/Washout (WRs) with percent diameter stenosis (%DS).

	W.TH	W.Ant	W.Inf	Ant Sten	Inf Sten	Avg Sten
W.TH	1.00	0.71	0.84	0.15	0.52	0.45
W.Ant	0.71	1.00	0.77	0.00	0.32	0.22
W.Inf	0.84	0.77	1.00	0.07	0.68	0.50
Ant Sten	0.15	0.00	0.07	1.00	0.21	0.75
Inf Sten	0.52	0.32	0.68	0.21	1.00	0.80
Avg Sten	0.45	0.22	0.50	0.75	0.80	1.00

W.TH = total washin/washout rate, W. Ant = anterior washin/washout rate, W. Inf = inferior washin/washout rate, Ant Sten = anterior percent diameter stenosis (%DS), Inf Sten = inferior %DS, Avg Sten = average %DS.

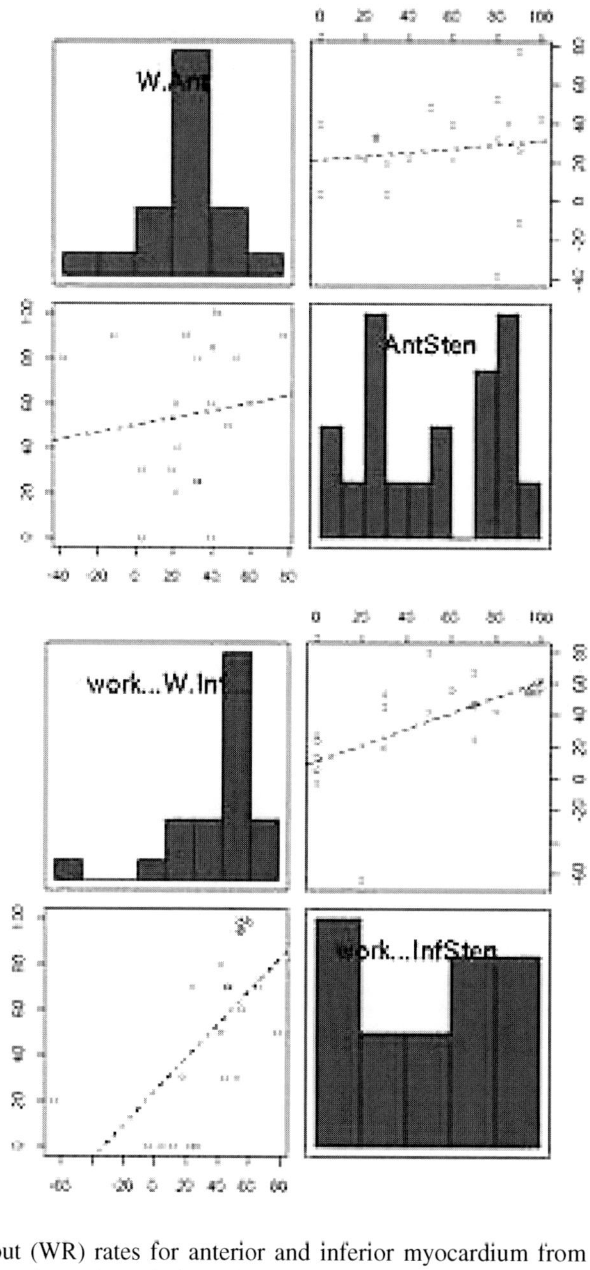

Figure 7. Washin/washout (WR) rates for anterior and inferior myocardium from static and dynamic imaging. These graphics show the relationship between washin/washout rates (WR) and percent diameter stenosis (% DS) reported from coronary angiography. Both graphics show a positive relationship between % DS and WR.

The strongest relationship was seen between W.TH and W. Ant (r=0.71, p<0.001) and W.TH and W. Inf (r=0.84, p<0.001). Furthermore, W.TH was significantly associated with %DS seen on coronary angiography, for Inf Sten (r=0.52, p<0.01) and with Avg Sten (r=0.45, p<0.05). W.Inf is highly correlated (r=0.68, p<0.001) with angiographically defined Inf Sten (%DS). When corrected for MII, the correlation between W.TH and Ant Sten was not as strong as that seen for Inf Sten, with a correlation of 0.15 (p=NS). The strongest ROI WR was noted for the inferior myocardium, where the W. Inf with the Inf Sten demonstrated a strong correlation (r=0.68, p<0.001) between W. Inf and the %DS of the artery supplying the inferior myocardium depending upon which artery (right or circumflex) was dominant. This relationship was less pronounced anteriorly. In an effort to determine if differences in WR anteriorly and inferiorly were partially influenced by the presence of MII, we then looked specifically at these ROIs and compared the relationship between WR and %DS in the presence or absence of prior MII. The relationship between W. Inf and Inf Sten did not change (r=0.68, p<0.001) independent of whether MII was 0, 1 or 2. When W. Ant was compared with Ant Sten, the relationship was greater if no (0) MII was present (r=0.34, p=NS), than if MII level 1 or 2 was present (r=0.29, p=NS). Figure 7 shows the graphic relationship between the anterior WRs and anterior %DS in the upper graphic and the relationship between inferior WRs and inferior % DS in the lower graphic. Figure 8 shows the differences noted when the subjects were split out depending upon the degree of MII present. Specifically, differences in WR post stress cannot be accounted for on the basis of MII (the ability of the myocyte to retain the isotope) alone, but does have some impact with the average of W.TH and the average MII correlating (r=0.60, p<0.005) significantly.

The Critical Finding of Washin (WR): Table 4 shows the specific information for the 22 individuals who underwent cardiac catheterization following the multiple study washin/washout (WR) analysis. Four (18%) of these 22 individuals studied demonstrated an increase in radioactive counts over time. Known as washin, these individuals are associated with (1) at least one critically narrowed artery supplying (2) a significant amount of viable myocardium at risk for MII if not treated promptly. An example of this is presented below.

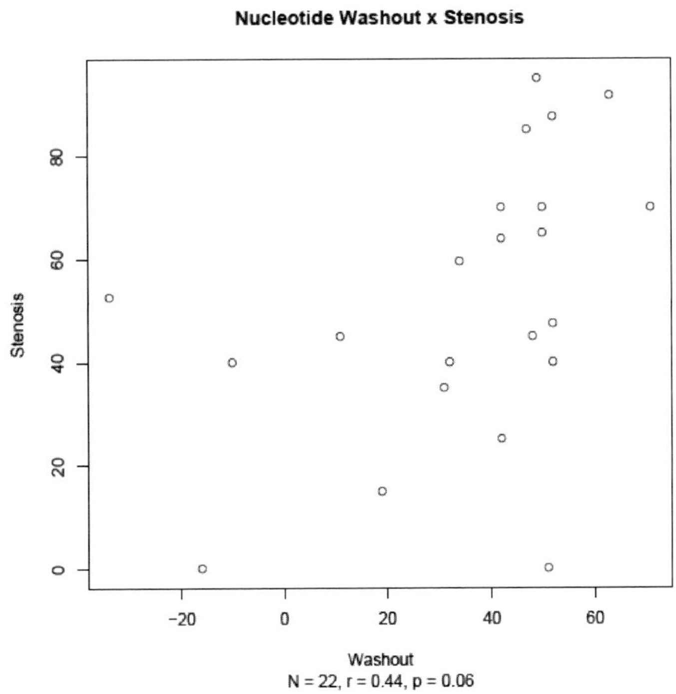

Figure 8. Continued on next page.

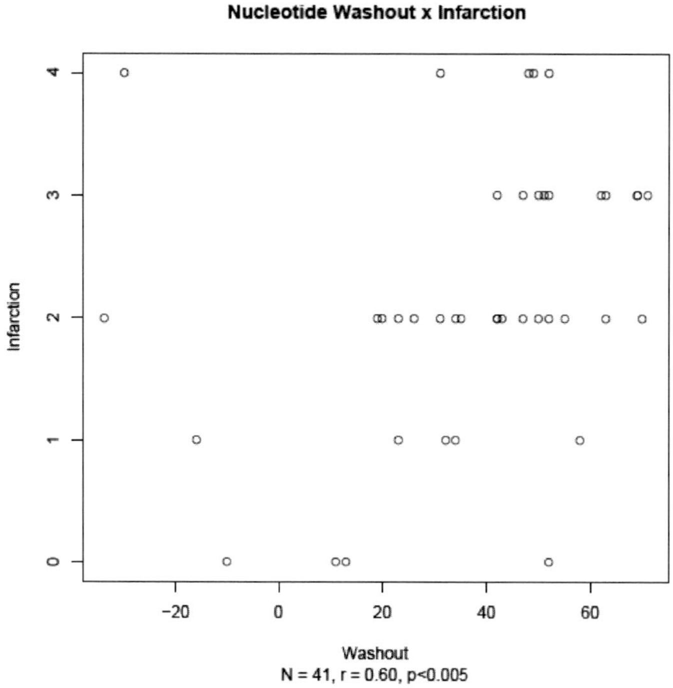

Figure 8. Differences in Washin/washout (WR) rates for anterior and inferior myocardium comparing those with and without myocardial infarction/injury (MII). These graphics show the relationship between washin/washout rates (WR) and percent diameter stenosis (% DS) reported from coronary angiography in individuals with ischemia only without MII and those with both ischemia and MII.

Table 4. Comparison of Washin/Washout (WR), left ventricular ejection fraction (LVEF), percent diameter stenosis (%DS) and presence of myocardial damage/injury.

ID	Iso	W.TH	W.Ant	W.Inf	H:L	EF.	AntSten	InfSten	NV	MI.Ant	MI.Inf
A	Mibi	42	19	54	2.2	60	30	98	3	0	2
E	Mibi	34	33	54	2.3	44	25	94	3	0	1
G	Mibi	50	32	55	2.9	64	80	60	2	0	2
H	Mibi	42	21	45	2.6	67	20	30	1	0	2
I	Mibi	51	39	28	2.3	51	0	0	0	1	2
J	Mibi	71	77	79	1.9	61	90	50	2	1	2
K	Mibi	32	-39	-4	2	52	80	0	2	0	1
M	Mibi	52	48	53	2.2	33	50	30	3	2	1
N	Mibi	19	3	23	2.1	64	30	0	0	0	2
O	Mibi	52	52	55	1.9	42	80	95	3	2	2
P	Mibi	31	3	24	1.8	59	0	70	2	2	2
Q	Mibi	49	-11	57	1.6	18	90	100	3	2	2
R	Mibi	-46	16	19	2.1	67	50	30	1	0	0
T	Mibi	-58	-100	-65	1.6	29	85	20	1	0	2
U	Mibi	0	0	4	2	48	0	0	0	0	1
A2	Mibi	47	42	47	2	50	100	70	3	1	2

Table 4. Continued

ID	Iso	W.TH	W.Ant	W.Inf	H:L	EF.	AntSten	InfSten	NV	MI.Ant	MI.Inf
B2	Mibi	42	21	42	2.3	48	60	80	3	1	2
C2	Mibi	52	32	66	.2.0	59	25	70	2	0	2
a	Myo	48	22	42	2.1	55	40	50	3	2	2
b	Myo	63	40	61	2	59	85	98	2	1	2
g	Myo	11	26	12	2.6	66	90	0	2	0	0
k	Myo	50	39	46	2.1	52	60	70	3	1	2

Iso=isotope used, Mibi=Sestamibi, Myo=Myoview, W.TH=Total washin/washout, W.Ant=Anterior washin/washout, W.Inf=Inferior washin/washout, H:L=Heart to Lung ratio, EF=Percent left ventricular ejection fraction, AntSten=percent diameter stenosis anteriorly, InfSten=percent diameter stenosis inferiorly, NV=number of epicardially diseased coronary arteries, MI. Ant=anterior infarction, MI. inf=inferior infarction.

Heart to Lung (H:L) ratios: The results of H:L, left ventricular ejection fraction (EF), total heart (W. TH) washin/washout, anterior (W. Ant) washin/washout, and inferior (W. Inf) washin/washout for all 41 individuals are shown in table 5. The total washin/washout was correlated with anterior ($r=0.71$, $p<0.001$) washin/washout and inferior ($r=0.84$, $p<0.001$) washin/washout. Finally, we restudied the question of H:L ratios and the presence or absence of disease with the individual findings noted in tables 4 and 5. The relationship between heart to lung (H:L) ratio was ($r=-0.38$, p=NS) when compared to the presence of anterior MII. While this relationship was NS, the relationship between left ventricular ejection fraction (EF) and anterior washout (W. Ant) was extremely significant ($r=0.46$, $p<0.002$).

Table 5. Comparison of Static Heart to Lung (H:L) ratios at Five Minutes post-stress and Left Ventricular Ejection Fraction (EF).

ID	Isotope	H:L	EF	W.TH	W.Ant	W.Inf
A	Mibi	2.2	60	42	19	54
B	Mibi	2.2	73	13	26	34
C	Mibi	2.1	25	35	-57	47
D	Mibi	1.5	46	26	-13	-8
E	Mibi	2.3	44	34	33	54
F	Mibi	1.7	63	58	48	51
G	Mibi	2.9	64	50	32	55
H	Mibi	2.6	67	42	21	45
I	Mibi	2.3	51	51	39	28
J	Mibi	1.9	61	71	77	79
K	Mibi	2	52	32	-39	-4
L	Mibi	2.2	45	23	6	21
M	Mibi	2.2	33	52	48	53
N	Mibi	2.1	64	19	3	23
O	Mibi	1.9	42	52	52	55
P	Mibi	1.8	59	31	3	24
Q	Mibi	1.6	18	49	-11	57
R	Mibi	2.1	67	-46	16	19

Table 5. Continued

ID	Isotope	H:L	EF	W.TH	W.Ant	W.Inf
S	Mibi	1.3	22	-13	-44	-15
T	Mibi	1.6	29	-58	-100	-65
U	Mibi	2	48	0	0	4
A2	Mibi	2	50	47	42	47
B2	Mibi	2.3	48	42	21	42
C2	Mibi	2.0	59	52	32	66
D2	Mibi	2.1	68	31	6	39
Aa1	Mibi	2.3	43	23	-40	9
a	Myo	2.1	55	48	22	42
b	Myo	2	59	63	40	61
c	Myo	2.1	60	69	66	74
d	Myo	2.1	41	55	40	50
e	Myo	2.4	57	20	-2	19
f	Myo	2	62	62	54	63
g	Myo	2.6	66	11	26	12
h	Myo	1.8	66	63	48	65
i	Myo	1.5	66	34	22	40
j	Myo	2.3	61	52	47	53
k	Myo	2.1	52	50	39	46
l	Myo	2	52	43	31	39
m	Myo	2.2	59	70	54	62
a2	Myo	1.6	51	47	18	42
b2	Myo	1.6	51	69	60	58

Iso=isotope used, Mibi=Sestamibi, Myo=Myoview, H:L=Heart to Lung ratio, EF=Percent left ventricular ejection fraction, W.TH=Total washin/washout, W.Ant=Anterior washin/washout, W.Inf=Inferior washin/washout.

Case Example of the Clinical Importance of Using Multiple Images Post-stress to Increase the Diagnostic Accuracy of Myocardial Perfusion Imaging. The Clinical Importance of Determining Washin & Washout: The ability to improve the results of a diagnostic study is of limited value if it does not result in improved patient care and management. Figures 2-6 represent the findings of a 58 year old gentleman who had previously undergone exercise stress, an echocardiogram, electrocardiogram and an echocardiographic stress test; all of which had been interpreted as "normal". The patient continued to experience exertional chest discomfort alleviated with rest. Both the findings of MPI at rest and those following adenosine stress are shown in figure 3, including both standard and AC images. While not shown here, there were no regional wall motion abnormalities[47,54] on the gated images which would suggest significant ischemia. The interpretation by the Boarded Nuclear Medicine physician was a "normal" study without evidence of infarction or ischemia. In an effort to be completely objective, no one else involved in this case noted ischemia or MII as being present on this final result. Figure 2 shows the initial isotope counts obtained 5 minutes post adenosine stress. When examined 55 minutes later the counts increased from 23,600 anteriorly to 30,470 (39% washin). The inferior counts had the expected 10% isotope count decay based upon the half-life (t-1/2) of Tc 99m. When the patient was taken to the cardiac catheterization laboratory following ST elevations in the anterior leads on the telemetry monitor and telemetry strips, he was shown to have an 80 %DS lesion at the ostium of his left anterior descending (LAD) artery, a long proximal (75 %DS) LAD lesion and an 80 %DS lesion at the ostium of his first obtuse marginal. The patient did quite well following placement of three drug eluting stents (DES) as shown in figure 6. The findings of the WR and coronary arteriography showed the need for immediate intervention which resulted in reducing patient morbidity and mortality and rescue of viable myocardium at risk.

Discussion

In 1953 Anger produced the first gamma image using a pin-hole in lead through which the image was projected on a scintillation screen and was developed on photographic film. Later the Anger circuit was developed and Kuhl and Edwards were the first to use this technology for tomography. The use of the Compton Effect, proposed by Everett, Fleming, Todd and Nightingale in 1977 added to this understanding and by 1983 the investigation into the Compton Camera began. Despite an enthusiastic start, much of the work since has focused on trying to improve the accuracy of MPI by developing agents with shorter half-life (t-1/2), narrower photopeak, and by improvements in computers and efforts to reduce attenuation effects by looking at AC using external sources, in this case Gadolinium, to assess differences due to body habitus. Despite these changes, most MPI interpretations of are visually qualitative. The physiologic assessment of ischemia on MPI has primarily been based upon a single image taken post stress after injection of a radioactive isotope (Tl-201, Teboroxime, Sestamibi, Myoview, et cetera). This approach has neither lead to significant improvements in the accuracy of MPI, based upon sensitivity and specificity, nor has it yielded the much sought after ability to define which artery is diseased or the amount of narrowing within the lumen of said artery, even though most patients and even many practitioners believe so. Hence, it has become known as "unclear" medicine. Yet, it is not the limitation of the technology; rather, that of the approach, which has resulted in this misconception and criticism. MPI and current day cameras have the ability to define the number of counts detected and to quantify this activity, allowing us to further define ROIs and better understand[9,10] the disease present not only in the larger epicardial arteries, but in the smaller arteries which cannot be seen by injection of contrast into an artery and subsequent imaging of that artery with fluoroscopy. This is simply a limit set by the physics of the wavelengths of fluoroscopy.

Recently investigators have begun to improve the results of MPI, not by using new isotopes (although this is happening), or by changing how we stress the patient (again this too is happening), but by using the tools we already have at our disposal to quantify the images and to look for information before us, but simply not noted. Like Sir Alexander Fleming we have only to look at the petri plates before us and ask what the camera is capable of seeing if we simply ask.

Investigations into H:L uptake[22,26-31], comparison of rest-stress ejection fractions[54] to unmask left main or triple vessel coronary artery disease have resulted in an improvement of our abilities to detect disease using Tc99m isotopes, but only after much delay in our understanding and investigations into the unique properties of these agents. Research has also demonstrated that, despite previous misperceptions, these Tc99m agents do not simply "stick" (with a decay rate of 10% over a 55 minute period of time) to the myocardium[2, 22, 26-35, 42,43] as was once thought. This limited approach is similar to that which once held back our understanding of the underlying inflammatory process which is the underlying cause of CAD resulting in the reduced ability of coronary arteries to dilate[7-10] to meet coronary flow demand. Just as we have come to understand that a coronary artery is more than just a simple conduit through which blood passes from point A to point B, so to do we now understand that coronary arteries are dynamic structures which can vary flow under a variety of circumstances influenced by inflammatory[5,6,9,10,19,20] changes within the arteries. These investigations have yielded a new era of understanding regarding the ability of these agents (Teboroxime, Sestamibi, Myoview, et cetera) using washin (an increase in isotope occurring in a region of myocardium over time) and washout (a greater than expected decrease in tracer occurring over time) to demonstrate the presence and severity of ischemia which cannot be detected by a single image of the heart at 60 minutes post stress. What is now apparent is that washin itself represents a unique situation detecting critically stenosed arteries supplying a significant region of myocardium at risk for MII. An increase in washout beyond the expected decay of 10% indicates the presence of ischemia which we can now detect, quantify and treat through a variety of approaches (risk factor modification, medical management, stenting/angioplasty, or if necessary coronary artery bypass surgery) increasing our ability to detect and treat disease, thereby, reducing patient morbidity, mortality and in the end costs.

Despite personal and institutional preferences to which type of stressor and which isotope should be used for MPI and under what circumstances, we found no differences between results obtained when people were stressed with EST, dobutamine or adenosine. Similarly there were no differences in the results seen with Sestamibi versus Myoview. This means, that independent of what a clinician or institution is using, our results indicate similar findings independent of the approach. Interpretation of ischemia by a Federal Employee Boarded in Nuclear Medicine yielded sensitivities of 67% and 53% depending upon whether the definition of CAD was one of 50% DS or 70% DS respectively. When looked at by ROI, the use of the single 60 minute image post stress correctly identified CAD requiring treatment in only half of the cases. In fact, much of the assessment of the presence of disease occurred without identifying the correct artery, as has been frequently noted in the past. The use of WR simply asks the question: Is there information we have been missing by not looking at multiple images post stress which could yield important physiologic information; thereby, unmasking ourselves to the information right in front of us, much as Sir Alexander Fleming did when he examined the petri plates before disposing of them?

The initial step in obtaining this information occurs with the assessment of W. TH., which represents an overall assessment of the heart. While the image on the screen appears to be two dimensional, it is exactly like taking a photograph. The image taken by the camera displays what we are looking at as if it were flat, but the mountains in the background are in the background. Similarly, while the image on the screen appears to be a flat slice of the heart, the quantitative assessment by the computer is nonetheless a collection of everything in front of, behind and within the plane of the heart which we appear to be looking at on the monitor or printed sheet. As such, W.TH is a collection of everything going on and as previously noted, provides us with a rapid assessment of Avg Sten ($r=0.45$, $p \leq 0.05$). This means that the first step in evaluating CAD is to look at W.TH.

Following the assessment of W.TH is the comparison of the total heart and total lung field counts as shown in Figure 2, from which H:L ratios are derived. The high correlations and statistical significance seen between W.TH and counts demonstrate that while counts may change from technologist to technologist, the use of identically sized ROIs to measure heart and lung counts, results in statistically reproducible WRs. We can therefore confirm the findings of Hurwitz[22] who noted that increased lung uptake of Sestamibi (and as we have established here, Myoview) at 4 minutes post stress is associated with greater ischemia. The WR and H:L ratio has been previously reported as extremely useful in predicting future CHF events in individuals with dilated cardiomyopathy[55] ; but only if this information is obtained as has been described above. As we have seen for the first time, W. Ant equals anterior ischemia and impaired wall motion with subsequent reduction in LVEF.

The routine interpretation of MPI has never been required to match the artery in question on the angiogram, to be deemed correct. In reality this is like a student accidentally answering a question correctly on an examination and being given full credit for getting the answer right. While we have all perhaps done this, it doesn't make it right. Finding disease on a MPI inferiorly (positive) while finding disease in the left anterior descending artery angiographically (the right coronary artery or circumflex artery supplies the inferior myocardium, depending upon vessel dominance) does not, in fact, identify the area of ischemia. Since this is after all the goal of MPI diagnostic imaging, it is no wonder that this has lead to the description of "nuclear" medicine (in this instance cardiology) as being referred to as "unclear" medicine. Results of coronary angiography are described (rightfully so) in artery specific terms, as was done in this study, and as such it is only appropriate that MPI be required to be reported in these same terms. In the subgroup of individuals (n=22) who underwent coronary angiography, 12 (55%) had regions described as being free of disease (false negatives, FNs) on the MPI which would have resulted in no change in treatment had it not been for the information obtained from the WR.

Following assessment of W.TH and evaluation of H:L ratios, we then turn our attention to more specific ROIs. The relationship between W. Inf and Inf Ste ($r=0.68$, $p \leq 0.01$) held up independent of whether MII was present or not. As we saw, the inferior region of the heart appears to be more prone to MII, possibly due to the limited number of vessels supplying it. The anterior region is less prone to MII perhaps in part because of the larger number of arteries supplying this region. We believe it is due to this increased number of arteries (including medium and smaller sized arteries which may not be detectable by angiography alone) that using the anterior ROI at only one site resulted in a lower correlation ($r=0.34$) with W. Ant, than did Inf Sten and W. Inf. This would also explain why there was a higher correlation between W.TH and Ant Sten indicating that more than one ROI should be analyzed anteriorly.

Diaphragmatic attenuation is a major problem noted by most clinicians, limiting interpretation of MPI. This was not corrected in our study by the use of AC, different isotopes or varying forms of "stress". It was; however, eliminated by the assessment of WR inferiorly when compared with Inf Stenosis on coronary angiography ($r=0.68$, $p \leq 0.01$). While the relationship between W.Ant and Ant Sten was not as significant, it was best ($r=0.34$) when only ischemia was present. This suggests that additional ROIs may be needed to more closely measure WR anteriorly due to the number of vessels supplying this region. Additionally, since we and others have clearly demonstrated that WR represents an active (not passive) physiologic process, we wonder what additional information regarding ischemia would be obtained by doing serial WRs beginning at 5 minutes and following those changes over time. As we have noted, the faster the WR, the greater the severity of ischemia and % DS. This is similar to the findings of Ono[32,33] who has demonstrated that the faster the WR, the more impaired the ability of the myocardium to retain Sestamibi under conditions of coronary vasospasm. These findings also raise the question as to whether resting images should be serially studied (multiple resting images) to determine if WR can distinguish between myocardial infarction, stunned and hibernating myocardium.

Finally, while our findings may be biased by the tendency to not catheterize patients with reportedly "negative" MPI reports, we did in fact begin catheterizing such patients based upon findings noted from WR after patients who did not receive interventions based upon the "negative" MPI reports (see figures 2-6), demonstrated persistent problems. The ability to more accurately detect disease may be of little or no value if it does not change the treatment of the patient or more importantly the outcome. The above results demonstrate the ability to more accurately define the presence and severity of CAD using WR by comparing multiple images obtained following stress. As we have seen, the more severe the disease, the less able the heart is to retain the isotope and this results in faster washout. However, we have also seen the opposite effect, viz. washin. When a major component of an epicardial artery is severely or critically narrowed and there is a significant amount of viable myocardium at risk, washin[40-42] is seen. This phenomena is not, or should not, be new to the reader. Like washin, 18-fluorodeoxyglucose (FDG) uptake demonstrated using PET imaging[49] shows increased uptake of FDG in regions of myocardium at risk (e.g. acute coronary syndrome, ACS) and appears to represent a similar setting. In fact, washin may be the only thing that is seen. Of the 41 people studied, 6 (15%) demonstrated washin, which as shown in the patient whose studies are displayed in figures 2-6, requires immediate intervention to avoid a bad outcome. This is a classic example of how patient diagnosis, treatment and management may all be improved by looking at the information we already have available to us if we only open the petri plate and look inside.

Conclusion

Standard MPI uses qualitative visual interpretation of images to Gestalt differences in isotope uptake to make a determination of the presence or absence of disease. Whether these images are interpreted using black and white or color formatted images remains (1) individual preference and (2) limited by visual interpretation. Just as coronary angiography has been criticized by limitations in visual interpretation[1,51] of %DS, so too is MPI. With the ability of modern computers to provide quantification of isotope from ROIs, it remains up to us to use this information in determining appropriate methods for measuring changes in isotope delivery and retention to improve the diagnostic accuracy and subsequent treatment of patients using MPI and washin/washout data. As we have clearly demonstrated, WR can provide more accurate diagnostic assessment of %DS which statistically correlate with the findings made in the cardiac catheterization laboratory, thereby improving the use of this non-invasive physiologic tool for the diagnosis, management and subsequent treatment of the patient with cardiomyopathy, Prinzmetal's angina, CHF and as we have now demonstrated, ischemic coronary artery disease. Further investigation is needed to determine if the utilization of WR during non-stressed (resting) studies can unmask differences between infracted, stunned and hibernating myocardium. Finally, these findings demonstrated a parabolic interactive model between coronary blood flow and cellular "uptake/release" of Technetium-99m tracers which more accurately detects coronary ischemia using a multiple post-stress imaging washin/washout model.

References

[1] Fleming RM, Kirkeeide RL, Smalling RW, Gould KL. Patterns in visual interpretation of coronary arteriograms as detected by quantitative coronary arteriography. *JACC* 1991;18:945-51.

[2] Taki J, Fujino S, Nakajima K, et al. 99mTc-Sestamibi retention characteristics during pharmacologic hyperemia in human myocardium: Comparison with coronary flow reserve measured by Doppler flowire. *J Nucl Med* 2001;42:1457-63.

[3] St. Goar FG, Pinto FJ, Alderman EL, Fitzgerald PJ, Stadius ML, Popp RL. Intravascular ultrasound imaging of angiographically normal coronary arteries: An in vivo comparison with quantitative angiography. *JACC* 1991;18:952-8.

[4] Fleming RM, Boyd L, Forster M. Unified Theory Approach Reduces Heart Disease and Recovers Viable Myocardium. 42nd Annual World Congress - International College of Angiology, San Diego, California, USA, June 29, 2000.

[5] Fleming RM. The Fleming Unified Theory of Vascular Disease: A Link Between Atherosclerosis, Inflammation, and Bacterially Aggravated Atherosclerosis (BAA). *Angiol* 2000; 51: 87-89.

[6] Fleming RM.: Chapter 64. *The Pathogenesis of Vascular Disease. Textbook of Angiology*. John C. Chang Editor, Springer-Verlag New York, NY. 1999, pp. 787-798.

[7] Kern MJ, Lerman A, Bech JW, et al. Physiological assessment of coronary artery disease in the cardiac catheterization laboratory: A scientific statement from the American Heart Association committee on diagnostic and interventional cardiac catheterization, council on clinical cardiology. *Circulation* 2006;114:1321-41.

[8] Maddahi J. Myocardial perfusion tracers in the detection and evaluation of coronary artery disease. 48th annual meeting of the society of nuclear medicine 2001.

[9] Fleming RM. Angina and coronary Ischemia are the result of coronary regional Blood Flow Differences. J Amer Coll Angiol 2003;1:127-42.

[10] Fleming RM., Boyd L., Forster M. Angina is Caused by Regional Blood Flow Differences - Proof of a Physiologic (Not Anatomic) Narrowing, Joint Session of the European Society of Cardiology and the American College of Cardiology, Annual American College of Cardiology Scientific Sessions, Anaheim, California, USA, 12 March 2000, 49th (Placed on internet www.prous.com for physician training and CME credit, April 2000.)

[11] Glover DK, Tuiz M, Edwards NC, et al. Comparison between 201Tl and 99mTc Sestamibi uptake during adenosine-induced vasodilation as a function of coronary stenosis severity. Circulation 1995;91:813-20.

[12] Sinusas AJ, Bergin JD, Edwards NC, et al. Redistribution of 99m-Tc-sestamibi and 201-Tl in the presence of a severe coronary artery stenosis. *Circulation*. 1994;89:2332-41.

[13] Dahlberg ST, Leppo JA. Physiologic properties of myocardial perfusion tracers. *Cardiol Clin* 1994;12:169-85.

[14] Beller GA, Sinusas AJ. Experimental studies of the physiologic properties of technetium-99m isonitriles. *Am J Cardiol* 1990;16:5E-8E.
[15] Hurwitz GA, Blais M, Powe JE, Champagne CL. Stress/injection protocols for myocardial scintigraphy with sestamibi and thallium-201: implications of early post-stress kinetics. *Nucl Med Commun* 1996;17:400-9.
[16] Husain SS. Myocardial perfusion imaging protocols: Is there an ideal protocol. J Nucl Med Tech 2007;35:3-9.
[17] Fleming RM., Kirkeeide RL, Taegtmeyer H, Adyanthaya A, Cassidy DB, Goldstein RA. A Comparison of Technetium 99-m Teboroxime Tomography to Automated Quantitative Coronary Arteriography and Thallium - 201 SPECT. *J Am Coll. Cardiol.* 1991;17:1297-1302.
[18] Parameswaran RV, Purantharan N, Prasad RD. Comparison of nitrate augmented 99mTc-Sestamibi infusion with nitrate augmented 99mTc-Sestamibi bolus injection for the detection of myocardial viability. *IJNM* 2006;21:36-40.
[19] Fleming RM. Using C-Reactive Protein as a Marker of Bacterially Aggravated Atherosclerosis in Acute Coronary Syndromes. *J Amer Coll Angiol* 2003;1:165-71.
[20] Fleming RM, Harrington GM. What is the relationship between myocardial perfusion imaging and coronary artery disease risk factors and markers of inflammation? *Angiology* 2008 [in press].
[21] Pace L, Catalano L, Del Vecchio S, et al. Washout of [99mTc] sestamibi in predicting response to chemotherapy in patients with multiple myeloma. *Q J Nucl Med Mol Imaging* 2005;49:281-5.
[22] Hurwitz GA, Ghali SK, Husni M, et al. Pulmonary uptake of Technetium-99m-Sestamibi induced by dipyridamole-based stress or exercise. *J Nucl Med* 1998;39:339-45.
[23] Hurwitz GA, Fox SP, Driedger AA, Willems C, Powe JE. Pulmonary uptake of sestamibi on early post-stress images: angiographic relationships, incidence and kinetics. *Nucl Med Commun* 1993;14;15-22. .
[24] Saha M, Forrest TF, Brown KA. Lung uptake of technetium-99m-sestamibi: relation to clinical, exercise, hemodynamic, and left ventricular function variables. *J Nucl Cardiol* 1994;1:52-6.
[25] Giubbini R, Bampini R, Milan E, et al. Evaluation of technetium-99m-sestamibi lung uptake: correlation with left ventricular function. *J Nucl Med* 1995;36:58-63.
[26] Sugiura T, Takase H, Toriyama T, et al. Usefulness of Tc-99m methoxyisobutylisonitrile scintigraphy for evaluating congestive heart failure. *J Nucl Cardiol* 2006;13:64 8.
[27] Kumita S, Seino Y, Cho K, et al. Assessment of myocardial washout of Tc-99m-sestamibi in patients with chronic heart failure: comparison with normal control. *Ann Nucl Med* 2002;16:237-42.
[28] Matsuo S, Nakae I, Tsutamoto T, Okamoto N, Horie M. A novel clinical indicator using Tc-99m sestamibi for evaluating cardiac mitochondrial function in patients with cardiomyopathies. *J Nucl Cardiol* 2007;14:215-20.
[29] Sugiura T, Takase H, Toriyama T, Goto T, Ueda R, Dohi Y. Usefulness of Tc-99m methoxyisobutylisonitrile scintigraphy for evaluating congestive heart failure. J Nucl Cardiol 2006;13:64-8.

[30] Ikawa M, Kawai Y, Arakawa K, et al. Evaluation of respiratory chain failure in mitochondrial cardiomyopathy by assessments of 99mTc-MIBI washout and 123I-BMIPP/99mTc-MIBI mismatch. *Mitochondrion* 2007;7:164-70.
[31] Meissner K, Sperker B, Karsten C, et al. Expression and localization of P-glycoprotein in Human Heart: Effects of Cardiomyopathy. *J Histochem Cytochem* 2002;50:1351-6.
[32] Ono S, Yamaguchi H, Takayama S, Kurabe A, Heito T. Rest delayed images on 99mTc-MIBI myocardial SPECT as a noninvasive screen for the diagnosis of vasospastic angina pectoris. Kaku Igaku 2002;39:117-24.
[33] Ono S, Yakeishi Y, Yamaguchi H, et al. Enhanced regional washout of technetium-99m-sestamibi in patients with coronary spastic angina. *Ann Nucl Med* 2003;17:393-8.
[34] Fukushima K, Momose M, Kondo C, et al. Myocardial kinetics of (201) Thallium, (99m) Tc-tetrofosmin, and (99m) Tc-sestamibi in an acute ischemia-reperfusion model using isolated rat heart. *Ann Nucl Med* 2007;21:267-73.
[35] VanBrocklin HF, Hanrahan SM, Enas JD, et al. Mitochondrial avid radioprobes. Preparation and evaluation of 7'(Z)-[125I]iodorotenone and 7'(Z)-[125I]iodorotenol. *Nucl Med Biol* 2007;34:109-16.
[36] Tanaka R, Nakamura T, Chiba S, et al. Clinical implication of reverse redistribution on 99mTc-sestamibi images for evaluating ischemic heart disease. *Ann Nucl Med* 2006;20:349-56.
[37] Liu Z, Johnson G 3rd, Beju D, Okada RD. Detection of myocardial viability in ischemic-reperfused rat hearts by Tc-99m sestamibi kinetics. *J Nucl Cardiol* 2001;8:677-86.
[38] Shin WJ, Miller K, Stipp V, Mazour S. Reverse redistribution on dynamic exercise and dipyridamole stress technetium-99m-MIBI myocardial SPECT. *J Nucl Med* 1995;36:2053-5
[39] Takeishi Y, Sukekawa H, Fujiwara S, et al. Reverse redistribution of technetium-99m-sestamibi following direct PTCA in acute myocardial infarction. *J Nucl Med* 1996;37:1289-94.
[40] Fujiwara S, Takeishi Y, Atsumi H, et al. Prediction of functional recovery in acute myocardial infarction: comparison between sestamibi reverse redistribution and sestamibi/BMIPP mismatch. *J Nucl Cardiol* 1998;5:119-27.
[41] Ayalew A, Marie PY, Menu P, et al. A comparison of the overall first-pass kinetics of thallium-201 and technetium-99m MIBI in normoxic and low-flow ischaemic myocardium. *Eur J Nucl Med* 2000;27:1632-40
[42] Richter WS, Cordes M, Calder D, Eichstaedt H, Felix R. Washout and redistribution between immediate and two-hour myocardial images using technetium-99m sestamibi. *Eur J Nucl Med* 1995;22:49-55.
[43] Meerdink DJ, Leppo JA. Myocardial transport of hexakis(2-methosyisobutyl isonitrile) and thallium before and after coronary reperfusion. *Circulation Research* 1990;66:1738-46.
[44] Ayalew A, Marie PY, Menu P, et al. 201 Tl and 99m Tc-MIBI retention in an isolated heart model of low-flow ischemia and stunning: Evidence of negligible impact of myocyte metabolism on tracer kinetics. *J Nucl Med* 2002;43:566-74.
[45] Takahashi N, Reinhardt CP, Marcel R, Leppo JA. Myocardial uptake of 99m Tc-tetrofosmin, Sestamibi, and 201 Tl in a model of acute coronary reperfusion. *Circulation* 1996;94:2605-13.

[46] Matsunari I, Haas F, Nguyen NTB, et al. Comparison of Sestamibi, Tetrofosmin, and Q12 Retention in Porcine Myocardium. *J Nucl Med* 2001;42:818-23.

[47] Calnon DA, Glover DK, Beller GA, et al. Effects of dobutamine stress on myocardial blood flow, 99m-Tc sestamibi uptake, and systolic wall thickening in the presence of coronary artery stenoses: implications for dobutamine stress testing. *Circulation* 1997;96:2353-60.

[48] Calnon DA, Ruiz M, Vanzetto G, et al. Myocardial uptake of 99mTc-N-NOET and 201 Tl during dobutamine infusion. *Circulation* 1999;100:1653-9.

[49] Fleming RM.: Chapter 31. *Nuclear Cardiology*: Its Role in the Detection and Management of Coronary Artery Disease *Textbook of Angiology*. John C. Chang Editor, Springer-Verlag New York, NY 1999, pp. 397-406.

[50] Fleming RM, Rose CH, Feldmann KM. Comparing a High Dose Dipyridamole SPECT Imaging Protocol with Dobutamine and Exercise Stress Testing Protocols. *Angiology* 1995;46(7):547-556

[51] Fleming RM, Gibbs HR, Swafford J. Using Quantitative Coronary Arteriography to Redefine SPECT Sensitivity and Specificity. *Am J Physiol. Imag*. 1992;7:59-65.

[52] Fleming RM, Detecting Coronary Artery Disease Using SPECT Imaging: A Comparison of Thallium-201 and Teboroxime. *Am J Physiol Imag* 1992;7(1):20-23.

[53] Personal communication with Dr. Robert Eckel, past president of the American Heart Association, Jan 2008.

[54] Fleming RM. A Tate-en-Tate Comparison of Ejection Fraction and Regional Wall Motion Abnormalities as Measured by Echocardiography and Gated Sestamibi SPECT. *Angiology* 2002;53:313-21.

[55] Toriyama T, Takase H, Sugiura T, et al. 99mTc-sestamibi scintigraphy in the prediction of cardiac events in patients with congestive heart failure. 7th International conference of Nuclear Cardiology-European Society of Cardiology 2005.

[56] Everett DB, Fleming JS, Todd RW, Nightingale JM. Gamma-radiation imaging system based on the Compton effect. *Proceedings of the IEEE* 1977;124:995-1000.

In: Heart Disease in Men
Editors: A.B. Todd and M.H. Mosley, pp. 101-123
ISBN: 978-1-60692-297-2

Chapter 4

DEPRESSION, SUICIDE RISK AND HEART DISEASE IN MEN

Maurizio Pompili[1,2,*], Marco Innamorati[1], Ilaria Cuomo[1], Giovanni Manfredi[1], Roberto Tatarelli[1] and David Lester[3]

[1]Department of Psychiatry – Sant'Andrea Hospital, University of Rome La Sapienza, Italy

[2]McLean Hospital, Belmont, MA - Harvard Medical School, Boston, MA, USA

[3]The Richard Stockton College of New Jersey, USA

Abstract

Depression strongly affects the quality of life of patients with heart diseases. Mood disorders in general, together with chronic medical conditions, result in a unique and additional impairment of patient functioning. Depression also increases the risk of morbidity and mortality related to cardiac disorders and may play an important role in the development of angina, hypertension, myocardial infarction, arrhythmias and sudden cardiac death. Lastly, depression may be linked with suicide. Studies on the link between heart disease and suicide risk are rare in the literature, But it appears that patients with coronary heart disease engage in more suicidal behavior independently of depression. A cross-sectional ecological study has reported that the use of calcium channel blockers (commonly prescribed in heart disease) could increase the risk of suicide. On the other hand, other researchers have found no increased risk of suicide associated with these drugs. Back in the 1960s, Farberow and colleagues studied 90 patients with cardiorespiratory illness: 45 patients who completed suicide and 45 nonsuicide controls. These authors found that the suicidal patients were more emotionally disturbed both before and while in the hospital. They were reported to be more hostile, anxious, agitated, apprehensive, depressed, and distressed over their illness than were the controls. These patients required more frequent hospitalization than the controls and had more difficult interpersonal relationships with the staff. They were called dependent–dissatisfied, a label already used by the authors for suicidal psychiatric patients to indicate the type of patient who was continually complaining, demanding, insisting, and controlling. These patients showed inflexibility and lack of adaptability, continually making demands on others regardless of their effect on them. They turned to hospital and staff for support, but

[*] E-mail: maurizio.pompili@uniroma1.it. tel. +39680345687. fax: +39680345342. Dr. Maurizio Pompili, Ospedale Sant'Andrea, Psichiatria, Via di Grottarossa, 1035-1039, 00189 Roma – Italy (Corresponding author)

consistently succeeded in alienating them with their insatiable demands for special attention. They seemed to need constantly repeated evidence of self-worth from outside sources in order to maintain their feelings of self-esteem. More recently, Pompili and colleagues explored suicidality and associated traits, such as hopelessness, in a sample of cardiac patients and controls. The authors found that patients with heart disease do not differ in these traits from control patients with other internal medicine disorders. Although their medical conditions were more serious than those of the control patients, this apparently had no impact on their hopelessness or suicidality. Men are generally at higher risk of suicide, but in this investigation, they were only slightly more hopeless than women. Implications regarding suicide risk and mood disorders in men are discussed

Introduction

Chronic illness, defined as any illness lasting 3 or more months (Stedman, 1995), is the largest cause of death in the world (Yach, Hawkes, Gould, & Hofman, 2004). Chronic illness is not only a biological process, it is a complex phenomenon involving psychological, social and economic aspects. Chronic illness is a cause of disability and lower wellbeing and is frequently associated with behavioural and emotional disorders (Feldman, Mayou, Hawton, Ardern, & Smith, 1987; Ramsey, Wright, Katz, Bielawska, & Katona, 1991). Depression is a highly frequent comorbid condition that increase the costs of care and worsens disability and outcome in physical diseases (Anderson, Freedland, Clouse, & Lustman, 2001; Egede, 2005; Feldman et al., 1987; Katon & Schulberg, 1992; Leichter & See, 2005; Myers et al., 1984; Rapp, Parisi, & Walsh, 1988; Scherrer et al., 2003). For example, Katon (2003) noted that, as one moves from community settings to primary-care settings to inpatient medical settings, the prevalence of major depression increases from 3%–5% to 5%–10% to 10%–14%. Zhang and colleagues (Zhang, Ye, Huang, Li, & Yang, 2008) studied the prevalence of depression in medical inpatients with different chronic diseases (cardiovascular disease, diabetes, and chronic pulmonary heart disease) and reported that 79% of patients were affected by depression (with almost 18% affected by moderate to severe depression). There were significant differences in the incidence of depression or different levels of depression among those with different diagnoses.

Major affective disorders and depression are highly associated with suicidal behavior, both in psychiatric and in medical settings (Conwell, Duberstein, & Caine, 2002; Pearson & Brown, 2000). Data indicate that more than two-thirds of completed suicides and suicide attempters have (mostly untreated) major depressive episodes at the time of the suicidal act (Coryell & Young, 2005). Harris and Barraclough (1994) searched reports of mortality studies for 63 medical disorders said to have an altered suicide risk. Their review indicated an increased risk of suicide in HIV/AIDS, malignant neoplasms as a group, head and neck cancers, Huntington's disease, multiple sclerosis, peptic ulcer, renal disease, spinal cord injury, and systemic lupus erythematosus. Inconclusive evidence for increased suicide risk was observed for amputation, heart valve replacement and surgery, disorders of the intestine (Crohn's disease, ileostomy, ulcerative colitis), hormone replacement therapy, alcoholic liver disease, neurofibromatosis, systemic sclerosis, and Parkinson's disease.

Juurlink (2004) studied the link among medical Illness and the risk of suicide in the elderly in a population-based case-control study set in Ontario (Canada) between 1992 and 2000. The authors focused on illnesses reported to be associated with an increased risk for suicide. Eleven of the 15 illnesses were associated with a significantly increased risk of suicide, with bipolar disorder, major depression, and severe pain associated with the largest increases in suicide risk. No increased risk was associated with gout, hypothyroidism, or glaucoma and, as expected, treatment for dyslipidemia was associated with a reduction in the risk for suicide. After adjustment for the presence of other illnesses, 11 conditions were found to be independent predictors of an increased risk for suicide: congestive heart failure (odds ratio [OR]: 1.36; 95% confidence intervals [95%CI]: 1.00-1.85), chronic lung disease (OR: 1.30; 95%CI: 1.06-1.58), hyperacidity syndromes (INSERT HERE), seizure disorder (OR: 2.41; 95%CI: 1.42-4.07), Parkinson's disease (OR: 1.11; 95%CI: 0.65-1.90), urinary incontinence (OR: 1.11; 95%CI: 0.65-1.89), psychoses and agitation (OR: 2.60; 95%CI: 1.93-3.50), depression (OR: 3.94; 95%CI: 3.27-4.75), anxiety and sleep disorders (OR: 3.22; 95%CI: 3.27-4.75); bipolar disorder (OR: 3.58; 95%CI: 1.57-8.18), moderate pain (OR: 1.24; 95%CI: 1.04-1.47) and severe pain (OR: 4.07; 95%CI: 2.51-6.59). Furthermore, the authors reported a strong association between the cumulative number of illnesses and the estimated relative risk of suicide. For example, patients with 3 illnesses were a 3 times more at risk of suicide (OR: 3.5; 95%CI: 2.9-4.2) than patients with no identified illness, and patients with 5 illnesses had about a 5-fold increase in risk (OR, 5.7; 95%CI: 4.4-7.4). Evans, Wang, Morris (2002) found that serious physical illness may be a stronger risk factor for suicide in men than in women.

Depression and suicide risk is often underdiagnosed by medical staff and general practitioners in patients with physical illness, especially in some population, e.g., frail elderly and adolescents. For example, Rapp, Walsh, and Parisi (1988) indicated that only 8.7% of inpatients with depression were correctly diagnosed as depressed by junior medical staff. Koenig, Meador, and Cohen (1988) reported that, among their sample of older inpatients identified as depressed, only for 20% of them had the junior medical staff documented the diagnosis in medical files. Even after the physician had been informed that comorbidity with major depression was possible in these patients, only 27% of the patients received a psychiatric consultation, and only 13% were given antidepressant medication. Zhang and colleagues (2008) reported only 16% of symptomatic depression was correctly diagnosed by medical physicians.

Suominen, Isometsa, Lonnqvist (2004) identified all consecutive suicide attempters treated in hospital emergency rooms in Helsinki, from January 1997 to January 1998, and found that, during the last 12 months before the attempt, most of the elderly suicide attempters had contact with primary health care staff, but only 4% had been diagnosed with a mood disorder although the rate of diagnoses rose to 57% after the attempt. Salib and Green (2003) found a high rate of suicide (38% and 16%, respectively, for men and women) with psychiatric morbidity but not known to clinical services. The situation can be related to irrational beliefs about suicide both among patients and family physicians. In fact, Stoppe et al. (1999) indicated that almost 20% of physicians interviewed said they would not talk about suicide to depressed individuals because either the patients would communicate suicidal intent themselves or because they feared inducing suicide by asking directly.

However, general practitioners are often the only health professionals who can be involved in the assessment and treatment of depressive disorders and suicide, especially for the elderly. In a previous paper, the present authors found that more than 40% of elderly suicides had sought a contact with their family physicians in the few months before their suicide. In contrast, as Cattell and Jolley (1995) reported, few elderly suicides have been in contact with psychiatric services. Therefore, education on the recognition, diagnosis and treatment of mood disorders and suicide risk is needed for general physicians.

The aim of the present study was to review the literature concerning depression and suicide risk in cardiovascular diseases, the leading cause of death in most Western, industrialized countries.

Material and Methods

We performed careful MedLine and PsycINFO searches from 1980 to 2008. The following search terms were used: "cardiopathic" OR "cardiovascular Diseases", suicid*, (which comprises suicide, suicidal, suicidality, and other suicide-related terms), and "depress*" (which comprises depression, depressive, and other depression-related terms). In addition, each category was cross-referenced with the others using the MeSH method (Medical Subjects Headings). Selection of papers suitable for this study allowed the inclusion only of those articles published in English peer-reviewed journals. Included were those studies that made an original contribution to the literature. A total of 210 articles were located through our search; the most relevant articles were selected for this overview.

Cardiovascular Disease and Depression

Numerous studies have identified an association between depression and cardiovascular disease (Barth, Schumacher, & Herrmann-Lingen, 2004; Booth-Kewley & Friedman, 1987; Carney et al., 1988; Empana et al., 2006; Glassman & Shapiro, 1998; Lett et al., 2004; Nicholson, Kuper, & Hemingway, 2006; Rozanski, Blumenthal, & Kaplan, 1999; Rutledge, Reis, Linke, Greenberg, & Mills, 2006; Stewart et al., 2003; Wulsin et al., 2005). Estimated rates of major depression vary between 20%–40% in patients with chronic heart failure (Barth et al., 2004; Konstam, Moser, & De Jong, 2005; Rutledge et al., 2006; van Melle et al., 2004), and are around 16%-18% in inpatients with myocardial infarction (Schleifer et al., 1989).

In patients with cardiovascular disease, depression is associated with higher short-term and long-term morbidity and mortality rates (Ahern et al., 1990; Barefoot et al., 1996; Carney & Freedland, 2003; Carney et al., 1988; Denollet et al., 1996; Dimsdale, Gilbert, Hutter, Hackett, & Block, 1981; Frasure-Smith, Lesperance, & Talajic, 1993; Jiang et al., 2001; Jiang et al., 2007; Ladwig, Kieser, Konig, Breithardt, & Borggrefe, 1991; Sherwood et al., 2007; Silverstone, 1987; van Melle et al., 2005), and poor quality of life. For example, Barefoot and colleagues (1996) investigated 1,250 patients with coronary artery disease for a follow-up time ranging up to 19 years. The authors reported that patients with moderate to severe depression at baseline, as measured with the Zung Depression Scale, had a 69% greater odds of cardiac death and a 78% greater odds of mortality from all causes than nondepressed; the risk being increased even after 10 years. However, some studies have reported negative results (Lane, Carroll, Ring, Beevers, & Lip, 2000, 2001; Mayou et al., 2000).

Nevertheless, even a subsyndromal depression must be carefully evaluated for treatment because almost 50% of patients with cardiovascular disease and mild depressive symptomatology may develop a major depression within the next 12 months after the index assessment (Hance, Carney, Freedland, & Skala, 1996).

Depression may also be considered a predictor of minor cardiac events. For example, Davis and colleagues (2008), using a population based approach, compared transition rates for patients with major depression with those for patients without major depression at several stages of cardiovascular disease progression. The authors reported that, among nearly 600,000 healthy members, those with major depression in the past year were 50% to 100% more likely than controls to develop hypertension or dyslipidemia. Rates were increased with a similar magnitude among patients with hypertension or dyslipidemia who subsequently developed either the other condition or coronary artery disease, and also among patients with hypertension and dyslipidemia who developed coronary artery disease or congestive heart failure.

Several authors have investigated the association among cardiovascular risk and single depressive symptoms. Lesperance and colleagues (1996) found that depression in heart disease patients was more strongly associated with death when sleep and appetite disturbances were excluded from the diagnostic criteria. Some authors have found that the cognitive and affective symptoms of the depressive disorder are better predictors of death than are the physical symptoms of depression (Anda et al., 1993; Appels & Otten, 1992; Barefoot et al., 2000; Everson et al., 1996; Irvine et al., 1999).

The adverse effects of depression in cardiovascular disease may be mediated by shared pathophysiological mechanisms. Several studies have indicated that patients with major depression have a reduced heart rate variability, reflecting altered autonomic tone (Carney et al., 1999; Carney et al., 1995; Dalack & Roose, 1990; Rechlin, Weis, Spitzer, & Kaschka, 1994; Rottenberg, Clift, Bolden, & Salomon, 2007; Taylor et al., 2006), a factor which is known to increase the risk of ventricular arrhythmias (Carney, Freedland, & Veith, 2005; Stein et al., 2000). For example, Mezzacapa and colleagues (2001) found that diminished vagal rebound during recovery from stress is associated with higher scores on standard risk factors for cardiovascular disease, and they suggested that increases in cardiac vagal control are crucial for restoring cardiovascular homeostasis. Rottenberg et al. (2003) found a lack of recovery of cardiac vagal control after crying for depressed individuals. Hallas and colleagues (2003) investigated the link among depression, blood pressure and heart rate variability in 22 patients who were preparing to receive coronary artery bypass graft surgery for the first time. The authors indicated that higher levels of anxiety and depression were predictive risk factors for reduced heart rate variability and increased blood pressure reactivity in response to mental stressors. De Jonge (2007) has suggested that only somatic depressive symptoms may be associated with lower heart rate variability. However, it should be noted that some studies have reported a nonsignificant association between depression and altered heart rate variability in patients with cardiovascular disease (Gehi, Mangano, Pipkin, Browner, & Whooley, 2005).

Pathophysiological mechanisms may also include increased hypothalamic-pituitary-adrenal function, sympathoadrenal hyperactivity, and excessive pro-inflammatory cytokine activation (Hughes, Watkins, Blumenthal, Kuhn, & Sherwood, 2004; Parissis, Fountoulaki, Paraskevaidis, & Kremastinos, 2005). Hyperactivity of the hypothalamic-pituitary-adrenocortical axis associated with depression can activate a cascade of effects and neurohormonal abnormalities: increased activity of the sympathetic nervous system, the release of catecholamines and serum cortisol (Banki, Karmacsi, Bissette, & Nemeroff, 1992; Brown, Varghese, & McEwen, 2004; Nemeroff et al., 1984), and an impaired feedback regulation of plasma cortisol. These abnormalities in turn contribute to surges in heart rate and blood pressure, increase the risk of atherosclerotic plaque rupture and acute coronary thrombosis, and result in irritability of the heart muscle, causing ventricular arrhythmias which may lead to ventricular fibrillation and cardiac arrest (Goldston & Baillie, 2008).

There is also evidence for a modulating role of the immune system in the interrelationship between depression and cardiovascular disease (Kop & Gottdiener, 2005; Musselman, Evans, & Nemeroff, 1998). Depressed patients have been shown to have elevated levels of markers such as interleukin-1 beta, interferon, and tumor necrosis factor alpha, which are proinflammatory cytokines involved in the nonspecific immune response (Miller, Stetler, Carney, Freedland, & Banks, 2002; Suarez, Krishnan, & Lewis, 2003). In contrast to activation of components involved in the nonspecific immune response, depressed patients show a blunted cell-mediated immune response (e.g., Natural killer cell activity), indicating immunosuppression (Hickie et al., 1995; Maes, 1995). The impaired immune response may cause cardiovascular risk both by influencing the activity of blood platelets and influencing the release and metabolism of several neurotransmitters, including dopamine (Jarskog, Xiao, Wilkie, Lauder, & Gilmore, 1997), norepinephrine (Kabiersch, del Rey, Honegger, & Besedovsky, 1988) and serotonin (Clement et al., 1997), all involved in sympathetic nerve outflow to the cardiovascular system (Huangfu, Hwang, Riley, & Guyenet, 1994).

Cardiovascular Disease and Suicide

Studies on the link between heart disease and suicide risk are rare in the literature. While Farberow et al. (1966) found no association between heart disease and suicide risk, more recently, Artero et al. (2006) found that patients with coronary heart disease engaged in more suicidal behavior independently of depression. Lindberg et al. (1998) carried out a cross-sectional ecologic study and reported that the use of calcium channel blockers (commonly prescribed in cardiopathies) could increase the risk of suicide. On the other hand, Gasse et al. (2000) investigated the same association and found no increased risk associated with these drugs. Farberow et al. (1970) studied 90 patients with cardiorespiratory illness: 45 patients who completed suicide and 45 nonsuicidal controls. These authors found that the suicidal patients were more emotionally disturbed both before and while in the hospital. They were reported to be more hostile, anxious, agitated, apprehensive, depressed, and distressed over their illness than were the controls. These patients required more frequent hospitalization than the controls and had more difficult interpersonal relationships with the staff. They were called *dependent–dissatisfied* patients, a label already used by the authors for suicidal psychiatric patients to indicate a patient who was continually complaining, demanding, insisting, and controlling (Farberow, Shneidman, & Neuringer, 1966). Such patients showed inflexibility and lack of adaptability, continually making demands on others regardless of their effect on them. They turned to hospital and staff for support, but consistently succeeded in alienating them with their insatiable demands for special attention. They seemed to need constantly repeated evidence of self-worth from outside sources to maintain their feelings of self-esteem.

Inoue and colleagues (2007) studied the causative factors of suicide among the elderly between 1996 and 2002 in Mie Prefecture in Japan. During the period, there were 842 suicides. The two major causative factors of suicide were "suffering from physical illness" and "psychiatric disorders". In particular, the three most frequent physical illnesses were cardiovascular disease, orthopedic disorder, and digestive organ disease. Recently, Pompili et al. (2007) compared 100 patients with heart disease and 100 control patients with other internal medicine disorders for suicidality and associated traits, such as hopelessness. The authors found that patients with heart disease, although showing a strong tendency to have more negative expectations for the future, did not differ from control patients in suicidal intent. Their more severe medical conditions apparently had no impact on their hopelessness or suicidality. Men were only slightly more hopeless than women.

Although, results regarding suicide in cardiovascular disease is mixed, clinician should screen patients for the presence of psychopathology and dysfunctional personality traits, such as impulsiveness and aggressiveness. Type-A Behavior Pattern (TABP), first conceptualized in the 1950's by Friedman and Rosenman (1974) in relation to the coronary-prone behaviour pattern, is characterized by high competitiveness, time urgency, and easily aroused hostility (Jenkins, Zyzanski, & Rosenman, 1979; Matthews & Haynes, 1986). Steinberg (1986) proposed a two dimensional model of TABP: a prosocial dimension (i.e., striving for achievement), and an antisocial dimension, characterized as impatience-aggression. There is considerable evidence that Type-A individuals are more affected by actual or threatened control loss and physical aggression (Brunson & Matthews, 1981; Bushman & Anderson, 1998; Carver & Glass, 1978; Glass, 1977; Rhodewalt & Davison, 1983). Innamorati and colleagues (2006) studied 340 university students, and reported that TABP aggressiveness and suicidal ideation were associated. Furthermore, hostility permitted a predictive model to be created with rules for classifying TABP individuals at a higher risk of suicide. Similarly, Dumais et al. (2005) found that impulsive-aggressive personality disorders and alcohol abuse/dependence were two independent predictors of suicide in major depression

Treatment for Comorbid Depression and Suicide Risk

Antidepressants

Research has shown poor outcomes for untreated depression after cardiovascular disease (Ladwig, Roll, Breithardt, Budde, & Borggrefe, 1994; Schleifer et al., 1989). However, when we have to treat depression in patients with cardiovascular disease, we have to consider both the safety and the efficacy of antidepressive treatments. The fundamental question regarding safety is whether antidepressive treatments increase cardiac morbidity and mortality. The question is quite complicated because treatments may increase or decrease cardiac risk as a consequence of the physiological changes associated with the resolution of a depressive episode or as a consequence of a direct or indirect side-effect not be related to the presumed antidepressant mechanism of action (Roose, 2003). The cardiovascular effects of a therapeutic plasma level of tricyclic antidepressants (TCA) has been extensively studied. Tricyclic antidepressants increase the heart rate by 11%, induce orthostatic hypotension that can result in falls and serious injuries, and slow cardiac conduction, which can result in 2-to-1 atrioventricular block in patients with preexisting bundle branch block. Tricyclics do not routinely have an adverse effect on ventricular function and also have significant antiarrhythmic activity (Roose, 2003). Studies also indicate that TCAs decrease all heart rate variability components (Roose, Dalack, & Woodring, 1991; Yeragani, 2000; Yeragani et al., 1991).

Furthermore, TCAs may be chosen in cases of suicidality because of their sedative effect, although clinicians have to constantly monitor adherence because overdoses with TCAs are associated with high risk of a fatal outcome (Goldsmith, Pellmar, Kleinman, & Bunney, 2002). Morgan et al. (2004) studied deaths from drug poisoning between 1993 and 2002, and reported that antidepressants were involved in 18% of the deaths, with TCAs accounting for 89% of these deaths. By contrast, selective serotonin reuptake inhibitors (SSRIs) accounted for around 6% of deaths by suicide, and other antidepressants, including venlafaxine, accounted only for around 3% of deaths by suicide.

A recent review of the literature on the safety of antidepressants in cardiac patients (Alvarez & Pickworth, 2003) confirmed the superior cardiovascular profile of SSRIs compared with TCAs. The cardiovascular effects of SSRIs include modest slowing of heart rate with rare hypotension, minimal effect on recumbent, sitting or standing blood pressure, and little electrocardiographic effect on the PR interval, QRS duration, or QT interval (Glassman, 1998). Rarely, SSRIs may stimulate coronary artery vasoconstriction yielding Prinzmetal's angina (Fricchione, Woznicki, Klesmer, & Vlay, 1993). Also SSRIs have an antiplatelet effect, normalizing elevated indices of platelet activation and aggregation in patients, which in turn may reduce the risk of ischemic events. However, the antiplatelet effect is not associated with the antidepressant effect (Roose, 2003; Serebruany et al., 2003).

Serotonin and Norepinephrine Reuptake Inhibitors (SNRI) presumably increase norepinephrine activity through the blockade of reuptake and may increase sympathetic tone resulting in increased QT variability (Roose, 2003). Venlafaxine has only a serotonergic effect at lower doses and both serotonin, norepinephrine and weak dopamine effect at higher doses (Harvey, Rudolph, & Preskorn, 2000; Muth et al., 1986; Thase, 1998). Other SNRIs have not been fully tested in depressed patients with cardiovascular disease and, in the absence of systematic study, it would be imprudent to consider these medications as proven safe in depressed patients with cardiovascular disease (Roose, 2003).

Mirtazapine should be used with caution in patients with coronary because it is associated with orthostatic hypotension in more than 5% of patients (Blier, 2001). Bupropion has dopamine and norepinephrine effects and may elevate blood pressure, and this vital sign should be monitored (Roose, Dalack, Glassman et al., 1991).

When considering suicide risk, other questions arise. First of all, does the antidepressant medication affect suicidal intent. For drug treatments prescribed for patients with higher suicide risk, the use of some antidepressants has been controversial. In recent years, the question shifted from whether antidepressants are beneficial for all patients with suicide risk to whether the use of antidepressants increases suicidal behavior in some patients. The risk-benefit ratio of antidepressants may be different between children or young adults and adults In October 2004, the US Food and Drug Administration (FDA) (US Food and Drug Administration, March 22, 2004) ordered pharmaceutical companies to add a black-box warning regarding the possible link between antidepressant treatment and suicidal ideation and behavior in children and adolescents. In England, the Medicines and Healthcare Products Regulatory Agency (MHRA) concluded that there was an increased risk of suicidal behaviours in this young age-group for SSRIs when compared with placebos (Medicines and Healthcare products Regulatory Agency, 2005). In December 2006, the FDA's Psychopharmacologic Drugs Advisory Committee recommended that the black-box warning be extended to include young adults and, in May 2007, the FDA asked drug manufacturers to revise their labels accordingly.

The data regarding suicidal profile of antidepressants derive both from ecological studies and controlled clinical trials. Several ecological studies have documented an overall reduction in suicide rate seen in some countries with the introduction of the newer antidepressants. In particular, it has been argued that the significant reduction in suicide rates among adolescents and adults in the US and other countries (Barbui, Campomori, D'Avanzo, Negri, & Garattini, 1999; Hall et al., 2003; Isacsson, 2000) has been a result of treatment with these drugs (Gibbons et al., 2007; Olfson, Shaffer, Marcus, & Greenberg, 2003). However, several confounding factors may explain the results, including changing socio-economic circumstances (Gunnell & Ashby, 2004). The direct link between antidepressants treatment and suicide risk has been studied more extensively using clinical trials, although most studies considered only acute treatments (8-12 weeks), and patients with higher suicide intent may have been screened out from the samples investigated. Thus, the utility of findings from meta-analyses as a basis for sound clinical practice and regulatory policy is limited by the low levels of "suicidal events" reported, even lower frequency of actual suicidal behaviors, and variable outcomes across trials and treatments Baldessarini 2006). Generally, clinical trials have produced mixed results when answering the question whether SSRIs increase suicide risk; but they are consistent with naturalistic studies (Leon et al., 1999) indicating an uncertainty about the consistency antidepressants in reducing suicide behavior.

Some studies (Jick, Kaye, & Jick, 2004) have found evidence in many patients of an increase in suicidal thoughts in the early stages of antidepressant treatment. The risk may be related to the delayed onset of the beneficial effects of antidepressant medications. At the beginning of treatment, mood often remains low, with prominent feelings of guilt and hopelessness, while energy and motivation increase. This may be related to the increase in suicidal thoughts. A similar situation can arise with patients who develop akathisia or increased anxiety due to a direct effect of some SSRIs and related drugs.

Teicher, Glod and Cole (1993) suggested nine mechanisms by which SSRIs may induce or exacerbate suicidal risk: 1) energizing depressed patients, 2) worsening their depression, 3) inducing akathisia, 4) inducing panic attacks, 5) switching patients to mania or hypomania, 6) causing insomnia and other sleep disorders, inducing an organic, obsessional state, 8) promoting personality disorders (borderline traits), and 9) producing neurological disturbances.

Henry and Demotes-Mainard (2006) proposed a different explanation of higher suicide rates in adolescents treated with SSRIs, that it is related either to misdiagnosis of bipolar disorders in this population or to the extremely broad meaning of the construct of depression. They argued that the amplitude of emotional reactivity and not sadness must be considered for defining subtypes of depression and for deciding upon the appropriate treatments.

When the use of antidepressants is recommended for the treatment of depressive symptoms, there are some key points to consider:

- Careful monitoring is needed when treatment is initiated with an antidepressant.
- Patients should be monitored regardless of the apparent severity of their depression.
- Patients started on antidepressants who are considered to be at an increased suicide risk or who are younger than 30 years should normally be seen at shorter intervals of time until the risk of suicide is no longer considered significant.

- A limited quantity of antidepressants should be prescribed, particularly in the initial stages of treatment with SSRIs. Signs of akathisia, suicidal ideation, and increased anxiety and agitation should be actively searched for.
- Clinicians should also advise patients of the risk of adverse events in the early stages of therapy and advise them to seek help promptly if these are at all distressing.
- Patients should also be warned about the risks of reducing or stopping the medication.
- In the event that a patient develops marked and/or prolonged akathisia or agitation while taking an antidepressant, the use of the drug should be reviewed.
- Toxicity in overdose for TCAs should be considered when choosing an antidepressant for patients at significant risk of suicide.
- When a patient with depression is assessed to be at a high risk of suicide, the use of additional support, such as more frequent direct contacts with primary care staff or telephone contacts, should be considered.
- Venlafaxine treatment should be initiated only by specialist mental health medical practitioners, including General Practitioners with a Special Interest in Mental Health.

Antypsychotics and Mood Stabilizers

In general, antipsychotic have significant cardiac side effects, especially with respect to conduction, rhythm and hypotension (Shah, Iqbal, White, & White, 2005). They can produce prolongation of the PR and QT intervals, ST segment depression, T wave changes, ventricular arrhythmias, and heart block. When administering a low potency neuroleptic along with an antiarrhythmic, electrocardiography should be used to monitor for conduction delays. When these agents are used together with antihypertensive agents, there is more chance of orthostatic hypotension (Shah et al., 2005). Haloperidol produces fewer of these effects and is, therefore, preferred in the presence of significant cardiac disease and after cardiac surgery (Stoudemire, Moran, & Fogel, 1991). However, intravenous administration may cause torsades de pointes (Hunt & Stern, 1995). Atypical antipsychotics may produce similar effects.

There is also evidence that atypical antipsychotics, particularly clozapine, approved by the FDA for the reduction of suicidal risk in schizophrenic patients, may contribute to a reduction in suicidality in patients with affective disorders ("Atypical antipsychotics for treatment of depression in schizophrenia and affective disorders. Collaborative Working Group on Clinical Trial Evaluations," 1998). Clozapine is a dibenzoxazepine with a strong affinity for D4-dopaminergic receptors and potent serotonergic, noradrenergic, histamine and cholinergic M2 receptor blocking ability. Clozapine may have cardiovascular side-effects (Merrill, Dec, & Goff, 2005). For example, the FDA compelled Novartis Pharmaceuticals to include a black-box warning for Clozaril (clozapine) regarding adverse cardiovascular effects. The back-box warning indicates that clozapine should be used with caution in patients with known cardiovascular and/or pulmonary disease, particularly in those with cardiac arrhythmias and conduction disturbances. In treatments with clozapine, orthostatic hypotension may represent a continuing risk, especially during the initial stage of the therapy. Therefore, upon initiation of clozapine therapy, it is recommended that therapy must be initiated with only 12.5 mg of clozapine once or twice daily. Tachycardia has been observed in approximately 25% of patients taking clozapine, with patients having an average increase in pulse rate of 10 to 15 bpm. Either tachycardia or hypotension may pose a serious risk for an individual with compromised cardiovascular function. A minority of clozapine-treated patients experience ECG repolarization changes, including S-T segment depression and flattening or inversion of T waves. Further, a higher incidence of myocarditis has been reported in clozapine-treated patients, with an odds risk 17-322 times greater than the general population, and an increased risk of fatal myocarditis with an odds risk 14-161 times greater than the general population. Finally, clozapine causes significant weight gain even in normal-weight patients, introducing a new cardiovascular risk (Feinstein, 2002). Because of all of these cardiovascular side-effects, clinicians ought to maintain a high degree of suspicion if signs or symptoms consistent with cardiac toxicity develop, and the drug should be stopped in patients with myocarditis, and interruption should be considered in patients with cardiomyopathy (Wooltorton, 2002).

In therapeutic doses, lithium exerts minimal cardiotoxicity in the majority of patients. It can be used safely in patients with cardiac disease if initiated at a low dose, increased gradually, and monitored carefully. Benign, reversible T wave changes (including inversion and flattening) are common with lithium administration and are not clinically significant (Shah et al., 2005). Clinically significant cardiovascular side effects of lithium may include sinus node dysfunction and increases in ventricular irritability. Rarely, lithium may worsen arrhythmias in patients with sinus node dysfunction (Steckler, 1994). Justo et al. (2005) investigated all published case report of torsade de pointes induced by psychotropic drugs in order to examine the prevalence of risk factors. they found concomitant use of more than one psychotropic drugs present in 30% of patients studied: of the 21 cases treated with two or more psychotropic drugs, 4 were treated with lithium. There are also a number of interactions with diuretics, some calcium channel blockers drugs, angiotensin, and methyldopa.

Antiepileptics as a group are considered reasonably safe drugs as far as their cardiac side effects and interaction with cardiovascular medications are considered. Cardiac effects, however, are relatively more common in the older anticonvulsive agents such as sodium valproate, and carbamezepine. When selecting those agents, clinicians must be aware of their inhibiting effect on the cytochrome P450 system; this effect may lead to elevated levels of the medication that prolong the QT interval and produce ventricular tachycardia (torsade de pointes) (Gutgesell et al., 1999). Furthermore, overdose with valproate has been shown to cause heart block. It can also lower the platelet count and fibrinogen levels and, therefore, can increase the prothrombin time (R. Davis, Peters, & McTavish, 1994).

Considering the anti-suicide properties of mood stabilizers, research supports the efficacy of long-term lithium treatment (Baldessarini, Pompili, & Tondo, 2006; Baldessarini, Tondo et al., 2006; Baldessarini, Tondo, & Hennen, 2003; Thies Flechtner, Muller Oerlinghausen, Seibert, Walther, & et al., 1996). Lithium is now considered to be the first-line treatment for reducing the risk of suicide (Grunze et al., 2002), but there is weaker evidence for the usefulness of anticonvulsants in preventing suicide (Goodwin et al., 2003; Thies Flechtner et al., 1996). Evidence emerging from clinical practice suggests that lithium may decrease suicide risk even in unipolar depression (Guzzetta, Tondo, Centorrino, & Baldessarini, 2007). Moreover, mood stabilizers reduce the agitation components of depressive-dysphoric states which often are correlated with impulsiveness and aggression and often found in those who are in a suicidal crisis (Baldessarini, Tondo et al., 2006). The role of mood-stabilizers appears to be the better remedy for the violent agitation that may precede suicide in bipolar disorders. Especially in mixed states, which may occur as a transitional condition when depression escalates into mania, the correct dosage of a mood stabilizer may determine whether or not an individual develops a high risk of suicide. Volatile and erratic moods associated with dysphoria and agitation should always lead clinicians to treat this condition carefully, monitoring suicide risk at all time.

Conclusions

Depression is a highly frequent comorbid condition that increase the costs of care and worsens disability and outcome in physical diseases (Anderson et al., 2001; Egede, 2005; Feldman et al., 1987; Katon & Schulberg, 1992; Leichter & See, 2005; Myers et al., 1984; Rapp, Parisi, & Walsh, 1988; Scherrer et al., 2003). For example, Zhang and colleagues (2008) indicated that around 79% of patients with chronic conditions are affected by different levels of depression In cardiovascular disease, rates of major depression are estimated between 20%–40% in patients with chronic heart failure (Barth et al., 2004; Konstam et al., 2005; Rutledge et al., 2006; van Melle et al., 2004), and around 16%-18% in inpatients with myocardial infarction (Schleifer et al., 1989). Depression is associated with higher short-term and long-term morbidity and mortality rates (Ahern et al., 1990; Barefoot et al., 1996; Carney & Freedland, 2003; Carney et al., 1988; Denollet et al., 1996; Dimsdale et al., 1981; Frasure-Smith et al., 1993; Jiang et al., 2001; Jiang et al., 2007; Ladwig et al., 1991; Sherwood et al., 2007; Silverstone, 1987; van Melle et al., 2005), including death from suicide. However, depression and suicide risk are often underdiagnosed by medical staff and general practitioners in patients with physical illness, especially in patients where physical complaints are the main form of communication with health professionals. For example, Rapp, Walsh, and Parisi (1988), and Koenig, Meador, and Cohen (1988) indicated that only 9% to 20% of inpatients with depression are correctly diagnosed as depressed by junior medical staff and, even after the physician had been informed that comorbidity with major depression was possible, few patients received a psychiatric consultation or antidepressant medication. The situation is still worse when we consider suicide. For example, Suominen, Isometsa, Lonnqvist (2004) identified all consecutive suicide attempters treated in hospital emergency rooms in Helsinki, from January 1997 to January 1998 and found that, during the last 12 months before the attempt, most elderly suicide attempters had contacts with primary health care, but only 4% had been diagnosed with a mood disorder although the rate of diagnoses rose to 57% after the attempt. This situation may be related to irrational beliefs about suicide among health professionals (Stoppe et al., 1999).

This means that programs to improve the skills of health professionals in identifying and treating depression and suicide risk are needed. In 1999, the US Surgeon General in the document "Call to action to prevent suicide" indicated as a major target as the improvement of the ability of primary care providers to recognize and treat depression, substance abuse and other major mental illnesses associated with suicide risk, an increase in referrals to specialty care when appropriate, and the institution of training for all health professional concerning suicide risk assessment, recognition, management and aftercare interventions (US Public Health Service, 1999).

Thus, it is important to educate primary care physicians about the association between certain physical illnesses and suicidal tendencies, and the appropriate selection and use of psychotropic medication for the treatment and prevention of psychiatric symptoms associated with suicidal behaviors when they present in primary care settings.

McManus et al. (2005) proposed a simple screening interview to detect most cases of depression in primary care. The interview was composed of two simple questions: "During the past month have you often been bothered by feeling down, depressed, or hopeless?" and "During the past month have you often been bothered by little interest or pleasure in doing things?". A yes answer to 1 of these 2 items was 90% sensitive and 69% specific for a diagnosis of depression. Alternatively, Dobbels (2002) proposed the use of self-report instruments (such as the Zung Depression Scale) to assess depression in primary care settings. However, screening and recognizing depression and suicide risk is not useful when this does not result in better treatment of depressed patients (Gilbody, House, & Sheldon, 2001).

Similarly, simple questions to assess self-injurious behavior may be extracted from the following list: in the last year (or six months) 1) "Have you felt tired of living and thought that life was not worth living?" 2) "Have you thought that, for yourself, your family, and your friends it would be better if you were dead?" 3) "Have you thought of harming yourself, but without dying?" 4) "Have you thought of ending your life?" 5) "Have you thought of a method for committing suicide?" 6) "Have you attempted suicide?"

When clinicians recognize that their patient is depressed, and that symptoms interfere with work, social relationship, or adherence to treatment, they must treat the depression or refer the patient to mental health professionals. When suicidal ideation and behaviour are present, clinicians must refer the patient as soon as possible to mental health professionals. Meanwhile, the use of additional support (such as more frequent direct face-to-face or telephone contacts) should be considered and, if treatment for depression is compulsory, they have to consider arguments for and against the use of TCAs, SSRIs or the newer SNRI antidepressants. Furthermore, patients should also be warned both about the risk of adverse events from the medication in the early stages of therapy, and about the risks of reducing or stopping the use of the medication.

References

Ahern, D. K., Gorkin, L., Anderson, J. L., Tierney, C., Hallstrom, A., Ewart, C., et al. (1990). Biobehavioral variables and mortality or cardiac arrest in the Cardiac Arrhythmia Pilot Study (CAPS). *The American journal of cardiology,* **66**(1), 59-62.

Alvarez, W., Jr., & Pickworth, K. K. (2003). Safety of antidepressant drugs in the patient with cardiac disease: a review of the literature. *Pharmacotherapy,* **23**(6), 754-771.

Anda, R., Williamson, D., Jones, D., Macera, C., Eaker, E., Glassman, A., et al. (1993). Depressed affect, hopelessness, and the risk of ischemic heart disease in a cohort of U.S. adults. *Epidemiology (Cambridge, Mass,* **4**(4), 285-294.

Anderson, R. J., Freedland, K. E., Clouse, R. E., & Lustman, P. J. (2001). The prevalence of comorbid depression in adults with diabetes: a meta-analysis. *Diabetes care,* **24**(6), 1069-1078.

Appels, A., & Otten, F. (1992). Exhaustion as precursor of cardiac death. *British Journal of Clinical Psychology,* **31** (Pt 3), 351-356.

Artero, S., Astruc, B., Courtet, P., & Ritchie, K. (2006). Life-time history of suicide attempts and coronary artery disease in a community-dwelling elderly population. *International journal of geriatric psychiatry,* **21**(2), 108-112.

Atypical antipsychotics for treatment of depression in schizophrenia and affective disorders. Collaborative Working Group on Clinical Trial Evaluations. (1998). *The Journal of clinical psychiatry,* **59** Suppl 12, 41-45.

Baldessarini, R. J., Pompili, M., & Tondo, L. (2006). Suicidal Risk in Antidepressant Drug Trials. *Archives of general psychiatry,* **63**(3), 246-248.

Baldessarini, R. J., Tondo, L., Davis, P., Pompili, M., Goodwin, F. K., & Hennen, J. (2006). Decreased risk of suicides and attempts during long-term lithium treatment: a meta-analytic review. *Bipolar disorders,* **8**(5 Pt 2), 625-639.

Baldessarini, R. J., Tondo, L., & Hennen, J. (2003). Lithium treatment and suicide risk in major affective disorders: update and new findings. *The Journal of clinical psychiatry,* **64** Suppl 5, 44-52.

Banki, C. M., Karmacsi, L., Bissette, G., & Nemeroff, C. B. (1992). CSF corticotropin-releasing hormone and somatostatin in major depression: response to antidepressant treatment and relapse. *Eur Neuropsychopharmacol,* **2**(2), 107-113.

Barbui, C., Campomori, A., D'Avanzo, B., Negri, E., & Garattini, S. (1999). Antidepressant drug use in Italy since the introduction of SSRIs: national trends, regional differences and impact on suicide rates. *Social psychiatry and psychiatric epidemiology,* **34**(3), 152-156.

Barefoot, J. C., Brummett, B. H., Helms, M. J., Mark, D. B., Siegler, I. C., & Williams, R. B. (2000). Depressive symptoms and survival of patients with coronary artery disease. *Psychosomatic medicine,* **62**(6), 790-795.

Barefoot, J. C., Helms, M. J., Mark, D. B., Blumenthal, J. A., Califf, R. M., Haney, T. L., et al. (1996). Depression and long-term mortality risk in patients with coronary artery disease. *The American journal of cardiology,* **78**(6), 613-617.

Barth, J., Schumacher, M., & Herrmann-Lingen, C. (2004). Depression as a risk factor for mortality in patients with coronary heart disease: a meta-analysis. *Psychosomatic medicine,* **66**(6), 802-813.

Blier, P. (2001). Pharmacology of rapid-onset antidepressant treatment strategies. *The Journal of clinical psychiatry,* **62** *Suppl* **15**, 12-17.

Booth-Kewley, S., & Friedman, H. S. (1987). Psychological predictors of heart disease: a quantitative review. *Psychological bulletin,* **101**(3), 343-362.

Brown, E. S., Varghese, F. P., & McEwen, B. S. (2004). Association of depression with medical illness: does cortisol play a role? *Biological psychiatry,* **55**(1), 1-9.

Brunson, B. I., & Matthews, K. A. (1981). The type A coronary-prone behavior pattern and reactions to uncontrollable stress: an analysis of performance strategies, affect, and attributions during failure. *Journal of personality and social psychology,* **40**(5), 906-918.

Bushman, B. J., & Anderson, C. A. (1998). Methodology in the study of aggression: integrating experimental and nonexperimental findings. In R. G. Geen & E. Donnerstein (Eds.), *Human Aggression: theories, research, and implications for social policy* (pp. 23–48). New York: Academic Press.

Carney, R. M., & Freedland, K. E. (2003). Depression, mortality, and medical morbidity in patients with coronary heart disease. *Biological psychiatry,* **54**(3), 241-247.

Carney, R. M., Freedland, K. E., & Veith, R. C. (2005). Depression, the autonomic nervous system, and coronary heart disease. *Psychosomatic medicine,* **67** *Suppl* **1**, S29-33.

Carney, R. M., Freedland, K. E., Veith, R. C., Cryer, P. E., Skala, J. A., Lynch, T., et al. (1999). Major depression, heart rate, and plasma norepinephrine in patients with coronary heart disease. *Biological psychiatry,* **45**(4), 458-463.

Carney, R. M., Rich, M. W., Freedland, K. E., Saini, J., teVelde, A., Simeone, C., et al. (1988). Major depressive disorder predicts cardiac events in patients with coronary artery disease. *Psychosomatic medicine,* **50**(6), 627-633.

Carney, R. M., Saunders, R. D., Freedland, K. E., Stein, P., Rich, M. W., & Jaffe, A. S. (1995). Association of depression with reduced heart rate variability in coronary artery disease. *The American journal of cardiology,* **76**(8), 562-564.

Carver, C. S., & Glass, D. C. (1978). Coronary-prone behavior pattern and interpersonal aggression. *Journal of personality and social psychology,* **36**(4), 361-366.

Cattell, H., & Jolley, D. J. (1995). One hundred cases of suicide in elderly people. *Br J Psychiatry,* **166**(4), 451-457.

Clement, H. W., Buschmann, J., Rex, S., Grote, C., Opper, C., Gemsa, D., et al. (1997). Effects of interferon-gamma, interleukin-1 beta, and tumor necrosis factor-alpha on the serotonin metabolism in the nucleus raphe dorsalis of the rat. *J Neural Transm,* **104**(10), 981-991.

Conwell, Y., Duberstein, P. R., & Caine, E. D. (2002). Risk factors for suicide in later life. *Biological psychiatry,* **52**(3), 193-204.

Coryell, W., & Young, E. A. (2005). Clinical predictors of suicide in primary major depressive disorder. *The Journal of clinical psychiatry,* **66**(4), 412-417.

Dalack, G. W., & Roose, S. P. (1990). Perspectives on the relationship between cardiovascular disease and affective disorder. *The Journal of clinical psychiatry,* **51** *Suppl,* 4-9; discussion 10-11.

Davis, J., Fujimoto, R. Y., Juarez, D. T., Hodges, K. A., & Asam, J. K. (2008). Major depression associated with rates of cardiovascular disease state transitions. *The American journal of managed care,* **14**(3), 125-128.

Davis, R., Peters, D. H., & McTavish, D. (1994). Valproic acid. A reappraisal of its pharmacological properties and clinical efficacy in epilepsy. *Drugs,* **47**(2), 332-372.

de Jonge, P., Mangano, D., & Whooley, M. A. (2007). Differential association of cognitive and somatic depressive symptoms with heart rate variability in patients with stable coronary heart disease: findings from the Heart and Soul Study. *Psychosomatic medicine,* **69**(8), 735-739.

Denollet, J., Sys, S. U., Stroobant, N., Rombouts, H., Gillebert, T. C., & Brutsaert, D. L. (1996). Personality as independent predictor of long-term mortality in patients with coronary heart disease. *Lancet,* **347**(8999), 417-421.

Dimsdale, J. E., Gilbert, J., Hutter, A. M., Jr., Hackett, T. P., & Block, P. C. (1981). Predicting cardiac morbidity based on risk factors and coronary angiographic findings. *The American journal of cardiology,* **47**(1), 73-76.

Dobbels, F., De Geest, S., Vanhees, L., Schepens, K., Fagard, R., & Vanhaecke, J. (2002). Depression and the heart: a systematic overview of definition, measurement, consequences and treatment of depression in cardiovascular disease. *Eur J Cardiovasc Nurs,* **1**(1), 45-55.

Dumais, A., Lesage, A. D., Alda, M., Rouleau, G., Dumont, M., Chawky, N., et al. (2005). Risk factors for suicide completion in major depression: a case-control study of impulsive and aggressive behaviors in men. *The American journal of psychiatry,* **162**(11), 2116-2124.

Egede, L. E. (2005). Effect of comorbid chronic diseases on prevalence and odds of depression in adults with diabetes. *Psychosomatic medicine,* **67**(1), 46-51.

Empana, J. P., Jouven, X., Lemaitre, R. N., Sotoodehnia, N., Rea, T., Raghunathan, T. E., et al. (2006). Clinical depression and risk of out-of-hospital cardiac arrest. *Archives of internal medicine,* **166**(2), 195-200.

Evans, J. M., Wang, J., & Morris, A. D. (2002). Comparison of cardiovascular risk between patients with type 2 diabetes and those who had had a myocardial infarction: cross sectional and cohort studies. *BMJ (Clinical research ed,* **324**(7343), 939-942.

Everson, S. A., Goldberg, D. E., Kaplan, G. A., Cohen, R. D., Pukkala, E., Tuomilehto, J., et al. (1996). Hopelessness and risk of mortality and incidence of myocardial infarction and cancer. *Psychosomatic medicine,* **58**(2), 113-121.

Farberow, N. L., McKelligott, J. W., & Cohen, S. (1970). Suicide among cardiovascular patients. In E. S. Shneidman, N. L. Farberow & R. E. Litman (Eds.), *The Psychology of Suicide* (pp. 368-384). New York: Science House.

Farberow, N. L., McKelligott, J. W., Cohen, S., & Darbonne, A. (1966). Suicide among patients with cardiorespiratory illnesses. *Journal of the American medical association,* **195**(6), 422-428.

Farberow, N. L., Shneidman, E. S., & Neuringer, C. (1966). Case history and hospitalization factors in suicides of neuropsychiatric hospital patients. *The Journal of nervous and mental disease,* **142**(1), 32-44.

Feinstein, R. E. (2002). Cardiovascular effects of novel antipsychotic medications. *Heart disease (Hagerstown, Md,* **4**(3), 184-190.

Feldman, E., Mayou, R., Hawton, K., Ardern, M., & Smith, E. B. (1987). Psychiatric disorder in medical in-patients. *The Quarterly journal of medicine,* **63**(241), 405-412.

Frasure-Smith, N., Lesperance, F., & Talajic, M. (1993). Depression following myocardial infarction. Impact on 6-month survival. *Journal of the American medical association,* **270**(15), 1819-1825.

Fricchione, G. L., Woznicki, R. M., Klesmer, J., & Vlay, S. C. (1993). Vasoconstrictive effects and SSRIs. *The Journal of clinical psychiatry,* **54**(2), 71-72.

Friedman, M., & Rosenman, R. H. (1974). *Type A behavior and your heart.* New York: Knopf.

Gasse, C., Derby, L. E., Vasilakis, C., & Jick, H. (2000). Risk of suicide among users of calcium channel blockers: population based, nested case-control study. *BMJ (Clinical research ed,* **320**(7244), 1251.

Gehi, A., Mangano, D., Pipkin, S., Browner, W. S., & Whooley, M. A. (2005). Depression and heart rate variability in patients with stable coronary heart disease: findings from the Heart and Soul Study. *Archives of general psychiatry,* **62**(6), 661-666.

Gibbons, R. D., Brown, C. H., Hur, K., Marcus, S. M., Bhaumik, D. K., & Mann, J. J. (2007). Relationship between antidepressants and suicide attempts: an analysis of the Veterans Health Administration data sets. *The American journal of psychiatry,* **164**(7), 1044-1049.

Gilbody, S. M., House, A. O., & Sheldon, T. A. (2001). Routinely administered questionnaires for depression and anxiety: systematic review. *BMJ (Clinical research ed,* **322**(7283), 406-409.

Glass, D. C. (1977). *Behavior patterns, stress and coronary heart disease*. Hillsdale: Erlbaum.

Glassman, A. H. (1998). Cardiovascular effects of antidepressant drugs: updated. *International clinical psychopharmacology,* **13** Suppl 5, S25-30.

Glassman, A. H., & Shapiro, P. A. (1998). Depression and the course of coronary artery disease. *The American journal of psychiatry,* **155**(1), 4-11.

Goldsmith, S. K., Pellmar, T. C., Kleinman, A. M., & Bunney, W. E. (Eds.). (2002). *Reducing suicide: A national imperative*. Washington, D.C.: Joseph Henry Press.

Goldston, K., & Baillie, A. J. (2008). Depression and coronary heart disease: a review of the epidemiological evidence, explanatory mechanisms and management approaches. *Clinical psychology review,* **28**(2), 288-306.

Goodwin, F. K., Fireman, B., Simon, G. E., Hunkeler, E. M., Lee, J., & Revicki, D. (2003). Suicide risk in bipolar disorder during treatment with lithium and divalproex. *Journal of the American medical association,* **290**(11), 1467-1473.

Grunze, H., Kasper, S., Goodwin, G., Bowden, C., Baldwin, D., Licht, R., et al. (2002). World Federation of Societies of Biological Psychiatry (WFSBP) Guidelines for Biological Treatment of Bipolar Disorders, Part I: Treatment of Bipolar Depression. *World J Biol Psychiatry,* **3**, 115 -124.

Gunnell, D., & Ashby, D. (2004). Antidepressants and suicide: what is the balance of benefit and harm. *BMJ (Clinical research ed,* **329**(7456), 34-38.

Gutgesell, H., Atkins, D., Barst, R., Buck, M., Franklin, W., Humes, R., et al. (1999). Cardiovascular monitoring of children and adolescents receiving psychotropic drugs: A statement for healthcare professionals from the Committee on Congenital Cardiac Defects, Council on Cardiovascular Disease in the Young, American Heart Association. *Circulation,* **99**(7), 979-982.

Guzzetta, F., Tondo, L., Centorrino, F., & Baldessarini, R. J. (2007). Lithium treatment reduces suicide risk in recurrent major depressive disorder. *The Journal of clinical psychiatry,* **68**(3), 380-383.

Hall, W. D., Mant, A., Mitchell, P. B., Rendle, V. A., Hickie, I. B., & McManus, P. (2003). Association between antidepressant prescribing and suicide in Australia, 1991-2000: trend analysis. *BMJ (Clinical research ed,* **326**(7397), 1008.

Hallas, C. N., Thornton, E. W., Fabri, B. M., Fox, M. A., & Jackson, M. (2003). Predicting blood pressure reactivity and heart rate variability from mood state following coronary artery bypass surgery. *Int J Psychophysiol,* **47**(1), 43-55.

Hance, M., Carney, R. M., Freedland, K. E., & Skala, J. (1996). Depression in patients with coronary heart disease. A 12-month follow-up. *General hospital psychiatry,* **18**(1), 61-65.

Harris, E. C., & Barraclough, B. M. (1994). Suicide as an outcome for medical disorders. *Medicine (Baltimore),* **73**(6), 281-296.

Harvey, A. T., Rudolph, R. L., & Preskorn, S. H. (2000). Evidence of the dual mechanisms of action of venlafaxine. *Archives of general psychiatry,* **57**(5), 503-509.

Henry, C., & J., D.-M. (2006). SSRIs, Suicide and Violent Behavior: Is there a Need for a Better Definition of the Depressive State? *Current Drug Safety,* **1**, 59-62.

Hickie, I., Hickie, C., Bennett, B., Wakefield, D., Silove, D., Mitchell, P., et al. (1995). Biochemical correlates of in vivo cell-mediated immune dysfunction in patients with depression: a preliminary report. *International journal of immunopharmacology,* **17**(8), 685-690.

Huangfu, D., Hwang, L. J., Riley, T. A., & Guyenet, P. G. (1994). Role of serotonin and catecholamines in sympathetic responses evoked by stimulation of rostral medulla. *The American journal of physiology,* **266**(2 Pt 2), R338-352.

Hughes, J. W., Watkins, L., Blumenthal, J. A., Kuhn, C., & Sherwood, A. (2004). Depression and anxiety symptoms are related to increased 24-hour urinary norepinephrine excretion among healthy middle-aged women. *Journal of psychosomatic research,* **57**(4), 353-358.

Hunt, N., & Stern, T. A. (1995). The association between intravenous haloperidol and Torsades de Pointes. Three cases and a literature review. *Psychosomatics,* **36**(6), 541-549.

Innamorati, M., Pompili, M., Ferrari, V., Cavedon, G., Soccorsi, R., Mancinelli, I., et al. (2006). Relationship Between Type-A Behavior Pattern, Aggression, and Suicide in Italian University Students. *Individual Differences Research,* **4**(3), 185-193.

Inoue, K., Tanii, H., Abe, S., Kaiya, H., Okazaki, Y., Nata, M., et al. (2007). Suicidal tendencies among the elderly in Mie Prefecture, Japan, between 1996 and 2002. *Legal Medicine,* **9**, 34-138.

Irvine, J., Basinski, A., Baker, B., Jandciu, S., Paquette, M., Cairns, J., et al. (1999). Depression and risk of sudden cardiac death after acute myocardial infarction: testing for the confounding effects of fatigue. *Psychosomatic medicine,* **61**(6), 729-737.

Isacsson, G. (2000). Suicide prevention--a medical breakthrough? *Acta psychiatrica Scandinavica,* **102**(2), 113-117.

Jarskog, L. F., Xiao, H., Wilkie, M. B., Lauder, J. M., & Gilmore, J. H. (1997). Cytokine regulation of embryonic rat dopamine and serotonin neuronal survival in vitro. *Int J Dev Neurosci,* **15**(6), 711-716.

Jenkins, C. D., Zyzanski, S. L., & Rosenman, R. H. (1979). *Jenkins Activity Survey Manual.* New York: Psychological Corporation.

Jiang, W., Alexander, J., Christopher, E., Kuchibhatla, M., Gaulden, L. H., Cuffe, M. S., et al. (2001). Relationship of depression to increased risk of mortality and rehospitalization in patients with congestive heart failure. *Archives of internal medicine,* **161**(15), 1849-1856.

Jiang, W., Kuchibhatla, M., Clary, G. L., Cuffe, M. S., Christopher, E. J., Alexander, J. D., et al. (2007). Relationship between depressive symptoms and long-term mortality in patients with heart failure. *American heart journal,* **154**(1), 102-108.

Jick, H., Kaye, J. A., & Jick, S. S. (2004). Antidepressants and the risk of suicidal behaviors. *Journal of the American medical association,* **292**(3), 338-343.

Justo, D., Prokhorov, V., Heller, K., & Zeltser, D. (2005). Torsade de pointes induced by psychotropic drugs and the prevalence of its risk factors. *Acta psychiatrica Scandinavica,* **111**(3), 171-176.

Juurlink, D. N., Herrmann, N., Szalai, J. P., Kopp, A., & Redelmeier, D. A. (2004). Medical illness and the risk of suicide in the elderly. *Archives of internal medicine,* **164**(11), 1179-1184.

Kabiersch, A., del Rey, A., Honegger, C. G., & Besedovsky, H. O. (1988). Interleukin-1 induces changes in norepinephrine metabolism in the rat brain. *Brain, behavior, and immunity,* **2**(3), 267-274.

Katon, W. (2003). Clinical and health services relationships between major depression, depressive symptoms, and general medical illness. *Biological psychiatry,* **54**(3), 216-226.

Katon, W., & Schulberg, H. (1992). Epidemiology of depression in primary care. *General hospital psychiatry,* **14**(4), 237-247.

Koenig, H. G., Meador, K. G., Cohen, H. J., & Blazer, D. G. (1988). Detection and treatment of major depression in older medically ill hospitalized patients. *International journal of psychiatry in medicine,* **18**(1), 17-31.

Konstam, V., Moser, D. K., & De Jong, M. J. (2005). Depression and anxiety in heart failure. *Journal of cardiac failure,* **11**(6), 455-463.

Kop, W. J., & Gottdiener, J. S. (2005). The role of immune system parameters in the relationship between depression and coronary artery disease. *Psychosomatic medicine,* **67** *Suppl* **1**, S37-41.

Ladwig, K. H., Kieser, M., Konig, J., Breithardt, G., & Borggrefe, M. (1991). Affective disorders and survival after acute myocardial infarction. Results from the post-infarction late potential study. *European heart journal,* **12**(9), 959-964.

Ladwig, K. H., Roll, G., Breithardt, G., Budde, T., & Borggrefe, M. (1994). Post-infarction depression and incomplete recovery 6 months after acute myocardial infarction. *Lancet,* **343**(8888), 20-23.

Lane, D., Carroll, D., Ring, C., Beevers, D. G., & Lip, G. Y. (2000). Effects of depression and anxiety on mortality and quality-of-life 4 months after myocardial infarction. *Journal of psychosomatic research,* **49**(4), 229-238.

Lane, D., Carroll, D., Ring, C., Beevers, D. G., & Lip, G. Y. (2001). Mortality and quality of life 12 months after myocardial infarction: effects of depression and anxiety. *Psychosomatic medicine,* **63**(2), 221-230.

Leichter, S. B., & See, Y. (2005). Problems that extend visit time and cost in diabetes care, 1: How depression may affect the efficacy and cost of care of diabetic patients. *Clinical Diabetes,* **23**, 53–54.

Leon, A. C., Keller, M. B., Warshaw, M. G., Mueller, T. I., Solomon, D. A., Coryell, W., et al. (1999). Prospective study of fluoxetine treatment and suicidal behavior in affectively ill subjects. *The American journal of psychiatry,* **156**(2), 195-201.

Lesperance, F., Frasure-Smith, N., & Talajic, M. (1996). Major depression before and after myocardial infarction: its nature and consequences. *Psychosomatic medicine,* **58**(2), 99-110.

Lett, H. S., Blumenthal, J. A., Babyak, M. A., Sherwood, A., Strauman, T., Robins, C., et al. (2004). Depression as a risk factor for coronary artery disease: evidence, mechanisms, and treatment. *Psychosomatic medicine,* **66**(3), 305-315.

Lindberg, G., Bingefors, K., Ranstam, J., Rastam, L., & Melander, A. (1998). Use of calcium channel blockers and risk of suicide: ecological findings confirmed in population based cohort study. *BMJ (Clinical research ed,* **316**(7133), 741-745.

Maes, M. (1995). Evidence for an immune response in major depression: a review and hypothesis. *Progress in neuro-psychopharmacology & biological psychiatry,* **19**(1), 11-38.

Matthews, K. A., & Haynes, S. G. (1986). Type A behavior pattern and coronary disease risk. Update and critical evaluation. *American journal of epidemiology,* **123**(6), 923-960.

Mayou, R. A., Gill, D., Thompson, D. R., Day, A., Hicks, N., Volmink, J., et al. (2000). Depression and anxiety as predictors of outcome after myocardial infarction. *Psychosomatic medicine,* **62**(2), 212-219.

McManus, D., Pipkin, S. S., & Whooley, M. A. (2005). Screening for depression in patients with coronary heart disease (data from the Heart and Soul Study). *The American journal of cardiology,* **96**(8), 1076-1081.

Medicines and Healthcare products Regulatory Agency. (2005, 29 September 2005). Overview of regulatory status and CSM advice relating to major depressive disorder (MDD) in children and adolescents including a summary of available safety and efficacy data. Retrieved May 25, 2008, from http://www.mhra.gov.uk/Safetyinformation/Safetywarningsalertsandrecalls/Safetywarningsandmessagesformedicines/CON019494

Merrill, D. B., Dec, G. W., & Goff, D. C. (2005). Adverse cardiac effects associated with clozapine. *Journal of clinical psychopharmacology,* **25**(1), 32-41.

Mezzacappa, E. S., Kelsey, R. M., Katkin, E. S., & Sloan, R. P. (2001). Vagal rebound and recovery from psychological stress. *Psychosomatic medicine,* **63**(4), 650-657.

Miller, G. E., Stetler, C. A., Carney, R. M., Freedland, K. E., & Banks, W. A. (2002). Clinical depression and inflammatory risk markers for coronary heart disease. *The American journal of cardiology,* **90**(12), 1279-1283.

Morgan, O., Griffiths, C., Baker, A., & Majeed, A. (2004). Fatal toxicity of antidepressants in England and Wales, 1993-2002. *Health Stat Q*(23), 18-24.

Musselman, D. L., Evans, D. L., & Nemeroff, C. B. (1998). The relationship of depression to cardiovascular disease: epidemiology, biology, and treatment. *Archives of general psychiatry,* **55**(7), 580-592.

Muth, E. A., Haskins, J. T., Moyer, J. A., Husbands, G. E., Nielsen, S. T., & Sigg, E. B. (1986). Antidepressant biochemical profile of the novel bicyclic compound Wy-45,030, an ethyl cyclohexanol derivative. *Biochemical pharmacology,* **35**(24), 4493-4497.

Myers, J. K., Weissman, M. M., Tischler, G. L., Holzer, C. E., 3rd, Leaf, P. J., Orvaschel, H., et al. (1984). Six-month prevalence of psychiatric disorders in three communities 1980 to 1982. *Archives of general psychiatry,* **41**(10), 959-967.

Nemeroff, C. B., Widerlov, E., Bissette, G., Walleus, H., Karlsson, I., Eklund, K., et al. (1984). Elevated concentrations of CSF corticotropin-releasing factor-like immunoreactivity in depressed patients. *Science (New York, N.Y,* **226**(4680), 1342-1344.

Nicholson, A., Kuper, H., & Hemingway, H. (2006). Depression as an aetiologic and prognostic factor in coronary heart disease: a meta-analysis of 6362 events among 146 538 participants in 54 observational studies. *European heart journal,* **27**(23), 2763-2774.

Olfson, M., Shaffer, D., Marcus, S. C., & Greenberg, T. (2003). Relationship between antidepressant medication treatment and suicide in adolescents. *Archives of general psychiatry,* **60**(10), 978-982.

Parissis, J. T., Fountoulaki, K., Paraskevaidis, I., & Kremastinos, D. (2005). Depression in chronic heart failure: novel pathophysiological mechanisms and therapeutic approaches. *Expert opinion on investigational drugs,* **14**(5), 567-577.

Pearson, J. L., & Brown, G. K. (2000). Suicide prevention in late life: directions for science and practice. *Clinical psychology review,* **20**(6), 685-705.

Pompili, M., Lester, D., Iliceto, P., Tatarelli, R., & Girardi, P. (2007). No increase in suicide risk among cardiopathic patients. *The American heart hospital journal,* **5**(2), 103-106.

Ramsey, R., Wright, P., Katz, A., Bielawska, C., & Katona, C. (1991). The detection of psychiatric morbidity and its effect on outcome in acute elderly medical admissions. *International journal of geriatric psychiatry,* **6**, 861–866.

Rapp, S. R., Parisi, S. A., & Walsh, D. A. (1988). Psychological dysfunction and physical health among elderly medical inpatients. *Journal of consulting and clinical psychology,* **56**(6), 851-855.

Rapp, S. R., Parisi, S. A., Walsh, D. A., & Wallace, C. E. (1988). Detecting depression in elderly medical inpatients. *Journal of consulting and clinical psychology,* **56**(4), 509-513.

Rechlin, T., Weis, M., Spitzer, A., & Kaschka, W. P. (1994). Are affective disorders associated with alterations of heart rate variability? *Journal of affective disorders,* **32**(4), 271-275.

Rhodewalt, F., & Davison, J., Jr. (1983). Reactance and the coronary-prone behavior pattern: the role of self-attribution in responses to reduced behavioral freedom. *Journal of personality and social psychology,* **44**(1), 220-228.

Roose, S. P. (2003). Treatment of depression in patients with heart disease. *Biological psychiatry,* **54**(3), 262-268.

Roose, S. P., Dalack, G. W., Glassman, A. H., Woodring, S., Walsh, B. T., & Giardina, E. G. (1991). Cardiovascular effects of bupropion in depressed patients with heart disease. *The American journal of psychiatry,* **148**(4), 512-516.

Roose, S. P., Dalack, G. W., & Woodring, S. (1991). Death, depression, and heart disease. *The Journal of clinical psychiatry,* **52** Suppl, 34-39.

Rottenberg, J., Clift, A., Bolden, S., & Salomon, K. (2007). RSA fluctuation in major depressive disorder. *Psychophysiology,* **44**(3), 450-458.

Rottenberg, J., Wilhelm, F. H., Gross, J. J., & Gotlib, I. H. (2003). Vagal rebound during resolution of tearful crying among depressed and nondepressed individuals. *Psychophysiology,* **40**(1), 1-6.

Rozanski, A., Blumenthal, J. A., & Kaplan, J. (1999). Impact of psychological factors on the pathogenesis of cardiovascular disease and implications for therapy. *Circulation,* **99**(16), 2192-2217.

Rutledge, T., Reis, V. A., Linke, S. E., Greenberg, B. H., & Mills, P. J. (2006). Depression in heart failure a meta-analytic review of prevalence, intervention effects, and associations with clinical outcomes. *Journal of the American College of Cardiology,* **48**(8), 1527-1537.

Salib, E., & Green, L. (2003). Gender in elderly suicide: analysis of coroners inquests of 200 cases of elderly suicide in Cheshire 1989-2001. *International journal of geriatric psychiatry,* **18**(12), 1082-1087.

Scherrer, J. F., Xian, H., Bucholz, K. K., Eisen, S. A., Lyons, M. J., Goldberg, J., et al. (2003). A twin study of depression symptoms, hypertension, and heart disease in middle-aged men. *Psychosomatic medicine,* **65**(4), 548-557.

Schleifer, S. J., Macari-Hinson, M. M., Coyle, D. A., Slater, W. R., Kahn, M., Gorlin, R., et al. (1989). The nature and course of depression following myocardial infarction. *Archives of internal medicine,* **149**(8), 1785-1789.

Serebruany, V. L., Glassman, A. H., Malinin, A. I., Atar, D., Sane, D. C., Oshrine, B. R., et al. (2003). Selective serotonin reuptake inhibitors yield additional antiplatelet protection in patients with congestive heart failure treated with antecedent aspirin. *Eur J Heart Fail,* **5**(4), 517-521.

Shah, S. U., Iqbal, Z., White, A., & White, S. (2005). Heart and mind: (2) psychotropic and cardiovascular therapeutics. *Postgraduate medical journal,* **81**(951), 33-40.

Sherwood, A., Blumenthal, J. A., Trivedi, R., Johnson, K. S., O'Connor, C. M., Adams, K. F., Jr., et al. (2007). Relationship of depression to death or hospitalization in patients with heart failure. *Archives of internal medicine,* **167**(4), 367-373.

Silverstone, P. H. (1987). Depression and outcome in acute myocardial infarction. *British medical journal (Clinical research ed,* **294**(6566), 219-220.

Steckler, T. L. (1994). Lithium- and carbamazepine-associated sinus node dysfunction: nine-year experience in a psychiatric hospital. *Journal of clinical psychopharmacology,* **14**(5), 336-339.

Stedman, T. L. (1995). *Stedman's Medical Dictionary: Illustrated in color* (26th ed.). Baltimore: Williams & Wilkins.

Stein, P. K., Carney, R. M., Freedland, K. E., Skala, J. A., Jaffe, A. S., Kleiger, R. E., et al. (2000). Severe depression is associated with markedly reduced heart rate variability in patients with stable coronary heart disease. *Journal of psychosomatic research,* **48**(4-5), 493-500.

Steinberg, L. (1986). Stability (and Instability) of Type A Behavior From Childhood to Young Adulthood. *Developmental Psychology,* **22**, 393-402.

Stewart, R. A., North, F. M., West, T. M., Sharples, K. J., Simes, R. J., Colquhoun, D. M., et al. (2003). Depression and cardiovascular morbidity and mortality: cause or consequence? *European heart journal,* **24**(22), 2027-2037.

Stoppe, G., Sandholzer, H., Huppertz, C., Duwe, H., & Staedt, J. (1999). Family physicians and the risk of suicide in the depressed elderly. *Journal of affective disorders,* **54**(1-2), 193-198.

Stoudemire, A., Moran, M. G., & Fogel, B. S. (1991). Psychotropic drug use in the medically ill. Part II. *Psychosomatics,* **32**(1), 34-46.

Suarez, E. C., Krishnan, R. R., & Lewis, J. G. (2003). The relation of severity of depressive symptoms to monocyte-associated proinflammatory cytokines and chemokines in apparently healthy men. *Psychosomatic medicine,* **65**(3), 362-368.

Suominen, K., Isometsa, E., & Lonnqvist, J. (2004). Elderly suicide attempters with depression are often diagnosed only after the attempt. *International journal of geriatric psychiatry,* **19**(1), 35-40.

Taylor, C. B., Conrad, A., Wilhelm, F. H., Neri, E., DeLorenzo, A., Kramer, M. A., et al. (2006). Psychophysiological and cortisol responses to psychological stress in depressed and nondepressed older men and women with elevated cardiovascular disease risk. *Psychosomatic medicine,* **68**(4), 538-546.

Teicher, M. H., Glod, C. A., & Cole, J. O. (1993). Antidepressant drugs and the emergence of suicidal tendencies. *Drug Saf,* **8**(3), 186-212.

Thase, M. E. (1998). Effects of venlafaxine on blood pressure: a meta-analysis of original data from 3744 depressed patients. *The Journal of clinical psychiatry,* **59**(10), 502-508.

Thies Flechtner, K., Muller Oerlinghausen, B., Seibert, W., Walther, A., & et al. (1996). Effect of prophylactic treatment on suicide risk in patients with major affective disorders: Data from a randomized prospective trial. *Pharmacopsychiatry,* **29**(3), 103-107.

US Food and Drug Administration, C. f. D. E. a. R. (March 22, 2004, May 2, 2007). FDA public health advisory: worsening depression and suicidality in patients being treated with antidepressant medications. Retrieved 6/13/2007, 2007, from http://www.fda.gov/cder/drug/antidepressants/AntidepressanstPHA.htm

US Public Health Service. (1999). *The Surgeon General's Call To Action To Prevent Suicide.* Retrieved. from http://www.surgeongeneral.gov/library/calltoaction/calltoaction.htm.

van Melle, J. P., de Jonge, P., Ormel, J., Crijns, H. J., van Veldhuisen, D. J., Honig, A., et al. (2005). Relationship between left ventricular dysfunction and depression following myocardial infarction: data from the MIND-IT. *European heart journal,* **26**(24), 2650-2656.

van Melle, J. P., de Jonge, P., Spijkerman, T. A., Tijssen, J. G., Ormel, J., van Veldhuisen, D. J., et al. (2004). Prognostic association of depression following myocardial infarction with mortality and cardiovascular events: a meta-analysis. *Psychosomatic medicine,* **66**(6), 814-822.

Wooltorton, E. (2002). Antipsychotic clozapine (Clozaril): myocarditis and cardiovascular toxicity. *Cmaj,* **166**(9), 1185-1186.

Wulsin, L. R., Evans, J. C., Vasan, R. S., Murabito, J. M., Kelly-Hayes, M., & Benjamin, E. J. (2005). Depressive symptoms, coronary heart disease, and overall mortality in the Framingham Heart Study. *Psychosomatic medicine,* **67**(5), 697-702.

Yach, D., Hawkes, C., Gould, C. L., & Hofman, K. J. (2004). The global burden of chronic diseases: overcoming impediments to prevention and control. *Journal of the American medical association,* **291**(21), 2616-2622.

Yeragani, V. K. (2000). Major depression and long-term heart period variability. *Depression and anxiety,* **12**(1), 51-52.

Yeragani, V. K., Pohl, R., Balon, R., Ramesh, C., Glitz, D., Jung, I., et al. (1991). Heart rate variability in patients with major depression. *Psychiatry Research,* **37**(1), 35-46.

Zhang, J., Ye, M., Huang, H., Li, L., & Yang, A. (2008). Depression of chronic medical inpatients in China. *Archives of psychiatric nursing,* **22**(1), 39-49.

In: Heart Disease in Men
Editors: A.B. Todd and M.H. Mosley, pp. 125-143
ISBN: 978-1-60692-297-2

Chapter 5

MAGNETICALLY SUPPORTED PERCUTANEOUS CORONARY INTERVENTIONS

Mark Patterson
Onze Lieve Voruwe Gasthuis, Amsterdam

Abstract

Magnetic navigation is the use of a magnetic field to actively re-orientate a magnetically-enabled wire or device. The field is directed by external magnets that are repositioned by a computer-controlled system. This young technology could lead to a significant evolution in the practice of coronary interventional procedures as it enhances or introduces 3 specific capabilities of exact tip orientation, computer-enhanced control and orientation of the magnetic field, and computer processing.

This chapter will describe the system, review current evidence and progress and potential future advances of this technology.

Section 1; Magnetic Navigation

Magnetic navigation is the use of a magnetic field to re-orientate a magnetically-enabled wire or device. The field is directed by external magnets that are moved by a computer-controlled system. Each function of the system is designed to improve wire steering. This young technology could improve percutaneous coronary interventional procedures as it gives an unprecedented improvement in 3 specific and complementary capabilities, namely precise tip adjustability, computer-enhanced, image-guided tip orientation, and computer–enhanced image processing. This chapter will explore the benefits that revolve around these three capabilities.

Although this technology is relatively new, it already appears that this system can equal, and even improve on, current conventional wire technique. The efficacy of this system is becoming evident at a point in time that is relatively soon after its regulatory approval. The current usability, combined with the exciting potential of future developments, could result in a formidable adjunct to PCI.

The System

The Stereotaxis Niobe Magnetic navigation system (MNS) is an advanced cardiology instrument control system for use in a hospital interventional suite. It is designed to enable physicians to complete more complex interventional procedures by providing image guided delivery of catheters and guidewires through the blood vessels and chambers of the heart to treatment sites, see figure 1.

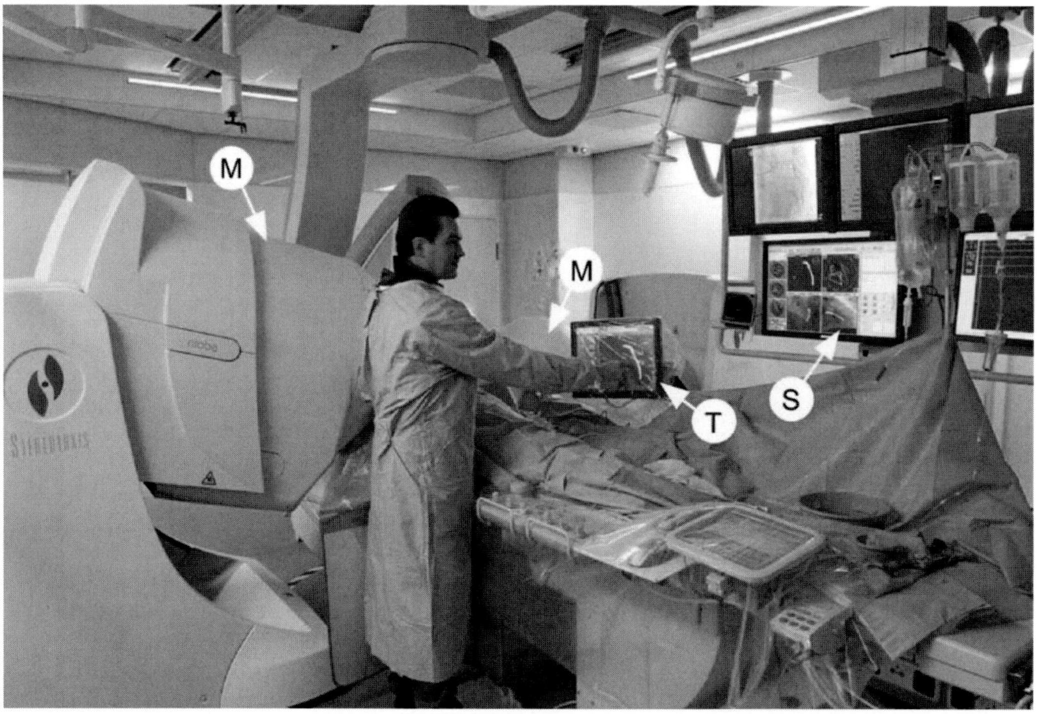

Figure 1. System in position for PCI. M indicates magnets in tilt position for better lateral movement of the image intensifier. T indicates touch screen interface to give real-time instruction to the MNS. S indicates in-lab main screen monitor.

The current system combines the Navigant™ Work Station that runs the computer software control for the Stereotaxis Niobe® magnet positioning system. This magnet positioning systems moves two large neodymium-iron-boron (Nd-B-Fe) magnets mounted on mechanical positioners, see figure 1. These result in an interacting magnetic field that produces a predictable vector at their midpoint. Magnetic moment is generated on a magnet when the applied field is offset from a magnet's principal magnetisation axis and this causes the magnet to align with the external field. The computer-controlled, externally-applied, magnetic field aligns a magnet on the working tip of the catheter or guidewire to govern the tip direction. The system obtained regulatory approval for use in humans in 2003.

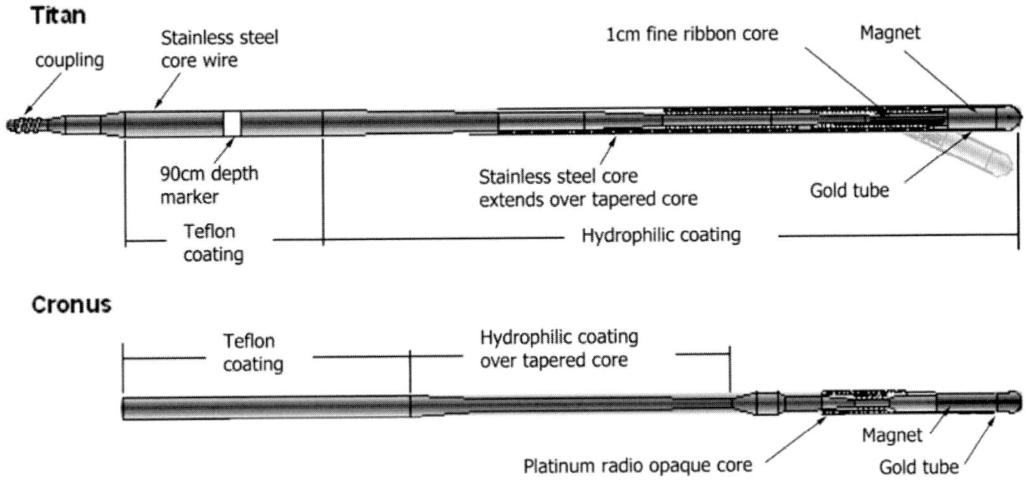

Figure 2. Schematic of the structure of the Titan Soft Support and Cronus wires.

The current list price for the Stereotaxis system is $1.9 million. The size of a typical modern Stereotaxis interventional suite is 770 square feet (72 square meters). The cost of magnetic shielding generally ranges from $50,000–$100,000 and consists of minimal common steel shielding in the walls, ceiling and floor. There is a range of magnetically enabled Stereotaxis 0.014" guidewires, see figure 2, that are priced at a marginal premium over conventional wires. All other PCI equipment is standard and compatible with the Stereotaxis guidewires and MNS.

Limitations of Conventional Manual Wire Manipulation

Traditionally 2D fluoroscopic images are interpreted using the training and anatomical knowledge of the physician to estimate and probe for the correct wire orientation to enable passage of the wire or device through a vessel. The tip of a conventional wire has a fixed angulation that is shaped before insertion. This tip is manipulated at a distance of approximately 1m by rotating the part of the wire that is external to the guiding catheter. Conventional manual wire manipulation is therefore a process of trial and error that is inherently limited by a number of problems.

First the wire direction is judged from the 2D image seen on a fluoroscopy screen image that is seldom at exactly 90° to the coronary vessel and therefore susceptible to foreshortening. Foreshortening can become problematic by hiding angulations and even the entire lesion.

Second, rotation of the shaft to redirect the fixed tip, seen in 2D, is imprecise as it is not possible to judge whether the tip is pointing into or out of the screen. While steering is generally easy in straightforward coronary anatomy, difficulty may occur in the multiple bends of a tortuous, calcified vessel that increases deformation of the wire, affecting wire rotation and therefore control.

Third, the conventional tip angle cannot be varied in cases where anatomy varies from straight segments to highly angulated segments and back again, thus a compromise tip angle has to be made. In simple anatomy this angle is often not crucial, and the wire can be passed distally easily. However in tortuous vessels with multiple angles, this compromise angle may not be suitable for all angles and this may result in the tip pointing inappropriately into the vessel wall.

These factors combine in tortuous and difficult anatomy to restrict wire delivery, increase use of irradiation, equipment and contrast and, in the worst case scenario, reduce procedural success.

Abilities Provided by the MNS

Magnetic navigation in percutaneous coronary intervention provides an unprecedented versatility that revolves around a number of capabilities.

Precise tip adjustability

As the magnetic field steers the front-end of the wire, the angulation of the tip can be exactly varied to the required angulation. This means that the tip can be kept co-axial to the vessel when crossing a straight segment and then directed at specific angles for tortuous bends or sharply angulated sidebranches. This control may help to prevent inadvertent sidebranch cannulation, facilitate the passage of extreme angulations or avoid dislodgement of friable material loosely attached to the wall e.g. in degenerated vein grafts or thrombus in acute lesions.

In addition, the magnetic field acts to stabilise the tip and tends to keep the tip pointing in the specified direction. This may reduce prolapse when resistance at the tip is encountered. This stabilisation of the tip at a certain angulation may improve the chance of the tip cleanly entering a tight lesion or a sidebranch.

Computer-enhanced, image-guided tip orientation

Orientation of the magnetic field in 3 dimensions is automatically achieved with the use of computer control. In practice this is done by using the preset vectors (standard 3D vectors derived from the average 3D direction of the coronary segment in 50 CT scans) or alternatively a patient-specific model from individually created 3 dimensional reconstructions of the patient's coronary arteries. This means that 3D information is integrated by the computer-adjusted magnetic field direction control to produce precise steering of the tip. Such 3D information may facilitate navigation in cases where the complexity may not be obvious on a 2D fluoroscopy screen.

Computer-enhanced image processing

The use of computers allows the production of digitalised images of the coronary arteries in great detail. These reconstructions can be made with the patient on the table or from previously acquired images. The fact that these images are digital allows post-processing that results in new ways to use the information giving new clinical applications such as the white-line overlay or the integration of MSCT.

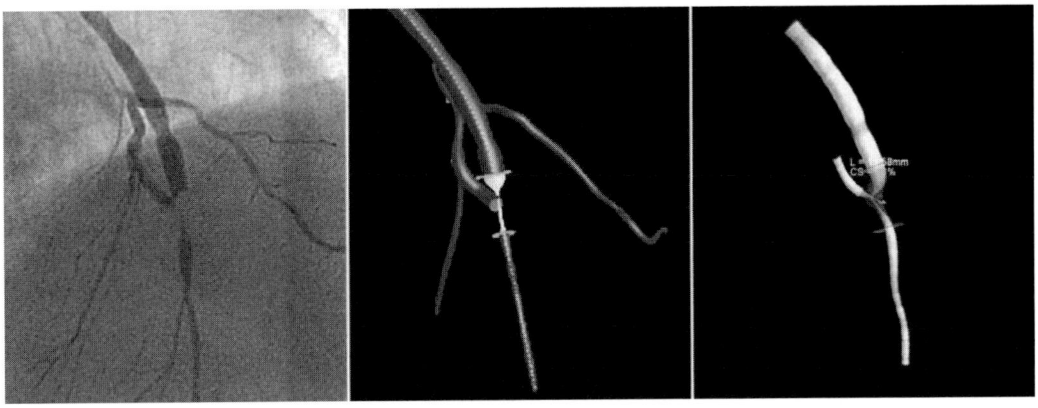

Figure 3. A severe lesion involving an anastomosis of a saphenous vein graft on a LAD. The left panel shows the angiographic image, the panel in the middle shows the Philips reconstruction and the right panel shows the Paeion reconstruction.

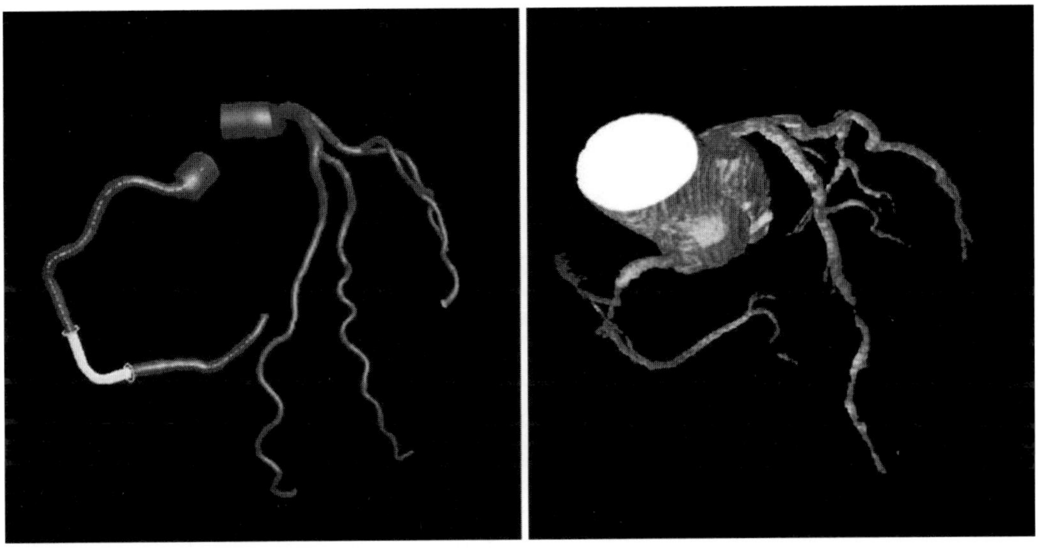

Figure 4. The left panel shows the coronary tree as extracted from MSCT by the Philips 3DCA system while the right panel shows the vessels extracted directly from CT by the Siemens package.

The production of a patient-specific, tailored vessel reconstruction is performed with dedicated reconstruction packages such as the Cardi-Op B software, (Paieon Medical Inc., Rosh Ha'ayin, Israel) integrated in the Navigant™ Work Station, and the 3DCA software on the stand-alone Interventional Tools workstation (Philips Medical Systems, Eindhoven, The Netherlands) (see figure 3). Both systems perform the reconstruction by triangulating points from 2 static images at different angulations at least 30° apart, but differ in that the Paeion system uses frames from 2 separate contrast injections at separate angles while the Philips system uses 2 frames from a single rotational acquisition. Frames are normally chosen in diastole to minimise movement artefact.

Current Applications of Post-Processing

Computed centre-line

This is derived from the calculated center-line of the reconstruction and is currently used in two ways.

First, the centre-line provides the patient-specific 3D trajectory of the vessel that is the basis for the magnetic field direction control used by the Niobe® system. The system sets the magnet positions to produce this magnetic field direction and therefore the direction that the tip of the magnetic wire will align itself to. The reconstruction therefore gives not only an individual reconstruction but also an individualized 3D direction for every point along that reconstruction.

Second, the centre-line is the basis of a white-line overlay that is projected onto the fluoroscopy screen. As the MNS has the data on the angulation and position of the image intensifier and table, this white-line overlay is orientated at the appropriate angulation for the fluoroscopic view and changes in real-time as the image intensifier moves. This gives the operator a permanently visible roadmap on the fluoroscopy screen that automatically adjusts to the angle of view to which he can compare either the shape of the wire or the contrast image.

MSCT integration

The introduction of patient-specific information from non-invasive, off-table investigations has obvious advantages. The use of MSCT can provide a complete coronary tree model for use during the procedure. With cardiac MSCT becoming both more accurate and more available in the ER for diagnosis, the possibility of reducing the on-table procedural burden of time and contrast use becomes more realistic.

This benefit not only applies to patent vessels but may be more valuable in the area of chronic total occlusion (CTO). First, MSCT can visualise the distal section of an occluded vessel to enable the wire to be steered in that direction. Second, the trajectory of the occluded segment may be visible. Third, information regarding the consistency of an occlusion or the surrounding tissue may be obtained e.g. for the extent of calcification. This information may be valuable in assessing the chance of success, choosing the strategy needed or directing the wire. However, the true benefit in CTO may only be realised when the loop can be fully closed with accurate tip localisation and dynamic mapping.

Summary of Potential Advantages

The system therefore gives a number of theoretical specific advantages to the PCI procedure that can be coupled with specific functionalities.

Navigation

Tip adjustment - *the ability to bend and direct the tip as requested, even to extreme angulations.*

Front-end steering - the avoidance of friction affecting manipulation.

Precision direction	- for steering along a path or for probing patterns.
3D orientation	- the ability to reliably use the third dimension during wire passage.
Wire stabilization	- the exact selection and maintenance of a direction along a vessel or into a sidebranch.
Lack of tip rotation	- tip direction becomes independent of friction on the shaft and the tip movements become more controlled
MSCT integration	- Computer-enhanced patient-specific 3D information.

Operator

White-line overlay	- a patient-specific visual map projected directly on the fluoroscopy screen
Endoluminal view	- an 'internal' view of the vessel that can be useful for sidebranch orientation.
MSCT integration	- missing vessel segments, extra-luminal details.

Procedure

Reduced irradiation	- reduced irradiation may occur from better navigation,
Reduced contrast	- contrast-sparing strategies using of diagnostic angiography films or MSCT for navigation.
Shorter procedures	- quicker and more efficient procedures not only benefit the patient but also the operator for example less irradiation or less time wearing protective lead coats

Conclusion

The system has a number of new capabilities that may bring advantages to a PCI procedure. Individually a specific advantage may not play a crucial role in each and every procedure but together may allow for smoother and less troubled wire passage. Ultimately magnetic navigation could potentially increase efficiency, reduce procedure time, facilitate the application of advanced technologies, decrease irradiation of the operators and thus better use hospital resources to lower overall hospital costs. The following section will review the current literature to assess whether there is support for these theoretical benefits and whether this is translated into a clinical benefit.

Section 2, Lessons from the Literature

Publications to Date Fall into a Number of Categories

Reviews

These articles have introduced and given an overview of the technology.[1,2] They have generally explored the currently evolving technique, describing the potential methods of utilisation and the situations where these may become useful. They have also introduced and previewed up-coming features and technology and speculated about the new areas where this technology may extend to the future such as remotely controlled procedures or stem cell injection.

Phantom Studies

These studies have looked at the use of the magnetic navigation in artificial phantoms to assess manoeuvrability and indicate which vessels might benefit the most. The earliest study used a 3 dimensional phantom with channels representing the LAD, Cx and RCA.[3] It was performed soon after regulatory approval, and with an early version of the software at a time when operators had had minimal experience with the system. It compared the speed (procedure time) and the amount of radiation (fluoroscopy time) needed to pass a wire, either conventional or magnetic, to a particular coronary segment. In most segments this early iteration of the system did not show improvement in navigating most segments but only suggested benefit in distal lesions such as the RDP with reductions in procedure time and fluoroscopy time. An additional part of the study examined the use of the system in stented bifurcations and suggested an advantage.

A later study used a 2 dimensional Perspex® model with 3 and 2mm channels to compare the effectiveness of conventional and magnetic wires in increasingly tortuous trajectories as well as comparing Interventionalists with different levels of experience.[4] This study showed that, while there was no significant advantage in more straightforward trajectories, magnetic navigation improved wire passage in the more tortuous trajectories. Furthermore in inexperienced hands the improved success rate was maintained in more complex lesions. This improved success rate was associated with a reduction in the number of wires needed to complete complex trajectories properly.

In conclusion, these phantom studies suggest a number of benefits and give some indication as to the areas where magnetic navigation may be particularly advantageous. First, there appeared to be particular benefit in tortuous trajectories with the suggestion that this technology may help in the treatment of bifurcation lesions. Second, there appeared to be improvement across all levels of experience. Third, there was a reduction in equipment use. However, phantom studies have the limitations of their artificial nature exemplified by their lack of movement, absence of stenoses, and an unnatural surface for wire passage and conclusions need to be drawn with caution and preferably should be mirrored by the findings of clinical studies.

Case Reports

The use of magnetic navigation has been described in a number of specific cases. Such case reports not only describe the feasibility of using the system in particular circumstances but also showcase the capabilities of the system.

An early case report demonstrated the ability to complete failed conventional procedures. In this case, a primary PCI had been performed conventionally but the bifurcation stenting procedure could not be completed with a kissing balloon dilatation as conventional wires would not cross into the sidebranch despite prolonged attempts.[5] Attempts to cannulate the sidebranch conventionally had produced an angiographically visible perivascular dissection parallel to the sidebranch. A further attempt to cannulate the sidebranch was performed later in the magnetic catheterisation suite. Here it proved relatively simple to cannulate the sidebranch and perform a kissing balloon dilatation. This led to a good angiographic result with obliteration of the perivascular dissection. This case not only demonstrated the ability to complete a case that could not be finished conventionally but also exemplified a possible advantage in bifurcation lesions where wire passage through the side of the stent was required, echoing the results of phantom studies.

It is clear that such navigation might be useful in complicated emergency procedures and this message was reinforced in a further primary PCI case.[6] In this primary PCI case procedure, material was more evident on one side of the vessel while crossing the lesion. The magnetic field was orientated to direct the wire away from the material. In addition, once flow was re-established, a bifurcation was seen. A bifurcation procedure was performed without incident. In this case the ability to steer the wire away from friable material and to steer without wire rotation (that would sweep around the circumference of a vessel and possibly dislodge material) could be an advantage in procedures where embolisation might be a risk such as primary PCI or diseased SVGs. In addition, the bifurcation proved easy to treat, again reinforcing a message about crossing a stent in a bifurcation.

A further demonstration of use in complex anatomy was described in a case that had proved resistant to conventional technique.[7] In this case 2 previous conventional procedures had failed despite the use of 5 catheters and 7 guidewires. A patient-specific 3D reconstruction was made from on-table angiography to give a tailored path from the LMS via the Cx to a remnant section of open vein graft and then on to the posterior descending branch of the RCA that filled retrogradely. While this did not prove to be a simple procedure, as it required an over-the-wire balloon and a support wire, it demonstrates the ability of the system to successfully navigate an extremely tortuous trajectory. In addition it also cautions that, while the wire may reach distal territories, new strategies to allow delivery of angioplasty materials may be needed.

The system has also been described in a difficult case of alcohol septal ablation to cannulate the septal when conventional wires had failed.[8] As it can occasionally prove problematic to enter septal branches, magnetic navigation may help to cross these extreme angulations. In this case there was a retroflexed 130° angulation of the origin of the septal artery that a number of conventional wires had failed to properly cannulate due to prolapse when attempting to advance more deeply. This case again demonstrates the ability of the system to navigate a single acute angulation that was impossible with conventional wires.

In conclusion these case studies demonstrate a number of points. They parallel the message from phantom studies regarding the usefulness of the system in bifurcation procedures, extreme angulations, and complex, tortuous anatomy. They show that the system is clinically useful in failed conventional cases, in primary PCI, and in cases where extreme care is necessary to avoid embolisation. However case reports are limited in that they are uncontrolled anecdotal reports that may have involved other factors than just the complexity of the lesion.

Technical Reports

There are a number of reports investigating the performance of technical aspects of the system predominantly focussing on the accuracy of the measuring ability of the system.[9,10]

These technical papers have both looked at the accuracy of calculated measurements of the dimensions of the reconstructions. In the first study, 22 angiographic images of precision-drilled plexiglass phantoms in pigs were compared both by the 3D reconstruction software (CardiOp-B™) and standard 2D software (CAAS II™). This showed that while there was good agreement of the 2 systems, underestimation was greater in the 3D system. A second study compared the 3D measurements with a newer 2D measurement system and showed a similar superiority of the 2D system. These results are not entirely surprising as the 3D reconstruction has been in development for a much shorter time than the 2D and in addition, it is important to realise that the 3D reconstruction software has been primarily designed to provide reconstructions rather than measurements. However the reports identify the interest in the potential of such 3D imaging technology and the emphasis on continued development of this software.

Feasibility Studies

The feasibility of the system has been described by a number of centres and at various stages since the system obtained regulatory approval.[11-14] A very early study examined general feasibility of passage of a wire in 68 lesions in 59 patients.[11] This study describes some of the very first experience and, even at this early stage, showed a reasonable success rate of 88% in crossing the lesion. Many of these procedures were completed with a conventional wire but it was noted that in 4 procedures the conventional wire failed and the magnetic wire succeeded, and that 3 of these failures were through the side of a stent into a jailed sidebranch, again paralleling results from the phantom and case studies. A second study at the same institution, also performed soon after system acquisition, compared crossing with a magnetic wire and then crossing-over to a conventional wire in 21 lesions.[12] This study included lesions described as having relatively simple and straightforward characteristics. The patients included were among the first 70 patients attempted at that institution. While on one hand, this study found significantly longer crossing times, more fluoroscopy and greater contrast use, on the other hand it showed a success rate for the magnetic wire of 90%. These latter 2 studies both used the first generation of magnetic wires and an early version of the navigation software and did not demonstrate a clear benefit.

A further study looked at a more difficult group of patients who were judged as difficult or impossible for conventional technique (primary attempt group, n = 46) or had failed conventionally (secondary attempt group, n = 13).[13] This study showed a reasonable success rate of 84% in the difficult (primary) group and a rate of 62%, well over half, in the conventional failure (secondary) group.

A further feasibility study has shown the initial experience of a center soon after system installation on a less-selected group of patients more representative of daily practice.[14] The success rates were again reasonably high at 86%. However an important note was highlighting of a problem with complex subtotal stenoses.

In conclusion, these feasibility studies show that the system is useable and gives reasonable success rates soon after system installation. However, there was no evidence of a clear superiority shown in these studies. However there has been some improvement with the newer generation of wires, newer software and more experience.

Comparative Studies

The OLVG Registry [15] study provides the first large single centre patient series describing the results obtained using magnetic navigation for PCI. This patient series included every patient treated by magnetic navigation from day 1. The procedures were examined by subdividing the first 320 patients into groups of 80 to examine issues such as a learning curve, and comparing the total group with historical controls. This center was deliberately organised with a small group of staff highly familiar with the system in order to examine issues related to optimisation of the start-up of system use.

In this fairly complex group of patients, success rates were high at 92% and procedural parameters were at least within the limits of usual practice. This study clearly showed a learning curve with improvements of over 50% in fluoroscopy time between the first group of 80 patients and the latest of the groups. An estimate of a learning curve of approximately 100 procedures was felt to be needed under these circumstances (small, dedicated team, routine use of the system in terms of regularity and use in all patient groups). This improvement appeared to be across the board with reduction in procedure and fluoroscopy times and less contrast use. The system had a high initial success rates and was highly applicable and safe in day-to-day practice. The system was used with the both transradial and femoral approaches.

An important point is the identification of inferior results in certain lesion types, such as CTO or severely eccentric tortuous lesions, and such lesions frequently needed to cross-over to dedicated angioplasty wires.

The comparison with historical controls showed no significant difference in fluoroscopy and procedural times but a reduction in contrast use. Moreover, in the MNS group significantly more lesions per patient were treated, while procedural and fluoroscopy times were within the same range as the single lesion stent control group.

In conclusion the system was shown to be feasible, effective and there appeared to be reduction in contrast, irradiation and consumables that was particularly evident in complex cases. A learning curve was demonstrated that has implications for the use of the system in other institutions.

Further analysis of this registry looked at particular sub groups with case matching to provide further insights into the effects. Cases have been matched for age, gender and vessel segment. In these case-matched groups, simple elective single vessel disease cases show a benefit with a reduction in contrast but no significant reduction in procedural or fluoroscopy time. However, complex cases show a significant improvement of all three of these parameters. The implications of this, if confirmed by randomised control trials could be significant with two particular points of interest. First, the ability to reduce contrast even in simple cases may have implications for procedures in groups at risk of contrast-induced nephropathy. Second, this demonstrated a greater advantage in complex anatomy, not just in terms of success or failure but also in reduction in time, irradiation and contrast. This suggests that this technology may give particular improvement in the performance of complex, difficult cases.

Stem Cell Injection

A possible development in stem cell delivery by intramyocardial injection may result from use of a magnetically-enabled, dedicated injection catheter, see figure 5.[1,15,17] This catheter has been shown to be effective in cell injection and accurate in targeting predefined segments.[16] The use of magnetic navigation may not only improve accuracy of delivery but may also enable better identification of suitable target areas as it allows easy, simultaneous electromechanical mapping with a combination of information derived on both movement (longitudinal linear shortening) and also electrical activity (unipolar voltage).

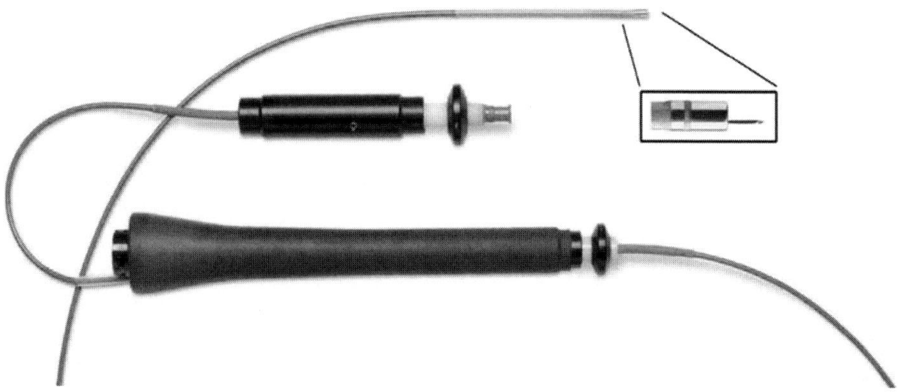

Figure 5. Stem cell delivery catheter combined with better electromechanical measurements.

Identification of Difficult Lesions

An important issue that emerges from review of the literature is the need for identification of the most appropriate lesions for magnetic navigation. A system that is based upon the 3D morphology of the vessel from 3D reconstruction has been described.[18] This examined the time needed to cross a lesion using a conventional wire and correlated this to various anatomical factors. A registry of procedures (awaiting publication) suggests that there was indeed a trend towards less influence and crossing times in vessels/lesions having high complexity scores. The ability to predict difficulty and a method of classifying and comparing complex procedures may help to define the patient population that would help derive the greatest benefit.

Summary of Points from the Literature

The system is both feasible and useable for clinical use in PCI.

Particular anatomy appears to derive particular benefit. These are tortuous segments, extreme angulation and bifurcations especially when crossing into sidebranches through a stent. These attributes clearly relate to complex or failed cases.

The literature indicates that use of magnetic navigation in such lesions may lead to benefit in terms of procedural time, fluoroscopy time and contrast use.

There appears to be a learning curve that may be optimised by the use of an defined, small group of users that regularly perform procedures. In addition early experience should not concentrate solely on difficult cases.

There may be a wider range of diverse clinical indications that may benefit from this technology such as alcohol septal ablation or the delivery of stem cells.

Limitations

Procedural

Initial use of the system can be time consuming due to of a lack of familiarity with what is a complex system that requires the isocenter position, moving the magnets into the correct position, and time to reconstruct. However, once there is an established routine, these manoeuvres become fluid and quick.

Care is suggested with intracardiac devices such as pacemakers and AICDs as the magnetic field may affect function. While no problems have been described thus far, the effect of a magnetic field on the device should be ascertained beforehand e.g. fixed rate pacing for pacemakers or inhibition of shock delivery for AICDs. Settings should be checked before and monitoring should be in place when the patient is brought into the magnetic field. A further device check is advisable after the procedure.

Software

The angiographic reconstructions still have a number of weaknesses. First, the reconstructions produced are susceptible to error if the diagnostic images are of poor quality. Angiographic images that are foreshortened in one or both views may severely underestimate the true angulation, a problem that is not infrequently seen in reconstructions of the LMS where the wire may not get enough angulation to turn into the appropriate major vessel. Second, the precision of the reconstructions is marginal. As seen with the technical reports, dedicated systems for measurement perform better then the systems used for navigation, this may have consequences and influence the accuracy of the models and therefore the accuracy of navigation. Third, the reconstructions are static and normally taken from diastolic frames. This has repercussions on passage of the wire at other phases of the cardiac cycle as the diastolic direction may be different to the direction in systole for the some point in the vessel.

On a minor level, the WLO is static and may be evident by a distracting scissoring of the WLO and the fluoroscopic image.

The software is constantly under development to optimize ergonomics.

Hardware

Wires

The wire-tip is a solid magnet that is 3 or 2mm long. Clearly, this does not have the flexibility of conventional wires that have a long history of development. This mainly leads to two problems.

Narrow channel angle grip

If calcium or tough scar tissue is present in an angulation it may prevent deflection of the tip and maintain an orientation that directs the tip into the vessel wall and into the intimal layer. It can be physically impossible for the solid inflexible wire tip to pass through a narrow, highly angulated channel, see figure 6. This may explain the results in sub-total and chronic total lesions that may involve sharp turns in calcified scarred tissue on a microscopic level.

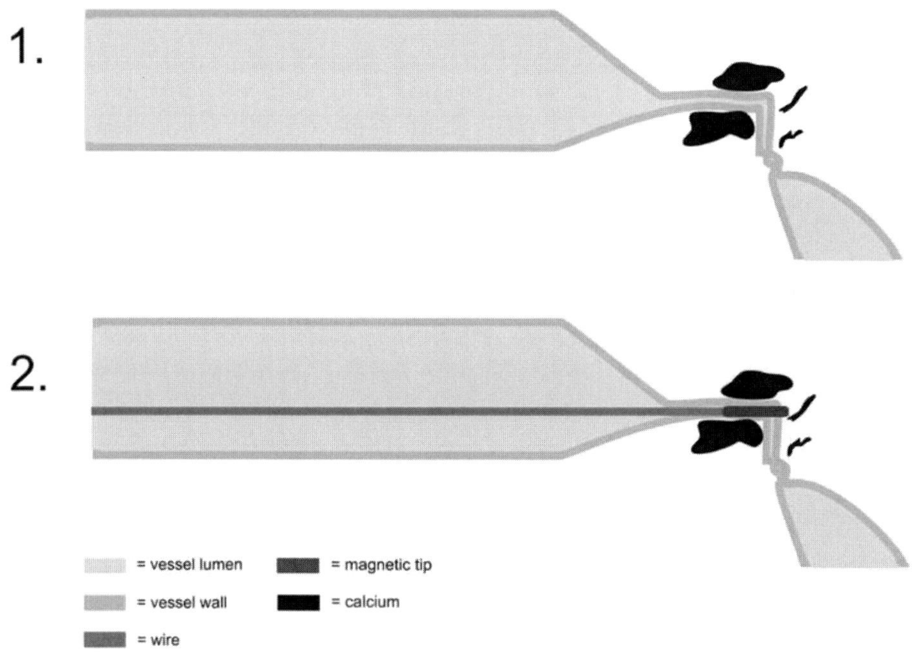

Figure 6. Schematic showing the wire tip attempting to turn a tight bend and being forced into the vessel wall.

Wire lock

The solid wire tip can become trapped behind stent struts or calcium. Traction on the wire will lead to a kink at the junction of wire and magnet and the wire becomes 'locked', see figure 7. At this point the risk of wire fracture becomes high. The problem can be avoided by ensuring correct tip orientation during the procedure and can be reversed by advancing the wire tip, possibly supported with a balloon to free the tip.

A range of new wires such as the Pegasus and multi-magnet wires may alleviate these problems.

Magnets

The magnetic field direction control is achieved by the movement of heavy solid external magnets on the positioners. The inertia of these magnets means that the response time is slow and, for example, is one factor against the development of dynamic roadmaps.

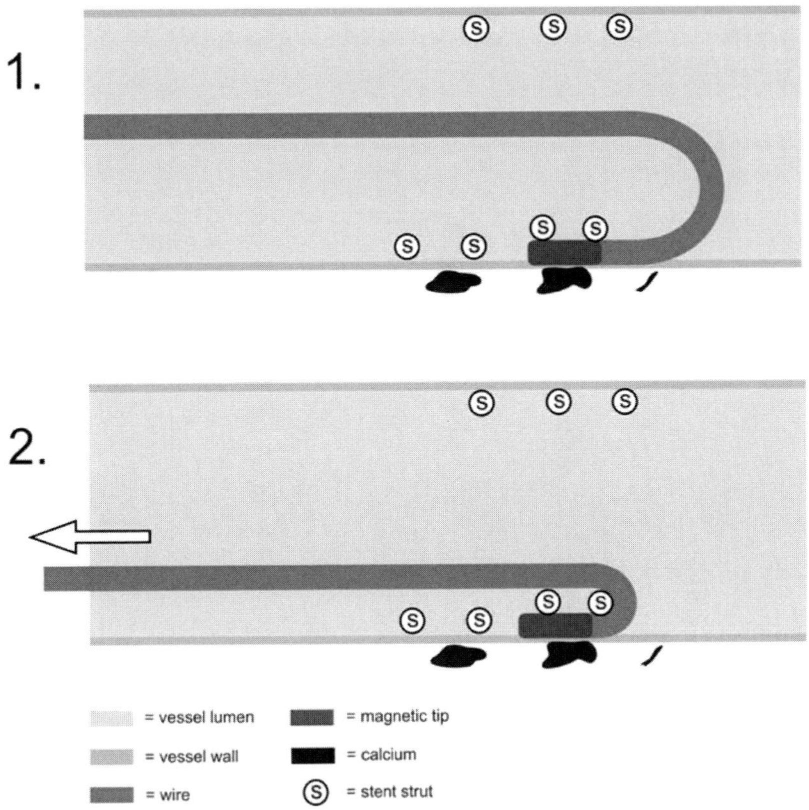

Figure 7. The two stage process of wire lock

Conclusion

New technology frequently suffers from slow uptake. This technology is relatively new with limited market penetration due to a combination of factors. This has resulted in this technology for PCI being restricted to a few pioneer institutions and results from factors such as the limited amount of evidence that is currently available due to the limited time since regulatory approval combined with the system cost and the investment in time and effort to learn the technique.

Section 3; Future Development

Clinical

Data is now accumulating from studies as to the possible clinical advantages of using the system and strategies to enhance the learning curve are developing.[14] More data is needed from randomised trials to convincingly show benefit and to identify which strategies, anatomy and patient groups can benefit the most. Methods for identifying, classifying and comparing complex procedures need further development

Technological

Future directions for research should include improvements in the software design and advancements in the hardware such as wire technology, RF ablation wire see figure 9 and remote control equipment, see figure 9.

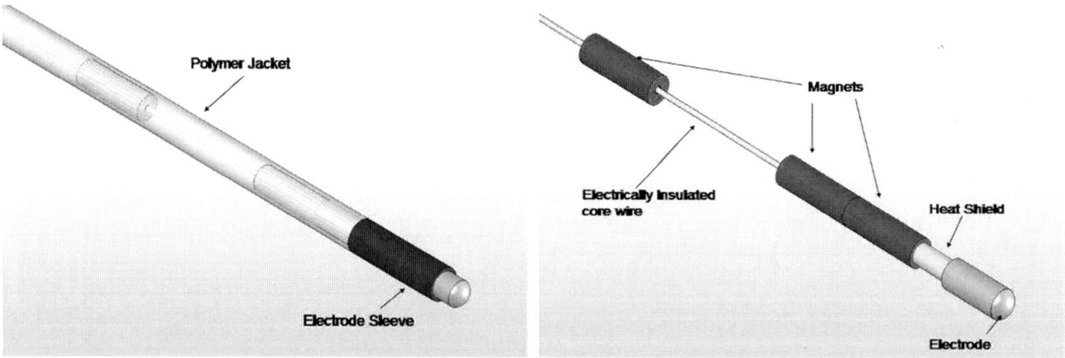

Figure 8. Magnetically controllable RF wire for hard and tough lesions.

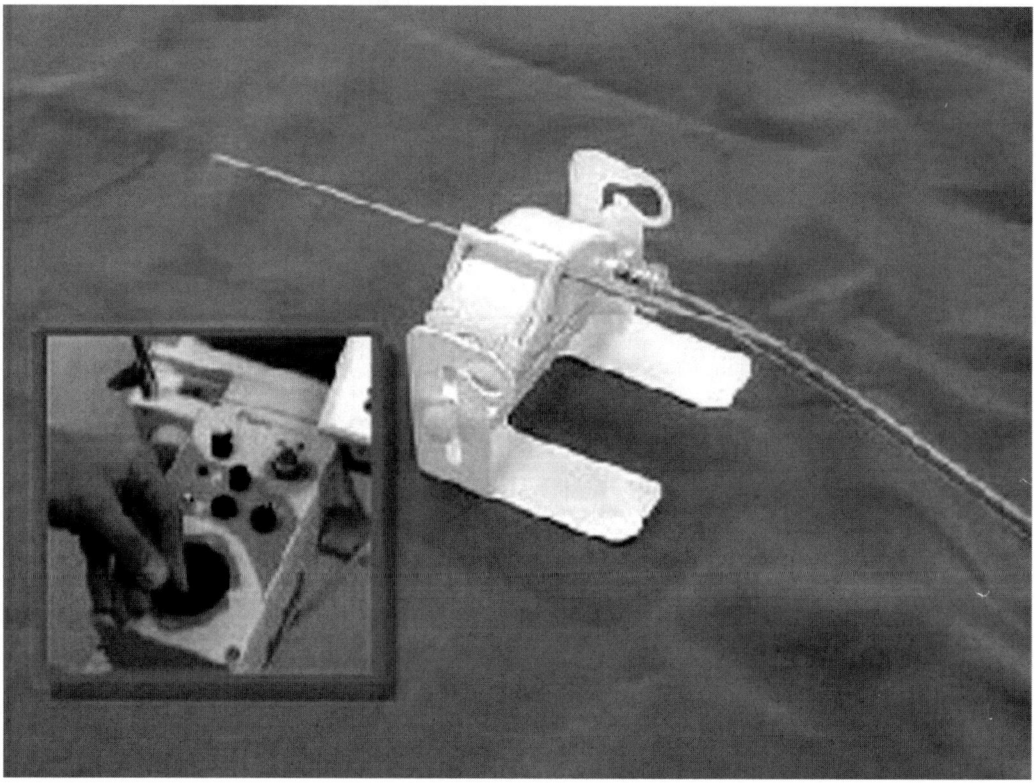

Figure 9. Remote control system.

Software developments include newer versions of the Navigant™ software. In particular, ease of use of current functions and improvements in integration are planned.

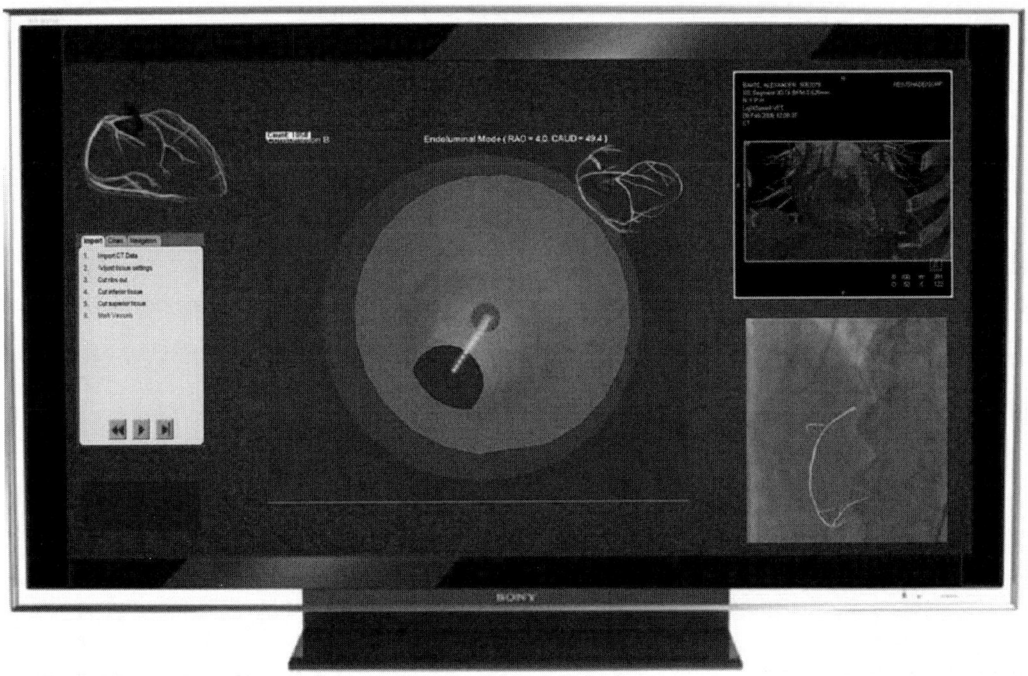

Figure 10. Odyssey screen.

Hardware projects in development include a magnetically controllable RF wire for hard and tough lesions, figure 8 remote control system, figure 9 and the Odyssey screen, figure 10.

Section 4; Conclusion

This new technology combines precise tip control, with image guided steering and the flexibility of computer enhancement. The 3D reconstruction of a virtual coronary artery can be performed in real-time while the patient is on the table during an interventional procedure. These images may not only give a better appreciation of the anatomy with regards to tortuosity but also give a volume-rendered model with the computer-calculated magnetic field direction control that allow magnetic navigation. These individualised, scale models supply the directions for deflecting the wire as it passes through the vessel.

The current advantages of this system in PCI include precise tip orientation, image-guided computer control and computer-enhanced image-processing. The current literature shows that there may be advantages of the system compared to conventional technique. Specifically, vessels with severe angulation(s), tortuousity, and particularly bifurcation that involve crossing stent struts may derive the greatest benefit. However, sub-total calcified lesions may prove less attractive with the current wire configuration. Identifying the appropriate classes of lesion may reinforce the benefit with respect to time, irradiation and contrast use that could have knock on effects on complications (such as contrast-induced renal dysfunction), the complexity of procedures (such as particularly complex or failed conventional procedures) and on new areas of intervention.

This new technology could transform the practice of interventional procedures with the introduction of computer enhanced imaging and guidance that revolves particularly around the production of 3D models.

Acknowledgement

The authors are grateful to Joep Maeijer for help with preparation of the images.

References

[1] Patterson MS, Schotten J, van Mieghem C, Kiemeneij F, Serruys PW. Magnetic navigation in percutaneous coronary intervention. *J Interv Cardiol* 2006;19:558–565.

[2] Ramcharitar S, Patterson MS, van Geuns RJ, van Miegham C, Serruys PW. Magnetic Navigation in Coronary Interventions. *Nat Clin Pract Cardiovasc Med* 2008 ;5(3):148-56.

[3] García-García H, Tsuchida K, Meulenbrug H, Ong ATL, van der Giessen WJ, Serruys PW. Magnetic navigation in a coronary phantom: Experimental results. *EuroIntervention* 2005;1:321–328.

[4] Ramcharitar S, Patterson MS, van Geuns RJ, van der Ent M, Sianos G, Welten GM, van Domburg RT, Serruys PW. A randomised controlled study comparing conventional and magnetic guidewires in a two-dimensional branching tortuous phantom simulating angulated coronary vessels. *Catheter Cardiovasc Intervention.* Catheter Cardiovasc Interv. 2007 Nov 1;70(5):662-8.

[5] Ramcharitar S, Patterson MS, van Geuns RJ, Serruys PW. Magnetic navigation system used successfully to cross a crushed stent in a bifurcation that failed with conventional wires. *Catheter Cardiovasc Interv* 2007;69:852–855.

[6] Riezebos RK, Patterson MS, Braat JH, Ramcharitar S, Serruys PW, Kiemeneij F. Primary Percutaneous Coronary Intervention using Magnetic Navigation. *Eurointervention* Web publication 2008. www.europcronline.com/eurointervention/authors/?authorId=1500.

[7] Patterson MS, Ramcharitar S. Serruys PW. Magnetically Supported PCI: success after failed surgery and conventional PCI. *Cath Lab Digest* 2007;15(3):1-14.

[8] Bach RG, Leach C, Milov SA, Lindsay BD. Use of magnetic navigation to facilitate transcatheter alcohol septal ablation for hypertrophic obstructive cardiomyopathy. *J Invasive Cardiol* 2006;18:E176–E178.

[9] Tsuchida K, van der Giessen WJ, Patterson M, Tanimoto S, García-García HM, Regar E, Ligthart JMR, Maugenest A-M, Maatrijk G, Wentzel JJ, Serruys PW. *In Vivo* Validation of A Novel Three-Dimensional Quantitative Coronary Angiography System (CardiOp-B): Comparison with A Conventional Two-Dimensional System (CAAS II) and with Special Reference to Optical Coherence Tomography. *Eurointervention* 2007; 3(1):
100-108.

[10] Ramcharitar S, Daeman J, Patterson MS, van Guens RJ, Boersma E, Serruys PW, van der Giessen WJ. The first direct in vivo comparison of two commercially available 3-

Dimensional Quantitative Coronary Angiography systems. *Cathet Cardiovasc Interv* 2008 Jan 1;71(1):44-50.

[11] Tsuchida K, Garcıa-Garcıa HM, Tanimoto S, Ong ATL, Ruchir S, van der Ent M, Sianos G, van der Giessen WJ. Feasibility and safety of guidewire navigation using a magnetic navigation system in coronary artery stenoses. *EuroIntervention* 2005;1:329–335.

[12] Tsuchida K, Garcia-Garcia HM, van der Giessen WJ, McFadden EP, van der Ent M, Sianos G, Meulenbrug H, Ong AT, Serruys PW. Guidewire navigation in coronary artery stenoses using a novel magnetic navigation system: First clinical experience. *Catheter Cardiovasc Interv* 2006;67:356–363.

[13] Atmakuri SR, Lev EI, Alviar C, Ibarra E, Raizner AE, Solomon SL, Kleiman NS. Initial experience with a magnetic navigation system for percutaneous coronary intervention in complex coronary artery lesions. *J Am Coll Cardiol* 2006; 47:515–521.

[14] Schneider MA, Hoch FV, Neuser H, Brunn J, Koller ML, Gietzen F, Schamberger R, Kerber S, Schumacher B. Magnetic-Guided Percutaneous Coronary Intervention Enabled by Two-Dimensional Guidewire Steering and Three-Dimensional Virtual Angioscopy: Initial Experiences in Daily Clinical Practice. *J Interv Cardiol.* 2008 Jan 28.

[15] Perin EC, Silva GV, Fernandes MR, Munger T, Pandey A, Sehra R, Talcott M, Bichard CJ, Creed J, Wong JWC, Oliveira OM, Zheng Y, Canals J, Cardoso CO, Patterson MS, Serruys PW. First experience with remote left ventricular mapping and transendocardial cell injection with a novel integrated magnetic navigation-guided electromechanical mapping system. *Eurointervention* 2007;3:142–148.

[16] Kiemeneij F, Patterson MS, Amoroso G, Laarman GJ, Slagboom T. Use of the Stereotaxis Niobe® Magnetic Navigation System for Percutaneous Coronary Intervention Using the Radial Approach: Results from 350 Consecutive Patients. *Cathet Cardiovasc Interv* 2008 Mar 1;71(4):510-6.

[17] Patterson MS, Duckers E, Ramcharitar S, Meliga E, van Weenen S, Maugenest A-M, Perin E, Serruys PW. Magnetically Supported Procedures and Cardiac Regeneration. *Eurointervention* Supplement 2007; 2(supp B), B42-B46.

[18] Patterson MS, Hoeks SE, Tanimoto S, van Mieghem C, Ramcharitar S, van Domburg RT, Serruys PW. A simple score for predicting prolonged crossing times to select patients who would benefit from a magnetic percutaneous coronary intervention. *European Heart Journal* , 2007; 28 ((Abstract Supplement P4762)):847-848.

[19] Patterson MS, Hoeks SE, Rijkenberg S, Ramchartar S, van Geuns RJ, Tanimoto S, van Domburg RT, Serruys PW. *Integration of 3D reconstruction in the SELection criteria for Excessive Crossing Times for Magnetically Supported Percutaneous Coronary Intervention.* SELECT-MP. Submitted to Eurointervention *in Press.*

In: Heart Disease in Men
Editors: A.B. Todd and M.H. Mosley, pp. 145-166
ISBN: 978-1-60692-297-2

Chapter 6

PSYCHOSOCIAL FUNCTIONING IN ADULTS WITH CONGENITAL HEART DISEASE: THE SAME IN MALES AS IN FEMALES?

***Elisabeth H.M. van Rijen*[1] *and Elisabeth M.W.J. Utens*[2]**

[1]Institute of Psychology, Erasmus University Rotterdam
Rotterdam, The Netherlands
[2]Department of Child and Adolescent Psychiatry, Erasmus MC - Sophia Children's Hospital, Rotterdam, The Netherlands

Abstract

As a result of dramatically improved survival rates for children with congenital heart disease, a new patient population of adults with congenital heart disease has emerged over the last decades. Since very little was known about long-term psychosocial outcomes in these patients, several studies have been done into the psychosocial functioning of adults with congenital heart disease.

For most of these studies, the main question has been whether psychosocial functioning of adults with congenital heart disease was comparable to that of their healthy peers from the general population. Within the population of adults with congenital heart disease, the effects of cardiac diagnosis and operative variables on psychosocial functioning have frequently been described. However, the effects of *gender* on psychosocial outcome in these patients have rarely been studied.

In most studies, no comparisons were made between male respectively female patients with same-sex persons from the general population, nor has the role of gender been explored directly between male versus female patients with congenital heart disease. This can be considered remarkable, since gender-differences in psychosocial functioning have been found in the general population. Therefore it seems unwarranted to assume that the psychosocial functioning of males with congenital heart disease will be comparable to that of female patients.

Introduction

Over the last decades, major advances in diagnostic and surgical techniques and medical treatment of Congenital Heart Disease (ConHD) have lead to dramatically higher survival rates in children with ConHD (Boneva et al., 2001). With more children with ConHD reaching adulthood, the population of adult patients with ConHD has rapidly increased. Since little was known about these patients' functioning and adjustment in adult life, several studies have been performed over the years into the psychosocial functioning of adults with ConHD. Most of these studies have compared the psychosocial functioning of ConHD adults with that of healthy peers. Also, the influence of medical variables (e.g. cardiac diagnoses, surgical techniques) on psychosocial outcome has been studied by several authors.

Although *gender differences* in emotional functioning are known to exist in the general population (Hofstra et al., 2000) and gender-specific normative data are available for many assessment instruments into emotional functioning (e.g. Achenbach, 1997; Aaronson et al., 1998), gender effects have, strangely enough, hardly been taken into account in studies into psychosocial functioning of adults with ConHD. Only few studies have compared male and female patients with same-sex persons from the general population (between-subject design), or have explored the role of gender directly between male and female patients with congenital heart disease (within-subject design). This can be considered remarkable, for several reasons. Firstly, as stated above, gender-differences in psychosocial functioning are well-known to exist in the general population. Secondly, gender differences are generally considered when evaluating medical outcomes of ConHD patients (e.g. Klitzner et al., 2006; Moons et al., 2006a). Thirdly, the consequences of ConHD for adult life might be different for males as for females. Adult life might present different barriers for male and female ConHD patients. Female ConHD patients can be concerned over and hampered by disease-specific uncertainties regarding the surgical scar, anticonception, pregnancy, etc (Van Rijen, 2003; Reid et al., 2008). Male ConHD patients may be hampered more by problems with employment, carreer or participation in sports., etc. It therefore seems unwarranted to assume that the psychosocial functioning of males with congenital heart disease will be comparable to that of female patients.

In this chapter, differences in psychosocial well-being between males and females with congenital heart disease that have been reported, will be discussed. Outcomes on psychosocial functioning that will be discussed include

I. emotional functioning, and
II. subjective health status and health-related quality of life.

Moreover, factors relating to

III. differences in psychosocial functioning between males and females with ConHD

will be discussed, such as body image; feelings regarding the surgical scar; relational, psychosexual, and reproductive issues; and styles of coping.

I. Emotional Functioning

Contradictory findings have been reported as to emotional functioning in adults with ConHD (Kovacs et al., 2005). Mostly negative outcomes have been found in this patient population (Brandhagen et al., 1991; Utens et al., 1998; Popelova et al., 2001; Bromberg et al., 2003; Van Rijen et al., 2005a; Geyer et al., 2006a). Some favorable outcomes regarding personality traits have been reported by Utens et al. (1994) and Van Rijen et al. (2003). Van der Rijken (2007) did not find any differences in the level of emotional and behavioral problems between an adult ConHD sample and a normative group. Cox et al. (2002) even found a low prevalence of psychopathology in adults with ConHD, but used orthopedic patients as a reference group.

In the section below, an overview of

1. long-term outcome of emotional functioning, and
2. gender-specific effects

will be given.

1. Long-term Outcome of Emotional Functioning

Differences in sample size, sample composition with regard to the type of ConHD, and assessment procedures (questionnaires, interviews), make it hard to compare the results from different studies. Table 1 provides an overview of different studies into emotional functioning of adults with ConHD, with a detailed description of study characteristics and results. The studies described all included heterogeneous samples with various types of ConHD. These studies can be divided into

1. comparisons with normative samples from the general population,
2. comparisons with somatic reference samples, and
3. ratings of psychiatric diagnostic criteria.

The findings of these studies will globally be discussed, followed by:

4. a summary of long-term outcome of emotional functioning.

1.1. Comparisons with Normative Samples from the General Population

Different types of instruments have been used to compare emotional functioning in adults with ConHD with that of healthy peers. Within the area of emotional functioning, these instruments have different scopes of measurement which can roughly be divided into

1. psychopathological symptoms,
2. emotional and behavioral problems, and
3. personality traits.

Table 1. Studies into emotional functioning of adults with ConHD (I)

Authors	Sample size (n)	Age range (in years)	Instrument	Rating of results (+/≈/-)[a]	Results
1.1. Comparisons with normative samples					
1.1.1. Psychopathological symptoms					
Brandhagen et al. (1991)	168	24-42	SCL-90-R	-	ConHD sample reported higher levels of obsessive compulsive thoughts, interpersonal sensitivity, depression, anxiety, hostility, phobic anxiety, paranoid ideation, and psychoticism, compared to a normative sample.
Bromberg et al. (2003)	22	19-60	BSI (global symptom index, and anxiety and depression subscales)		27.3% of the ConHD sample reported pathological emotional functioning.
Geyer et al. (2006a)	361	14-45	BSI	-	ConHD sample reported higher levels of somatization, obsessive compulsive thoughts, interpersonal sensitivity, anxiety, hostility, and paranoid ideation, compared to a normative sample.
1.1.2. Emotional and behavioral problems					
Utens et al. (1998)	166	19-25	YASR	-	Proportions of ConHD patients scoring in the psychopathological range were higher than those in the general population, which was mainly due to scores of 22-25-year-old-males.
				-/+	ConHD patients reported more problems on only 2 out of 7 problem areas: more somatic complaints and more strange behavior and ideas (including obsessions and hallucinations) compared to a normative group.
Van Rijen et al. (2005a)	251	20-32	YASR	-	Proportions of ConHD patients scoring in the psychopathological range were higher than those in the general population.
				-	ConHD patients reported more somatic complaints compared to a normative group.
			YABCL	-	Proportions of ConHD patients scoring in the psychopathological range were higher than those in the general population.
				-	ConHD patients show more anxious or depressed behavior, withdrawn behavior, somatic complaints, thought problems, attention problems, intrusive behavior, and aggressive behavior, compared to a normative group.

Table 1. Continued

Authors	Sample size (n)	Age range (in years)	Instrument	Rating of results (+/≈/-)[a]	Results
Van der Rijken et al. (2007)	48	18-27	YASR	≈	No differences in emotional and behavioral problems were found between a ConHD sample and normative sample.
1.1.3. Personality traits					
Utens et al. (1994)	278	18-35	DPQ	+	ConHD patients reported fewer feelings of hostility and neuroticism and a higher self-esteem compared to a normative sample.
Van Rijen et al. (2003)	362	20-46	DPQ	+	ConHD patients reported fewer feelings of hostility and neuroticism and a higher self-esteem compared to a normative sample
1.2. Comparisons with somatic reference samples					
Cox et al. (2002)	87	17-73	HADS	+	ConHD patients obtained more favorable scores compared to a reference group of orthopedic patients, with borderline significance.
			GHQ	+	ConHD patients obtained more favorable scores compared to a reference group of orthopedic patients.
1.3. Ratings of psychiatric diagnostic criteria					
Horner et al. (2000)	29	26-56	Interview DSM-III-R criteria		4 out of 29 ConHD patients met the criteria for a major depressive disorder, and 5 out of 29 ConHD patients were diagnosed with panic disorder.
Popelova et al. (2001)	32	19-64	Zung's Questionnaire		Depression was found in 34% of the ConHD patients.
Bromberg et al. (2003)	22	19-60	Interview DSM-IV-criteria		27.3% of the ConHD sample met the criteria for a depressive episode and 9.1% met the criteria for a anxiety disorder.

Note. ConHD = Congenital heart disease, SCL-90-R = Symptom-Checklist-90-Revised, BSI = Brief Symptom Inventory, YASR = Young Adult Behavior Checklist, YABCL = Young Adult Behavior Checklist, DPQ = Dutch Personality Questionnaire, HADS = Hospital and Anxiety Questionnaire, GHQ = General Health Questionnaire, DSM = Diagnostic and Statistical Manual

[a] +: results of ConHD sample are more favorable than those of a normative group.

≈: results of ConHD sample are similar to those of a normative group.

-: results of ConHD sample are less favorable than those of a normative group.

1.1.1. Psychopathological Symptoms

Brandhagen et al. (1991) used the *Symptom Checklist-90-Revised (SCL-90-R*; Derogatis, 1977), a self-report instrument which can be used to assess a broad range of psychological problems and symptoms of psychopathology. Geyer et al. (2006a) used a shortened version of the SCL-90, namely the *Brief Symptom Inventory (BSI*; Derogatis & Melisaratos, 1983). Both Brandhagen et al. (1991) and Geyer et al. (2006a) found that ConHD patients showed a large variety and elevated levels of psychopathological symptoms, compared to normative samples. Bromberg et al. (2003), who studied a sample of ConHD patients with no apparent symptoms of depression or anxiety, also found pathological emotional functioning on the BSI.

1.1.2. Emotional and Behavioral Problems

Several studies used the *Young Adult Self-Report* (*YASR*; Achenbach, 1997), a self-report questionnaire, which contains syndrome scales and two broad-band groupings of syndromes: internalizing problems (anxious, depressed and withdrawn behavior) and externalizing problems (intrusive, delinquent and aggressive behavior). Utens et al. (1998) and Van Rijen et al. (2005a) both found increased levels of emotional and behavioral problems in adult ConHD patients, compared to normative groups. In the study of Van Rijken et al. (2007) no differences on the YASR were reported between a sample of adult ConHD patients and a normative sample. Van Rijen et al. (2005a) also used the *Young Adult Behavior Checklist* (*YABCL*; Achenbach, 1997), an instrument parallel to the YASR, to be completed by an other informant who is familiar with the ConHD patient (e.g. parent or spouse). On these other-informant reports of the patients' emotional and behavioral problems (YABCL), differences between the ConHD patient sample and the normative group were even more pronounced compared to the self-reports (YASR).

1.1.3. Personality Traits

Utens et al. (1994) and Van Rijen et al. (2003) used the *Dutch Personality Questionnaire* (*DPQ*; Luteijn et al., 1985) to assess personality traits in their cohort. In both studies, the ConHD patients showed favorable outcomes on the personality traits neuroticism, self-esteem and hostility, compared to a normative sample.

Since emotional and behavioral problems were found in this same cohort (Utens et al., 1998, Van Rijen et al., 2005a), these favorable outcomes are quite remarkable. The difference between the emotional and behavioral outcomes, assessed by the YASR and YABCL and the personality trait-outcomes, found on the DPQ can be explained by the way items are formulated in the questionnaires concerned. The DPQ contains more globally formulated items concerning abstract personality traits, whereas the YASR and YABCL contain more concrete items concerning observable emotional and behavioral problems. Possibly overcompensation and denial, which have been suggested for adults with ConHD (Utens et al., 1994; Van Rijen et al., 2005a), underlie the favorable outcomes as to the personality traits, while the existence of concrete emotional and behavioral problems is more difficult to deny.

1.2. Comparisons with a Somatic Reference Sample

Cox et al. (2002) used the *Hospital Anxiety and Depression Scale* (HADS; Zigmond & Snaith, 1983) and the *General Health Questionnaire* (*GHQ*; Goldberg, 1985), a more global (self-report) screening device for minor (non-psychotic) disorders. On both instruments, more favorable outcomes were found for the ConHD patient sample compared to a reference sample of orthopedic patients.

These favorable findings might partly be explained by the relatively high prevalence of psychological problems in the reference sample of orthopedic patients, since these patients are frequently referred after traumatic events (e.g. traffic accidents), which might lead to psychological sequelae. Finding an appropriate comparison sample is a challenge in studies concerning patients with ConHD (Miatton et al., 2006). The advantage of somatic reference samples is that they have some experiences (e.g. hospitalizations) in common with ConHD patients, so that e.g. psychological problems can more easily be attributed to specific medical experiences (e.g. open heart surgery). However, somatic samples may differ from each other in many aspects, and comparisons between them do not provide any information about the patients' functioning in comparison to the general population. Moreover, relative small comparison samples encompass the risk of finding chance findings, whereas larger normative groups have the strength to be more representative for the general population.

1.3. Ratings of Psychiatric Diagnostic Criteria

In stead of comparing emotional functioning of adult ConHD patients with that of normative or somatic reference samples, some studies performed ratings of psychiatric diagnostic criteria to establish which and how many patients could be diagnosed with specific mental disorders.

Popelova et al. (2001) used *Zung's questionnaire* (Zung, 1965), a self-rating instrument that focuses specifically on depression, and found that in about one third of a sample of cyanotic ConHD patients, depression was found to be present.

In two studies (Horner et al., 2000; Bromberg et al., 2003), a structured interview was used to determine how many ConHD patients met respectively the *DSM-III-R or DSM-IV (Diagnostic and Statistical Manual) criteria of psychiatric illnesses*. Both studies (Horner et al., 2000; Bromberg et al., 2003) identified depressive and anxiety disorders in adults with ConHD.

1.4. A Summary of Long-term Outcome of Emotional Functioning

In conclusion, different emotional and behavioral outcomes have been reported in adults with ConHD, varying from no difference with normative groups, to positive findings on personality traits, but mostly elevated levels of problems have been reported, among which are internalized problems (anxiety, depression, interpersonal difficulties or withdrawn behavior), externalized problems (hostility, intrusive and aggressive behavior), and even symptoms that may indicate psychotic disorders (see Table 1).

In our opinion screening and treatment for psychopathology in adult patients with ConHD, should be provided at an early stage, since at younger age these symptoms appear to be less persistent and better treatable (Van Rijen et al., 2005a). Congenital cardiologists should have the opportunity to refer patients with psychosocial problems to psychologists who are specialized in this very unique field.

2. Gender-specific Effects

Although gender differences in prevalence of emotional difficulties have been reported for several of the above mentioned instruments (e.g. GHQ (Koeter & Ormel, 1991), SCL-90 (Hafkenscheid, 1993), YASR (Achenbach, 1997)), in studies regarding patients with ConHD, gender effects have been neglected. Of the studies mentioned above, Utens et al. (1994, 1998), Van Rijen et al. (2003, 2005a), Geyer et al. (2006a), and Van der Rijken et al. (2007) did study gender differences in emotional functioning of adults with ConHD.

Regarding psychopathological symptoms, Geyer et al. (2006a) made no direct comparison between male and female patients, but compared male and female patients separately with same-sex peers from a normative group. ConHD females in the age of 14 to 24 years showed no differences in psychopathological symptoms compared to normative peers. In the age of 25 to 35 years, higher interpersonal sensitivity, anxiety and aggression were reported in ConHD females compared to normative peers. ConHD females in the age of 36 to 45 years showed higher reports of obsessive compulsive thoughts and paranoid ideation compared to the normative group. In contrast, ConHD males reported more problems compared to normative peers in all of these areas (interpersonal sensitivity, anxiety, aggression, obsessive compulsive thoughts, paranoid ideation) over all age groups. Moreover, higher reports of somatization, depression, phobic anxiety and psychoticism were also observed in two or three age groups for ConHD males in comparison to normative peers.

With respect to behavioral and emotional problems, Utens et al. (1998) found that significantly more 22 to 25 year old male ConHD patients scored in the clinical range compared to same sex- and same age peers from the general population. Van Rijen et al. (2005a) found that significantly more young female patients (aged 20 to 27 years) scored in the clinical range compared to same sex- and same age peers from the general population, according to both the self- and other informant report. In both studies of Utens et al. (1998) and Van Rijen et al. (2005a), differences between ConHD males and ConHD females on the self-reports of emotional and behavioral problems appeared to be in the same direction as in the general population (e.g. higher reports of delinquent behavior in males, higher reports of somatic complaints in females). However, regarding the other-informant reports of emotional and behavioral problems in the ConHD patients (filled in by someone familiar to the patient), ConHD males scored more favorably than ConHD females on attention problems, intrusive behavior and externalizing problems, whereas in the reference group, the reversed situation was observed (Van Rijen et al., 2005a). Van der Rijken (2007) who also used the YASR, found no differences between male and female ConHD patients.

Regarding personality traits, both Utens et al. (1994) and Van Rijen et al. (2003) found, in accordance with gender differences reported in the reference group, higher complaints of neuroticism in ConHD females compared to ConHD males. Moreover, Van Rijen et al. (2003) found lower self-esteem in ConHD females, compared to ConHD males.

In summary, except for one study that did not find any gender differences between ConHD males and ConHD females (Van der Rijken, et al., 2007), perhaps due to a small sample size, studies that looked into gender differences in larger samples (Utens et al., 1994; Utens et al., 1998; Van Rijen et al., 2003, Van Rijen et al., 2005a; Geyer et al., 2006a) did find differences in emotional functioning between ConHD males and ConHD females. However, the observed gender differences are not all in the same direction. Compared to normative groups, Utens et al. (1998) found higher reports of emotional and behavioral problems in young ConHD males, Van Rijen et al. (2005a) found higher problem levels in young ConHD females, and Geyer et al. (2006a) found higher levels of psychopathological symptoms in both ConHD females and ConHD males, however far more pronounced in ConHD males. In accordance with the general population, ConHD males showed somewhat more favorable outcomes on personality traits compared to ConHD females (Utens et al., 1994; Van Rijen et al., 2003). Results on gender differences in emotional functioning in ConHD adults have thus far been inconclusive.

II. Subjective Health Status and Health-Related Quality of Life

The last decades, next to morbidity and mortality, subjective health status and health-related quality of life have become important outcome measures to evaluate the efficacy of medical interventions. The way patients themselves experience and evaluate their health subjectively can be very determining for their well-being (Kamphuis et al., 2002).

In the field of research that is generally referred to as "quality of life", "subjective health status" and "health-related quality of life" are often used as equivalents but a clear distinction should be made between these concepts. Subjective health status refers to the patient's perception and assessment of his or her state of abilities and actual, more objective problems in functioning , whereas health-related quality of life can be considered a multidimensional construct, which refers to the patient's subjective evaluation, personal feelings and emotional reaction to this state of abilities.

Subjective health status and health-related quality of life have frequently been studied in patients with ConHD. Although some studies have reported serious restrictions in different domains of subjective health status or health-related quality of life in adults with ConHD (Kamphuis et al., 2002; Lane et al., 2002; Simko & McGinnis, 2003; Rose et al., 2005), other studies found that, besides possible physical limitations, the perceived health of adult ConHD patients further was comparable or sometimes even better than that of the general population (Saliba et al., 2001; Daliento et al., 2005; Van Rijen et al., 2005b; Moons et al., 2006b). In Table 2, studies in this area are categorized by their domains of assessment, which were qualified as either subjective health status, or health-related quality of life. The findings of these studies regarding:

1. long-term outcome of subjective health status, and
2. long-term outcome of health-related quality of life,

will globally be discussed (a more detailed description of study characteristics and specific results is given in Table 2), and will be followed by:

3. a summary of long-term outcome of subjective health status and health-related quality of life,

and a discussion on:

4. gender specific effects.

Table 2. Studies into subjective health status and health-related quality of life of adults with ConHD (II)

Authors	Sample size (n)	Age range (in years)	Instrument	Rating of results (+/≈/-)[a]	Results
1. Subjective health status					
Saliba et al. (2001)	67	17-49	Duke Health Profile	≈	ConHD sample reported physical, mental, social, general, and perceived health, comparable to a reference group from the general population.
Kamphuis et al. (2002)	78	18-32	SF-36	-	ConHD sample reported more limitations in physical activities due to health problems, more limitations in usual role activities due to physical health problems, lower vitality and lower general health perceptions, compared to a reference group from the general population.
Lane et al. (2002)	276	16-85	SF-36	-	ConHD patients with inoperable conditions reported a lower subjective health status than the general population on all SF-36 domains.
				-	ConHD patients deemed surgically cured also reported a lower subjective health status compared to the general population on nearly all SF-36 domains, except for bodily pain.
Simko & McGinnis (2003)	124	18-59	SIP	-	ConHD sample reported poorer psychosocial and physical health compared to a matched control group.
Immer et al. (2005)	154	14-72	SF-36	≈	The total sample of ConHD patients showed normal reports of subjective health status, comparable to a matched control group.
				-	A sub-sample of patients with complete AV-canal defect reported more limitations in physical activities due to health problems and more limitations in usual role activities due to emotional problems.
Daliento et al. (2005)	54	mean age: 32 years	SF-36	-	ConHD sample reported more limitations in physical activities due to health problems, compared to a reference group from the general population.
Rose et al. (2005)	111	mean age: 33 years	WHOQOL-Bref	-	ConHD sample reported more restrictions as to physical health and to a lesser extent as to psychological health compared to a reference group from the general population.
Van Rijen et al. (2005b)	349	20-46	SF-36	-	ConHD sample reported more limitations in physical activities due to health problems, compared to a reference group from the general population.
				+	ConHD sample reported fewer limitations in social activities due to physical or emotional problems, fewer limitations in usual role activities due to emotional problems and less bodily pain compared to a reference group from the general population.

Table 2. Continued

Authors	Sample size (n)	Age range (in years)	Instrument	Rating of results (+/≈/-)[a]	Results
Moons et al. (2006b)	404	18-56	LAS	+	ConHD sample reported more favorable outcome compared to a matched control group of healthy peers.
			SWLS	+	ConHD sample reported more favorable outcome compared to a matched control group of healthy peers.
2. Health-related quality of life					
Kamphuis et al. (2002)	78	18-32	TAAQOL	-	ConHD sample reported lower health-related quality of life regarding gross motor functioning and vitality, compared to a reference group from the general population.
Bol Raap et al. (2007)	28	-	TAAQOL	-	ConHD sample reported lower health-related quality of life regarding cognitive functioning and sleep, compared to a reference group from the general population.
Moons et al. (2006b)	404	18-56	CHD-TAAQOL (analysis on item-level)	-	TAAQOL-items that referred to specific symptoms, doctor visits, diet recommendations, and physical limitations, were more distressing for the ConHD patients than for a matched control group.
Moons et al. (2007)	441	18-57	CHD-TAAQOL (subscale sexual activity)	+	ConHD sample reported less sexual problems regarding the items 'not enjoying having sex', and 'worrying about your sex life', compared to a matched control group.
				-	ConHD sample reported more distress regarding 'worrying about your sex life', compared to a matched control group.

Note. ConHD = Congenital heart disease, Sf-36 = Short Form Health Survey, SIP = Sickness Impact Profile, WHOQOL-Bref = Shortened version of the Quality of Life Questionnaire of the World Health Organization, LAS = Linear Analog Scale, SWLS = Satisfaction with Life Scale, TAAQOL = TNO-AZL Quality of Life instrument, CHD-TAAQOL = Congenital Heart Disease - TNO-AZL Quality of Life instrument.

[a.] +: results of ConHD sample are more favorable than those of a normative group.
≈: results of ConHD sample are similar to those of a normative group.
-: results of ConHD sample are less favorable than those of a normative group.

1. Long-term Outcome of Subjective Health Status

Several studies into adults with ConHD used the *Short Form Health Survey* (*SF-36*; Ware & Sherbourne, 1992), a self-report questionnaire for subjective health status (e.g. Kamphuis et al., 2002; Lane et al., 2002; Immer et al., 2004; Daliento et al., 2005; Van Rijen et al., 2005b). The SF-36 assesses eight health concepts: limitations in physical activities due to health problems, limitations in social activities due to physical or emotional problems, limitations in usual role activities due to physical health problems, limitations in usual role activities due to emotional problems, bodily pain, general mental health, vitality, and general health perceptions.

Kamphuis et al. (2002), who studied a sample of adult patients operated for complex ConHD (e.g. by Senning, Mustard, or Rastelli procedures) found significantly more limitations, particularly in physical functioning, compared to the general population. Lane et al. (2002) used the SF-36 in a sample of ConHD patients representing treatment categories that varied from 'surgically cured' to 'inoperable'. Patients with inoperable conditions reported a lower subjective health status than the general population on all domains, but, surprisingly, patients deemed surgically cured also reported a lower subjective health status. In a sample of ConHD patients with various cyanotic and acyanotic diagnoses, Immer et al. (2005) found normal reports of subjective health status, comparable to the general population for the total sample, except for a sub-sample of patients with complete AV-canal defect, who reported more limitations. Daliento et al. (2005) found a higher report of limitations in physical activities in a sample of adults with repaired Tetralogy of Fallot, but furthermore a subjective health status that was comparable to the general population. In a sample of patients with various types of ConHD, Van Rijen et al. (2005b) found more physical limitations, but also more favorable reports of subjective health status compared to the general population.

A large variety of self-report questionnaires encompassing subjective health status has been used in other studies into adults with ConHD (e.g. Saliba et al., 2001; Simko & McGinnis, 2003; Rose et al., 2005, Moons et al., 2006b). Saliba et al. (2001), who used the *Duke Health Profile* (Parkerson et al., 1990), found that the subjective health status of patients with univentricular hearts was similar to that of the normal population. Simko & McGinnis (2003) used the *Sickness Impact Profile* (Damiano, 1996), an instrument which measures the way that sickness changes daily behavior and activities, and found higher dysfunction in a sample of ConHD patients with cyanotic as well as acyanotic diagnoses, compared to a matched control group. Rose et al. (2005) applied the *shortened version of the Quality of Life Questionnaire of the World Health Organization* (*WHOQOL-Bref*; The WHOQOL-Group, 1998), and also found a high report of restrictions in a sample of patients with various diagnoses of ConHD. Moons et al. (2006b) reported more favorable subjective health status in sample of patients with various diagnoses of ConHD, compared to a matched control group on both a *Linear Analog Scale* (*LAS*) and the *Satisfaction with Life Scale* (*SWLS*; Diener et al., 1985).

2. Long-term Outcome of Health-related Quality of Life

In contrast to the above mentioned instruments, which measure subjective health status, the *TNO-AZL Quality of Life instrument* (*TAAQOL*; Fekkes et al., 2001) assesses health-related quality of life. That is, the TAAQOL not only measures the patient's perception of functioning, but also the patient's personal feelings regarding their functioning. The TAAQOL measures health-related quality of life in 12 domains: gross motor functioning, fine motor functioning, pain, sleeping, cognitive functioning, social functioning, daily activities, sexual activity, vitality, happiness, depressive moods and aggressiveness. Kamphuis et al. (2002) and Bol Raap et al. (2007) used the TAAQOL in samples of patients with respectively complex ConHD and repaired ventricular septal defects and reported impaired health-related quality of life on different domains. Moons et al. (2006b) compared their patient sample including various diagnoses of ConHD with a matched control group on the *Congenital Heart Disease TNO-AZL Quality of Life instrument* (*CHD-TAAQOL*; Kamphuis et al., 2004; a disease-specific version of the TAAQOL for ConHD patients) at item level. CHD-TAAQOL-items that were more distressing for the ConHD patients than for the control group referred to specific symptoms, doctor visits, diet recommendations, and physical limitations. In another study, Moons et al. (2007) focused on 5 (global) items of the CHD-TAAQOL-scale 'sexual activity' within the same cohort. The ConHD patients reported fewer sexual problems than did healthy controls, but if problems occurred, patients reported more distress regarding worries about their sex lives.

3. A Summary of Long-term Outcome of Subjective Health Status and Health-Related Quality of Life

In summary, reduced subjective health status and health-related quality of life has frequently been reported in adults with ConHD, reflecting limitations in physical health as well as limitations in emotional functioning. Experiencing limitations regarding health is not restricted to patients with the most severe diagnoses, but is also seen in patients with relatively mild ConHD.

As to limitations in emotional functioning, we already recommended early screening and psychological treatment for adult patients with ConHD. As to limitations in physical functioning, monitored physical training might help patients (with poor physical condition) to feel more secure about their bodily function.

4. Gender-specific Effects

Gender differences have been reported for several of the above mentioned instruments (e.g. SF-36 (Aaronson et al., 1998), WHOQOL (Masthoff et al., 2005)). Although several studies took gender differences into account, by either correcting for gender by including it as a covariate in statistical analyses (Kamphuis et al., 2002; Bol Raap et al., 2007), or using a gender-matched control group (Simko & McGinnis, 2003; Immer et al., 2004; Moons et al., 2006b), only few studies made direct comparisons between males and females with ConHD regarding their subjective health status or health-related quality of life (Van Rijen et al., 2005b; Moons et al., 2007).

Van Rijen et al. (2005b) found that ConHD males reported better performance in physical activities, less interference with normal social activities, better mental health and better vitality compared to ConHD females.

In the study of Moons et al. (2007), sexual problems like 'not enjoying having sex', 'being insecure about having sex', and 'not being aroused while having sex', occurred more often in ConHD females than in ConHD males. Moreover, ConHD females experienced more distress from 'being insecure about having sex' than ConHD males.

In both the study of Van Rijen et al. (2005b) and that of Moons et al (2007) gender differences in subjective health status and health-related quality of life were in favor of ConHD males. These gender differences are in line with those found in the general population, but indicate nonetheless that gender is an important indicator of subjectively perceived health in ConHD patients.

III. Differences in Psychosocial Functioning between Males and Females with Congenital Heart Disease

It is remarkable that effects of gender on the two domains of psychosocial functioning discussed, namely emotional functioning respectively health status and health-related quality of life, have had so little attention until now.

Comparing outcomes of ConHD males with those of ConHD females directly, showed results mainly in favor of ConHD males. Whereas patterns of reduced subjective health status and health-related quality of life in ConHD females are overall in line with gender differences found in the general population, the findings concerning emotional and behavioral problems show a different picture. Here, Van Rijen et al. (2005a) found that, in contrast to self-reports, the other-informant reports of emotional and behavioral problems revealed that female ConHD patients showed more attention problems, intrusive behavior and externalizing problems compared to male patients, while in the general population, the reserved situation was observed.

Studies that compared male and female patients with same sex peers from the general population have yielded less consistent results. Higher reports of problems in emotional functioning in both ConHD males (Utens et al., 1998, Geyer et al., 2006a) and ConHD females (Van Rijen et al., 2005a; Geyer et al., 2006a), have been reported.

Since only few studies have studied gender differences in psychosocial functioning of adults with ConHD, it is hard to draw firm conclusions. Both male as female adults with ConHD, might be hampered in psychosocial functioning, compared to healthy peers. In comparison to ConHD males, psychosocial problems seem to be more prevalent in ConHD females. Partially, this could reflect gender differences in the general population, however some psychosocial problems might be enlarged or specific for ConHD females. In the sections below,

1. factors related to gender-specific effects
2. in adults with congenital heart disease will be discussed, which will be concluded by a our final answer to the question:

"Psychosocial functioning, the same in males as in females?"

1. Factors Related to Gender-specific Effects

Males and females with ConHD may face different obstacles in adulthood, which will have a differential impact on emotional adjustment. In the section below, the following factors, related to gender-specific effects in psychosocial functioning of adults with congenital heart disease, will be discussed:

1. body image,
2. feelings regarding the surgical scar,
3. relational, psychosexual, and reproductive issues,
4. styles of coping.

1.1. Body Image

ConHD is often reflected in visual signs as to the patient's physical appearance. Surgical scars or bluish coloring of the skin from cyanosis may have a negative impact on the patient's body image (Gantt, 1992; Kovacs et al., 2005). As a result of these visible signs adults with ConHD can be hampered in their strive to be considered "normal" and "the same as others" (Claessens et al., 2005; Tong et al., 1998). Geyer et al. (2006b) found that the perception of body image was a stronger predictor for psychopathological symptoms reported in adult ConHD patients, compared to limitations of activity and impaired cardiac performance. Geyer et al. (2006b) evaluated negative aspects of body image (rejection of the body) as well as positive aspects (vitality). Rejection of the body was found to have strong effects on a wide range of psychopathological symptoms for both male as female ConHD patients, however more pronounced in ConHD males. Lack of vitality was primarily associated with psychopathological symptoms in ConHD females. Geyer et al. (2006b) suggested that different underlying problems such as perception of the body as deficient and injured in ConHD males, and to a lesser extent, lack of vitality in ConHD females, may be responsible for increased levels of psychopathology in respectively males and females with ConHD.

1.2. Feelings Regarding the Surgical Scar

Open heart operations often leave considerable scars on the patients' chests. Adults have been reported to dislike or feel restricted by the scar (Van Rijen et al., 2004a; Crossland et al., 2005) or to try to conceal the scar by clothing or cosmetics (Horner et al., 2000; Crossland et al., 2005; Kantoch et al., 2006). Negative feelings regarding the surgical scar have a negative impact on emotional and behavior problems (van Rijen et al., 2004a) and feelings of self-esteem and self-confidence (Kantoch et al. 2006) in adults with ConHD. In the study by Van Rijen et al. (2004a), 40.5% of female patients and 18.9% of male patients reported to feel restricted by the scar. In the study of Kantoch et al. (2006) 62% of the male patients and 53% of the female patients reported being disfigured by the scar (difference not statistically significant). However, more female than male patients reported a negative impact from the scar on self-confidence and self-esteem (respectively 23% vs. 13%, and 25 vs. 15%; difference not statistically significant). Overall, ConHD females seem to be particularly bothered by the surgical scar. Since thoracic scars are unfavorably situated on the chest, they may be a source of uncertainties and discomfort when entering sexual relationships (Gantt, 1992).

1.3. Relational, Psychosexual, and Reproductive Issues

Young adults with ConHD less often live on their own and tend to live longer with their parents compared to normal peers (Kokkonen and Paavilainen., 1992; Utens et al., 1994; Simko et al., 2006). Favorable outcome as to marital status has been reported in adults with ConHD (Ternestedt et al., 2001; Nieminen et al., 2003; Van Rijen et al., 2003; Sairanen et al., 2005; Simko et al., 2006), however some studies found that patients with ConHD get married less often, or get married at a later age (Kokkonen and Paavilainen., 1992; Gersony et al., 2003). Offspring rates in adults with ConHD overall are lower of that of healthy peers (Gersony et al., 2003; Nieminen et al., 2003; Sairanen et al., 2005). Adults with ConHD seem to start families at a later age (Van Rijen et al., 2003). Gersony et al. (1993) found no differences in offspring rates or marital status between male and female ConHD patients.

Young adults with ConHD have been found to be less sexual active, compared to healthy peers (Uzark et al., 1989; Reid et al., 2008). Reid et al. (2008) found that more young adult ConHD females compared to young adult ConHD males were sexual active. This result is in line with rates of sexual behavior reported in chronically ill youth (Suris and Parera, 2005). In the study of Moons et al. (2007) discussed previously (see: Subjective health status and health-related quality of life, Gender-specific effects), ConHD females reported more sexual problems (not enjoying or being aroused during sex, being insecure) and, if problems were present, higher distress as a result of sexual problems, compared to ConHD males.

Young females with ConHD are often concerned about matters as fertility, pregnancy, birth control and genetic transmission (Gantt, 1992; Simko et al., 2006; Reid et al., 2008). Often, ConHD females are very poorly informed about reproductive matters, which leave them with lots of uncertainties (Gantt, 1992; Hargrove et al., 2005). Rogers et al. (2007) found that many ConHD females received poor or no advice about contraception or pregnancy risks from the treating physician.

There is a general tendency for reproduction to be more important for ConHD women than ConHD men at this point in their lives (Reid et al., 2008) Reid et al. (2008) found that female ConHD patients were more concerned compared to male ConHD patients about the risk that any future children might have ConHD, and about their fertility. Especially females with complex ConHD had the highest levels of concerns regarding their fertility, as well as concerns about harmful effects of pregnancy on their own health and their ability to carry a child to term.

Overall, adults with ConHD may show a delay in starting a family life and appear to be less sexual active. Especially ConHD females are at risk for problems regarding sexual function and uncertainties regarding reproductive issues.

1.4. Styles of Coping

As discussed above, patients with ConHD encounter a lot of challenges in adult life. Not all patients respond in the same way to problems they face. Styles of coping, that is personal ways of dealing with problems, can differ widely among patients with ConHD. Van Rijen et al. (2004b) studied styles of coping in a large cohort of ConHD patients. Overall, styles of coping were found to be comparable to those of peers in the general population. Female ConHD patients, however, showed less active problem solving compared to normative females. On the contrary, male ConHD patients showed more favorable styles of coping compared to normative males, such as more seeking of social support, less passive reaction patterns, and less expression of negative emotions. ConHD males seem to have more favorable styles of coping to their disposal than ConHD females, and might therefore be better equipped to deal with the disease-related struggles in adult life.

2. "Psychosocial Functioning, the Same in Males as in Females?"

From the scarce data on gender-specific effects discussed above the picture arises that, overall, ConHD females experience more problems regarding psychosocial functioning compared to ConHD males.

A closer look into the results reveals that female patients may encounter different obstacles in adult life, compared to male patients, with consequently increased levels of problems. Overall, females with ConHD feel more restricted by the surgical scar, have more sexual problems and distress, experience more concerns about reproductive issues and show less favorable styles of coping, compared to male patients. Males with ConHD may feel more disfigured by the scar (but not more restricted), and negative attitudes towards their physical appearance (rejection of the body) may have a larger impact on their emotional functioning, compared to female patients.

In a previous study (Van Rijen et al., 2005a), we suggested that (young) females with ConHD can experience disease-specific uncertainties regarding sexual relationships, offspring, etc., which may put ConHD females more at risk for emotional problems than ConHD males. This explanation is supported by the theoretical model of Cyranowski et al.(2000), who states that females have a preference for close emotional communication, intimacy and responsiveness within interpersonal relationships and develop a sense of self in relation to others, whereas males are more focused on personal autonomy. According to Cyranowski et al. (2000), this difference between sexes explains why females are more likely than males to get depressed when faced with negative life events with interpersonal consequences.

In adulthood, ConHD females may particularly feel hampered by the ConHD when entering sexual relationships (especially when they feel restricted by the surgical scar) and feel concerned about pregnancy-related issues. ConHD males may be at risk for emotional maladjustment when their feelings of autonomy are threatened, e.g. by a distorted body image, or for example when reduced physical abilities limit them in their professional career. As previously suggested by Geyer et al. (2006b), it is evident that different (emotional and physical) processes influence the level of psychosocial problems in respectively male and female adults with ConHD.

Conclusion

In this chapter, gender differences in psychosocial functioning of adults with ConHD were reviewed. Both males and females with ConHD may experience problems in their emotional functioning, subjective health status, or health-related quality of life, compared to healthy peers. However, female patients with ConHD overall seem more hampered in their psychosocial functioning compared to male patients with ConHD.

Different problems may underlie psychosocial problems in respectively female and male ConHD patients. For females with ConHD, these problems may include feeling restricted by the surgical scar, experiencing sexual problems and distress, having concerns about reproductive issues and disposing of less adequate styles of coping. For males with ConHD, having a distorted body image may have a larger impact on their psychosocial functioning.

Implications for Future Research

Since ConHD can have such different impact on adult life for male and female patients, we strongly suggest that effects of gender on long-term psychosocial functioning should be investigated more extensively in future research. Gender-specific effects should not only be studied by comparing males and females with same-sex persons from the general population (between-subject designs), but also by direct comparisons between male and female ConHD patients (within-subject designs), to evaluate the role of gender next to other predictors and correlates of psychosocial functioning.

Implications for Clinical Practice

In assessing the patients' subjective health status and overall well-being, special attention should be given to restrictions young ConHD females experience as to the scar, sexual functioning, fertility status, birth control, pregnancy risks, heritability, and abilities to raise their children.

Sensitive disease-specific patient education on these topics is very important and may relief uncertainties, misconceptions and unnecessary burdens or limitations. It is the more important to discuss these issues since many female patients appear to be poorly informed about these matters. As to entering sexual relationships, subjective restrictions due to the scar should be evaluated instead of the more objective, esthetical aspects. Regarding styles of coping, psychological counseling may enhance more active coping so that particularly ConHD female patients may feel more in control of their situation.

References

Aaronson, N. K., Muller, M., Cohen, P. D. A., Essink-Bot, M. L., Fekkes, M., Sanderman, R., Sprangers, M. A. G., te Velde, A., & Verrips, E. (1998). Translation, validation, and norming of the Dutch language version of the SF-36 Health Survey in community and chronic disease populations. *Journal of Clinical Epidemiology,* **51**(11), 1055-1068.

Achenbach, T. M. (1997). *Manual for the Young Adult Self-Report and Young Adult Behavior Checklist.* Burlington: University of Vermont, Department of Psychiatry.

Bol Raap, G., Meijboom, F. J., Kappetein, A. P., Galema, T. W., Yap, S-C., Bogers, A. J. J. C. (2007). Long-term follow-up and quality of life after closure of ventricular septal defect in adults. *European Journal of Cardio-thoracic Surgery,* **32**, 215-219.

Boneva, R. S., Botto, L. D., Moore, C. A., Yang, Q., Correa, A.., & Erickson J. D. (2001). Mortality associated with congenital heart defects in the United States: Trends and racial disparities, 1979-1997. *Circulation,* **103**, 2376-2381.

Brandhagen, D. J., Feldt, R. H., & Williams, D. E. (1991). Long-term psychologic implications of congenital heart disease: a 25-year follow-up. *Mayo Clinic Proceedings,* **66**(5), 474-479.

Bromberg, J. I., Beasley, P. J., D'Angelo, E. J., Landzberg, M., & DeMaso, D. R. (2003). Depression and anxiety in adults with congenital heart disease: a pilot study. *Heart & Lung,* **32**, 105-110.

Claessens, P., Moons, P., Dierckx de Casterlé, B., Cannaerts, N., Budts, W., Gewillig, M. (2005). What does it mean to live with a congenital heart disease? A qualitative study on the lived experiences of adult patients. *European Journal of Cardiovascular Nursing,* **4**, 3-10.

Cox, D., Lewis, G., Stuart, G., & Murphy, K. (2002). A cross-sectional study of the prevalence of psychopathology in adults with congenital heart disease. *Journal of Psychosomatic Research,* **52**(2), 65-68.

Crossland, D. S., Jackson, S. P., Lyall, R., Hamilton, J. R. L., Hasan, A., Burn, J., & O'Sullivan, J. J. (2005). Patient attitudes to sternotomy and thoracotomy scars. *Thoracic and Cardiovascular Surgeon,* **53**(2), 93-95.

Cyranowski, J. M., Frank, E., Young, E., & Shear, M. K. (2000). Adolescent onset of the gender difference in lifetime rates of major depression: a theoretical model. *Archives of General Psychiatry,* **57**(1), 21-27.

Daliento, L., Mapelli, D., Russo, G., Scarso, P., Limongi, F., Iannizzi, P., Melendugno, A., Mazzotti, E., & Volpe, B. (2005). Health related quality of life in adults with repaired tetralogy of Fallot: psychosocial and cognitive outcomes. *Heart,* **91**, 213-218.

Damiano, A. M. (1996). *The Sickness Impact Profile User's Manual and Interpretation Guide.* Boston, Mass: Medical Outcomes Trust.

Derogatis, L. R., & Melisaratos, N. (1983). The Brief Symptom Inventory: an introductory report. *Psychological Medicine,* **13**, 595-605.

Derogatis, L. R. (1992). *SCL-90-R, administration, scoring & procedures manual-II for the R(evised) version and other instruments of the Psychopathology Rating Scale Series.* Townson: Clinical Psychometric Research Inc.

Diener, E., Emmons, R. A., Larsen, R. J., Griffin, S. The satisfaction with life scale. *J Personality Assessment,* **49**, 71-75.

Fekkes, M., Kamphuis, R. P., Ottenkamp, J., Verrips, E., Vogels, T. G., Kamphuis, M., & Verloove-Vanhorick, S. P. (2001). Health-related quality of life in young adults with minor congenital heart disease. *Psychology and Health,* **16**, 239-250.

Gantt, L. T. (1992). Growing up heartsick: The experiences of young women with congenital heart disease. *Health Care for Women International,* **13**(3), 241-248.

Gersony, W. M., Hayes, C. J., Driscoll, D. J., Keane, J. F., Kidd, L., O'Fallon, W. M., Pieroni, D. R., Wolfe, R. R., & Weidman, W. H. (1993). Second natural history study of congenital heart defects. Quality of life of patients with aortic stenosis, pulmonary stenosis, or ventricular septal defect. *Circulation,* **87**(2 Suppl), I52-65.

Geyer, S., Hessel, A., Kempa, A., Zoege, M., Norozi, K., Wessel, A., & Albani, C. (2006a). Psychological symptoms and body image in patients after surgery for congenital heart disease: comparisons between patients and general population samples. *Psychother Psych Med,* **56**, 425-431.

Geyer, S., Norozi, K., Zoege, M., Kempa, A., Buchhorn, R., & Wessel, A. (2006b). Psychological symptoms in patients after surgery for congenital heart disease. *Cardiology in the Young,* **16**, 540-548.

Goldberg, D. (1985). Identifying psychiatric illness among general medical patients. *British Medical Journal,* **291**, 161-163.

Hafkenscheid, A. (1993). Psychometric evaluation of the Symptom Checklist (SCL-90) in psychiatry inpatients. *Personality and Individual Differences,* **14**, 751-756.

Hargrove, A., Penny, D. J., & Sawyer, S. M. (2005). Sexual and reproductive health in young people with congenital heart disease: A systematic review of the literature. *Pediatric Cardiology,* **26**, 805-811.

Hofstra, M. B., Van der Ende, J., & Verhulst, F. C. (2000). Continuity and change of psychopathology from childhood into adulthood: a 14-year follow-up study. *Journal of the American Academy of Child and Adolescent Psychiatry,* **39**(7), 850-858.

Horner, T., Liberthson, R., & Jellinek, M. S.(2000). Psychosocial profile of adults with complex congenital heart disease. *Mayo Clinic Proceedings,* **75**, 31-36.

Immer, F. F., Althaus, S. M., Berdat, P. A., Saner, H., & Carrel, T. P. (2005). Quality of life and specific problems after cardiac surgery in adolescents and adults with congenital heart disease. *European Journal of Cardiovascular Prevention and Rehabilitation,* **12**(2), 138-143.

Kamphuis, M., Ottenkamp, J., Vliegen, H. W., Vogels, T., Zwinderman, K. H., Kamphuis, R. P., & Verloove-Vanhorick, S. P. (2002). Health related quality of life and health status in adult survivors with previously operated complex congenital heart disease. *Heart,* **87**(4), 356-362.

Kamphuis, M., Zwinderman, K. H., Vogels, T., Vliegen, H. W., Kamphuis, R. P., Ottenkamp, J., et al. (2004). A cardiac-specific health-related quality of life module for young adults with congenital heart disease: Development and validation. *Quality of Life Research,* **13**, 735-745.

Kantoch, M. J., Eustace, J., Collins-Nakai, R. L., Taylor, D. A., Boisvert, J. A., Lysak, P. S. The significance of cardiac surgery scars in adult patients with congenital heart disease. *Kardiologia Polska,* **64**, 51-56.

Klitzner, T. S., Lee, M., Rodriguez, S., & Chang, R. K. (2006). Sex-related disparity in surgical mortality among pediatric patients. *Congenital Heart Disease,* **1**(3), 77-88.

Koeter, M. W. J., & Ormel, J. (1991). *General Health Questionnaire. Nederlandse bewerking. Handleiding.* Lisse: Swets & Zeitlinger.

Kokkonen, J., & Paavilainen, T. (1992). Social adaptation of young adults with congenital heart disease. *International Journal of Cardiology,* **36**(1), 23-29.

Kovacs, A. H., Sears, S. F., & Saidi, A. S. (2005). Biopsychosocial experiences of adults with congenital heart disease: review of the literature. *American Heart Journal,* **150**, 193-201.

Lane, D. A., Lip, G. Y. H., & Millane, T. A. (2002). Quality of life in adults with congenital heart disease. *Heart,* **88**(1), 71-75.

Luteijn, F., Starren, J., & van Dijk, H. (1985). *Manual for the Dutch Personality Questionnaire, revised version. Handleiding bij de NPV, herziene uitgave.* Lisse: Swets & Zeitlinger B.V.

Masthoff, E. D., Trompenaars, F. J., Van Heck, G. L., Hodiamont, P. P., De Vries, J. (2005). Validation of the WHO Quality of Life assessment instrument (WHOQOL-100) in a population of Dutch adult psychiatric outpatients. *European Psychiatry,* **20**, 465-473.

Miatton, M., De Wolf, D., François, K., Thiery, E., & Vingerhoets, G. (2006). Neurocognitive consequences of surgically corrected congenital heart defects: a review. *Neuropsychological Review,* **16**, 65-85.

Moons, P., Van Deyk, K., Dedroog, D., Troost, E., & Budts, W. (2006a). Prevalence of cardiovascular risk factors in adults with congenital heart disease. *European Journal of Cardiovascular Prevention and Rehabilitation,* **13**, 612-616.

Moons, P., Van Deyk, K., De Bleser, L., Marquet, K., Raes, E., De Geest, S., & Budts, W. (2006b). Quality of life and health status in adults with congenital heart disease: a direct comparison with healthy counterparts. European *Journal of Cardiovascular Prevention and Rehabilitation,* **13**(3), 407-413.

Moons, P., Van Deyk, K., Marquet, K., De Bleser, L., Budts, W.,& De Geest, S. (2007). Sexual functioning and congenital heart disease: Something to worry about? *International Journal of Cardiology,* **121**, 30-35.

Nieminen, H., Sairanen, H., Tikanoja, T., Leskinen, M., Ekblad, H., Galambosi, P., Jokinen, E. (2003). Long-term results of pediatric cardiac surgery in Finland: Education, employment, marital status, and parenthood. *Pediatrics,* **112**, 1345-1350.

Parkerson, G. R., Broadhead, W. E., & Tse, C. K. (1990). The Duke health profile. A 17-item measure of health and dysfunction. *Medical Care,* **28**, 1056-1072.

Popelova, J., Slavik, Z., & Skovranek, J. (2001). Are cyanosed adults with congenital cardiac malformations depressed? *Cardiology in the Young,* **11**, 379-384.

Reid, G. J., Siu, S. C., McCrindle, B. W., Irvine, M. J., & Webb, G. D. (2008). Sexual behavior and reproductive concerns among adolescents and young adults with congenital heart disease. *International Journal of Cardiology,* **125**, 332-338.

Rogers, P., Mansour, D., Mattinson, A., & O'Sullivan, J. J. (2007). A collaborative clinic between contraception and sexual health services and an adult congenital heart disease clinic. *J Fam Plann Reprod Health Care,* **33**(1), 17-21.

Rose, M., Köhler, K., Köhler, F., Sawitzky, B., Fliege, H., Klapp, B. F. (2005). Determinants of the quality of life of patients with congenital heart disease. *Quality of Life Research,* **14**, 35-43.

Sairanen, H. I., Nieminen, H. P., Jokinen, E. V. (2005). Late results and quality of life after pediatric cardiac surgery in Finland: a population-based study of 6,461 patients with follow-up extending up to 45 years. *Pediatric Cardiac Surgery Annual,* **8**, 168-172.

Saliba, Z., Butera, G., Bonnet, D., Bonhoeffer, P., Villain, E., Kachaner, J., Sidi, D., & Iserin, L. (2001). Quality of life and perceived health status in surviving adults with univentricular heart. *Heart,* **86**(1), 69-73.

Simko, L. C., & McGinnis, K. A. (2003). Quality of life experienced by adults with congenital heart disease. *AACN Clinical Issues,* **14**(1), 42-53.

Simko, L. C., McGinnis, K. A., Schembri, J. (2006). Educational needs of adults with congenital heart disease. Journal *of Cardiovascular Nursing,* **21**(2), 85-94.

Suris, J. C., & Parera, N. (2005). Sex, drugs and chronic illness: health behaviours among chronically ill youth. *European Journal of Public Health,* **15**, 484-488.

Ternestedt, B. M., Wall, K., Oddsson, H., Riesenfeld, T., Groth, I., & Schollin, J. (2001). Quality of life 20 and 30 years after surgery in patients operated on for tetralogy of Fallot and for atrial septal defect. *Pediatric Cardiology,* **22**(2), 128-132.

The WHOQOL Group (1998). Development of the World Health Organization WHOQOL-BREF Quality of Life Assessment. *Psychological Medicine,* **28**, 551-558.

Tong, E. M., Sparacino, P. S., Messias, D. K., Foote, D., Chesla, C. A., Gillis, C. L. (1998). Growing up with congenital heart disease: the dilemmas of adolescents and young adults. *Cardiology in the Young,* **8**(3), 287-289.

Utens, E. M. W. J., Verhulst, F. C., Erdman, R. A. M., Meijboom, F. J., Duivenvoorden, H. J., Bos, E., Roelandt J. R. T. C. & Hess, J. (1994). Psychosocial functioning of young adults after surgical correction for congenital heart disease in childhood: A follow-up study. *Journal of Psychosomatic Research,* **38**(7), 745-758.

Utens, E. M., Versluis-Den Bieman, H. J., Verhulst, F. C., Meijboom, F. J., Erdman, R. A., & Hess, J. (1998). Psychopathology in young adults with congenital heart disease. Follow-up results. *European Heart Journal,* **19**(4), 647-651.

Uzark, K., VonBargen-Mazza, P., & Messiter, E. (1989). Health education needs of adolescents with congenital heart disease. *Journal of Pediatric Health Care,* **3**(3), 137-143.

Van der Rijken, R. E. A., Maassen, B. A. M., Walk, T. L. M., Daniëls, O. & Hulstijn-Dirkmaat, G. M. (2007). Outcome after surgical repair of congenital cardiac malformations at school age. *Cardiology in the Young,* **17**, 64-71.

Van Rijen, E. H. M. (2003). *Psychosocial aspects of congenital heart disease in adulthood. A longitudinal cohort study of 20-33 years follow-up.* PhD thesis, Erasmus University Rotterdam, Rotterdam.

Van Rijen, E. H. M., Utens, E. M. W. J., Roos-Hesselink, J. W., Meijboom, F. J., Van Domburg, R. T., Roelandt, J. R. T. C., Bogers, A. J. J. C., & Verhulst, F. C. (2003). Psychosocial functioning of the adult with congenital heart disease: a 20-33 years follow-up. *European Heart Journal,* **24**(7), 673-683.

Van Rijen E. H. M., Utens E. M. W. J., Roos-Hesselink J. W., Meijboom F. J., Van Domburg R. T., Roelandt J. R. T. C., Bogers, A. J. J. C., & Verhulst, F. C. (2004a). Medical predictors for psychopathology in adults with operated congenital heart disease. *European Heart Journal,* **25**, 1605-1613.

Van Rijen E. H. M., Utens E. M. W. J., Roos-Hesselink J. W., Meijboom F. J., Van Domburg R. T., Roelandt J. R. T. C., Bogers, A. J. J. C., & Verhulst, F. C. (2004b). Styles of coping and social support in a cohort of adults with congenital heart disease. *Cardiology in the Young,* **14**, 122-130.

Van Rijen, E. H. M., Utens, E. M. W. J., Roos-Hesselink, J. W., Meijboom, F. J., Van Domburg, R. T., Roelandt, J. R. T. C., Bogers, A. J. J. C., & Verhulst, F. C. (2005a). Longitudinal development of psychopathology in an adult congenital heart disease cohort. *International Journal of Cardiology,* **99**, 315-323.

Van Rijen, E. H. M., Utens, E. M. W. J., Roos Hesselink, J. W., Meijboom, F. J., Van Domburg, R. T., Roelandt, J. R. T. C., Bogers, A. J. J. C., & Verhulst, F. C. (2005b). Current subjective state of health, and longitudinal psychological well-being over a period of 10 years, in a cohort of adults with congenital cardiac disease. *Cardiology in the Young,* **15**, 168-175.

Ware, J. E., & Sherbourne, C. D. (1992). The MOS 36-item short-form health survey (SF-36). Conceptual framework and item selection. *Medical Care,* **30**, 473-483.

Zigmond, A., & Snaith, R. P. (1983). The hospital anxiety and depression scale. *Acta Psychiatrica Scandinavia,* **67**, 361-370.

Zung, W. W. K. (1965). *A self-rating depression scale. Archives of General Psychiatry,* **12**, 63-70.

In: Heart Disease in Men
Editors: A.B. Todd and M.H. Mosley, pp. 167-182
ISBN: 978-1-60692-297-2

Chapter 7

THE USE OF CARDIOVASCULAR BIOMARKERS FOR THE ASSESSMENT OF HEART DISEASE IN MEN

David C. Gaze

Clinical Blood Sciences, Department of Chemical Pathology,
St George's Healthcare NHS Trust, London, United Kingdom, SW17 0QT

Abstract

Cardiovascular disease (CVD) is the leading cause of death in the Western World. CVD is not a disease of old age: evidence from autopsy studies demonstrated the presence of atheroma in coronary arteries in children as young as seven years old. CVD does not occur in isolated succinct episodes but occurs as a continuous spectrum, from initiation of atheroma formation, destabilization, development of cardiac ischemia through to cellular necrosis and cardiac dysfunction. The symptomatic part of the disease spectrum is known as the acute coronary syndrome (ACS). ACS is due to the rupture or erosion of atheroma. This produces, depending on its size, surrounding vascular anatomy and the degree of collateral vessels present, a mismatch between oxygen supply and demand resulting in tissue ischemia. This may progress to cardiomyocyte necrosis, known as a myocardial infarction (MI). Post-MI survival results in remodelling of the myocardium and the development of cardiac failure. A number of blood-borne biomarkers are available which can aid in the diagnosis of all of disease stages: the risk assessment of developing CVD, assessing the risk of plaque rupture, diagnosis and prognosis of ACS and the subsequent assessment of myocardial dysfunction.

The most challenging stage with respect to biomarkers and one of current research focus is the detection of cardiac ischemia. A number of potential ischemia markers have been investigated. However, to date, only one, ischemia-modified albumin (IMA) has been clinically validated. The problem associated with developing an ischemia marker is that there is currently no reference standard for diagnosis. This is problematic when assessing the sensitivity and specificity of any candidate biomarker. Measurement of the cardiac structural proteins, the troponins is now recognised as the gold standard test for detection of myocardial necrosis. The sensitive nature of these tests has also revealed that myocardial necrosis is also found in a range of other clinical situations, including trauma, pulmonary embolism, renal failure, multiple organ failure or in cases of arduous physical exercise. This highlights the need to assess biomarker status in conjunction with the clinical picture at presentation. The natriuretic peptides, in particular the B-type and its N-terminal pro-hormone cleaved subunit are diagnostic and prognostic in both acute ACS and detecting post infarction myocardial dysfunction. The role of the B type natriuretic peptides in detection of cardiac failure, both acute and chronic, is well defined. Their role in ACS remains the subject of further studies.

Introduction

Cardiovascular disease (CVD) is the leading cause of mortality in the Western World. The majority of CVD cases are due to acute myocardial infarction (AMI) [1]. The rates of CVD are higher than for any cancer or other non-CVD disease. Although epidemiologically CVD remains the biggest health burden, the rates of CVD are declining. Recent data from the Centre for Disease Control [2] for mortality up to 2005 has demonstrated a reduction in CVD since 1999 by 25 percent. A similar reduction of 24% has also been demonstrated for strokes. Similar data from the United Kingdom Office of National Statistics has sown a rapid fall in circulatory based diseases since the early 1980's [3]. Similar data exists for other countries in Europe [4]. Whilst the trends show promise, in part due to recent therapeutic and interventional advances in cardiology; the incidence of the causative risk factors that contribute to a higher risk of development of CVD, including smoking and obesity remain either steady or are increasing. The long term effect of this may be an upward trend in the number of cases of CVD.

CVD does not occur in isolated distinct episodes but is a disease process associated with the development of atheromatous lesions in the coronary arteries. This process occurs over decades rather than months or years. In recent years and now the focus of major research efforts, the inflammatory processes involved in development of atheroma are being understood. In the majority of cases, CVD is only diagnosed in the latter stages of atheroma development when the initial lesion has ruptured or eroded causing thrombosis or embolism. The ensuing effect is tissue hypoxia, irreversible ischemia and cellular necrosis. These stages are known clinically as the acute coronary syndrome and include unstable angina and AMI.

The laboratory plays an important role in the identification and management of CVD patients. Biomarkers can be used to assess the four major stages of CVD progression:

1) The risk assessment of developing CVD
2) Assessing the risk of plaque rupture
3) The diagnosis and prognosis of ACS
4) Assessment of myocardial dysfunction

Broadly speaking these biomarkers fall into two categories; a) those which are available widely in clinical chemistry laboratories and can be performed with high quality assays on large automated instruments and b) the more specialized or novel biomarkers which are analytical and clinically more difficult to measure and interpret. One prevailing concept of biomarker development is the difficulty in successfully transferring from lab based *in-vitro* studies into routine clinical practice. This pathway can take years of research and is heavily dependent on the disease prevalence in the population of study.

Many biomarkers seem promising in basic science studies when they are assessed in a disease group and compared to a control group. As will be demonstrated, even in clinical trial situations, the effectiveness of the biomarker may be over estimated due to the tight control of patient selection criteria to define the disease and controls as worst and best cases alike. Often biomarkers fail to perform adequately as diagnostic or prognostic tools in the routine clinical setting as the disease prevalence is far lower than in the clinical trial setting. None the less, a number of biomarkers have successfully transferred from the lab bench to the bed side and along with other diagnostic modalities form a decision making pathway for the diagnosis and management of patients with CVD.

Gender differences between the prevalence of heart disease exist. Life expectancy is slightly lower for men than women. In the United Kingdom, the life expectancy at birth of males and females is 77 and 81 years respectively. For the United States of America it is 75 and 80 respectively [5]. Globally, CHD is responsible for 6.8% of disability adjusted life years in men and 5.3% in women [6]. Rates of CHD are decreasing in developed countries but transitional countries or those in developing world are experiencing an increase in rates of CHD. This is due to improved life expectancy, socio-economic and lifestyle changes as a result of urbanization.

In the UK in 2006, there were slightly more deaths due to CVD in women than in men (table 1). There was an exponential increase in the number of deaths from CVD with age for both males and females. Women view heart disease as less of a health burden than breast cancer, yet heart disease is the leading cause of death in women >25 years old. It is responsible for higher mortality in this gender group than either breast or cervical cancer. Only 13% of women think heart disease is a health threat. This is in part driven by the concentration of basic science and clinical research on males. There are gender differences between the symptoms of myocardial infarction. Whilst males often show the classical symptoms of chest, arm and neck pain and shortness of breath, women often report nausea, fatigue and dizziness. This presents as a major problem to the emergency services or attending physicians in the emergency room.

Table 1. Mortality due to coronary heart disease. Number of deaths in men and women at different ages in both the United Kingdom in 1996

	Number of deaths from CVD by gender and age (years)						
	All	**<35**	**35-44**	**45-54**	**55-64**	**65-74**	**>75**
Men	94,987	358	1521	4254	10,068	19,276	59,320
Women	102,780	315	634	1537	3892	11,279	85,123
Total	197,797	663	2155	5791	13,960	30,555	144,443

Development of Atherosclerosis

Plaque Development

The atherosclerotic plaque until recently was thought to be a product of a lipid-storage disease, consisting of proliferative smooth muscle, cholesterol and cholesterol esters encapsulated in a fibrotic cap. It is now accepted that the process of atherogenesis, includes complex inflammatory processes which interact with the lipid accumulation process to produce a localized highly inflammatory response. Biochemical signals from the inflammatory milieu attract other blood-derived cells which in turn activate other cellular mechanisms. The resulting effect is both localized and systemic alteration to the biology of the vascular system.

Initiation of atheroma formation is a result of genetic predisposition and environmental influences. Autopsy studies of children and young adults have shown the presence of lipid laden macrophage (foam cells) in pre-pubescent children. 15% of 16-19 year olds have pre-atheromatous or atheromatous lesions [7]. Risk factors for the development of CHD are multifactorial and fall into two main groups (table 2): those that are constant (nature) which are predetermined genetically and those that are modifiable, commonly known as lifestyle or environmentally associated (nurture) risk factors. Modification of these risk factors by simple lifestyle alteration or therapeutic intervention for hyperlipidaemia, hypertension or diabetes can alter the progression of atherosclerosis and CAD. Initial clinical examination of the CVD patient includes risk factor assessment and this is the primary area of life-style modification to alter CVD progression.

Hyperlipidaemia is a complex pathological process derived from both genetic predisposition and lifestyle. High total serum cholesterol, elevated LDL/VLDL and a reduced HDL is a lipid 'signature' for CVD development [8].

Table 2. Risk factors associated with the development of cardiovascular disease

Constant risk factors	Modifiable risk factors
Age	Hyperlipidaemia
Gender	Hypertension
Family history of CAD	Obesity (abdominal)
Personal history of CAD	Smoking
Diabetes Mellitus type I	Excessive alcohol consumption
Elevated homocysteine	Diabetes Mellitus type II
Elevated haemostatic factors	Sedentary lifestyle
	Low antioxidant levels
	Infection

At the level of the coronary artery, lipid and collagen accumulation occurs following the initial chemical or mechanical insult to the smooth endothelial cell lining [9]. Lesions develop primarily at bifurcations in arteries where there is a disturbance to the laminar flow of blood. The disruption can cause localized hypercoagulation and intimal damage. The juvenile atheroma appears as yellow discoloured streaks on the endothelial wall lining. If allowed to progress, the intimal layer thickens due to an increase in the number of smooth muscle cells and the depositon of connective tissue. Calcification and fibrosis occurs at the end point of development. The plaques now appear raised and white to the naked eye (figure 1). The bulging of the plaque causes further disruption to laminar flow.

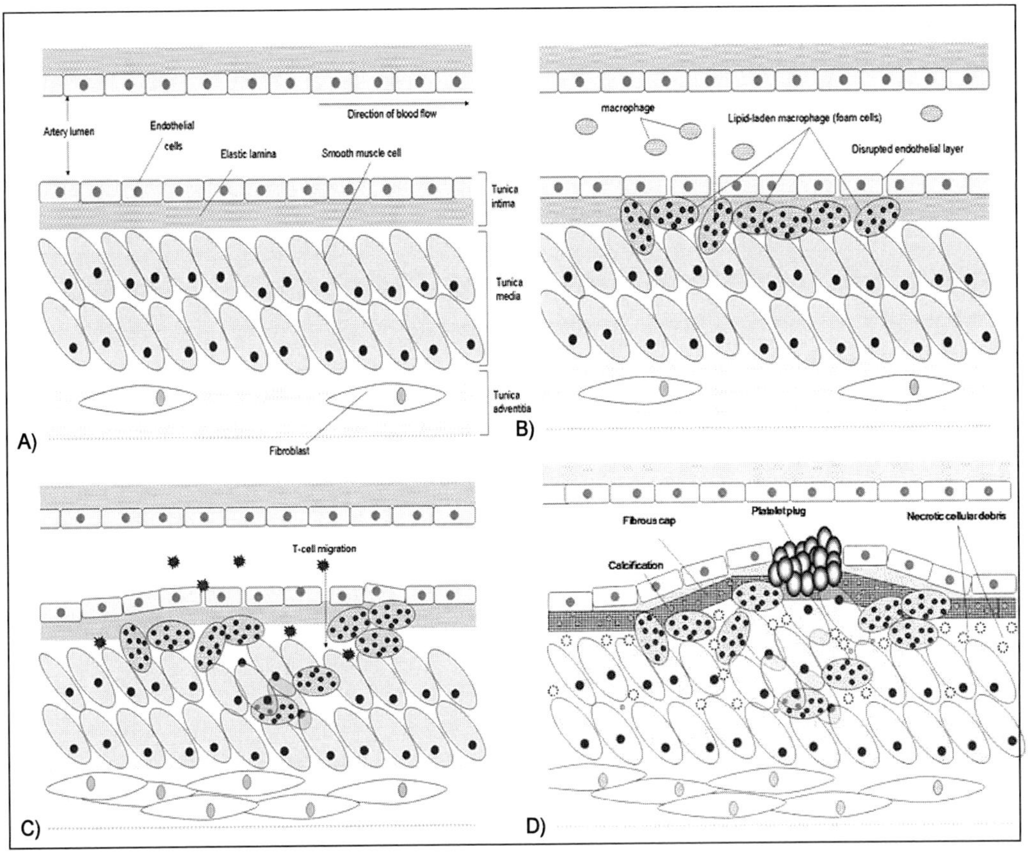

Figure 1. Pathophysiology of atherosclerosis. A) Pathogenesis of atheroma is initiated with damage to the endothelial lining of the artery. Cholesterol rich LDL particles enter the intimal layer. B) Macrophage accumulate oxidised lipid independently of the LDL receptor mechanism, resulting in formation of raised fatty streaks. C) Macrophage release lipid and cytokines into the intimal space. Cytokines stimulate intimal cell proliferation, which then secrete collagen, which initiates fibrosis. The lesion is appears raised and yellow (lipid plaque). As the lesion develops, the medial layer atrophies and the elastic lamina is disrupted. D) Collagen forms a fibrous cap that appears hard and white (fibrolipid plaque). The plaque contains macrophage laden with lipid as well as free lipid. The endothelium is now fragile, often ulcerating at weak points like the shoulder of the cap. Platelet aggregation and thrombosis can occur. This lesion is responsible for narrowing the lumen of the artery and distal embolisation of a piece of this thrombus can totally occlude smaller arteries.

Plaque Destabilization and Rupture

The internal environment of the plaque contains inflammatory cells which express various chemokines and cytokines which act as chemotactic attractants for other cell types. The plaque is now vulnerable with thinning of the fibrous cap, especially at the shoulder regions which are rich in foam cells and T cells. The T cells produce interferon gamma (IFN-γ) which inhibits the production of matrix by smooth muscle cells. Intrinsic (composition and structural features) and extrinsic (mechanical forces) of the plaque contribute to the rupture of the fibrous cap of the atheroma [10]. Protease enzymes are released from macrophages which degrade extracellular matrix material. The plaque centre is now necrotic with an excess of inflammatory mediators. Small vessels may grow into the plaque from the medial lining and provide an entry route further exacerbating the inflammatory process [11].

Biomarkers of Cardiovascular Disease

Biomarkers of Plaque Development and Progression

Serum total cholesterol and lipoproteins such as oxidised low density lipoprotein (LDL), small dense LDL and intermediate density lipoprotein are atherogenic. The laboratory repertoire common for the determination of plaque development and progression include the measurement of apolipoprotein b and the calculation the cardio-protective high density lipoprotein. Other lipid components such as small dense LDL and intermediate density lipoprotein which are particularly atherogenic can be measured but this is not common in the clinical laboratory setting. Lipoprotein (a) (Lp(a)) contains a central core of LDL which is covalently bonded to a polypeptide chain of apolipoprotein a. This peptide shares sequence homology with plasminogen and has been proposed as a mechanism linking plaque rupture and the development of thrombosis.

The biggest single cause of plaque initiation and inflammation is modified and oxidised LDL [12]; however plaque development, progression and destabilisation is multifactorial. Numerous enzyme linked immunosorbent assay (ELISA) exist for modified and oxidised LDL however many have not made the transition to immunoassay or automated clinical chemistry analysers. Therefore their use in the clinical setting is somewhat prohibited. A large number of studies have been performed using modified and oxidised LDL assays [13], however when this is translated to routine clinical use in the general chest pain population, the diagnostic and prognostic efficiency of the marker is questionable [14].

Homocysteine is a risk biomarker for the development and progression of CVD. Homocysteine is a sulphur containing amino acid closely related to methionine and cystine. A high plasma homocysteine concentration is associated with disruptive damage to the endothelium. In vitro studies have demonstrated that homocysteine can induce direct damage to endothelial cells, increase platelet activity, increase collagen synthesis, smooth muscle cell proliferation and has pro-coagulant effects.

Biomarkers of Plaque Stability

Endothelial injury results in chemotactic recruitment of mononuclear cells within the plaque. Interleukin-6 (IL-6) concentrations are increased in patients at risk of with established CVD as well as those who have an acute coronary syndrome. Kinetically, IL-6 rises and falls rapidly but produces an acute phase response. This in turn initiates the production of acute phase reactants such as C-reactive protein (CRP) and serum amyloid A protein (SAA).

CRP is a hepatically derived pentraxin of 23KDa. CRP has a long plasma half-life and is now understood to be a mediator as well as a marker of atherothrombotic disease [15]. The primary use of CRP is as a marker of infection, during which concentrations can be 100-fold higher than the limits of normal. In CVD patients, values are typically in the range 0-3 mg/L.

Due to the recent development of sensitive assays, which can accurately report below 5 mg/L, highly sensitive CRP has been demonstrated to be a strong predictor of future cardiovascular events. Sensitive CRP has demonstrated better predictive power for adverse cardiac events than low density lipoprotein (LDL) cholesterol [15]. A large number of studies have demonstrated that CRP is related to the risk of subsequent cardiac events in both patients with and without pre-existing CVD.

Plasma CRP concentrations of <1, 1 to 3, and >3mg/L correspond to low, moderate, and high-risk groups for future cardiovascular events. Individuals with LDL cholesterol below 1.3g/L who have CRP levels >3mg/L represent a high-risk group often missed in clinical practice [14]. The addition of CRP to standard cholesterol evaluation may provide an improvement to global risk prediction and monitoring compliance with preventive intervention. Currently CRP is used as a risk predictor for primary prevention intervention. The use of aspirin is associated with a reduction in CRP concentrations and subsequent lower CVD event rate. The use of statin therapy (HMG-CoA reductase inhibitors) for hypercholesterolaemia is also associated with a reduction in CR, suggesting statins themselves also exert an anti-inflammatory effect.

Whilst IL-6 may be a more sensitive marker for CVD prediction, it is less readily available in clinical chemistry laboratories as a routine assay and is harder to measure due to analyte stability and storage conditions.

Lipoprotein-associated phospholipase A2 (Lp-PLA_2) is an intracellular phospholipase which hydrolyzes phospholipids in cellular membranes. Attached to LDL, it is responsible for the hydrolysis of oxidised phospholipid in the LDL molecule [16]. Using immunohistochemical staining with monoclonal antibodies, it has been demonstrated that juvenile plaques show less staining for Lp-PLA_2 than rupture-prone or ruptured plaques [17]. In patients with cardiovascular metabolic syndrome, modification of Lp-PLA_2 through treatment of obesity, hyperlipidaemia and diabetes mellitus (Lp-PLA_2 is independent of insulin resistance), who would otherwise be at intermediate risk of a future cardiac event has shown promise [18]. To date, this marker has not been established on an automated clinical chemistry analyser.

Biomarkers of Plaque Rupture

The classical view of plaque rupture is increasing size of the plaque causing luminal narrowing. It is known that approximately 80% of plaques that cause an ACS event are not flow limiting stenoses. Markers of coagulation are raised in the ACS patient and these include prothrombin fragment 1 and 2 and factor VIIa. Thrombin/antithrombin complex is often elevated and associated with increased plasma cardiac troponin. Inflammatory cells contribute to plaque rupture [19]. Foam cells derived from macrophages congregate in the shoulder region of the vulnerable plaque. At this time, the foam cells express matrix metalloproteinase enzymes (MMPs). These proteolytic enzymes can inactivate zymogens (proMMP) enzymes as well as angiotensin II. A number of MMPs are syntesised and relased by macrophage. These include interstitial collegnase (MMP-1), gelatinase enzymes (MMP-2 and MMP-9) and stromelysin (MMP-3). MMP-1 expression is increased by oxidised LDL IFN-γ, IL-1 and tumour necrosis factor alpha (TNF-α) [20].

Biomarkers of Cardiac Ischemia

The detection of cardiac ischemia prior to myocardial infarction is both a major diagnostic and therapeutic challenge, especially in the emergency room setting. The detection of cardiac ischaemia prior to myocyte necrosis gives rise to the development of potential therapeutic (pharmacological or invasive) interventions to limit or prevent the extent of irreversible damage caused by cell necrosis. A plethora of candidate markers have been proposed as an ischemia marker, including whole blood choline and unbound free fatty acids however only one has been made the translational step from a basic science investigation into a fully developed FDA and CE marked commercial assay. This is known as ischemia modified albumin (IMA®).

A reduction in oxygen supply versus demand by the tissue results in ischaemia, due to the surrounding acidosis and the generation of free radicals. Copper and zinc ions, normally bound to proteins in the plasma are released from protein binding sites to circulate in the free form [21-23]. The N-terminus of albumin binds transition metals such as, Co^{2+}, Ni^{2+} and Cu^{2+} ions [24]. The N-terminus however, is susceptible to biochemical alteration [25]. Following a period of ischaemia, a reduction in the ability of albumin to bind cobalt is apparent. This is the basis of the albumin cobalt-binding test (ACB® test) for IMA [26,27].

IMA alone has a diagnostic sensitivity of 82% with 46% specificity if measured in the first three hours of presentation to the ED [28]. The combination of a positive ECG, cTnT (>0.05 μg/L) and IMA however demonstrated a 95% sensitivity for diagnosis of ACS. In a study of 538 patients admitted to a chest pain evaluation unit, admission measurement of IMA plus cTnT had 100% sensitivity for prediction of a final diagnosis of AMI [29].

Although the assay has been cleared for *in vitro* diagnostic use, two problems remain to be resolved with IMA. First is the exact mechanism by which IMA is generated and the relationship to the underlying pathophysiological mechanisms during ischemia. The second is the assay format; Very low albumin levels [30,31] and the presence of co-existing lactic acidosis affect assay performance [30]. Finally samples need to be analysed within a STAT fashion due to the instability of IMA [32].

Biomarkers of Cardiomyocyte Necrosis

Historically markers of cardiac necrosis have focused on the cytosolic enzymes [33] such as aspartate transaminase (AST), lactate dehydrogenase (LD), creatine kinase (CK), its MB isoenzyme (CK-MB) and small proteins such as the respiratory protein myoglobin. Whilst these markers proved initially useful, they are not tissue specific as they are expressed in varying concentrations in both skeletal and cardiac tissue. The need to distinguish between skeletal muscle and myocardial damage is paramount, not only in clinical presentations of suspected acute coronary syndromes but in cases of exercise induced skeletal muscle myopathy.

Clinical cardiology and emergency medicine have undergone a radical change in diagnostic test utilisation for acute cardiac chest pain patients since the introduction of the cardiac troponins (cTn), cardiac troponin T (cTnT) and I (cTnI). These biomarkers offer superior sensitivity and specificity to the 'classical' enzymes and myoglobin. The evidence for the superiority of cTn has been reflected in the redefinition of acute myocardial infarction

(AMI) by a joint committee of the European Society of Cardiology/American College of Cardiology [34]. This consensus document defines any increase in cardiac troponin T or I above the 99th percentile of a healthy reference population as indicative of myocardial cell necrosis [34]. Furthermore, small increases in cardiac troponin above the 99th percentile can direct clinical decision-making and guide appropriate therapeutic or invasive coronary intervention [34,35].

Markers of cardiac cell necrosis can be split into those located in the cytoplasm of the cell and those that form the structural apparatus which control muscle contraction. The cytosolic component contains myoglobin, LD, CK, CKMB as well as fatty acid binding protein (FABP). The structural compartment consists of the troponin proteins troponin T and troponin I. Troponins have tissue specific isoforms cardiac troponin T (cTnT) and cardiac troponin I (cTnI) and are expressed uniquely in myocardial cells, whilst predominantly structural both cardiac troponins (cTn) have a small unbound cytosolic fraction (between 6% and 8% for cTnT and 2.8%-8.3% for cTnI) [36]. The location of the markers of cardiac necrosis and schematic of release from cells during ischaemia and infarction are shown in figure 2.

The measurement of cardiac troponin is now considered the "Gold Standard" test for myocardial necrosis [34]. Although there may be a role for measurement of cytosolic markers such as myoglobin and the MB isoenzyme of creatine kinase (CKMB), cTnT and cTnI measurement should be used to diagnose AMI [35-36]. The reason for the dominant position of troponin measurement is due to the sensitivity and specificity of the test and the evidence base for outcome prediction.

The sensitivity of any biochemical test is dependant on its ability to discriminate between the normal and abnormal state. A test that is elevated in all patients with a condition and is normal in all controls will have a sensitivity of 100%. Sensitivity is influenced by the background level of signal in the normal state and is referred to as noise. This in turn is compared to the change of signal in the abnormal state, known as the signal to noise ratio. It was presumed that the circulating concentration of cTn in apparently healthy people was absolute zero, due to the intracellular location of the proteins. With the advent of more sensitive immunoassay methods the current commercial cTn assays demonstrate a background level in the circulation that appears to be determined by the detection limit of the assay. Although there may be a background level of cTn in the circulation, this is undetectable in the majority of cases by the assays currently commercially available. Elevation occurs only where there is myocardial damage. The combination of low background noise with cardiospecificity means that although in absolute terms the amount of cTn released is less than the amount of CKMB, the ability to detect it is much greater, and the signal to noise ratio is much higher.

Using cTn specific assay, it has been demonstrated that elevations of the cardiac isoform do not occur where there is pure skeletal muscle trauma [37,38]. In a study of 696 apparently healthy individuals aged 18-84 years, of which 45% were male, two commercial cTnI assays have demonstrated a gender difference, with a higher upper limit of normal in males. The other five cTnI assays and the cTnT assay tested did not demonstrate a gender difference. In the same population, CKMB mass was significantly higher in males compared to females. [39].

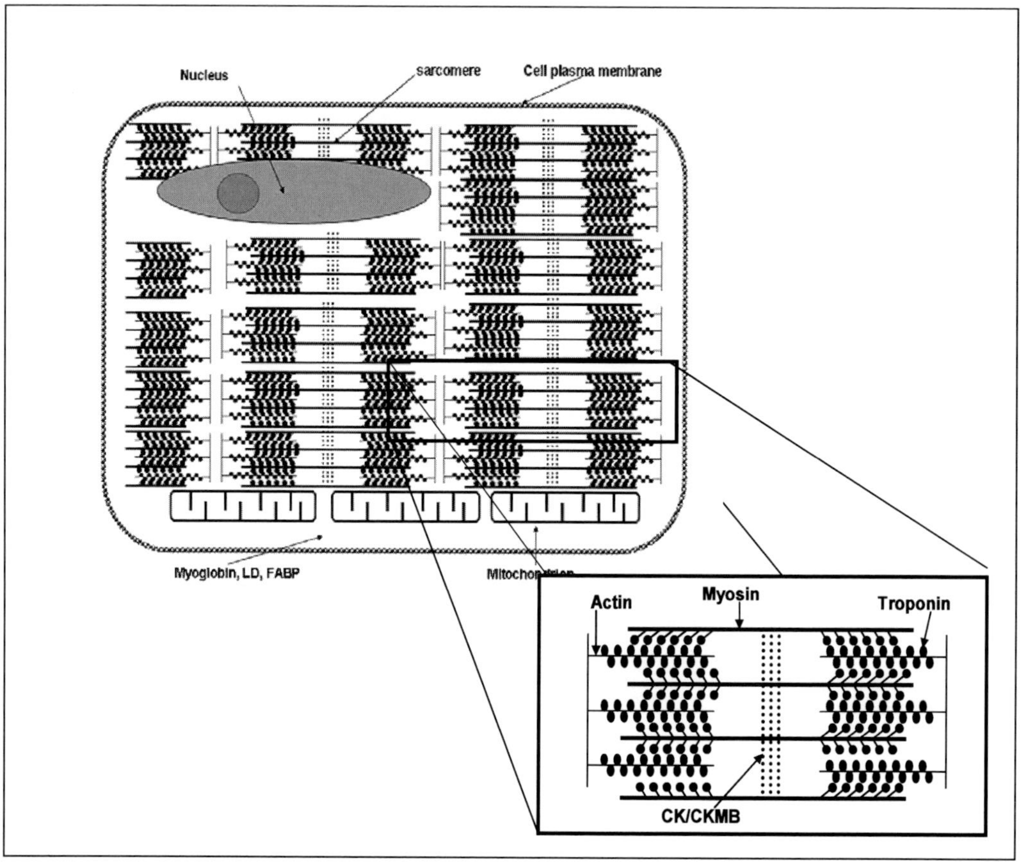

Figure 2. Schematic diagram of a cardiomyocyte. Cardiac cells are similar to skeletal muscle; however contain numerous mitochondria supplying the energy for a continuous heartbeat. The sarcoplasm is divided into myofibrils (enlargement box). The myofibril contains the muscle proteins, actin, myosin, tropomyosin and the troponin complex, although a minor percentage of all bound proteins exist in the cytoplasm. Creatine kinase contributes to the M band. Myoglobin, lactate dehydrogenase (LD) and fatty acid binding protein (FABP) are diffusely located within the cytoplasm of the cell.

Clinical studies of cTn have concentrated on the diagnostic and prognostic utility of the assays. Initial studies showed that cTnT could be detected in a significant proportion of patients who were classed as having unstable angina using the conventional World Health Organisation (WHO) criteria for myocardial infarction. In these studies, both short term and long term follow up showed that an elevated troponin was associated with an increased risk of cardiac event [40,41].

Determination of cTn is by immunoassay. For both cTnT and cTnI, several generations of assay have existed and have been comprehensively reviewed [36]. The measurement technology utilising electrochemiluminescence for cTnT is supplied by only one manufacturer (Roche Diagnostics) due to patent restrictions on the antibodies selected for the assay. Measurement of cTnI however is available on a range of immunoassay platforms from different manufacturers. Due to a lack of assay standardisation both for a common calibrator and for antibody selection, comparison between methods is often problematic. Despite this, a similar series of studies for the different cTnI methods has shown that cTnI elevation predicts adverse cardiac events in patients with unstable angina [42-45]. The use of cTnT and cTnI determinations results in approximately reclassification of 33% of unstable angina patients into patients who have suffered an MI.

In a study of 1865 patients derived from three therapeutic interventional studies on AMI of which 34% were female, the differential expression of cardiac biomarkers for each gender were assessed. Men showed a predominance of elevated CKMB and cTn, however women demonstrated elevated CRP and b type natriuretic peptide (see biomarkers of cardiac dysfunction section). The prognostic utility of the biomarkers examined were similar in both genders. The use of a combined multimarker approach identified a greater proportion of women considered to be high-risk. Women who were all biomarker negative demonstrated improved outcome if treated with a conservative rather than invasive strategy [46].

Biomarkers of Cardiac Dysfunction

Survival rates following AMI are increasing for both genders. Survival improvement is primarily due to a combination of early diagnosis and a rapid therapeutic or invasive intervention to open occluded vessels and to salvage myocardium. Patients with some degree of damaged myocardium however further develop cardiac failure. Cardiac failure is a pathophysiological state in which an abnormality of cardiac function is responsible for the failure of the heart to pump blood at a rate commensurate with the requirements of the metabolising tissues [47]. Cardiac failure affects 0.4-2% of the population and the age adjusted mortality due to cardiac failure is increasing [47]. There is a 50% survival rate four years after diagnosis [48]. Currently, the clinical diagnostic methodologies available are inadequate due to poor sensitivity and specificity. There is heavy reliance on the identification of heart failure from symptoms, ECG changes and/or chest x-ray diagnosis. The 'gold standard' for diagnosis of cardiac failure is currently cardiac imaging technology including echocardiography or magnetic resonance imaging; however these are often expensive and not always routinely available. A blood borne marker of cardiac dysfunction is therefore highly desirable.

B type natriuretic peptide (BNP) is a hormone secreted predominantly by ventricular wall myocytes in response to increased ventricular stretch. It is not stored following production, but is under constant renewal by transcription and translation of mRNA. A prohormone proBNP is produced within the myocyte. This prohormone is cleaved by the enzyme corin to give the active portion of the molecule, B type natriuretic peptide (BNP) and the N terminal portion of the hormone, NTproBNP. Both are available as routine biomarker assay tests on a range of immunoassay platforms. The half-life of the active BNP is short (20 minutes) compared to that of the NTproBNP (120 minutes).

Measurements of NTproBNP and BNP are used in the diagnosis of suspected acute or chronic cardiac failure. It has been demonstrated that the measurement of BNP/NTproBNP allows exclusion with a high certainty of left ventricular systolic dysfunction (LVSD) in patients presenting to primary care with symptoms suggestive of heart failure, mainly shortness of breath. [49-55]. It has been suggested, therefore, that BNP/NTproBNP measurement should be used as the "gold standard" test for the detection of ventricular dysfunction. In a prospective randomised trial of diagnosis based on BNP with conventional clinical diagnosis in 452 patients, the diagnostic pathway including BNP produced reduction in hospital stay; stay in intensive care and lower cost but with equivalent mortality [56].

The role of BNP/NTproBNP in patients presenting with ACS however remains more uncertain. Studies have shown that measurement of NTproBNP/BNP on admission in both selected and unselected suspected ACS patients can be used to predict outcome. A study of 2525 patients enrolled in a clinical trial (OPUS-TIMI 16) with a mixed population of ST segment elevation MI (STEMI), non ST segment elevation MI (NSTEMI) and unstable angina pectoris (UAP) showed that quartiles of BNP concentrations were predictive of survival. There was a 9% mortality rate in the highest quartile compared with less than 1% in the lowest quartile at 10 months follow up. The population was dichotomised into those with BNP above or below the cut point of 80 pg/L. An elevated BNP $\geq$80pg/mL showed a significantly greater risk of death, heart failure or MI both at 30 days and at 10 months [57]. In a study of 666 patients admitted with AMI, BNP and NTproBNP were measured 24-96 hours from symptom onset. Subsequent death or heart failure was predicted by BNP/NTproBNP levels even when ejection fraction exceeded 40% [58]. BNP/NTproBNP measurements have been combined with other biomarkers including CRP and cTn [59] or cTn alone [60]. Measurements of NTproBNP /BNP provide additive information under these circumstances with the worst prognosis seen when the greatest number of biomarkers are elevated.

Conclusion

Cardiac biomarkers are integral to the diagnosis of CVD at every stage of disease progression from plaque formation through to acute cardiac cell necrosis and cardiac dysfunction. In the acute setting, cardiac biomarkers have evolved from an adjunct test to front line assays with the advent of cTn and natriuretic peptides which all offer immense diagnostic and prognostic potential and offer additional resource in patient management. It should be noted that cTn are markers of myocardial cell damage and not a marker of AMI *per sae*, which remains a clinical diagnosis within the appropriate clinical context Elevation of cTn occurs in a range of other conditions associated with non-ACS cardiac damage and include surgical intervention, drug- and toxin- induced cardiotoxitcy and renal failure [61]. The elevations in these groups carry prognostic significance.

References

[1] World Health Organisation. WHO-MONICA Project, Myocardial infarction and coronary deaths in the World Health Organisation Monica Project. Registration procedures, event rates and case-fatality rates in 38 populations from 21 countries in 4 continents. *Circulation* 1994;90:583-

[2] Kung HC, Hoyert DL, Xu JQ, Murphy SL. Deaths: Final data for 2005. *National vital statistics reports*; vol 56 no 10. Hyattsville, MD: National Center for Health Statistics. 2008.

[3] Office of National Statistics 2001; General Register Office Edingburgh; General Register office, Northern Ireland.

[4] World Health Organization 2004. (www.who.ch) Last accessed 15th July 2008.

[5] *Life tables for WHO Member States*. Geneva, World Health Organization, 2006 (http://www.who.int/whosis/database/life_tables/life_tables.cfm). Last accessed 15th July 2008.

[6] Mackay J, Mensah G, Eds. The Atlas of Heart Disease and Stroke. World Health Organisation, 2004. Found also at (www.who.int/cardiovascular_diseases/resources/atlas/en/). Last accessed 22nd July 2008.

[7] Stary HC: Lipid and macrophage accumulations in arteries of children and the development of atherosclerosis. *Am. J. Clin. Nutr.* 2000 Nov;72(5 Suppl):1297S-1306S.

[8] Luis AJ. Atherosclerosis. *Nature* 2000;407:233-241.

[9] Gertz SD, Roberts WC. Haemodynamic sheer force in rupture of coronary arterial atherosclerotic plaques. *Am. J. Cardiol.* 1990;66:1368-1372.

[10] Arroyo LH, Lee RT: Mechanism of plaque rupture: mechanical and biological interatctions. *Cardiovasc. Research* 199;41:369-375.

[11] Moultan KS, Folkman J. in *Molecular Basis of Cardiovascular disease* (ed. Chen KR) Saunders, Philadelphia, 1999. p393-410.

[12] Davis MJ. Is it all plaque rupture? In. Challenges in Acute Coronary Syndromes (eds. DeBono D, Sobel BE) *Blackwell Science* 2001. p3-17.

[13] Khuseyinova N, Joenig W. Lipoprotein-associated phospholipase A2 and other lipid-related biomarkers in cardiovascular disease. In *Cardiovascular Biomarkers: Pathophysiology and Disease Management* (ed. Morrow DA), Humanna Press, Totowa, NJ 2006. p519-542.

[14] Gaze DC, Sinha M, Kaski JC, Collinson PO. Oxidised low density lipoprotein is a poor short term event marker in acute coronary syndrome patients who present to the emergency department. *Clin. Chem.* 2006;52:A128.

[15] Ridker, PM: Clinical Application of C-Reactive Protein for Cardiovascular Disease Detection and Prevention. *Circulation* 2003;107:363-369.

[16] Macphee CH, Moores KE, Boyd HF, Dhanak D, Ife RJ, Leach CA et al. Lipoprotein-associated phospholipase A_2, platelet-activating factor acetylhydrolase, generates two bioactive products during the oxidation of low density lipoprotein: use of a novel inhibitor. *Biochem. J.* 1999;338:479-487.

[17] Kolodigie FD, Burke AP, Skorija KS, Ladich E, Kutys R, Makuria AT et al. Quantitation and distribution of lipoprotein-associated phospholipase A_2 protein expression in the natural progression of human coronary artery atherosclerosis. *Atheroscler. Thromb. Vasc. Biol.* 2006;26:2523-2529.

[18] Anderson JL: Lipoprotein-Associated Phospholipase A2: An Independent Predictor of Coronary Artery Disease Events in Primary and Secondary Prevention. *Am. J. Cardiol.* 2008;101(suppl):23F-33F.

[19] Galis ZS, Sukhova GK, Kranzhofer R, Clark S, Libby P> Macrophage foam cels from experimental atheroma constutively prodcuce matrix degrading proteinases. *Proc. Natl. Acad. Sci. USA* 1995;92:402-6.

[20] Rajavashisth TB, Liao JC, Galis ZS, Tripathi S, Laufs U, Tripathi J, Chai NN, Xu XP, Jovinge S, Shah PK, Libby P: Inflammatory cytokines and oxidized low density lipoproteins increase endothelial cell expression of membrane type-1-matirx metalloproteinase. *J. Biol. Chem.* 1999;274:11924-9.

[21] Chevion M, Jiang Y, Har-El R, Berenshtein E, Uretzky G, Kitrossky N. Copper and iron are mobilized following myocardial ischemia: possible predictive criteria for tissue injury. *Proc. Natl. Acad. Sci. USA* 1993;90:1102-6.

[22] Cobbe SM,.Poole-Wilson PA. The time of onset and severity of acidosis in myocardial ischaemia. *J.Mol.Cell Cardiol.* 1980;12:745-60.

[23] McCord JM. Oxygen-derived free radicals in postischemic tissue injury. *N. Engl. J. Med.* 1985;312:159-63.

[24] Sadler PJ, Tucker A, Viles JH. Involvement of a lysine residue in the N-terminal Ni2+ and Cu2+ binding site of serum albumins. Comparison with Co2+, Cd2+ and Al3+. *Eur. J. Biochem.* 1994;220:193-200.

[25] Chan B, Dodsworth N, Woodrow J, Tucker A, Harris R. Site-specific N-terminal auto-degradation of human serum albumin. *Eur. J. Biochem.* 1995;227:524-8.

[26] Bar-Or D, Lau E, Winkler JV. A novel assay for cobalt-albumin binding and its potential as a marker for myocardial ischemia-a preliminary report. *J. Emerg. Med.* 2000;19:311-5.

[27] Bar-Or D, Winkler JV, Vanbenthuysen K, Harris L, Lau E, Hetzel FW. Reduced albumin-cobalt binding with transient myocardial ischemia after elective percutaneous transluminal coronary angioplasty: a preliminary comparison to creatine kinase-MB, myoglobin, and troponin I. *Am. Heart J.* 2001;141:985-91.

[28] Sinha MK, Roy D, Gaze DC, Collinson PO, Kaski JC. Role of "Ischemia Modified Albumin", a new biochemical marker of myocardial ischaemia, in the early diagnosis of acute coronary syndromes. *Emerg. Med. J.* 2004;21:29-34.

[29] Collinson PC, Gaze DC, Bainbridge K, Morris F, Morris B, Price A, Goodacre S: Utility of admission cardiac troponin and 'Ischemia Modified Albumin' measurements for rapid evaluation and rule out of suspected acute myocardial infarction in the emergency department. *Emerg. Med. J.* 2006;23:256-261.

[30] Zapico-Muniz E, Santalo-Bel M, Merce-Muntanola J, Montiel JA, Martinez-Rubio A, Ordonez-Llanos J. Ischemia-modified albumin during skeletal muscle ischemia. *Clin. Chem.* 2004;50:1063-5.

[31] Gaze DC, Crompton L, Collinson PO: Ischemia-modified albumin cocentrations should be interpreted with caution in patients with low serum albumin concentrations. *Med. Princ. Pract.* 2006;15:3212-324.

[32] Gaze DC, Crompton L, Collinson PO: Sample stability of Ischameia modified albumin (IMA) as assessed by the Albumin Cobalt Binding (ACB^{TM}) test. *Clin. Chem.* 2003;49:A40.

[33] Gaze, DC, Collinson PO. Cardiac troponins as biomarkers of drug- and toxin-induced cardiac toxicity and cardioprotection. *Expert Opin. Drug Metab. Toxicol.* 2005;1:715-725.

[34] Alpert, JS, Thygesen K, Antman, E, Bassand, JP et al: Myocardial infarction redefined - a consensus document of the Joint European Society of Cardiology/American College of Cardiology Committee for the Redefinition of Myocardial Infarction. *J. Am. Coll. Cardiol.* 2000;36:959-69.

[35] Braunwald E, Antman EM, Beasley JW, Califf RM, Cheilin MD, Hochman JS, et al: ACC/AHA guidelines for the management of patients with unstable angina and non-ST segment elevation myocardial infarction: executive summary and recommendations. A report of the American College of Cardiology/ American Heart Association task force

on practice guidelines (Committee on the management of patients with unstable angina). *J. Am. Coll. Cardiol.* 2000;36:970-1062.

[36] Collinson PO, Boa FG, Gaze DC: Measurement of cardiac troponins. *Ann. Clin. Biochem.* 2001;38:423-449.

[37] Collinson PO, Chandler HA, Stubbs PJ, Moseley DS, Lewis D, Simmons MD: Measurement of serum troponin T, creatine kinase MB isoenzyme, and total creatine kinase following arduous physical training. *Ann. Clin. Biochem.* 1995;32:450-453.

[38] Collinson, PO, Stubbs, PJ, Kessler, AC: Multicentre Evaluation of Routine Immunoassay Of Troponin T Study. *Heart* 2003;89:280-286.

[39] Apple FS, Quiest HE, Doyle PJ, Otto AP, Murakami MM: Plasma 99th Percentile Reference Limits for Cardiac Troponin and Creatine Kinase MB Mass for Use with European Society of Cardiology/American College of Cardiology Consensus Recommendations. *Clin. Chem.* 2003;49:1331-1336.

[40] Hamm CW, Ravkilde J, Gerhardt W, Jorgensen P, Peheim E, Ljungdahl L, et al: The prognostic value of serum troponin I in unstable angina *N. Engl. J. Med.* 1992;327:146-150.

[41] Stubbs P, Collinson P, Moseley D, Greenwood T, Noble M: Prospective study of the role of cardiac troponin T in patients admitted with unstable angina. *Br. Med. J.* 1996;313:262-264.

[42] Antman EM, Tanasijevic MJ, Thompson B, Schactman M, McCabe CH, Cannon CP et al: Cardiac-specific troponin I levels to predict the risk of mortality in patients with acute coronary syndromes. *N. Engl. J. Med.* 1996;335:1342-1349.

[43] Galvani M, Ottani F, Ferrini D, Ladenson JH, Destro A, Baccos D, et al: Prognostic influence of elevated values of cardiac troponin I in patients with unstable angina. *Circulation* 1997;95:2053-2059.

[44] Luscher MS, Thygesen K, Ravkilde J, Heickendorff L. Applicability of cardiac troponin T and I for early risk stratification in unstable coronary artery disease. TRIM Study Group. Thrombin Inhibition in Myocardial Ischemia. *Circulation* 1997;96:2578-2585.

[45] Collinson PO, Wiggins N, Gaze DC: Clinical Evaluation of the ACS:180 cardiac troponin I assay. *Ann. Clin. Biochem.* 2001;38:509-519.

[46] Wiviott SD, Cannon CP, Morrow DA, Murphy SA, Gibson M, McCabe CH et al: Differential Expression of Cardiac Biomarkers by Gender in patients with Unstable Angina/Non-ST-Elevation Myocardial Infarction: a TACTICS-TIMI 18 (Treat Angina with Aggrastat and determine Cost of Therapy with an Invasive or Conservative Strategy-Thrombolysis In Myocardial Infarction 18) substudy. *Circulation.* 2004;109:580-586.

[47] Remme WJ, Swedberg K: Task Force for the Diagnosis and Treatment of Chronic Heart Failure, European Society of Cardiology *Eur. Heart J.* 2001, 22, 1527-1560.

[48] Cowie MR, Zaphiriou A: Management of Chronic Heart Failure *Br. Med. J.* 2002; 325:422-425.

[49] McDonagh TA, Robb SD, Murdoch DR, Morton JJ, Ford I, Morrison CE, et al: Biochemical detection of left ventricular systolic dysfunction. *Lancet* 1998;351:9-13.

[50] McDonagh TA, Morrison CE, Lawrence A, Ford I, Tunstall-Pedoe H, McMurray JJ et al: Symptomatic and asymptomatic left ventricular systolic dysfunction in an urban population. *Lancet* 1997;350:829-833.

[51] Cowie MR, Struthers AD, Wood DA, Coats AJ, Thompson SG, Poole-Wilson PA et al. Value of natriuretic peptides in assessment of patients with possible new heart failure in primary care. *Lancet* 1997;350:1349-1353.

[52] Zaphiriou A, Robb S, Murray-Thomas T, Mendez G, Fox K, McDonagh T, et al: The diagnostic accuracy of plasma BNP and NTproBNP in patients referred from primary care with suspected heart failure: results of the UK national natriuretic peptide study. *Eur. J. Heart Fail.* 2005;7:537-541.

[53] Hobbs FD, Davis RC, Roalfe AK, Hare R, Davies MK, Kenkre JE. Reliability of N-terminal pro-brain natriuretic peptide assay in diagnosis of heart failure: cohort study in representative and high risk community populations. *Br. Med. J.* 2002;324:1498-1503.

[54] Hobbs FD, Davis RC, Roalfe AK, Hare R, Davies MK: Reliability of N-terminal proBNP assay in diagnosis of left ventricular systolic dysfunction within representative and high risk populations. *Heart* 2004;90:866-870.

[55] Groenning BA, Raymond I, Hildebrandt PR, Nilsson JC, Baumann M, Pedersen F: Diagnostic and prognostic evaluation of left ventricular systolic heart failure by plasma N-terminal pro-brain natriuretic peptide concentrations in a large sample of the general population. *Heart* 2004;90:297-303.

[56] Mueller C, Scholer A, Laule-Kilian K, Martina B,Schindler C, Buser P, et al: Use of B-type natriuretic peptide in the evaluation and management of acute dyspnea. *N. Engl. J. Med.* 2001;345:1014-1021.

[57] de Lemos JA, Morrow DA, Bentley JH, Omland T, Sabatine MS, McCabe, CH, et al: The prognostic value of B-type natriuretic peptide in patients with acute coronary syndromes. *N. Engl. J. Med.* 2001;345:1014-1021.

[58] Richards AM, Nicholls MG, Espiner EA, Lainchbury JG, Troughton RW, Elliott J, et al: B-type natriuretic peptides and ejection fraction for prognosis after myocardial infarction. *Circulation* 2003;107:2786-2792.

[59] Sabatine MS, Morrow DA, de Lemos JA, Gibson CM, Murphy SA, Rifai N, et al: Multimarker approach to risk stratification in non-ST elevation acute coronary syndromes: simultaneous assessment of troponin I, C-reactive protein and B-type natriuretic peptide. *Circulation* 2002, 105, 1760-1763.

[60] Jernberg T, Stridsberg M, Venge P, Lindahl B: N-terminal pro-brain natriuretic peptide on admission for early risk stratification of patients with chest pain and no ST-segment elevation. *J. Am. Coll. Cardiol.* 2002;40:437-445.

[61] Collinson PO, Gaze DC: Biomarkers of Cardiovascular Damage. *Med. Princ. Pract.* 2007;16:247-261.

In: Heart Disease in Men
Editors: A.B. Todd and M.H. Mosley, pp. 183-200
ISBN: 978-1-60692-297-2

Chapter 8

IMMUNE RESPONSES TO HEAT SHOCK PROTEINS IN CHRONIC PERIODONTITIS AND CORONARY HEART DISEASE

A. Hasan, D. Sadoh and M. Foo
Department of Periodontology, King's College London Dental,
Institute at Guy's, King's College and St Thomas',
Hospitals, London, UK

Abstract

Coronary heart disease (CHD) shares a number of features with chronic periodontitis (CP) including risk factors such as smoking and diabetes; an aetiopathogenesis implicating a number of microbial species, as well as chronic inflammation. However, the link between these two conditions remains unclear. The prevalence of CHD increases with age and is higher in males than females. CP is a chronic inflammatory condition which destroys the supporting tissues of teeth and also increases in prevalence with age. Immune responses against heat shock proteins (HSP) can be cross-reactive among bacterial and human antigens. There is evidence that microbial HSP65 and human HSP60 is involved in periodontal disease and CHD and may therefore provide a mechanistic link between CP and CHD. The aim of this study is to investigate immune responses to the human HSP60 and microbial HSP65 in patients with CP and CHD and relate these to the level of inflammation. We collected serum samples from 100 male subjects divided into 4 groups, each matched for age: (a) Healthy control group with minimal gingivitis, (b) CP, (c) CHD with gingivitis (d) CHD with CP. ELISA was used to determine the levels of serum anti-HSP and C-reactive protein (CRP) in the 4 groups. Peripheral blood mononuclear cells were also isolated from these 4 groups and stimulated with HSPs. Significant lymphoproliferation was seen in CHD with or without CP when stimulated with human HSP60. CRP and serum anti-human HSP60 IgG were elevated in the patients groups compared to the healthy control group, but not serum anti-microbial HSP 65 IgG,. In view of the potential confounding effects of smoking in CP and CHD, a group of current smokers (n=24) were also recruited to investigate whether smoking affects HSP immune responses.There was no significant difference in HSP-induced lymphoproliferation between smokers and non-smokers in any of the four groups. There was a significant correlation between CRP and lymphoproliferative responses to Human HSP60.

This study shows that serum anti-human HSP60 IgG and serum CRP are raised in CHD with or without CP. In CHD with or without CP, serum CRP levels correlated significantly with human HSP60-induced lymphoproliferation, but not with anti-HSP antibody levels.

Introduction

Cardiovascular disease arising as a result of atherosclerosis is a major cause of death in western societies and has been associated with periodontal disease (Beck et al 1996, DeStefano et al 1993). Both atherosclerosis and chronic periodontitis share risk factors, most relevantly smoking, and this has led some groups to conclude that shared risk factors are acting as confounders and that there is no link between the two conditions (Hujoel et al 2001); however further evidence for an association continue to appear in the literature (Desvarieux et al 2005).

The periodontium in the diseased state is a complex polymicrobial niche (Lang et al 1998). Over 300 species of bacteria have been isolated and characterised from plaque deposits (Moore & Moore 1994). In 1mg of dental plaque, more than 10^8 bacteria are present (Lang et al 1998). In a neglected dentition, common oral hygiene procedures may result in bacteraemias with consequent systemic inflammation (Carroll & Sebor 1980, Silver et al. 1977).

Chronic periodontitis (CP) is an inflammatory disease characterised by connective tissue destruction and bone resorption. The aetiology of CP is associated with a number of bacteria, autoimmunity or microbial cross-reactivity (Listgarten et al 2003). There is evidence from cross-sectional studies implicating *Porphyromonas gingivalis, Tannerella forsythia* as well as other microbial species including Gram-negative and Gram-positive bacteria, some of which are unculturable (Kumar et al 2003). These findings support the hypothesis that the aetiology of CP is polymicrobial. Serum concentration of CRP, a marker of systemic inflammation, is raised in patients with chronic periodontitis (Amar et al 2003, Buhlin et al 2003}.

HSPs are the most highly conserved group of proteins known in phylogeny with respect to biochemical function, mode of regulation and structure (Ellis 1995, Jindal et al 1989, Thole et al 1988). They are expressed in all eukaryotic and prokaryotic cells including Gram-positive and Gram-negative bacteria (Ellis 1995). The high degree of homology between microbial and human HSPs has led to the hypothesis that tissue damage can occur as a result of cross-reactivity between bacterial and human HSPs. Humoral and T cell response to HSPs have been demonstrated in CP (Hasan et al 2005, Buhlin et al 2003, Tabeta et al 2000, Lopatin et al 1999, Schett et al 1997a, Ando et al 1995).

Chronic infection may also play a role in coronary heart disease (CHD) (Danesh et al 1997, Zhu et al 2000, Saikku et al 1988). As well as DNA from *Chlamydia pneumoniae,* studies have also demonstrated the presence of DNA from periodontotopathic organisms such as *Porphyromonas gingivalis, Tannerella forsythia,* and *Actinobacillus actinomycetemcomitans* in atheromatous plaques (Ford et al 2005, Haraszthy et al 2000). Furthermore, antibodies to periodontal pathogens are associated with CHD (Pussinen et al 2003).

Animal models provide evidence for shared pathogenic mechanisms between atherosclerosis and periodontitis. When apolipoprotein-E-deficient (-/-) mice are immunized with a major periodontopathogen, *Porphyromonas gingivalis,* thereby increasing the burden of pathogen, atherogenesis was enhanced (Ford et al 2007). Host HSP could be detected in atherosclerotic lesions and lesion progression correlated with anti-GroEL antibody levels suggesting that molecular mimicry between GroEL and host HSP60 is involved (Ford et al 2007).

Many studies have focused on identifying a single pathogen, however it has been postulated that the risk factor is the cumulative pathogen burden rather than mono-infections (Epstein 2002). Given the wide range of microbial species implicated in both conditions, a role for HSPs seems probable and in CHD has been suggested by a number of findings: autoantibodies to microbial HSP65 have been shown to mediate macrophage lysis (Schett et al 1997b) and endothelial cytotoxicity (Schett et al 1995) and mucosal administration of microbial HSP65 reduced the presence of atherosclerosis and inflammation in the aortic arch of LDL receptor deficient mice (Maron et al 2002).

The objectives of this investigation are to determine whether serum anti HSP60/65 IgG and IgA are associated with chronic periodontitis and/or CHD in male Caucasian patients and to determine if inflammation, as reflected by CRP levels, correlates with these immune responses.

Material and Methods

Subjects

Patients with CP and CHD were recruited from the department of Periodontology at Guy's, King's and St Thomas's Institute and the Coronary Care Unit St Thomas's Hospital (Table 1). All subjects were male caucasians, aged between 35 and 69 years of age and had at least 15 standing teeth. CHD patients with angiographic evidence of atherosclerosis but no history of myocardial infarction or previous heart bypass operation were recruited. A small number of smokers were also recruited and matched in age and condition to the 4 groups (Table 2). Subjects were excluded from the study if they had systemic disease including diabetes mellitus, recurrent aphthous stomatitis and autoimmune disease, a history of malignancies, previous treatment for periodontitis, or a history of antibiotic therapy within the past six months prior to recruitment .

Subjects were allocated into

(1) Healthy control with minimal gingivitis group
(2) Chronic periodontitis only group (CP)
(3) CHD group with minimal gingivitis(CHD-G)
(4) CHD group with Chronic Periodontitis (CHD-CP).

In each subject, probing depths and recession of all teeth (rounded down to the nearest millimetre) were determined using a William's probe. Recession was measured as the distance from the cemento-enamel junction to the gingival margin. Measurements were rounded down to the nearest mm from 6 sites: mesio-buccal, mid-buccal, disto-buccal, mesio-lingual, mid-lingual and disto-lingual, probing attachment loss was then calculated as the sum of probing pocket depth and recession.

Table 1. Clinical data and optical densities at 1:100 for serum IgA antibodies to human HSP60 and microbial HSP65 of patients showing median (interquartile range).

Group & Number of patients	Healthy controls n=25	CP n=25	CHD-G n=25	CHD-CP n=25
Age (years) ANOVA p=0.239	48.0 (44-58)	49.0 (43-53)	52.0 (48-56)	54.0 (50-55)
Probing attachment level (mm)	0.9 (0.8-1.0)	3.2 (2.8-4.2)	1.0 (0.8-1.2)	3.2 (2.4-4.8)
Anti-microbial HSP65 IgA ANOVA p=0.362	0.38 (0.28-0.54)	0.33 (0.24-0.66)	0.30 (0.24-0.41)	0.47 (0.27-0.75)
Anti-human HSP60 IgA ANOVA p=0.559	0.62 (0.41-1.07)	0.58 (0.43-0.84)	0.50 (0.36-0.76)	0.53 (0.37-0.94)

Table 2. Clinical data from smokers in each of the 4 groups. showing median (interquartile range).

Present Smokers	Healthy controls n=6	CP n=6	CHD-G n=6	CHD-CP n=6
Age (yrs) ANOVA P=0.331	47 (43-57)	48 (44-51)	50 (47-52)	53 (47-51)
Probing attachment level (mm) p=0.3	0.8 (0.7-1.0)	3.0 (2.7-4.1)	0.9 (0.7-1.1)	3.0 (2.2-4.3)

Periodontitis was defined as probing attachment loss ≥4mm in at least 4 teeth and healthy control group as probing attachment loss < 2mm in all teeth. Probing attachment loss was calculated as the sum of the probing depth and recession. Ethical committee approval was obtained (code no 98/12/04) and subject consent obtained. 50ml of venous blood were withdrawn from each subject before periodontal probing or angiography.

HSP

Recombinant HSP65 derived from *Mycobacterium bovis* was prepared at the National Institute of Public Health and Environmental Protection, Bilthoven, the Netherlands and used at a predetermined optimal concentration of 10μg/ml. Human HSP60 was purchased from Stressgen (Victoria, Canada). The two HSPs were detoxified using Detoxi-gel columns

(Pierce, Oxford, UK) and the endotoxin level was determined by Limulus Amoebocyte Lysate assay (Sigma-Aldrich, Poole, Dorset, UK). The concentration of endotoxin was <0·007 U/μg or 7 pg endotoxin/μg for both HSPs.

Serum ELISA Measurements

Antibodies to the HSP (human HSP60 and microbial HSP65) were detected by enzyme-linked immunosorbent assay. 96-well flat-bottomed polystyrene microtitre plates were coated (Immulon 4 HBX USA) with HSP60 (Stressgen, Victoria, Canada) or microbial HSP65 diluted (1μg/ml) with phosphate buffered saline (PBS, pH 7.4) and left overnight at room temperature. HSPs were detoxified using Detoxigel columns (Pierce, Oxford, UK) and the endotoxin level was determined by Limulus Amoebocyte Lysate assay Sigma-Aldrich, Poole, Dorset, UK). Uncoated sites were then blocked with 0.5% wt/vol BSA (Sigma-Aldrich Irvine U.K.) in PBS (200μl/well) for 60 minutes at room temperature. In addition, human sero-negative and sero-positive samples were identified by running the whole series of patient serum samples and obtaining the most positive and negative samples as positive and negative controls respectively. Serum from rabbits previously immunised with microbial HSP65 and human HSP60 (kindly provided by Dr L Bergmeier and Dr A Hasan, KCL Dental Institute, London) was also used as positive control. Serum samples obtained from patients including positive and negative controls were then diluted as follows in PBS containing 0.5% BSA and 0.05% tween 20; 2 fold dilution of serum at 1:100 for anti-human HSP60 IgG, anti-microbial HSP 65 IgG and anti-HSP60 IgA, 2 fold dilution of serum at 1:50 for anti-microbial HSP65 IgA. 100μl of each diluted sample or positive/negative control were then added in duplicates to each well and serially diluted to 1:6400, except for anti-microbial HSP65 IgA which had a final dilution of 1:3200.

Plates were then incubated at room temperature for 2 hours and washed 4 times with PBS containing 0.05% Tween 20. Secondary antibody goat anti-human IgG, or IgA Fc specific, alkaline phosphatase conjugates (Sigma-aldrich, U.K.) were diluted in diluent buffer to an optimal concentration. 100μl were then added to each well and incubated at room temperature for 2 hours. Anti-human IgG alkaline phosphatase conjugate was used at 1:2000. Anti-human IgA alkaline phosphatase conjugate was used at 1:1000 for detection of serum anti-human HSP60 IgA and at 1:500 for the detection of serum anti- microbial HSP65 IgA. Plates were then washed 4 times with wash buffer and were developed with para-nitrophenylphosphate in diethanolamine buffer (pH 9.8) at room temperature. The absorbance was determined using a microplate reader (Anthos 2001, Anthos labtec instruments U.K.) for IgG, and (Opsys MR DYNEX technologies) for IgA at 405nm with wavelength correction at 620nm. Inter-assay variation was monitored using a standard positive serum in each assay (Direskeneli et al 1996). The variation of the titre of this positive serum was within one dilution step.

Separation of Cells

Peripheral blood mononuclear cells (PBMC) were separated from blood by density gradient centrifugation and cultured as described previously (Pervin et al 1993). Briefly, 10^5 cells were cultured in RPMI with or without antigens, including ovalbumin (Sigma, Poole, UK) as an unrelated protein control, in quadruplicate in 96-well round-bottomed plates for 6 days. Cells were cultured in RPMI-1640 and 10% autologous serum for 1 h at 37 °C in 5% CO^2. In the final 6 h of culture the cells were pulsed with [3H]-thymidine (0·5 μCi or 18·5 mBq per well; Amersham International, Amersham, UK). The results were assessed by calculating the stimulation index (SI), which is the ratio of antigen-stimulated to antigen-unstimulated cultures (Pervin et al 1993).

Detection of C-reactive Protein by ELISA

50μL of pre-diluted standard and blank were added to a 96 well plate precoated with anti-serum CRP IgG (Kalon Biological Ltd). Serum samples were diluted 1:1000 with assay diluent (Kalon Biological Ltd) and dispensed in duplicates to designated wells in CRP precoated plates. The Plate was then incubated at room temperature for 60 minutes. Plates were washed 4 times with wash buffer (Kalon Biological Ltd). 100μL of CRP tracer (affinity purified sheep anti-CRP labelled with alkaline phosphatase, Kalon Biological Ltd U.K) were then dispensed to each well and incubated uncovered for 30 minutes at room temperature. Plates were washed again 4 times with washing buffer (Kalon Biological Ltd, U.K).

100μl of substrate solution (4-nitrophenylphosphate in substrate buffer Kalon Biological Ltd) were then dispensed to each well and incubated at room temperature for 30 minutes. The reaction was stopped with 100μl of (120g/L) sodium hydroxide. Optical densities were read at 405nm with micoplate reader (Anthos 2001, Anthos labtec instruments U.K.). A standard curve was constructed with standard points and curve fitted with four parameter logistic curve fitting software. Test serum values were then read off the standard curve.

Statistical Method

Kruskal-Wallis ANOVA test was used to assess differences between the groups. ELISA for serum anti-HSP IgG or IgA was analysed by using data consisting of optical density readings for the performed test. The mean optical density was then analysed at 1:100. The significance level was set at $p<0.05$. Post-ANOVA pair wise comparisons between the healthy with CP group; healthy with CHD-G group CP, and with CHD-CP group was carried out using the Mann-Whitney U test, using the Bonferroni correction test to set the significance level at $p<0.02$. Inter-relationships between serum anti-HSP60 IgG and serum CRP levels were tested using Spearman ranked correlation coefficients (r_s). Non-parametric data is displayed in graphs as median (1st and 3rd quartile, minimum, maximum).

Results

Clinical Data

We recruited 120 patients (non-smokers) divided into 4 groups, The median (interquartile range) age of the subjects in the control group was 48 (44-58) years, in the CP group 49 (43-53) years, in the CHD-G group 52 (48-56) and in the CHD-CP group 54 (50-55) and there was no statistically significant difference between the groups, (ANOVA $p=0.239$, Table 1). In order to investigate the effect of smoking on lymphoproliferative responses, we recruited a small number of current smokers (Table 2). The current smokers were matched for age, gender, and disease status with non-smokers from the 4 groups. There were no significant differences in the age and periodontal status of non-smokers in each of the 4 groups when compared with smokers in the 4 groups (p>0.05).

For the non-smokers, the median (interquartile range) probing attachment level in the control group was 0.9 (0.8-1.0) mm, in the CP group 3.2 (2.8-4.2) mm, in the CHD-G group 1.0 (0.8-1.2) mm and in the CHD-CP group 3.2 (2.4-4.8) mm (Table 1). In view of the confounding effect of smoking in studies associating periodontitis to cardiovascular disease, the data from smokers and non-smokers have been kept separate in all figures and tables.

IgA Antibodies to Microbial HSP65 and Human HSP60

The OD at 1:100 dilution of serum for anti-microbial HSP65 IgA was 0.38 (0.28-0.54) in the control group, 0.33 (0.24-0.66) in the CP group, 0.30 (0.24-0.41) in the CHD-G group and 0.47 (0.27-0.75) in the CHD-CP group, and was not significant ANOVA, p=0.362 (Table 1). Similarly, there was no difference in serum anti-human HSP60 IgA in the 4 groups (Table 1). The median (interquartile range) OD at 1:100 dilution of serum was 0.62 (0.41-1.07) in the control group, 0.58 (0.43-0.84) in the CP group, 0.50 (0.36-0.76) in the CHD-G group, and 0.53 (0.37-0.94), or in the CHD-CP group ANOVA (p=0.559) (Table 1).

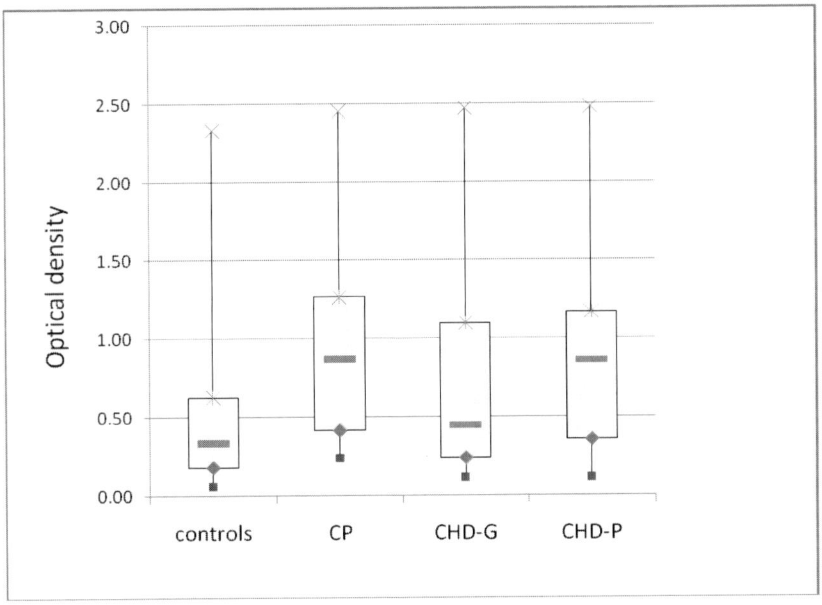

Figure 1. Boxplots showing median, interquartile range, minimum and maximum OD for serum anti-microbial HSP65 IgG in 4 groups of patients The median (interquartile range) OD of 1:100 dilution of serum for anti-human HSP60 IgG was 0.26 (0.17-0.34) in the control group, 0.87 (0.42-1.27) in the CP group, 0.33 (0.24-1.1) in the CHD-G group and 0.86 (0.36-1.17) in the CHD-CP group and this was statistically significant by ANOVA (p<0.001) (figure 2). Post-ANOVA analysis revealed a significant difference between the controls and the CP group (p<0.001). There was also a significant difference between the control and the CHD-G group (p=0.019), but no significant difference between the chronic periodontitis and the CHD-CP group (p=0.907).

IgG Antibodies to Microbial HSP65 and Human HSP60

The median (interquartile range) optical density at 1:100 dilution of serum for anti-microbial HSP65 IgG was 0.34 (0.17-0.63) in the control group, 0.46(0.25-0.85) in the CP group, 0.35 (0.23-0.71) in the CHD-G group and 0.59 (0.2-0.94) in the CHD-CP group (Figure 1). There was no significant difference amongst the 4 groups in serum anti-HSP65 IgG titres by ANOVA (p=0.661).

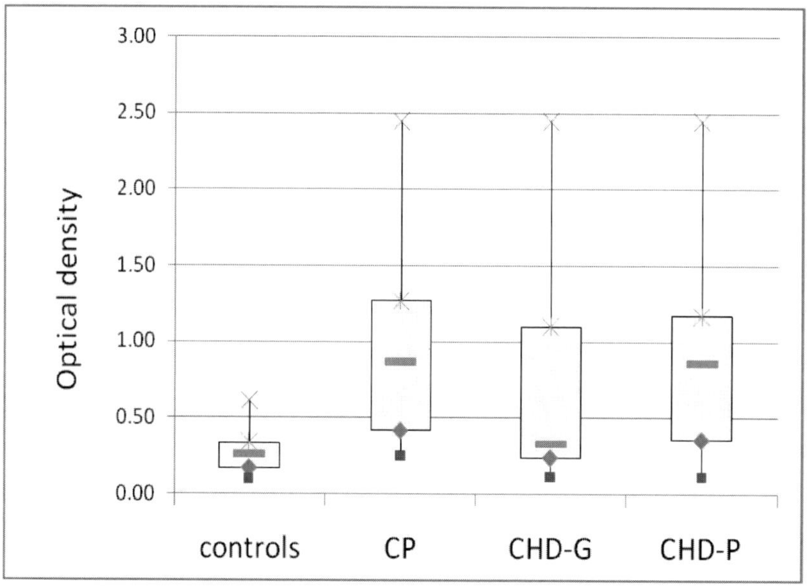

Figure 2. Boxplots showing median, interquartile range, minimum and maximum OD for serum anti-human HSP60 IgG in 4 groups of patients

Serum levels of anti-microbial HSP65 IgG were significantly associated with serum levels of anti-human HSP60 IgG in only 2 groups: the CP group (r_s= 0.538, p= 0.005) and the CHD-G group (r_s =0.524, p=0.007) (Table 3). No statistically significant relationship was revealed between serum anti-microbial HSP 65 IgG and serum anti-human HSP60 IgG in the control group (r_s=0.005, p=0.983) and the CHD-CP group (r_s=0.255, p=0.219) (Table 3).

Table 3. Correlation between serum anti-human HSP60 IgG and serum CRP levels to serum anti-microbial HSP 65 IgG

		anti-microbial HSP65 IgG	CRP
Control	r_s	0.005	0.115
n=25	p	0.983	0.583
CP	r_s	#0.538	-0.194
n=25	p	*0.005	0.352
CHD-G	r_s	#0.524	-0.099
n=25	p	*0.007	0.637
CHD-CP	r_s	0.255	#0.417
n=25	p	0.219	*0.038

significant correlation coefficient (r_s) * Significant p value

Lymphoproliferative Responses to Human HSP60 in Smokers and Non-smokers

The results of the lymphoproliferative assays are expressed as stimulation indices (the ratio of antigen-stimulated to unstimulated cultures). An analysis of smokers and non-smokers in each group yielded no significant differences in lymphoproliferative responses between any of the four groups (figure 3). All patient groups responded significantly to human HSP60, in contrast to the healthy controls which yielded a median (interquartile range) stimulation index of 2.0 (0.45) ($p<0.001$). Smoking does not appear to influence HSP60-induced proliferation in CP or CHD. In all groups of non-smokers except the controls, HSP proliferative responses correlated with CRP levels ($p<0.02$).

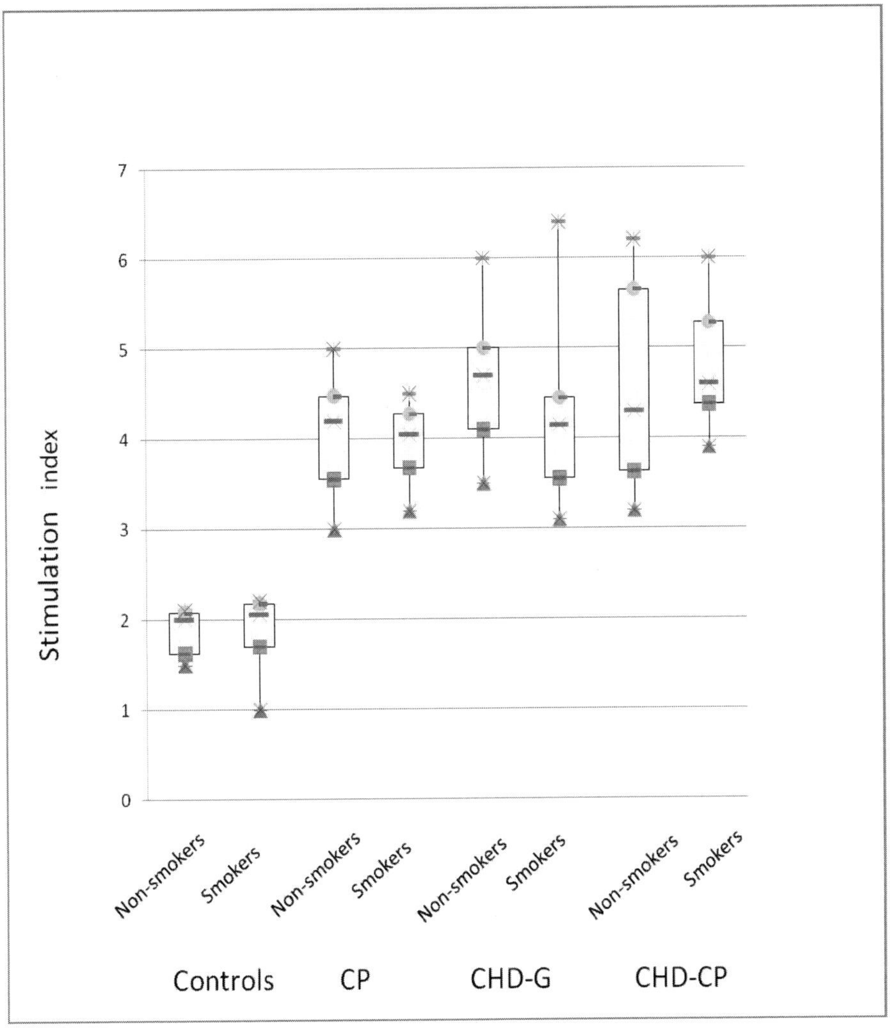

Figure 3. Boxplots showing median, interquartile range, minimum and maximum stimulation index of Human HSP60-induced lymphoproliferative responses in non-smokers and smokers (n=6 for each group). CP and CHD with or without CP responded significantly to HSP60 (ANOVA $p<0.001$)

CRP

The median (interquartile range) of serum CRP levels in the 4 groups was 0.64 (0.18-1.86) mg/L in the control group, 1.27 (1.01-2.83) mg/L in the CP group, 2.15 (1.03-2.94) in the CHD-G group and 2.0 (1.31-3.78) in the CHD-CP group (figure 4). There was a statistically significant difference amongst the groups by ANOVA (p=0.002). Post-ANOVA analysis revealed significant differences between the control group compared to the CP group (p=0.007) and the control group compared with the CHD-G group (p=0.001). However there was no significant difference between the CP compared with the CHD-CP group (p=0.383). It is tempting to interpret this to mean that CP influences CRP levels, however we do not have data on whether these responses may fluctuate with time, and what other innate or adaptive mechanisms determine the outcome; nor do we know how this impacts on CHD.

Serum CRP levels are not significantly associated with serum anti-human HSP60 IgG levels in the control group (r_s =0.115, p=0.583), in the CP group (r_s =-0.194, p=0.352) and in the CHD-G group (r_s =-0.099, p=0.637) (Table 3). However in the CHD-CP group there was an association between serum CRP levels and serum anti-human HSP60 IgG levels (r_s =0.417, p= 0.038) (Table 3).

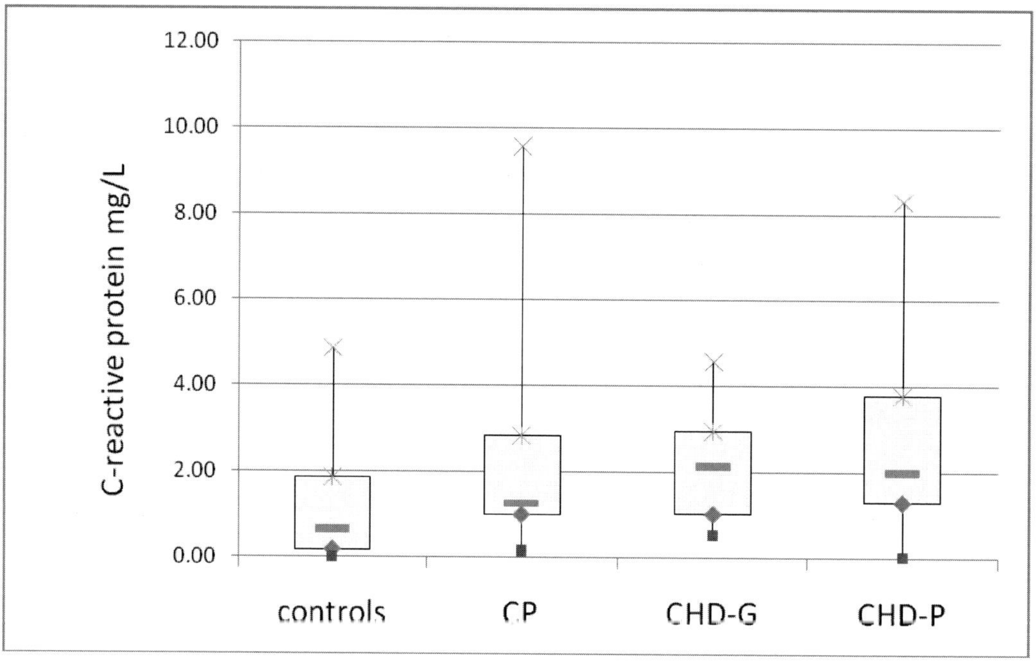

Figure 4. Boxplots showing median, interquartile range, minimum and maximum level of serum C-reactive protein amongst the 4 groups of patients

Discussion

The results show that serum anti-human HSP60 IgG but not serum anti-microbial HSP65 IgG was elevated in patients with chronic periodontitis compared to the control group. No significant differences were noted in the level of serum anti-human HSP60 IgA and serum anti-microbial HSP65 IgA between the control group and patients with chronic periodontitis. These findings contrast with a study showing an elevation of serum anti-HSP65 IgG (Schett et al 1997a) and another study showing depression of serum anti-HSP65 IgA with no difference in serum anti-human HSP60 IgG and serum anti-microbial HSP 65 IgG in CP patients compared to the control group (Buhlin et al 2003). However these studies are difficult to compare directly as there are significant differences in demographical and clinical parameters. In one of these studies the patient group had a mean age of 37.5 ± 12.6 years range 26-65 years (Schett et al 1997); with this age range it is likely that more than one form of periodontitis was included. Our study included only patients with moderate-advanced chronic periodontitis or gingival health/mild gingivitis. The median age (interquartile range) of our patients with chronic periodontitis is 49 (43-53). Younger aged patients with advanced periodontitis may represent a different diagnostic category or a different spectrum of response from older patients suffering from chronic periodontitis (Ranney 2000), and may mount different immune responses (Gunsolley et al 1990).

The recruitment of patients who are undergoing treatment for chronic periodontitis (Buhlin et al 2003) is problematic and may yield conflicting results as treatment of CP has a modulating effect on humoral immune responses to HSP (Yamazaki et al 2004) and instrumentation may immunise patients with plaque antigens. To minimise the confounding effect of treatment in our results we recruited untreated cases.

Our findings are in agreement with studies where the mean ages of untreated chronic periodontitis were similar (Tabeta et al 2000, Lopatin et al 1999). These studies demonstrated a significant elevation in serum anti-human HSP 60 IgG compared to a control group (Tabeta et al 2000). Serum anti-microbial HSP65 IgG levels were either similar (Lopatin et al 1999) or elevated (Tabeta et al 2000) in chronic periodontitis patients compared to control patients.

It was important to match our patients for age, as clearly both CP and CHD occur with increasing frequency in older populations. In addition, the diagnosis of periodontal diseases is unfortunately age-dependent, so the distinction between early onset forms of periodontitis and chronic adult periodontitis becomes harder to establish when patients present at the age of 30-35. Until the behaviour of the disease can be determined it is difficult to be certain the correct diagnosis has been made without resorting to special tests and culture studies. We were therefore careful to match the age of patients to those presenting at the Coronary care unit, rather than those attending a Periodontal clinic where the patients tend to be three decades younger.

In this study whilst we demonstrated a statistically significant elevation in serum anti-human HSP60 IgG in the CHD-G group, there was no statistical difference in serum anti-microbial HSP65 IgG. A number of studies have demonstrated elevation in serum anti-microbial HSP65 IgG in patients with CHD (Ciervo et al 2002, Mahdi et al 2002, Prohászka et al 2001, Birnie et al 1998, Hoppichler et al 1996, Xu et al 1993) which was sustained over a number of years (Xu et al 1999) and predicted cardiovascular events (Veres et al 2002, Xu et al 1999). Most of these studies analysed subjects aged 60 years or over (Veres et al 2002, Ciervo et al 2002, Mahdi et al 2002, Xu et al 1999, Hoppichler et al 1996, Xu et al 1993) or did not include a healthy control group (Birnie et al 1998). Furthermore, the periodontal status of these patients was not determined. When a younger age group (less than 60 yrs old) was analysed for anti-HSP65 IgG, no significant difference was found compared with the control group (Xu et al 1993). In studies where the age group was comparable to our study, serum anti-HSP60 IgG was demonstrated to be elevated in the patient group compared to control

(Bason et al 2003, Burian et al 2003, Prohászka et al 2001, Zhu et al 2001). Additionally, serum antibodies from these patients recognised human HSP60 peptide fragments (Bason et al 2003, Wysocki et al 2002). Older subjects have been shown to be more prone to chronic infections resulting in an increase in markers of inflammation including anti-microbial HSP65 (Kiechl et al 2001). The presence of anti-microbial HSP65 antibodies may reflect the cumulative effect of infections which increases with age. However this is still compatible with the hypothesis that cross-reactivity between microbial HSP65 and human HSP60 may lead to tissue damage in CP and CHD (Mayr et al 1999).

Serum anti-human HSP60 IgA when present with *Chlamydia pneumoniae* has been identified as a risk factor for future coronary events in patients who were initially healthy (Huittinen et al 2003, Huittinen et al 2002). Whilst we found there was no statistically significant difference in serum anti-human HSP60 IgA or serum anti-microbial HSP65 IgA between the control and the CHD-G group, it remains to be established whether antibody levels remain elevated or fluctuate in relation to intercurrent infections. It is clearly important to determine how innate, humoral and cellular immune responses change with time, infection, or coronary events in CP or CHD.

Cross reactivity between anti-microbial HSP65 antibodies and human HSP60 antibodies has been suggested to mediate macrophage lysis (Schett et al 1997b) and endothelial damage (Schett et al 1995). Serum anti-microbial HSP65 have been shown to recognise specific epitopes on human HSP60 in subjects with atherosclerosis (Perschinka et al 2003). In our study there was a moderate correlation between serum anti-human HSP60 IgG and serum anti-microbial HSP65 IgG in patients with CP and CHD-G, and therefore the possibility of cross-reactivity still exists. Shared epitopes within human HSP60 may help account for the association between CP and CHD and reveal a mechanistic link for tissue destruction. Once the epitopes recognised in CP and CHD have been mapped, the role of T and B cell epitopes in relation to inflammatory and anti-inflammatory responses can be elucidated.

Smoking is a risk factor for chronic periodontitis and CHD (Genco et al 2002). In addition smoking has been suggested to be a confounding variable in the association of CP with CHD (Hujoel et al 2000). Smoking is known to modulate immune response and in chronic periodontitis there is a direct correlation between serum cotinine levels and serum levels of intracellular adhesion molecule- a risk factor for CHD (Palmer et al 1999). Exposure of human monocytes and endothelial cells to freshly prepared filtrates of tobacco smoke induces expression of the inducible HSP70 (Vayssier-Taussat et al 2001). The role of smoking on the cellular and humoral immune responses to HSP in patients with chronic periodontitis and CHD has not been fully elucidated although, exposure to smoking reduces the release of TNF-α in human alveolar macrophages (Yamaguchi et al 1993) and PBMC (Ryder et al 2002). We found no difference between smokers and non-smokers in any of the subject groups suggesting that at least HSP-induced proliferation is not affected by smoking. It however remains to be determined how smoking affects HSP-induced T cell responses and inflammatory cytokine production in CHD and CP.

Serum CRP levels in patients with CP and CHD when compared to a healthy control group were significantly elevated. Previous studies have shown that serum CRP levels are elevated in CP (D'Aiuto et al 2004, Buhlin et al 2003, Ide et al 2003). Cross-sectional studies have shown that CRP levels are also raised in patients with angiographically recorded coronary heart disease (Garcia-Moll et al 2000, Rifai et al 1999) and in patients with symptoms of angina but normal coronary angiogram (Cosin-Sales et al 2003). In a prospective multiple risk factor intervention trial CRP was found to be an independent risk factor for coronary heart disease mortality in healthy but high risk individuals (Kuller et al 1996). Furthermore, CRP could be used to predict the risk of acute myocardial infarction and mortality of patients with angiographically recorded coronary heart disease (Bickel et al 2002, Zebrack et al 2002).

No significant correlation was shown between CRP and serum anti-HSP60 IgG levels in subjects, except in the CHD-CP group. This is in agreement with previous reports in the literature which do not demonstrate significant relationship between CRP and serum anti-human HSP60 levels (Veres et al 2002, Zhu et al 2001). These conflicting findings may simply reflect the complex nature of innate immunity and its diverse relationships to both inflammatory and anti-inflammatory mechanisms.

Conclusion

This study demonstrated that serum anti-human HSP 60 IgG but not serum anti-microbial HSP65 IgG is elevated in patients with CP with or without CHD indicating there are autoantibodies to human HSP60 in CP and CHD and together with our previous findings of autoimmune T cell response to human HSP provides further support for cross-reactivity in the pathogenesis of CP and CHD. Serum CRP levels were also significantly raised in the patient groups but there was no significant relationship between serum CRP levels with serum anti-human HSP60 IgG levels. If we are to determine successfuly whether the association between CP and CHD is real, HSP-induced inflammatory and anti-inflammatory mechanisms need to be further elucidated in relation to innate immunity.

References

Amar, S., Gokce, N., Morgan, S., Loukideli, M., Van Dyke, T.E. & Vita, J.A. (2003) Periodontal disease is associated with brachial artery endothelial dysfunction and systemic inflammation. *Arteriosclerosis, thrombosis, and vascular biology*, **23**, 1245-1249.

Ando, T., Kato, T., Ishihara, K., Ogiuchi, H. & Okuda, K. (1995) Heat shock proteins in the human periodontal disease process. *Microbiology and immunology*, **39**, 321-327.

Badersten A., Nilveus R, Egelberg J. (1981) Effect of nonsurgical periodontal therapy. I. Moderately advanced periodontitis. *Journal of clinical periodontology*, **1**, 57-72.

Bason, C., Corrocher, R., Lunardi, C., Puccetti, P., Olivieri, O., Girelli, D., Navone, R., Beri, R., Millo, E., Margonato, A., Martinelli, N. & Puccetti, A. (2003) Interaction of antibodies against cytomegalovirus with heat-shock protein 60 in pathogenesis of atherosclerosis. *Lancet*, **362**, 1971-1977.

Beck J. Garcia R. Heiss G. Vokonas PS. Offenbacher S. (1996) Periodontal disease and cardiovascular disease. *Journal of Periodontology*. **67**(10 Suppl):1123-37

Bickel, C., Rupprecht, H.J., Blankenberg, S., Espiniola-Klein, C., Schlitt, A., Rippin, G., Hafner, G., Treude, R., Othman, H., Hofmann, K.P. & Meyer, J. (2002) Relation of markers of inflammation (C-reactive protein, fibrinogen, von Willebrand factor, and leukocyte count) and statin therapy to long-term mortality in patients with angiographically proven coronary artery disease. *The American journal of cardiology*, **89**, 901-908.

Birnie, D.H., Holme, E.R., McKay, I.C., Hood, S., McColl, K.E. & Hillis, W.S. (1998) Association between antibodies to heat shock protein 65 and coronary atherosclerosis. Possible mechanism of action of Helicobacter pylori and other bacterial infections in increasing cardiovascular risk. *European heart journal*, **19**, 387-394.

Buhlin, K., Gustafsson, A., Pockley, A.G., Frostegard, J. & Klinge, B. (2003) Risk factors for cardiovascular disease in patients with periodontitis. *European heart journal*, **24**, 2099-2107.

Burian, K., Kis, Z., Virok, D., Endresz, V., Prohaszka, Z., Duba, J., Berencsi, K., Boda, K., Horvath, L., Romics, L., Fust, G. & Gonczol, E. (2001) Independent and joint effects of antibodies to human heat-shock protein 60 and Chlamydia pneumoniae infection in the development of coronary atherosclerosis. *Circulation*, **103**, 1503-1508.

Carroll, G.C. & Sebor, R.J. (1980) Dental flossing and its relationship to transient bacteremia. *Journal of periodontology*, **51**, 691-692.

Ciervo, A., Visca, P., Petrucca, A., Biasucci, L.M., Maseri, A. & Cassone, A. (2002) Antibodies to 60-kilodalton heat shock protein and outer membrane protein 2 of Chlamydia pneumoniae in patients with coronary heart disease. *Clinical and diagnostic laboratory immunology*, **9,** 66-74.

Cosin-Sales, J., Pizzi, C., Brown, S. & Kaski, J.C. (2003) C-reactive protein, clinical presentation, and ischemic activity in patients with chest pain and normal coronary angiograms. *Journal of the American College of Cardiology*, **41**, 1468-1474.

Danesh, J., Collins, R. & Peto R. (1997) Chronic infections and coronary heart disease: is there a link? *Lancet*, **350**, 430-436.

D'Aiuto, F., Parkar, M., Andreou, G., Suvan, J., Brett, P.M., Ready, D. & Tonetti, M.S. (2004) Periodontitis and Systemic Inflammation: Control of the Local Infection is Associated with a Reduction in Serum Inflammatory Markers. *Journal of dental research*, **83**, 156-160.

DeStefano F. Anda RF. Kahn HS. Williamson DF. Russell CM. (1993) Dental disease and risk of coronary heart disease and mortality. *BMJ*. **306**(6879):688-91

Desvarieux M. Demmer RT. Rundek T. Boden-Albala B. Jacobs DR Jr. Sacco RL. Papapanou PN. (2005) Periodontal microbiota and carotid intima-media thickness: the Oral Infections and Vascular Disease Epidemiology Study (INVEST). *Circulation*. **111**(5):576-82

Direskeneli, H., Hasan, A., Shinnick, T., Mizushima, R., van der Zee, R., Fortune, F., Stanford, M.R. & Lehner, T. (1996) Recognition of B-cell epitopes of the 65 kDa HSP in Behcet's disease. *Scandinavian journal of immunology*, **43**, 464-471.

Ellis RJ Stress proteins as molecular chaperones. (1995) In *Stress proteins in medicine,* eds. Willem V.E., Douglas B. Y & Mercel, D . 1st edition., pp. 1-26. Inc New york, Basel, Hong Kong.

Epstein SE. (2002) The multiple mechanisms by which infection may contribute to atherosclerosis development and course. *Circulation Research*. **90**(1):2-4

Ford PJ. Gemmell E. Hamlet SM. Hasan A. Walker PJ. West MJ. Cullinan MP. Seymour GJ. (2005) Cross-reactivity of GroEL antibodies with human heat shock protein 60 and quantification of pathogens in atherosclerosis. *Oral Microbiology & Immunology*. **20**(5):296-302

Ford PJ. Gemmell E. Timms P. Chan A. Preston FM. Seymour GJ. (2007) Anti-P. gingivalis response correlates with atherosclerosis. *Journal of Dental Research.* **86**(1):35-40

Garcia-Moll, X., Zouridakis, E., Cole, D. & Kaski, J.C. (2000) C-reactive protein in patients with chronic stable angina: differences in baseline serum concentration between women and men. *European heart journal*, **21**, 1598-1606.

Genco, R., Offenbacher, S. & Beck, J. (2002) Periodontal disease and cardiovascular disease: epidemiology and possible mechanisms. *The Journal of the American Dental Association*, **133** Suppl, 14S-22S.

Gunsolley, J.C., Tew, J.G., Gooss, C., Marshall, D.R., Burmeister, J.A. & Schenkein, H.A. (1990) Serum antibodies to periodontal bacteria. *Journal of periodontology*, **61**, 412-419.

Haraszthy, V.I., Zambon, J.J., Trevisan, M., Zeid, M. & Genco, R.J. (2000) Identification of periodontal pathogens in atheromatous plaques. *Journal of periodontology*, **71**, 1554-1560.

Hasan A, Sadoh D, Palmer R, Foo M, Marber M and Lehner T (2005) The immune responses to human and microbial heat shock proteins in periodontal disease with and without coronary heart disease, *Clinical & Experimental Immunology*, **142**(3)585-594

Hoppichler, F., Lechleitner, M., Traweger, C., Schett, G., Dzien, A., Sturm, W. & Xu, Q. (1996) Changes of serum antibodies to heat-shock protein 65 in coronary heart disease and acute myocardial infarction. *Atherosclerosis*, **126**, 333-338.

Hujoel, P.P., Drangsholt, M., Spiekerman, C. & Derouen, T.A. (2000) Periodontal disease and coronary heart disease risk. *The journal of the American Medical Association*, **284**, 1406-1410.

Hujoel PP. Drangsholt M. Spiekerman C. Derouen TA.(2001) Examining the link between coronary heart disease and the elimination of chronic dental infections. *Journal of the American Dental Association.* **132**(7):883-9

Huittinen T, Leinonen M, Tenkanen L, Manttari M, Virkkunen H, Pitkanen T, Wahlstrom E, Palosuo T, Manninen V& Saikku P. (2002). Autoimmunity to human heat shock protein 60, Chlamydia pneumoniae infection, and inflammation in predicting coronary risk. *Arteriosclerosis, thrombosis, and vascular biology*, **22**, 431-437

Huittinen, T., Leinonen, M., Tenkanen, L., Virkkunen, H., Manttari, M., Palosuo, T., Manninen, V. & Saikku, P. (2003) Synergistic effect of persistent Chlamydia pneumoniae infection, autoimmunity, and inflammation on coronary risk. *Circulation*, **107**, 2566-2570.

Ide, M., McPartlin, D., Coward, P.Y., Crook, M., Lumb, P. & Wilson, R.F. (2003) Effect of treatment of chronic periodontitis on levels of serum markers of acute-phase inflammatory and vascular responses. *Journal of clinical periodontology*, **30**, 334-340.

Jindal S. Dudani AK. Singh B. Harley CB. Gupta RS. (1989) Primary structure of a human mitochondrial protein homologous to the bacterial and plant chaperonins and to the 65-kilodalton mycobacterial antigen. *Molecular & Cellular Biology.* **9**(5):2279-83.

Kiechl, S., Egger, G., Mayr, M., Wiedermann, C.J., Bonora, E., Oberhollenzer, F., Muggeo, M., Xu, Q., Wick, G., Poewe, W. & Willeit, J. (2001) Chronic infections and the risk of carotid atherosclerosis: prospective results from a large population study. *Circulation*, **103**, 1064-1070.

Kuller, L.H., Tracy, R.P., Shaten, J. & Meilahn, E.N. (1996) Relation of C-reactive protein and coronary heart disease in the MRFIT nested case-control study. Multiple Risk Factor Intervention Trial. *American journal of epidemiology*, **144**, 537-547.

Kumar PS. Griffen AL. Barton JA. Paster BJ. Moeschberger ML. Leys EJ. (2003) New bacterial species associated with chronic periodontitis. *Journal of Dental Research.* **82**(5):338-44,

Lang PN, Mombelli A & Attström R (1998) Dental Plaque and Calculus. In *Clinical Periodontology and Implant Dentistry,* eds. Lindhe, J., Karring, T. & Lang, N.P.. 3rd edition. p.102-137. *Copenhagen: Munksgaard..*

Listgarten MA. Loomer PM. (2003) Microbial identification in the management of periodontal diseases. A systematic review. *Annals of Periodontology.* **8**(1):182-92

Lopatin, D.E., Shelburne, C.E., Van Poperin, N., Kowalski, C.J. & Bagramian, R.A. (1999) Humoral immunity to stress proteins and periodontal disease. *Journal of periodontology,* **70**, 1185-1193.

Mahdi, O.S., Horne, B.D., Mullen, K., Muhlestein, J.B. & Byrne, G.I. (2002) Serum immunoglobulin G antibodies to chlamydial heat shock protein 60 but not to human and bacterial homologs are associated with coronary artery disease. *Circulation,* **106**, 1659-1663.

Maron, R., Sukhova, G., Faria, A.M., Hoffmann, E., Mach, F., Libby, P. & Weiner, H.L. (2002) Mucosal administration of heat shock protein-65 decreases atherosclerosis and inflammation in aortic arch of low-density lipoprotein receptor-deficient mice. *Circulation,* **106**, 1708-1715.

Mayr, M., Metzler, B., Kiechl, S., Willeit, J., Schett, G., Xu, Q. & Wick, G. (1999) Endothelial cytotoxicity mediated by serum antibodies to heat shock proteins of Escherichia coli and Chlamydia pneumoniae: immune reactions to heat shock proteins as a possible link between infection and atherosclerosis. *Circulation,* **99**, 1560-1566.

Moore, W.E. & Moore, L.V. (1994) The bacteria of periodontal diseases. *Periodontology* 2000, 5, 66-77.

Palmer, R.M., Scott, D.A., Meekin, T.N., Poston, R.N., Odell, E.W. & Wilson, R.F. (1999) Potential mechanisms of susceptibility to periodontitis in tobacco smokers. *Journal of periodontal research,* **34**, 363-369.

Perschinka, H., Mayr, M., Millonig, G., Mayerl, C., Van der Zee, R., Morrison, S.G., Morrison, R.P., Xu, Q. & Wick, G. (2003) Cross-reactive B-cell epitopes of microbial and human heat shock protein 60/65 in atherosclerosis. *Arteriosclerosis, thrombosis, and vascular biology,* **23**, 1060-1065.

Pervin K. Childerstone A. Shinnick T. Mizushima Y. van der Zee R. Hasan A. Vaughan R. Lehner T. (1993) T cell epitope expression of mycobacterial and homologous human 65-kilodalton heat shock protein peptides in short term cell lines from patients with Behcet's disease. *Journal of Immunology.* **151**(4):2273-82

Prohaszka, Z., Duba, J., Horvath, L., Csaszar, A., Karadi, I., Szebeni, A., Singh, M., Fekete, B., Romics, L. & Fust, G. (2001) Comparative study on antibodies to human and bacterial 60 kDa heat shock proteins in a large cohort of patients with coronary heart disease and healthy subjects. *European journal of clinical investigation,* **31**, 285-292.

Pussinen, P.J., Jousilahti, P., Alfthan, G., Palosuo, T., Asikainen, S. & Salomaa, V. (2003) Antibodies to periodontal pathogens are associated with coronary heart disease. *Arteriosclerosis, thrombosis, and vascular biology,* **23**, 1250-1254.

Ranney, R.R. (1993) Classification of periodontal diseases. *Periodontology* 2000 , 2, 13-25.

Rifai, N., Joubran, R., Yu, H., Asmi, M. & Jouma, M. (1999) Inflammatory markers in men with angiographically documented coronary heart disease. *Clinical chemistry*, **45**, 1967-1973.

Ryder, M.I., Saghizadeh, M., Ding, Y., Nguyen, N. & Soskolne, A. (2002) Effects of tobacco smoke on the secretion of interleukin-1beta, tumor necrosis factor-alpha, and transforming growth factor-beta from peripheral blood mononuclear cells. *Oral microbiology and immunology*, **17**, 331-336.

Saikku, P., Leinonen, M., Mattila, K., Ekman, M.R., Nieminen, M.S., Makela, P.H., Huttunen, J.K. & Valtonen, V. (1988) Serological evidence of an association of a novel Chlamydia, TWAR, with chronic coronary heart disease and acute myocardial infarction. *Lancet*, **2,** 983-986.

Schett, G., Metzler, B., Kleindienst, R., Moschen, I., Hattmannsdorfer, R., Wolf, H., Ottenhoff, T., Xu, Q. & Wick, G. (1997a) Salivary anti-hsp65 antibodies as a diagnostic marker for gingivitis and a possible link to atherosclerosis. *International archives of allergy and immunology*, **114**, 246-250.

Schett, G., Metzler, B., Mayr, M., Amberger, A., Niederwieser, D., Gupta, R.S., Mizzen, L., Xu, Q. & Wick, G. (1997b) Macrophage-lysis mediated by autoantibodies to heat shock protein 65/60. *Atherosclerosis*, **128**, 27-38.

Schett, G., Metzler, B., Kleindienst, R., Amberger, A., Recheis, H., Xu, Q. & Wick, G. (1999) Myocardial injury leads to a release of heat shock protein (hsp) 60 and a suppression of the anti-hsp65 immune response. *Cardiovascular research*, **42**, 685-695.

Silver, J.G., Martin, A.W. & McBride, B.C. (1977) Experimental transient bacteraemias in human subjects with varying degrees of plaque accumulation and gingival inflammation. *Journal of Clinical Periodontology*, **4**, 92-99.

Tabeta, K., Yamazaki, K., Hotokezaka, H., Yoshie, H. & Hara, K. (2000) Elevated humoral immune response to heat shock protein 60 (hsp60) family in periodontitis patients. *Clinical and experimental immunology*, **120**, 285-293.

Thole JE, Hindersson P, de Bruyn J, Cremers F, van der Zee J, de Cock H, Tommassen J, van Eden W, van Embden JD. (1988) Antigenic relatedness of a strongly immunogenic 65 kDA mycobacterial protein antigen with a similarly sized ubiquitous bacterial common antigen. : *Microbial pathogenesis* **4**(1):71-83

Vayssier-Taussat, M., Camilli, T., Aron, Y., Meplan, C., Hainaut, P., Polla, B.S. & Weksler, B. (2001) Effects of tobacco smoke and benzo[a]pyrene on human endothelial cell and monocyte stress responses. *American journal of physiology. Heart and circulatory physiology*, **280**, H1293-H1300.

Veres, A., Fust, G., Smieja, M., McQueen, M., Horvath, A., Yi, Q., Biro, A., Pogue, J., Romics, L., Karadi, I., Singh, M., Gnarpe, J., Prohaszka, Z. & Yusuf, S. (2002) Relationship of anti-60 kDa heat shock protein and anti-cholesterol antibodies to cardiovascular events. *Circulation*, **106**, 2775-2780.

Wysocki, J., Karawajczyk, B., Gorski, J., Korzeniowski, A., Mackiewicz, Z., Kupryszewski, G. & Glosnicka, R. (2002) Human heat shock protein 60 (409-424) fragment is recognized by serum antibodies of patients with acute coronary syndromes. *Cardiovascular pathology*, **11**, 238-243.

Xu, Q., Willeit, J., Marosi, M., Kleindienst, R., Oberhollenzer, F., Kiechl, S., Stulnig, T., Luef, G. & Wick, G. (1993) Association of serum antibodies to heat-shock protein 65 with carotid atherosclerosis. *Lancet*, **341**, 255-259.

Xu, Q., Kiechl, S., Mayr, M., Metzler, B., Egger, G., Oberhollenzer, F., Willeit, J. & Wick, G. (1999) Association of serum antibodies to heat-shock protein 65 with carotid atherosclerosis : clinical significance determined in a follow-up study. *Circulation*, **100** , 1169-1174.

Yamaguchi, E., Itoh, A., Furuya, K., Miyamoto, H., Abe, S. & Kawakami, Y. (1993) Release of tumor necrosis factor-alpha from human alveolar macrophages is decreased in smokers. *Chest*, **103**, 479-483.

Yamazaki, K., Ueki-Maruayama, K., Honda, T., Nakajima, T. & Seymour, G.J. (2004) Effect of periodontal treatment on the serum antibody levels to heat shock proteins. *Clinical Experimental Immunology*, **135**, 478-482.

Zebrack, J.S., Anderson, J.L., Maycock, C.A., Horne, B.D., Bair, T.L. & Muhlestein, J.B. (2002) Usefulness of high-sensitivity C-reactive protein in predicting long-term risk. *The American journal of cardiology*, **89**, 145-149.

Zhu, J., Quyyumi, A.A., Rott, D., Csako, G., Wu, H., Halcox, J. & Epstein, S.E. (2001) Antibodies to human heat-shock protein 60 are associated with the presence and severity of coronary artery disease: evidence for an autoimmune component of atherogenesis. *Circulation*, **103**, 1071-1075.

In: Heart Disease in Men
Editors: A.B. Todd and M.H. Mosley, pp. 201-218
ISBN: 978-1-60692-297-2

Chapter 9

THE ROLE OF DRUG ELUTING STENTS: FACTS AND FICTION 2008

*Marco Balducelli**
Cardiac catheterization laboratory, Ospedale S. Maria delle Croci
Viale Randi 5, 48100 Ravenna, Italy

Abstract

Since the introduction of drug eluting stents (DES) in the treatment of coronary artery disease in 2002, many randomized clinical trials (RCTs) have been published. At the same time, as often is the case in medicine, utilization of these devices has grown far beyond the approved indications derived from RCTs (on-label). The DES employment in the "real world" scenario generated several registry studies intended to deem their actual safety and efficacy. Only a couple of years after the DES introduction in the market, reports arose about serious safety concerns. Cases of fatal late stent thrombosis began to appear in the literature and thorough revision of DES implant follow up were accomplished. Some researchers reported about an apparent excess in late mortality of patients who were treated with a DES more than 12 months before. As a result, many interventional cardiologists panicked and began to reduce consistently their utilization of DES. Like a wave in a sea storm generates and then is destroyed by the following calm, the same is happening for DES use in interventional cardiology. Stimulated by these alarming calls several other investigators began to report the results of wide national or regional registries that contradicted the previous catastrophic and hurried conclusions. Complete endothelization is often delayed and sometimes never totally accomplished after DES. This is due to the non selective action of drugs blocking cellular replication of endothelial cells, essential to the integrity of all biological processes and the prevention of clot formation and, probably, of polymers to which the drugs are attached and that are not biocompatible. Such intrinsic limitation of the DES is magnified in cases of difficult anatomic conditions (implant in small vessels, bifurcation stenosis, chronic total occlusions etc.) and probably also in particular unfavourable clinical substrates (diabetes, acute myocardial infarction), namely in all the so-called "off-label" indications. Paradoxically, it is particularly in these clinical and anatomic conditions that the potential of DES advantage over conventional treatment could display at the most. To solve these problems DES are changing in terms of different mechanical and biological solutions ultimately aimed at removing their weaknesses and sometimes even changing the philosophy of the device (as for

* E-mail address: ra.hocardioemo@ausl.ra.it. Phone: +39 0544 286068. Fax: +39 0544 285424.

the biodegradable stent approach). At the same time cardiologists are looking for a real comprehension of patients' peculiarities that must be the guide to find the most appropriate and tailored solutions as in most other fields in medicine.

Percutaneous Coronary Revascularization

It was in the late 70's that PCI was introduced in the clinical practice. Although initially adversed by the surgeons and, in general, by the gatekeepers of tradition, percutaneous coronary intervention, in the initial form of balloon PTCA gained consensus and began to grow at a progressively faster pace. Its main advantage over by-pass surgery was the far lesser degree of invasiveness and, as a consequence, the easier acceptance by the patients. Effectiveness was sufficiently high and so it was safety even though incidents and necessity to cross over to surgery was not negligible. With the refining of techniques and the great aid of specifically dedicated technology, the dependence from the surgical stand-by progressively disappeared. However long term efficacy of PCI was greatly impaired by recurrences (in up to 40% of cases). Soon it became sufficiently evident that the process of restenosis at the site of balloon angioplasty was caused by an abnormally strong reparative process (neo-endothelization) together with a mechanical recoil of the dilated vessel (Fig.1). The main

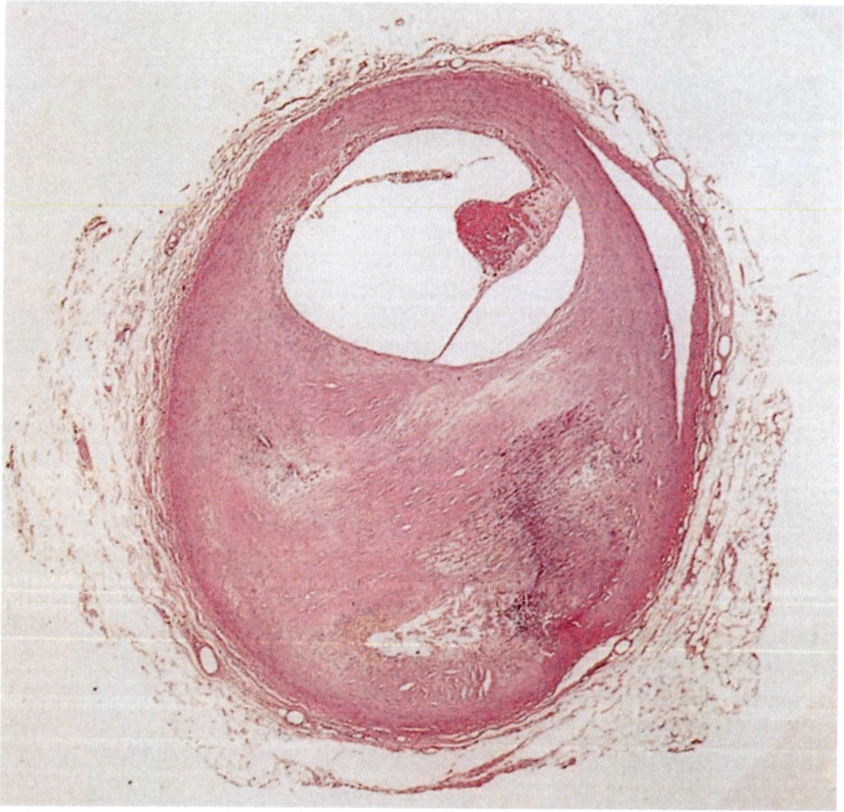

Figure 1. Restenosis: istopathological appearance of restenotic process with wide neointimal tissue occupying the vessel lumen.

actors of the hyperplastic response are the smooth muscle cells that are recruited from the media with a chemotactic signal and then made actively replicating and secreting collagen to form a consistent acellular medium. This new myointimal tissue is the core of the restenosis occupying the lumen and hindering a normal flow. Together with this hyperplastic process, an inflammatory response to the initial damage caused by balloon inflation was evident, sometimes being a concause of thrombus formation. The mechanical process of vessel recoil was also evident after balloon dilatation, especially in case of hard plaques and very eccentric lesions. Several different pharmacological approaches to solve this problem were undertaken but almost all failed or were only marginally successful.

Coronary Stents

Metallic endoprostheses i.e. stents were a first strong advance in the battle against restenosis in the early 90's. They just eliminated completely the mechanical recoil of the vessel wall after dilation of stenotic segments offering a scaffold able to resist also the wear of the continuous movement of the vessel at each heart beat (Figure 2). It was soon apparent that they overcame balloon angioplasty in terms of efficacy reducing restenosis rate by 25-33%. However, even if improvement in design, alloy selection, miniaturization of struts made possible to access difficult coronary anatomies and treat complex lesions not affordable in the balloon era, the restenosis was still a significant drawback of the procedure. Histological examination in the experimental animal and in humans, post-mortem, revealed an even bigger proliferative response in respect to that elicited by balloon PCI. This has been attributed to the deeper injury caused by the metallic prosthesis into the vessel wall. So it was again time to fight the battle against restenosis in a new setting and with adequate means.

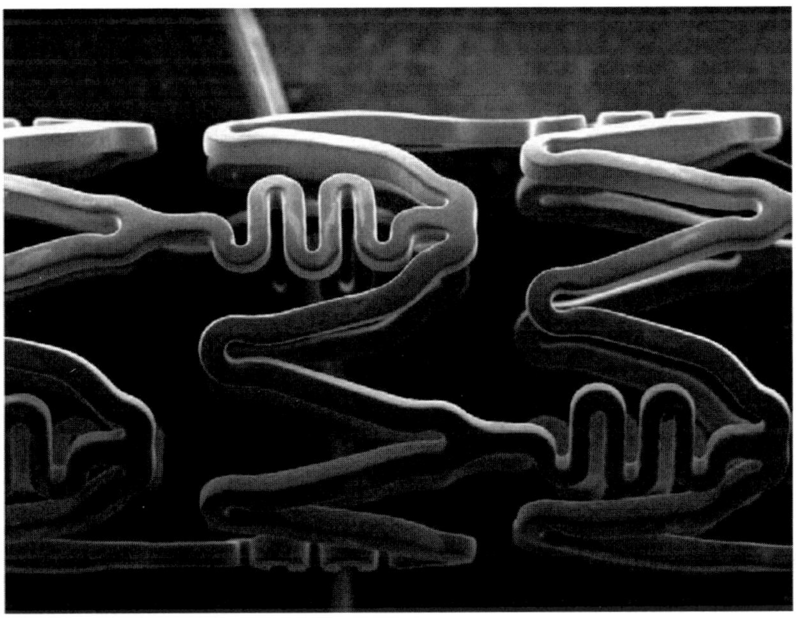

Figure 2. A bare metal stent at high magnification: note the thin metal struts with a wave-shaped design.

Drug-Eluting Stents

The next advance in the interventional field was even more revolutionary since it combined the advantages of mechanical support of the metallic devices with the antiproliferative effects of specific drugs carried directly to the plaque site (Fig. 3). This solution seemed to represent the Columbus' egg deemed to reduce the occurrence of in-stent restenosis and the need for subsequent target vessel revascularization compared with bare-metal stents. The principal mechanism of action of the drug-eluting stents is the controlled release (via a polymer carrier on the stent) of an antiproliferative or immunomodulatory compound that accumulates locally and inhibits the proliferative process responsible for restenosis. Initial first-in-man studies demonstrated dramatic suppression of neointimal hyperplasia, and randomized clinical trials of drug-eluting stents (Table 1) eventually demonstrated 70% or greater reductions in the rate of target lesion revascularization compared with bare-metal stents, an effect that was consistently observed across all patient and lesion subgroups. However, the benefit of drug-eluting stents may have been overestimated because these trials involved routine angiographic follow-up and the use of "thick-strut" bare-metal stents in the bare-metal stent control groups [10].

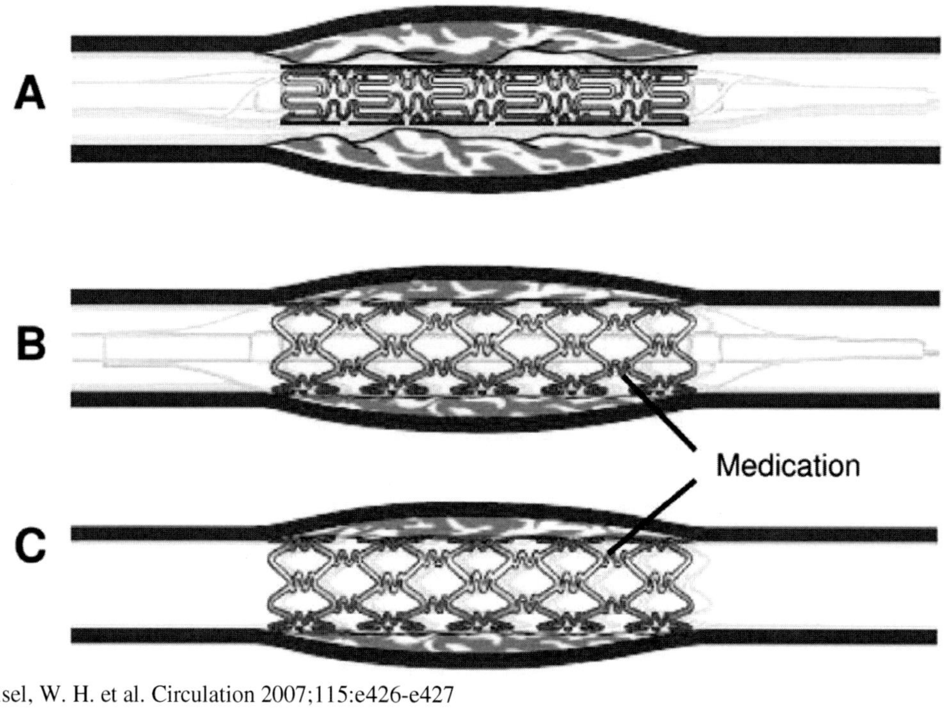

Maisel, W. H. et al. Circulation 2007;115:e426-e427

Figure 3. Cartoon with deployment of a drug eluting stent (adapted from Maisel, W. H. et al. Circulation 2007;115:e426-e427).

Table 1. Clinical Events in Pivotal Trials of Sirolimus- and Paclitaxel-Eluting Stents (adapted from Jeremias, A. et. al. Ann Intern Med 2008;148:234-238)

Table 1. **Clinical Events in Pivotal Trials of Sirolimus- and Paclitaxel-Eluting Stents***

Study (Reference)	Target Lesion Revascularization†, %		Stent Thrombosis, %		Myocardial Infarction, %		Total Mortality, %		Major Adverse Cardiac Events, %	
	DES	BMS	DES	BMS	DES	BMS	DES	BMS	DES	BMS
Sirolimus-eluting stent trials										
RAVEL (1)	0.0	22.9	0.0	0.0	3.3	4.2	1.7	1.7	5.8	28.8
SIRIUS (2)	4.1	16.6	0.4	0.8	2.8	3.2	0.9	0.6	7.1	18.9
Canadian SIRIUS (3)	4.0	18.0	2.0	2.0	2.0	4.0	0.0	0.0	4.0	18.0
European SIRIUS (4)	4.0	20.9	1.1	0.0	4.6	2.3	1.1	0.6	8.0	22.6
Paclitaxel-eluting stent trials										
TAXUS I (5)	0.0	10.0	0.0	0.0	0.0	0.0	0.0	0.0	3.0	10.0
TAXUS II (6)	4.2	14.4	0.7	0.0	3.1	5.3	0.0‡	0.8‡	10.4	21.8
TAXUS IV (7)	3.0	11.3	0.6	0.8	3.5	3.7	1.4‡	1.1‡	8.5	15.0
TAXUS V (8)	8.6	15.7	0.7	0.7	5.4	4.6	1.3‡	1.4‡	15.0	21.2
TAXUS VI (9)	6.8	18.9	0.5	1.3	8.2	6.2	0.0	0.9	16.4	22.5

* BMS = bare-metal stent; DES = drug-eluting stent; RAVEL = Randomized Study with the Sirolimus-Coated Bx Velocity Balloon-Expandable Stent in the Treatment of Patients with De Novo Native Coronary Artery Lesions; SIRIUS = Study of the Sirolimus-Eluting Balloon-Expandable Stent in the Treatment of Patients with De Novo Native Coronary Artery Lesions.
† Repeated revascularization within the stent and 5 mm proximal and distal to the stent.
‡ Cardiac mortality.

"Off-Label" Use of Drug-Eluting Stents

The pivotal clinical trials were for the most part restricted to low-risk patient and lesion subsets that are not completely representative of those seen in routine clinical practice. Specifically, the "on-label" indications for use of drug-eluting stents include only symptomatic patients with ischemic disease due to a single de novo lesion less than 30 mm in native coronary arteries, with a reference vessel diameter of 2.5 to 3.5 mm. Because the use of bare-metal stents in more complex lesion and patient subgroups is typically associated with higher rates of restenosis, many interventionalists have hypothesized that the efficacy of drug-eluting stents may be more pronounced in this population, with greater absolute reductions in repeated revascularization. Initial data from some of the pivotal randomized studies that included more complex lesion subsets have demonstrated this benefit [8]. Additional studies are emerging about the use of drug-eluting stents for various "off-label" indications, including acute myocardial infarction (MI), chronic total occlusion, in-stent restenosis, diffuse disease, saphenous vein grafts, bifurcation lesions, and left main coronary artery stenting. In addition, several ongoing registries have provided "real-world" data that show favorable long-term outcomes and statistically significant reductions in major adverse cardiac events [11]. More recently data have become available on long-term follow up of patients treated with bare metal and drug eluting stents for "off label" indications [12,13]. Patients with complex angiographic disease (including chronic total occlusions, vein graft disease, and bifurcation lesions) were not included in the RCTs, nor were those with multivessel coronary artery disease or urgent acute coronary syndromes. These patients are all represented in the 2 registries. Both studies indicate higher acute and late ischemic complication rates among patients receiving drug-eluting stents for off-label compared with on-label indications.

Safety of Drug-Eluting Stents: The Concern and the Fiction

The more pronounced inflammatory response documented after DES deployment in autopsy studies may be the trigger for a delayed and incomplete vascular healing and the subsequent formation of coronary aneurisms, late acquired stent malapposition and/or be the cause of late stent thrombosis (LST). Camenzind proposed a possible pathophysiologic explanation for LST. (1) an abnormal vessel wall lining (eg, incomplete endothelialization), (2) an abnormal blood-flow pattern (eg, slow flow), and (3) altered blood constituents (eg, increased blood thrombogenicity) may favor intravascular thrombus formation.

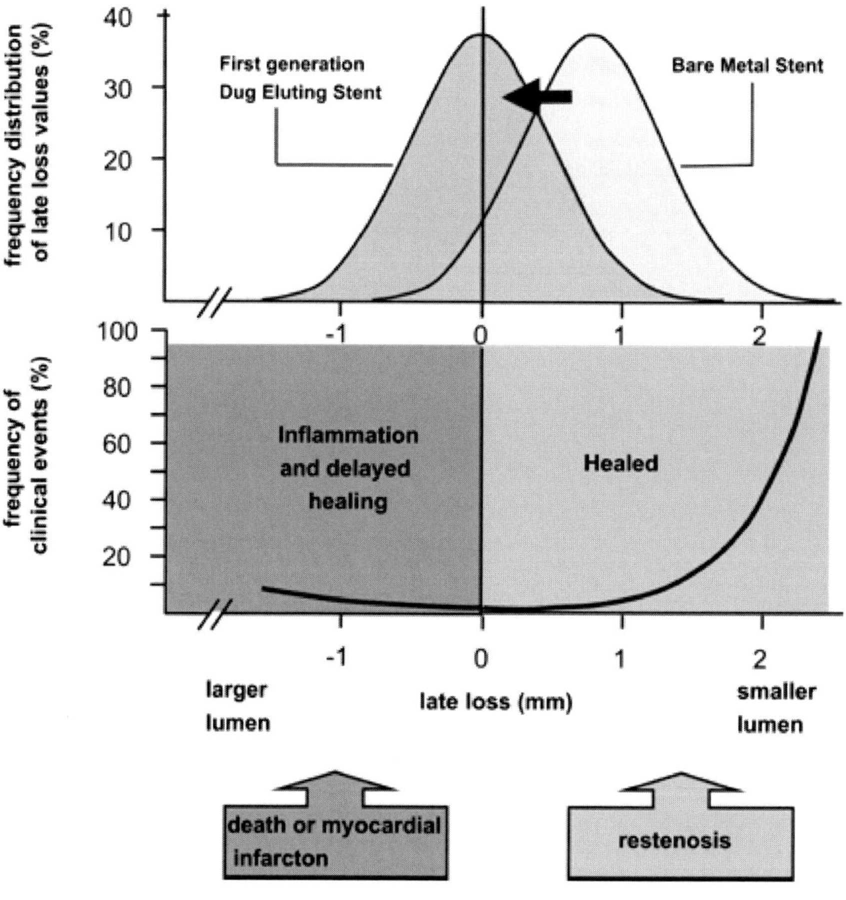

Figure 4. J shaped relationship between drug eluting stent restenosis and thrombosis and late luminal loss at follow up (from Camenzind et al., Circulation. 2007;115:1440-55).

On the basis of these pathological observations and of subsequent confirmation by others, Camenzind proposed a link between the antirestenosis effect or healing response measured by late loss (LL) at the follow up and clinical events [LST and in-stent restenosis (ISR)] after DES implantation depicatble as a J-shaped curve relationship: Both negative and high LL are linked to an excess in clinical events (Fig. 4) [14]. LST is rare (flatter portion of the J curve) and more likely to occur in the patient population with negative LL (larger lumen by angiography as a result of delayed healing or nonhealing). Repeat revascularization is frequent (steeper portion of the J curve) and occurs more often as the LL values increase (smaller angiographic lumen as a result of exuberant healing and neointimal growth). Any increase in the population with negative LL is expected to increase the absolute number of patients potentially subject to LST .

A first meta-analysis suggested a statistically significant 2.4% increased risk for death or MI compared with bare-metal stents [14] .Another meta-analysis demonstrated a statistically significant increase in noncardiac mortality at 2 to 3 years among patients receiving the sirolimus-eluting stent [15]. Even if criticized for methodological pitfalls, these publications caused a worlwide panic about the long-term safety of drug-eluting stents. An initial analysis of an observational registry of Swedish patients reported additional adverse outcomes, indicating an increase in mortality with drug-eluting stents that became apparent 6 months after the procedure [16], and other recent studies have reported the development of coronary aneurysms 6 to 21 months after drug-eluting stent implantation [17].

Drug Eluting Stent Thrombosis: The Facts

On the basis of the currently available data from clinical trials [2, 7] and registries [12,13,18], the overall rate of subacute stent thrombosis, defined as thrombosis occurring 24 hours to 30 days after stent implantation, appears to be similar for bare-metal and drug-eluting stents. However, several studies indicate a small but measurable increase in the rate of late stent thrombosis (thrombosis occurring 30 days to 1 year after stent implantation) in patients receiving drug-eluting stents, with an estimated incidence of 0.2% to 0.5% per year [19]. One trial even showed an incidence of late stent thrombosis of 1.4% in the drug-eluting stent group versus 0.8% in the bare-metal stent group [20]. Although these rates appear to be unusually high (even in the bare-metal stent group), in the aggregate, these data suggest an increased rate of late stent thrombosis in patients receiving drug-eluting stents. Stent thrombosis occurred more commonly among the patients receiving drug-eluting stents for off-label indications, and this finding remains after adjustment for dual antiplatelet therapy, suggesting an independent risk contribution of receiving a drug-eluting stent for an off-label indication [12,13].

Individual patient data from the major randomized trials have subsequently been analyzed to specifically address the incidence of stent thrombosis with drug-eluting stents at 4-year follow-up. Overall, the frequency of protocol-defined stent thrombosis did not statistically differ with drug-eluting stents (1.2% for sirolimus-eluting stents versus 0.6% for bare-metal stents [$P = 0.20$]; 1.3% for paclitaxel-eluting stents versus 0.9% for bare-metal stents [$P = 0.30$]) [21]. However, when very late stent thrombosis events (occurring >1 year after stent implantation) were analyzed separately, an increase in events was observed with sirolimus-eluting stents (5 events vs. 0 events with bare-metal stents; $P = 0.025$) and paclitaxel-eluting stents (9 events vs. 2 events; $P = 0.028$). Given the high incidence of death and MI associated with stent thrombosis, the expected mortality and MI rates should in theory be elevated in patients with drug-eluting stents. However, most studies (including meta-analyses of the studies on which these analyses were based) have found no statistically significant difference in death and MI even after years of follow-up [21–23]. Does the small but measurable increase in late stent thrombosis not translate into an increased rate of death and MI ?

Some clinician think that unlike native coronary artery disease, in which plaque rupture with subsequent thrombus formation can lead to acute MI and death, restenosis due to gradual hyperplasia of neointima cannot result in acute coronary syndromes, and instead is a "stable," nonfatal condition associated only with recurrent angina and myocardial ischemia. Recently this hypothesis has been questioned, because approximately 10% of patients with restenosis have acute MI as their presenting symptom [24]. and 8.9% of patients have a totally occluded vessel at angiography (19% of whom present with ST-segment elevation MI). Another explanation for the lack of an association between possible increases in late stent thrombosis and other end points, such as death or MI, is the different stent thromboses definitions employed in the pivotal randomized trials and in the more recent studies and registries.

Indeed, in an analysis based on a new definition of stent thrombosis proposed by the Academic Research Consortium that counted all events regardless of past revascularization, the occurrence of stent thrombosis on an intention-to-treat basis was similar with drug-eluting and bare-metal stents at 4 years of follow-up [25]. Even with the inclusion of possible stent thrombosis (which represents the most inclusive definition), the thrombosis rate was almost identical between the 2 groups.

It is however difficult to know exactly the incidence of drug eluting stent thrombosis and specifically designed trials are unlikely to be done. For instance, if one were to design an adequately powered clinical trial to demonstrate even a doubling of the stent thrombosis rate with drug-eluting stents, the trial would have to enroll approximately 8000 patients to adequately detect a 50% relative increase (1% absolute increase) in the rate of stent thrombosis, assuming a baseline rate of 2% in the group with bare-metal stents. In comparison, all 9 major randomized trials comparing sirolimus-eluting stents with paclitaxel-eluting stents enrolled a total of 5261 patients, and thus the available published data remain greatly underpowered to address the comparative stent thrombosis incidence.

The Dilemma between Randomized Clinical Trials and the “Real World” Registries

Clinicians are puzzled by the conflicting results of RCTs and registries and even more dazzled by the different interpretations of data coming from meta-analysis. Almost every day new publications in relevant and widely read medical journals shed a personal light on this enigma, not always producing a beneficial effect on comprehension of the situation. Every clinician rely on his personal experience and on evidence-.based medicine. The dilemma becomes clear when everyday practice is somewhat different from published results. What do we have to trust? Medicine is a science with a strong empiric component and interventional cardiology is not an exception to this general rule. It is tentative and iterative and not always physician learn from other’s past errors and do want to experience them by their own. Stent thrombosis, particularly when very late, two or three years after the procedure, is something very disturbing for the clinician (and the patient too, obviously) both for the immediate clinical consequences, being fatal in many cases, and for the implications that come along with it. This is a iatrogenic disease, something that would have not happened in the natural history of the patient, at least not at that site, and that is highly unpredictable, despite its recognized predictors. All the process that has led to the first stent implant must be reviewed in search for errors and the regret is very likely to be the feeling that hits the interventionalist at that time. Do we have to trade a better quality of life for a definite, even if small, adjunctive risk of death when we use a drug eluting stent?

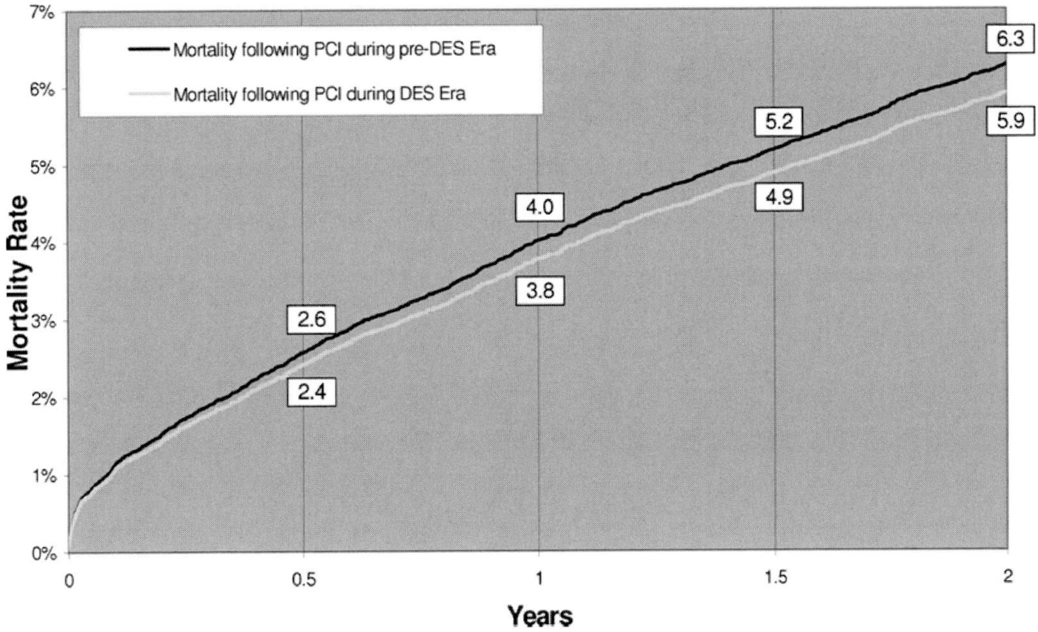

Figure 5. Mortality after PCI in the pre-DES and post-DES era (from Hannan et., Circulation 2008; 117(16):2071-78).

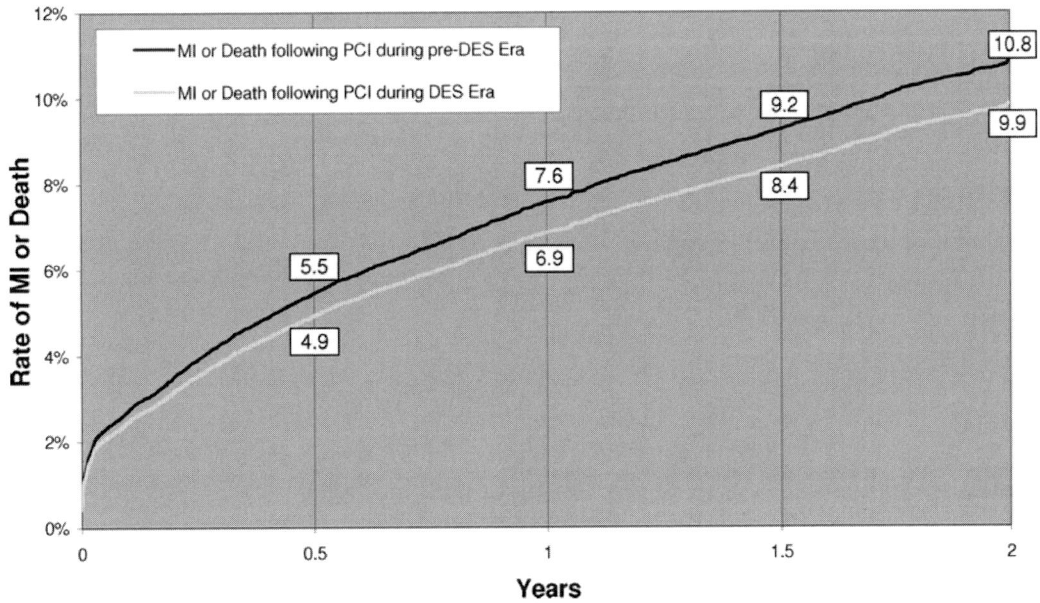

Figure 6. Incidence of myocardial infarction and mortality after PCI in the pre-DES and post-DES era (from Hannan et., Circulation 2008; 117(16):2071-78).

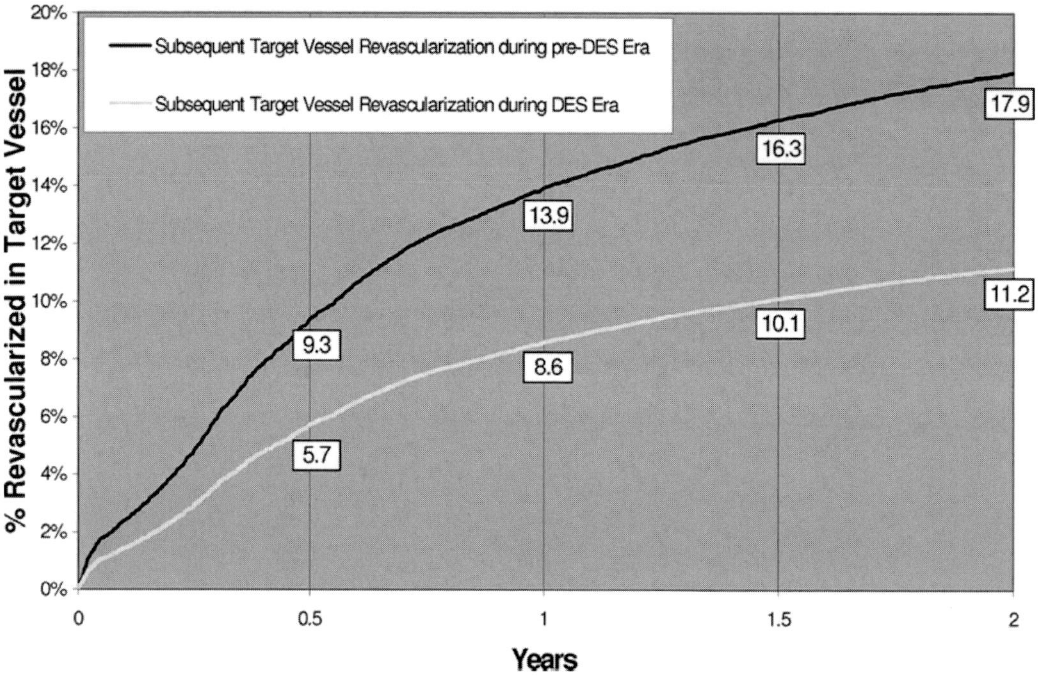

Figure 7. Incidence of target vessel revascularization (TVR) after PCI in the pre-DES and post-DES era (from Hannan et., Circulation 2008; 117(16):2071-78).

The highest-quality evidence is attributed to multiple RCTs—or a single large RCT—that have sufficient size (ie, provide adequate power) to observe or exclude meaningful treatment effects, are conducted in representative patient populations, have relevant clinical end points, and are analyzed appropriately. Such trials are best performed when the science is mature, so that the intervention is stable enough to be tested in large cohorts to detect events of rare frequency (usually less than 10%—as now applies for all end points in PCI). By their very design, RCTs are limited because they provide only a snapshot of a disease and a population and because they frequently exclude the sickest patients. Moreover given a significant heterogeneity in the definition of the "so called" major adverse cardiovascular events among RCTs, results in terms of safety if not efficacy, may be widely questioned [26]. Observational studies complement RCTs and are especially valuable for examining the uptake of a new therapy into broader community practice and including groups that have not been adequately studied in trials. These types of studies can provide valuable practice information regarding quality of care, unusual adverse effects, uptake beyond the populations studied, and comparative effectiveness. What do we have now in the DES field in 2008? A large observational Italian registry (REAL) on more than 10.000 patients (allcomers) showed 2 years adjusted death and MI free-survival rates superimposed for DES and BMS reassuring a good safety profile and, at the same time, confirmed adequate efficacy in preventing TVR [27]. We also have different meta-analysis [21-23, 25] all giving the same re-assuring message on clinical safety. A recent observational study on outcome of stent PCI in the pre-DES and post-DES eras shows similar mortality rates after the introduction of DES but with a lower incidence of MI and a net advantage in TVR and TLR [28] (Fig. 5-7).

The Net Clinical Benefit

The net clinical benefit of any medical device or pharmaceutical agent is defined by its beneficial properties relative to its adverse effects. When the net effect is being considered, however, the relative clinical benefit must be weighed against the severity of the adverse effects. In the case of drug-eluting stents, the clinical benefit is the relative reduction in revascularization by approximately 50% to 70% across most lesion subsets (translating into an absolute reduction of 5% to 20%, depending on patient and lesion characteristics). This benefit must be weighed against a possible absolute increase in late stent thrombosis by approximately 0.5%, although the confidence intervals around this latter estimate remain wide in the absence of a large number of events. The number needed to treat to prevent 1 restenosis event ranges from 5 to 20, whereas the number needed to harm (causing 1 excess event of stent thrombosis) is 200. Of note, because stent thrombosis is a more dire event than restenosis in general, the directionality and magnitude of the net clinical effect of drug-eluting stents are influenced not only by the number needed to treat or the number needed to harm but also by the differing clinical consequences of each competing risk.

Subgroup analyses from all clinical trials and numerous registries have demonstrated that implantation of drug-eluting stents reduces angiographic and clinical restenosis to a similar extent in all analyzed patient and lesion subgroups [2, 7]. In fact, higher-risk patients may experience a greater absolute reduction in revascularization because of their higher baseline risk for restenosis. Given that the rate of serious adverse events (death and MI) has not been demonstrated to differ from that for bare-metal and considering that drug-eluting stents are very effective in the reduction of repeated revascularization, the net clinical benefit of drug-eluting stents appears to be favorable [21–23]. A meta-analysis of all randomized trials comparing drug-eluting stents with bare-metal stents (as well as head-to-head trials comparing sirolimus-eluting stents with paclitaxel-eluting stents) demonstrated similar mortality rates for all groups [29]. It remains clear, however, that the use of a bare-metal stent if either the frequency of restenosis is low or its clinical consequences are limited, may be the best choice for many patients. In addition, multiple studies have shown that the single most important predictor of stent thrombosis is the premature discontinuation of antiplatelet therapy, with a dramatic increase in stent thrombosis seen in patients taken off therapy [18]. Currently, uninterrupted dual-antiplatelet therapy (typically consisting of aspirin and clopidogrel) is recommended for at least 30 days after implantation of bare-metal stents and for a minimum of 1 year after implantation of drug-eluting stents. Consequently, it is critical that before stent implantation, all patients be evaluated for their ability to continuously receive and tolerate dual antiplatelet therapy [30]. Also, all patients should receive optimal medical therapy, including anti-ischemic therapy (such as long-acting metoprolol or isosorbide mononitrate) and aggressive therapy to decrease low-density lipoprotein cholesterol levels and increase high-density lipoprotein cholesterol levels, as either an adjunct to percutaneous coronary intervention or as an initial strategy in asymptomatic patients or carefully selected patients with symptoms of low-risk stable angina [31]. Moreover when looking at events in patients treated with DES, especially the long-term ones, one should not forget that the natural history of atherosclerosis and ischemic heart disease can account for most "hard" events such as death an MI, and that a single intervention, i.e. DES, may not be sufficient to alter this process especially in the sickest patients. It is not surprising at all that other factors such as diabetes, especially when not sufficiently controlled by a proper pharmacological regimen, may account for most of the clinical events in patients receiving drug eluting stents and that clinical results may be inferior to those expected on the basis of reported RCT's.. In a large observational study on the use of DES in diabetic patients the use of DES was associated with a non significant adjusted 21% relative risk reduction of major adverse events at 2 years, largely attributable to a reduction in the risk of TVR [32].

New Strategies in the Development of Drug Eluting Stents

Further studies are ongoing to test other types of drugs that can favour a rapid healing of the artery without increasing the proliferative response or, in alternative, eliminate the need of a carrier (polymer) which is potentially harmful. Stent-based drug delivery has been accomplished by three distinct mechanisms: bio-absorbable polymeric stents can be loaded with a drug that is eluted slowly over time; metal stents can have a drug bound to their surface or embedded within macroscopic fenestrations or microscopic nano-pores, thus providing more rapid drug delivery; metal stents coated with an outer layer of polymer (bio-absorbable or non-bio-absorbable) can be drug-loaded, thus providing more controlled and sustained drug delivery, which might allow more effective drug-tissue interactions. Recent experimental data [33] suggest that stent strut configuration directly determines the pattern and degree of drug delivery achieved by the stent. After deployment of even highly soluble and rapidly diffusing drugs, homogeneous drug delivery throughout the vessel with uniform concentration at various depths of the vessel wall is not achieved. Therefore stent designs that maintain regular strut spacing despite expansion in various anatomical circumstances will provide the most regular and predictable drug delivery. For drugs with wide toxic-to-therapeutic window, such as members of the sirolimus family, regularity of strut spacing might be less important and adequate doses can be applied to the stent surface so that, despite broad variability in the location of delivery, an adequate dose is uniformly released. On the other hand, drugs with narrower toxic-to-therapeutic ratios, such as paclitaxel, might suffer from inadequate dosing at sites where stent struts lie far apart and possibly from over-therapeutic or toxic dosing at sites where stent struts bunch together owing to vessel curvature or asymmetric expansion. Several other "next-generation" DES are currently under investigation. The Endeavor™ stent from Medtronic (Medtronic Inc., Minneapolis, MN, USA), which uses the non-erodible polymer phosphorylcholine to release the sirolimus analogue ABT-578, is the first DES to use a non-stainless steel alloy as the foundation for a polymer-coated DES, i.e. the thin-strut cobalt-chromium alloy (Driver). A novel approach is constituted by the XIENCE V™ stent from Abbott, Illinois, USA, which uses a highly deliverable metallic stent platform and a bio-stable acrylic coating for drug encapsulation and release, with the potential benefit of the restriction to the abluminal (outer) surface of each strut (so that drug and polymer are not exposed to the flowing blood in the arterial lumen) and the eventual degradation of the polymer to carbon dioxide and water, which are free of any toxic byproducts. Thus, the stent design guarantees the complete elimination of the drug from the stent over a finite period of time without drug retention, potential cause of late adverse events months to years after implantation.

The strategy of minimizing stent struts and polymer thickness to aid re-endothelization seems to be a good path to follow as results of studies such the SPIRIT trials with the everolimus eluting Xience V (Abbott Vascular) DES are being reported. together with those of the zotarolimus Endeavor stent (Medtronic). Several clinical conclusions can be drawn by the results of all these experiences. First of all the severely delayed or empaired re-endothelization seen with the first generation of DES (Cypher or sirolimus DES and Taxus or paclitaxel DES) requires prolonged dual antiplatelet therapy. Secondly late loss should not be the only discriminator of superiority among DES. Third, arterial healing is an equally important end-point and preclinical models may be the best way to evaluate this. Fourth, confirmation of safety of these devices requires long-term follow-up (3-5 years). Novel methods for stent based drug-delivery are under investigation. They comprehend direct coating to non-modified surface, methods of surface modification such as depot/drug reservoirs, macroporous, microporous and nanoporous stents. The latter are often ceramic stents with metallic deposition techniques to obtain a very thin and uniform coating. New stategies are also methods of chemical attachment and novel polymer often bioabsorbable. The new frontiers of DES are thin-struts cobalt-chromium alloy platforms with safer drug-polymer coating, biodegradable polymers with special designs allowing multiple drug carrier capability, surface modifications with drug delivery without use of polymers and bioabsorbable stents. All of these experiences together with the improvement in stent engineering are likely to improve long term efficacy and safety of drug eluting stents in the next few years.

One of the areas of research is the search for endothelium friendly coverings. Endothelial derived substances such as prostacyclin and NO are known to inhibit platelet aggregation, smooth muscle cell proliferation and local inflammatory responses, and have known protective effects on cells. Therefore, they may act to protect the vessel against injury and promote regeneration of a functional endothelium. Because these compounds are produced naturally by the endothelium, they have potentially less deleterious side effects than existing approaches. Local stent-based release of the prostacyclin analogue, iloprost, in combination with the thrombin inhibitor hirudin, reduced neointima formation in pig and sheep coronary arteries [34]. Stents coated with the NO donor, sodium nitroprusside, have had mixed results to date. One study failed to demonstrate a reduction in neointima in a pig coronary artery model [35]. However, recently a reduction in neointima was achieved in a pig carotid artery model [36].

There is growing evidence that oxidative stress and the subsequent imbalance in the production of damaging reactive oxygen species play a significant role in the response to stent insertion, and ultimately in the process of neointima development. By reducing oxidative stress, antioxidants can protect the endothelium against dysfunction and encourage endothelialisation. A number of trials with oral delivery of antioxidants such as probucol and its analogue AGI-1067 have demonstrated beneficial effects in reducing constrictive remodelling of the vasculature following PCI [37]. A phosphorylcholine coated stent releasing the antioxidant, carvedilol, reduced neointima formation by 42% in a pig model of in-stent restenosis [38].

Oestrogen is well known for its protective effects on the cardiovascular system. In pigs it inhibits smooth muscle cell proliferation and migration. However, it may represent a significant advance on existing DES because it also stimulates endothelial cell proliferation and migration [39]. This prospect has led to the development of a phosphorylcholine-coated stent providing release of 17-beta-oestradiol. Clinical trials of this technology have demonstrated the safety of this device with no deaths or thromboses at six months [40].

However, in a subsequent study, no beneficial effect on angiographic restenosis at six months was observed, compared with a phosphoryl-choline coated stent alone [41].

Vascular endothelial growth factor (VEGF) is released by endothelial cells to promote angiogenesis of the vasculature. Although its promotion of endothelial cell repair makes it an attractive option, it is also associated with increases in smooth muscle cell proliferation and migration. This potentially nonselective stimulation of angiogenesis may represent a drawback. In one clinical study, local catheter based delivery of a gene, which promotes the synthesis of VEGF, failed to demonstrate a reduction in restenosis [42], although the low overall restenosis rates in each arm of this study made differences difficult to observe. However, a phosphoryl-choline-coated stent releasing a VEGF gene has produced promising results in a rabbit iliac artery model. An increase in the rate of endothelialisation was observed in addition to an increase in the lumen diameter [43].

Seeding endothelial cells onto vascular prostheses is appealing because these cells would then be able to release various substances to limit neointima formation. Progress in this area has been limited to date because of the time required to grow a sufficient number of cells and the limited adherence of these cells to the artery surface during dynamic flow conditions. Endothelial cells have been grown within polymer matrices, which can be subsequently implanted to encourage vascular repair following injury [44]. Surface coating with plasma protein such as fibronectin, which contains specific endothelial cell binding sites, is known to increase the rate of endothelial cell growth on artificial surfaces [45]. More recently, neointima formation in rabbit arteries was reduced by the injection of fibrin glue that contained thrombin and endothelial cells into the artery immediately following angioplasty [46] However, significant obstacles remain such as the source and seeding time of endothelial cells before application in a clinical setting can be considered.

The discovery of endothelial progenitor cells and their potential role in re-endothelialisation following injury may provide an opportunity for the next generation DES. By releasing a specific peptide, which binds endothelial progenitor cells, from a polymer coated stent it has been shown that endothelialisation can be significantly improved. A consequent reduction in the neointimal area was also observed [47].A similar approach has been evaluated clinically, which has demonstrated the potential of this "prohealing" approach [48]. In this study, a covalently coupled polysaccharide coating has been used in combination with a CD34 antibody for endothelial progenitor cell capture. No thrombosis was reported at six months despite cessation of clopidogrel anti-platelet therapy after one month, although no reduction in neointima formation was observed. Further improvements to this stent system are underway, including increasing the stability of the antibodies by producing the coating in a dry form, which removes the need for rinsing prior to use. Similarly, the bioactivity of the antibody coating has been enhanced by using a lower level of gamma irradiation (<15 kGy) in the sterilisation process. Taken together, these modifications have improved endothelial progenitor cell capture rate in vitro and may enhance the performance of the stent in subsequent trials.

Conclusion

Numerous studies and registries have demonstrated that when used for "on-label" indications, drug-eluting stents are effective at reducing restenosis and the need for repeated revascularization in all patient subgroups and lesion types, without an increase in late MI or excess mortality. However, there are few overall safety data from adequately controlled trials on the use of drug-eluting stents for "off-label" indications. Larger prospective studies with adequate power to detect small differences in stent thrombosis, MI, and mortality rates are required to address these issues definitively. In the meantime, all patients should undergo rigorous screening before coronary intervention to assess their ability to tolerate uninterrupted dual antiplatelet therapy for a minimum of 3 to 6 months and preferably 1 year, as suggested by the Society for Cardiovascular Angiography and Interventions [49]. In addition, all patients should receive optimal medical therapy as either an adjunct to percutaneous coronary intervention or as an initial strategy in asymptomatic patients or carefully selected patients with symptoms of low-risk stable angina [31]. Present and future advancements in stent design and novel techniques of drug delivery are likely to overcome some of the problems currently encountered with the first and second generations of DES and we can be reasonably optimistics about science defeating fiction after 2008.

References

[1] Morice MC, Serruys PW, Sousa JE, Fajadet J, Ban Hayashi E, Perin M, et al. RAVEL Study Group. A randomized comparison of a sirolimus-eluting stent with a standard stent for coronary revascularization. *N Engl J Med.* 2002;346:1773-80.

[2] Moses JW, Leon MB, Popma JJ, Fitzgerald PJ, Holmes DR, O'Shaughnessy C, et al. SIRIUS Investigators. Sirolimus-eluting stents versus standard stents in patients with stenosis in a native coronary artery. *N Engl J Med.* 2003;349:1315-23.

[3] Schampaert E, Cohen EA, Schlüter M, Reeves F, Traboulsi M, Title LM, et al. C-SIRIUS Investigators. The Canadian study of the sirolimus-eluting stent in the treatment of patients with long de novo lesions in small native coronary arteries (C-SIRIUS). *J Am Coll Cardiol.* 2004;43:1110-5.

[4] Schofer J, Schlüter M, Gershlick AH, Wijns W, Garcia E, Schampaert E, et al. E-SIRIUS Investigators. Sirolimus-eluting stents for treatment of patients with long atherosclerotic lesions in small coronary arteries: double-blind, randomised controlled trial (E-SIRIUS). *Lancet.* 2003;362:1093-9.

[5] Grube E, Silber S, Hauptmann KE, Mueller R, Buellesfeld L, Gerckens U, et al. TAXUS I: six- and twelve-month results from a randomized, double-blind trial on a slow-release paclitaxel-eluting stent for de novo coronary lesions. *Circulation.* 2003;107:38-42

[6] Colombo A, Drzewiecki J, Banning A, Grube E, Hauptmann K, Silber S, et al. TAXUS II Study Group. Randomized study to assess the effectiveness of slow- and moderate-release polymer-based paclitaxel-eluting stents for coronary artery lesions. *Circulation.* 2003;108:788-94.

[7] Stone GW, Ellis SG, Cox DA, Hermiller J, O'Shaughnessy C, Mann JT, et al. TAXUS-IV Investigators. A polymer-based, paclitaxel-eluting stent in patients with coronary artery disease. *N Engl J Med.* 2004;350:221-31.

[8] Stone GW, Ellis SG, Cannon L, Mann JT, Greenberg JD, Spriggs D, et al. TAXUS V Investigators. Comparison of a polymer-based paclitaxel-eluting stent with a bare metal

stent in patients with complex coronary artery disease: a randomized controlled trial. *JAMA*. 2005;294:1215-23

[9] Dawkins KD, Grube E, Guagliumi G, Banning AP, Zmudka K, Colombo A, et al. TAXUS VI Investigators. Clinical efficacy of polymer-based paclitaxel-eluting stents in the treatment of complex, long coronary artery lesions from a multicenter, randomized trial: support for the use of drug-eluting stents in contemporary clinical practice. *Circulation*. 2005;112:3306-13.

[10] Tung R, Kaul S, Diamond GA, Shah PK. Narrative review: drug-eluting stents for the management of restenosis: a critical appraisal of the evidence. *Ann Intern Med.* 2006;144:913-9.

[11] Lemos PA, Serruys PW, van Domburg RT, Saia F, Arampatzis CA, Hoye A, et al. Unrestricted utilization of sirolimus-eluting stents compared with conventional bare stent implantation in the "real world": the Rapamycin-Eluting Stent Evaluated At Rotterdam Cardiology Hospital (RESEARCH) registry. *Circulation*. 2004;109:190-5

[12] Win HK, Caldera AE, Maresh K, et al, EVENT Registry Investigators. Clinical outcomes and stent thrombosis following off-label use of drug-eluting stents. *JAMA*. 2007;297:2001-2009.

[13] Beohar N, Davidson CJ, Kip KE, et al. Outcomes and complications associated with off-label and untested use of drug-eluting stents. *JAMA*. 2007;297:1992-2000.

[14] Camenzind E, Steg PG, Wijns W. Stent thrombosis late after implantation of first-generation drug-eluting stents: a cause for concern. *Circulation*. 2007;115:1440-55; discussion 1455

[15] Nordmann AJ, Briel M, Bucher HC. Mortality in randomized controlled trials comparing drug-eluting vs. bare metal stents in coronary artery disease: a meta-analysis. *Eur Heart J.* 2006;27:2784-814.

[16] Lagerqvist B, James SK, Stenestrand U, Lindback J, Nilsson T, Wallentin L, SCAAR Study Group. Long-term outcomes with drug-eluting stents versus bare-metal stents in Sweden. *N Engl J Med*. 2007;356:1009-19.

[17] Bavry AA, Chiu JH, Jefferson BK, Karha J, Bhatt DL, Ellis SG, et al. Development of coronary aneurysm after drug-eluting stent implantation [Letter]. *Ann Intern Med.* 2007;146:230-2.

[18] Jeremias A, Sylvia B, Bridges J, Kirtane AJ, Bigelow B, Pinto DS, et al. Stent thrombosis after successful sirolimus-eluting stent implantation. *Circulation*. 2004;109:1930-2.

[19] Urban P, Gershlick AH, Guagliumi G, Guyon P, Lotan C, Schofer J, et al. e-Cypher Investigators. Safety of coronary sirolimus-eluting stents in daily clinical practice: one-year follow-up of the e-Cypher registry. *Circulation*. 2006;113:1434-41

[20] Pfisterer M, Brunner-La Rocca HP, Buser PT, Rickenbacher P, Hunziker P, Mueller C, et al. BASKET-LATE Investigators. Late clinical events after clopidogrel discontinuation may limit the benefit of drug-eluting stents: an observational study of drug-eluting versus bare-metal stents. *J Am Coll Cardiol*. 2006;48:2584-91.

[21] Stone GW, Moses JW, Ellis SG, Schofer J, Dawkins KD, Morice MC, et al. Safety and efficacy of sirolimus- and paclitaxel-eluting coronary stents. *N Engl J Med.* 2007;356:998-1008.

[22] Spaulding C, Daemen J, Boersma E, Cutlip DE, Serruys PW. A pooled analysis of data comparing sirolimus-eluting stents with bare-metal stents. *N Engl J Med.* 2007;356: 989-97

[23] Kastrati A, Mehilli J, Pache J, Kaiser C, Valgimigli M, Kelbaek H, et al. Analysis of 14 trials comparing sirolimus-eluting stents with bare-metal stents. *N Engl J Med.* 2007;356:1030-9.

[24] Chen MS, John JM, Chew DP, Lee DS, Ellis SG, Bhatt DL. Bare metal stent restenosis is not a benign clinical entity. *Am Heart J.* 2006;151:1260-4.

[25] Mauri L, Hsieh WH, Massaro JM, Ho KK, D'Agostino R, Cutlip DE. Stent thrombosis in randomized clinical trials of drug-eluting stents. *N Engl J Med.* 2007;356:1020-9.

[26] Kip EK, Hollabaugh RN, Marroquin OC, Williams DO. The problems with composite end points in cardiovascular studies. *JACC.* 2008;51:701-7

[27] Marzocchi A, Saia F, Piovaccari G et al. Long-Term Safety and Efficacy of Drug-Eluting Stents: Two-Year Results of the REAL (REgistro AngiopLastiche dell'Emilia Romagna) Multicenter Registry. *Circulation.* 2007;115(25):3181-88

[28] Hannan EL, Racz M, Holmes DR, Walford G, Sharma S, Katz S, Jones R, King SB III. Comparison of Coronary Artery Stenting Outcomes in the Eras Before and After the Introduction of Drug-Eluting Stents. *Circulation* 2008; 117(16):2071-78

[29] Stettler C, Wandel S, Allemann S, Kastrati A, Morice MC, Schömig A, et al. Outcomes associated with drug-eluting and bare-metal stents: a collaborative network meta-analysis. *Lancet.* 2007;370:937-48

[30] Spertus JA, Kettelkamp R, Vance C, Decker C, Jones PG, Rumsfeld JS, et al. Prevalence, predictors, and outcomes of premature discontinuation of thienopyridine therapy after drug-eluting stent placement: results from the PREMIER registry. *Circulation.* 2006;113:2803-9.

[31] Boden WE, O'Rourke RA, Teo KK, Hartigan PM, Maron DJ, Kostuk WJ, et al. COURAGE Trial Research Group. Optimal medical therapy with or without PCI for stable coronary disease. *N Engl J Med.* 2007;356:1503-16.

[32] Ortolani P, Balducelli M, Marzaroli P et al. Two-year Clinical Outcomes with Drug-Eluting Stents for Diabetic Patients with De Novo Coronary Lesions. Results from a Real-World Multicenter Registry. Circulation

[33] Hwang CW, Wu D, Edelman ER. Physiological transport forces govern drug distribution for stent-based delivery. *Circulation* 2001;104:600-5.

[34] E. Alt et al., "Inhibition of Neointima Formation After Experimental Coronary Artery Stenting: a New Biodegradable Stent Coating Releasing Hirudin and the Prostacyclin Analogue Iloprost," *Circulation,***101**,1453–8 (2000).

[35] J.H. Yoon et al., "Local Delivery of Nitric Oxide from an Eluting Stent to Inhibit Neointimal Thickening in a Porcine Coronary Injury Model," *Yonsei Med.J.,***43**,242–51 (2002).

[36] D. Hou et al., "Stent-Based Nitric Oxide Delivery Reducing Neointimal Proliferation in a Porcine Carotid Overstretch Injury Model," *Cardiovasc.Intervent.Radiol.,***28**,60–5 (2005).

[37] J.C. Tardif et al., "Prevention of Restenosis with Antioxidants: Mechanisms and Implications," *Am.J.Cardiovasc.Drugs,***2**,323–34 (2002)

[38] W. Kim et al., "Effect of Anti-Oxidant (Carvedilol and Probucol) Loaded Stents in a Porcine Coronary Restenosis Model," *Circ.J.,***69**,101–6 (2005).

[39] P. Geraldes et al., "Specific Contribution of Estrogen Receptors on Mitogen-Activated Protein Kinase Pathways and Vascular Cell Activation," *Circ.Res.*,**93**,399–405 (2003).
[40] Abizaid et al., "First Human Experience with the 17-Beta-Estradiol-Eluting Stent: The Estrogen and Stents To Eliminate Restenosis (EASTER) Trial," *J.Am. Coll. Cardiol.*, **43**, 1118–21 (2004).
[41] F. Airoldi et al., "17-Beta-Estradiol Eluting Stent Versus Phosphorylcholine-Coated Stent for the Treatment of Native Coronary Artery Disease," *Am. J. of Cardiol.*,**96**,664–7 (2005).
[42] M. Hedman et al., "Safety and Feasibility of Catheter-Based Local Intracoronary Vascular Endothelial Growth Factor Gene Transfer in the Prevention of Postangioplasty," *Circulation*,**107**,2677–83 (2003).
[43] D.H. Walter et al., "Local Gene Transfer of phVEGF-2 Plasmid by Gene-Eluting Stents: An Alternative Strategy for Inhibition of Restenosis," *Circulation*,**110**,36–45 (2004).
[44] H.M. Nugent, E.R. Edelman, "Endothelial Implants Provide Long-Term Control of Vascular Repair in a Porcine Model of Arterial Injury," *J. Surg. Res.*,**99**,228–34 (2001).
[45] N. Kipshidze et al., "Role of the Endothelium in Modulating Neointimal Formation: Vasculoprotective Approaches to Attenuate Restenosis after Percutaneous Coronary Interventions," *J.Am.Coll.Cardiol.*,**44**,733–9 (2004).
[46] N. Kipshidze et al., "Endoluminal Reconstruction of the Arterial Wall with Endothelial Cell/Glue Matrix Reduces Restenosis in an Atherosclerotic Rabbit," *J.Am.Coll.Cardiol.*, **36**,1396–403 (2000).
[47] R. Blindt et al., "A Novel Drug-Eluting Stent Coated with an Integrin-Binding Cyclic Arg-Gly-Asp Peptide Inhibits Neointimal Hyperplasia by Recruiting Endothelial Progenitor Cells," *J.Am.Coll.Cardiol.*,**47**,1786–95 (2006).
[48] J. Aoki et al., "Endothelial Progenitor Cell Capture by Stents Coated with Antibody Against CD34: the HEALING-FIM (Healthy Endothelial Accelerated Lining Inhibits Neointimal Growth-First In Man) Registry," *J.Am.Coll.Cardiol.*,**45**,1574–9 (2005).
[49] Hodgson JM, Stone GW, Michael Lincoff A, Klein L, Walpole H, Bottner R, et al. Society for Cardiovascular Angiography and Interventions. Late stent thrombosis: considerations and practical advice for the use of drug-eluting stents: a report from the Society for Cardiovascular Angiography and Interventions Drug-eluting Stent Task Force. *Catheter Cardiovasc Interv.* 2007;69:327-33.

In: Heart Disease in Men
Editors: A.B. Todd and M.H. Mosley, pp. 219-241
ISBN: 978-1-60692-297-2

Chapter 10

DOSE INDIVIDUALIZATION OF DRUGS BASED ON BODY COMPOSITION

Michael Barras [1,2] ***and Bruce Green*** [1,3]
[1]University of Queensland, Brisbane, Australia
[2] Mater Hospital, Brisbane, Australia
[3]Model Answers Pty Ltd, Brisbane, Australia

Abstract

The effect of body composition on the disposition of drugs is an important topic for clinicians due to the escalating prevalence of obesity. In the United States alone, approximately 25% of adults are obese (body mass index ≥30 kg/m^2) and 65% are either overweight or obese (body mass index ≥25 kg/m^2). This discernable growth in obesity is directly correlated with morbidity and mortality from cardiovascular disease. Nevertheless, only a limited number of studies have evaluated the impact of obesity-associated physiological changes on the time course of drug effect.

For many drugs, a dose approved for use in normal-weighted subjects is unlikely to result in the desired pharmacodynamic response if given to obese subjects. However, there are few guidelines that can aid the clinician to choose an optimal dose for the obese population. This knowledge deficit can be partly attributed to the exclusion of obese subjects from clinical trials, but also because there has not been a suitable body size descriptor to allow dose adjustment across a wide range of body compositions. The effect of body composition on drug disposition, drug response, and therefore patient outcomes is particularly pertinent in cardiovascular medicine where excessive drug exposure results in adverse drug events, and suboptimal drug exposure leads to clinical failure.

To help ensure drug exposure in the obese is similar to normal-weighted subjects, maintenance doses of drugs need to be chosen based upon some metric that is correlated with drug clearance. Adipose tissue has little metabolic activity and is therefore unlikely to contribute towards a drug's clearance (CL) while lean body weight (LBW) encapsulates 99% of the body's metabolic processes and is therefore intuitively more likely to be representative of a drug's CL. Dosing regimens adjusted by LBW rather than total body weight (TBW) are therefore more likely to result in comparable exposures across the spectrum of body compositions.

Recently, the hypothesis that drug CL is correlated with LBW rather than TBW has sparked interest in the development of novel individualized dose strategies in the field of cardiology. The benefits of dose individualization are well established in contemporary cardiovascular pharmacotherapy, and essential for drugs with a narrow therapeutic index; for example digoxin, warfarin and unfractionated heparin. This chapter discusses concepts and evidence for drug dosing based upon LBW, principally in the obese population. We discuss historical methods to improve dosing across body compositions; recent advances and future directions with a focus on strategies significant to cardiovascular disease.

1. Introduction

Prevalence of Obesity

The number of people worldwide that are overweight or obese has now reached epidemic proportions. Approximately 1.6 billion adults are now classified as overweight with at least 400 million obese [1]. The World Health Organisation (WHO) estimates that by 2015 approximately 2.3 billion adults will be overweight and more that 700 million will be obese [1]. In the United States (US) approximately 66% (134 million) of adults aged 20 and older are either overweight or obese and 31% (64 million) are obese [2]. Three million adults are now morbidly obese [3].

The problem is not isolated to the US. In the United Kingdom (UK), 43% of men and 33% of women are overweight with an additional 22% of men and 23% of women obese [4]. A government paper released in 2007 predicts that 40% of Britons will be obese by 2025 with an associated cost of 46 billion pounds a year by 2050 [5]. Similar data are reported in Australia, where 60% of adults aged 25 or over are obese or overweight and 21% are obese [6].

The prevalence of obesity appears to increase with age with 27% of men and 31% of women between 16 to 24 years of age classified as overweight or obese. This rises to 79% of men and 71% of women by age 55 to 64 [6]. Children are not immune to the "growing" epidemic, with nearly 20% of 2 to 10 year olds expected to be obese by 2010 [5]. In 2006 almost 2 million UK school children were overweight and 0.7 million were obese. This equates to approximately 25% of girls and 20% of boys considered to have unhealthy weights [7]. In the US, from 1999-2002, 17% of children were overweight or obese [8].

The Definition of Obesity

Obesity is characterized anatomically by an abnormal increase in the proportion of fat cells, mainly in the viscera and subcutaneous tissues of the body. It is typically defined using body mass index (BMI), which is an index of weight-for-height, calculated by dividing total body weight (TBW) in kilograms by the square of their height (HT) in meters (equation 1). The WHO categorizes BMI based on the relationship between BMI and mortality [1]. These categories are listed in table 1.

$$BMI(kg/m^2) = \frac{TBW(kg)}{HT^2(m)} \qquad \text{Eq.1.}$$

Whilst the WHO has used BMI as a marker for health status, it is not without its limitations. BMI does not differentiate between weight from muscle and adipose tissue (fat) with comparable BMI's often representing dissimilar body compositions. Given this disparity, waist circumference has become increasingly popular as a metric to define disease risk such as coronary heart disease (CHD). This is a useful addition to BMI as abdominal fat mass may vary greatly within a narrow range of total body fat or BMI. Individuals with a waist circumference ≥ 94 cm in men and ≥ 80 cm in women have an increased risk of CHD. Measurements ≥ 102 cm in men and ≥ 88 cm in women are defined as a "substantial increased risk" [1].

Table 1. The World Health Organisation (WHO) classification of body size using Body Mass Index (BMI) in Caucasian adults [1]

Category	BMI range (kg/m^2)
Underweight	< 18.5
Normal Weight	18.5 to 24.99
Overweight	25 to 29.99
Obese class I	30 to 34.99
Obese class II	35 to 39.99
Obese Class III*	≥ 40

* The term morbid obesity is synonymous with the definition of obese class III.

2. Obesity and Its Relationship with Coronary Heart Disease (CHD)

The American Heart Association and College of Cardiology guidelines for secondary prevention in CHD lists obesity (BMI ≥ 30 kg/m^2) as a major modifiable cardiovascular risk factor that is associated with an increased risk of morbidity and mortality [9]. While the number of people with other risk factors for CHD such as smoking, increased blood pressure and elevated cholesterol have fallen or remained static over the past 10 years, the prevalence of obesity and type 2 diabetes have both been rising [9].

The link between obesity and CHD is compelling. About 30% of subjects who have had an acute myocardial infarct have a BMI of 25 or greater and approximately 5% of deaths from CHD are due to obesity [4]. The risk of developing Type II diabetes, hypertension and dyslipidemia increase from a BMI of 21 [9] with approximately 90% of people who develop Type 2 diabetes having a BMI > 23 [10, 11]. Similarly, it has been reported that 85% of subjects with hypertension have a BMI > 25 [11]. It has been proposed that a 25% decrease in the prevalence of obesity would reduce mortality from CHD by 1.2% and 1.4% for men and women respectively [4].

Obesity is linked to other cardiovascular diseases such as heart failure with approximately 14% and 11% of diagnoses in men and women respectively attributable to obesity [12]. Obesity also increases the risk of stroke, atrial fibrillation, venous thromboembolism and metabolic syndrome [13], indicating that the effects of obesity on cardiovascular function are multi-factorial [14]. Other diseases such as dementia, some cancers, arthritis and depression have all been linked to obesity [11].

What is also of note is the time scale of CHD events. In one study, adults who were obese during middle age (31-64 years) but otherwise healthy, had a 43% greater increased risk of hospitalization or death from CHD compared to subjects of normal body weight after a mean follow up of 32 years [15]. This confirmed previous data indicating the negative impact of obesity on life expectancy [16]. The future prevalence of CHD is likely to be higher than expected with over 1 million children in Europe considered obese with conditions highly correlated with CHD [7].

Relevance to Clinicians

Many clinicians might ask the question: "Is knowledge of drug dosing principles in the obese population relevant to cardiovascular medicine?" In addition to the increasing prevalence of obesity and obesity related diseases, there is also evidence that clinician workload and prescribing rate is increasing in this population. A retrospective analysis in 2005 discovered that a higher percentage of cardiovascular drugs are prescribed for the obese when compared to normal-weighted subjects. Similarly, length of treatment was longer, clearly indicating that clinicians need increasingly detailed knowledge about suitable dose selection for the obese population [17]. Unfortunately, product labels for most drugs provide little or no direction for the prescriber.

3. The Concept of Dose Individualization

The "one dose fits all" paradigm of drug dosing is hopefully being replaced by strategies aimed at delivering "individualized therapy" to patients. Dose individualization has the potential to improve drug efficacy and minimize adverse events, hence optimizing patient care and reducing health-care costs due to suboptimal dosing.

Dose individualization strategies can broadly be categorized into three methods: dosing based on a covariate or characteristic such as the subject's weight, for example low-molecular-weight heparin (LMWH) dosing on a mg per kg dosing; empiric/protocol based dosing to a desired pharmacodynamic (PD) response, for example warfarin dosing based on INR; dosing aimed at a concentration or a therapeutic range that has been shown to have optimal clinical outcomes, for example digoxin and heart failure.

In addition to these individualized methods, a fixed (or flat) dose strategy where all patients receive the same dose remains the most common form of drug dosing proposed by the industry today.

Fixed Dosing

Fixed dosing strategies are common in contemporary cardiovascular medicine. Relevant examples include clopidogrel (75mg daily) and aspirin (150mg daily) for the prevention of thromboembolic disease, spironalactone (25mg daily) for the treatment of heart failure and hydrochlorothiazide (12.5mg daily) for the treatment of hypertension. Fixed dosing can often be highly effective, which has been demonstrated with aspirin where the anti-platelet effect does not appear to be significantly influenced by demographic characteristics. .

Covariate Dosing

For many drugs, however, large variations in pharmacokinetic (PK) and PD response exist between subjects. The cause of this between subject variability (BSV) may be due to weight, age, genetics, environmental factors, concurrent diseases or interacting drugs. It could also be unknown in which case dose individualization based on patient demographics would be fruitless. Where there is clear evidence that covariates describe some of the BSV, dose individualization using this method should be encouraged to help normalize drug exposure across a range of different populations.

Doses normalized by a subject's renal function or TBW are the most frequently used methods of dose individualization in cardiology. Drugs such as enoxaparin [18], unfractionated heparin (UFH) [19], bivalirudin [20], abciximab [21] and tirofiban [22] are all dosed using a microgram or milligram per kg strategy.

Dosing to a Specific Response

For some drugs, initial dosing can be made using either a fixed or covariate dosing method with subsequent dose adjustments made secondary to a PD response. Examples of fixed dosed drugs include the calcium channel blocking agents nifedipine and verapamil which can be subsequently dose adjusted according to heart rate or blood pressure. Drugs that are initially dosed using covariates (TBW) include dobutamine and dopamine which are then titrated to a desired cardiac or renal output. In both cases, drug concentration is not considered, with the PD response alone driving dose selection.

Dosing to a Concentration or Therapeutic Range

Whilst covariate based dosing can account for some variability between subjects, and therefore help normalize drug exposure, in many cases unknown sources of variability remain for which covariate based dosing fails to normalize exposure sufficiently. In these cases, drug dosing can be adjusted to target a defined concentration range that seeks to maximize effectiveness and minimize toxicity. Examples of drugs used in cardiology include digoxin, perhexiline, amiodarone and UFH. Methods to target a defined concentration range are commonly termed Therapeutic Drug Monitoring (TDM). Following blood sampling, a suitable dose is recommended based upon an individual's concentration. The dose adjustment can be made given some knowledge of the individuals PK parameters which should help ensure the next concentration is within a range that has a higher probability of effectiveness and less chance of toxicity. TDM has often been criticized as the target range is usually designed for the 'typical' population and does not target a specific concentration suited to the individual, primarily as the parameters describing the individual's PD response are typically unknown.

The unexplained variability in the relationship between a concentration and response may be large enough to warrant further adjustment in dosing. Target Concentration Intervention (TCI) based upon an individual's response is a new dose individualization strategy where population PK models are used to optimize therapy to a target concentration not a therapeutic range [23]. If a target concentration is known that maximizes an individual's response (or minimizes an adverse response such as bleeding), PK models can be used to determine an appropriately tailored dose (and dose interval) using the individual's PK parameters. This method has been applied to drugs such as the aminoglycosides [24] and some chemotherapeutic agents [25]. It is anticipated that future research using these methods will develop in cardiovascular medicine. The advantages of population PK modeling are discussed in further detail in section 5.

4. Selecting Optimal Drug Doses for the Obese

The Impact of Obesity on PK

PK encompasses the pathways of drug absorption, distribution, elimination and of importance, the rate at which these processes occur. To produce a PD effect, a drug must be present in sufficient concentrations for an appropriate period of time at its site of action. PD defines the relationship between the concentration and the effect of the drug on the body. The term 'effect' can be used to describe a variety of observable responses to a drug. For example, the beta-receptor blocker metoprolol, reduces heart rate, thereby causing a decrease in blood pressure (which may in turn determine the subjects' survival). Heart rate, blood pressure and survival are all considered 'observable effects'.

To produce an optimal PD response in the obese subject, drug exposure should be normalized to that of a normal weighted subject who was typically recruited in the drug development process. To do this requires an understanding of how obesity influences the PK, which represents a challenge from a mechanistic perspective with further research necessary to fully understand these processes. We do not provide a detailed review summarizing PK-PD research for specific drugs in the obese population as this is beyond the scope of this chapter. Clinicians are encouraged to read references [26 to 29] for additional information. For the purposes of this chapter, we limit our discussion to drug dosing principles and introduce new ideas that could change the global framework of drug dosing in obesity. Specifically, we have limited our discussion to the two primary PK parameters of interest essential to understand how to dose drugs across a population that might include the obese. These two PK parameters are the volume of distribution (V) and clearance (CL). We will not discuss absorption which has currently not been shown to be significantly modified in the presence of obesity [26].

V is a PK parameter related to structural aspects of the body, which quantifies the apparent volume in which a drug would theoretically distribute. Drugs that are hydrophilic generally have a high plasma concentration relative to dose and a smaller V. In contrast, drugs that are lipophilic distribute more freely into adipose tissue which results in lower plasma concentrations and a larger V. Hydrophilic drugs such as the LMWHs typically remain in plasma resulting in a V that is correlated with a measure of LBW. In contrast, V is more likely to be correlated with TBW for a drug that is lipid soluble [27-29].

The impact of obesity on V appears to primarily depend upon the lipophilicity of the drug. Maximum blood flow into fat is estimated to be 25–30 ml/minute/100 g of tissue, which accounts for less than 5% of cardiac output, implying that hydrophilic drugs should not be significantly influenced by excess adipose tissue [26]. Alternatively, highly lipophilic drugs distribute extensively into adipose tissue, resulting in a larger V. Examples include the benzodiazepines such as midazolam or diazepam, where V may increase 10-fold in obese individuals [26]. Drugs with a high V often require "loading doses" to "fill" the compartments in which the drug is distributed. Once an appropriate loading dose is administered, the clinician needs to ensure a constant dose-rate to maintain steady state plasma concentrations. Maintenance dose-rate is entirely dependent upon the PK parameter CL.

CL represents the functional capacity of the body and is the sum of both metabolism and excretion. It is defined as the volume of blood (or plasma) from which a drug is completely removed per unit time (usually reported as L/hr). Adipose tissue has little metabolic activity whereas LBW encapsulates 99% of the body's metabolic processes, which is representative of drug CL [30]. As the obese have an excess fat mass and an accompanying but significantly smaller increase in LBW, CL of drugs are expected to increase in a non linear fashion with TBW (refer section 6). As CL determines the maintenance dose of drugs, the clinician should consider how body composition impacts dosing in obese subjects rather than TBW.

Apart from a select few drugs such as androgens and estrogens where there is some evidence of metabolism by adipose tissue [31], merely increasing the dose for obese subjects based on TBW cannot be scientifically justified. What is required is a descriptor of body size that normalizes CL across a wide range of body compositions. A variety of body size descriptors already exist in the literature although it is only recently that a mechanistic descriptor has been developed that has the capability to dose drugs across individuals with ranges of body composition [32].

Body Size Descriptors

The purpose of this section is to provide a brief overview and critique of commonly used body size descriptors that clinicians might base drug dosing upon, and further discuss the limitations of dosing based on TBW in the obese subject. The most common body size descriptors presented in the literature include body mass index (BMI), body surface area (BSA), ideal body weight (IBW), fat-free mass (FFM), lean body weight (LBW), and predicted normal weight (PNWT) (Table 2). Others such as adjusted body weight (ABW) and percent of ideal body weight (%IBW) are seldom used.

Table 2. Traditional descriptors of weight and commonly used formulae (note other formulae may exist)*

Name	Formula
Body mass index (BMI)	$\frac{TBW(kg)}{HT(m)^2}$, kg/m^2
Body surface area (BSA) [35]	TBW (kg) $^{0.425}$ × HT (cm)$^{0.725}$ × 0.007184, m^2
Ideal body weight (IBW) [33]	45.4 + 0.89 × (HT (cm) − 152.4) + 4.5 (if male), kg
Fat-free mass (FFM) [66]	0.285 × TBW (kg) + 12.1 × HT (m)^2 for males, kg 0.287 × TBW (kg) + 9.74 × HT (m)^2 for females, kg

Table 2. Continued

Name	Formula
Predicted normal weight (PNWT)[37]	$1.57 \times \text{TBW(kg)} - 0.0183 \times \text{BMI (kg/m}^2) \times \text{TBW(kg)} - 10.5$ for males, kg $1.75 \times \text{TBW(kg)} - 0.0242 \times \text{BMI (kg/m}^2) \times \text{TBW(kg)} - 12.6$ for females, kg
LBW (males) [32]	$\frac{9270 \times TBW(kg)}{6680 + 216 \times BMI(\text{kg/m}^2)}$, kg
LBW (females)	$\frac{9270 \times TBW(kg)}{8780 + 244 \times BMI(\text{kg/m}^2)}$, kg

* TBW refers to total body weight, HT refers to height.

Traditional Body Size Descriptors

The most common body size descriptor used for dosing is TBW. Dosing by TBW is certainly the easiest method practically which is probably why it is often the method of choice for dose individualization. A dose per kilogram on the product label is however often assumed to be TBW by the clinician as alternative body size descriptors, apart from BSA in oncology, are rarely defined. Dosing for normal weighted subjects based on TBW is usually a scientifically justified method of dose individualization as TBW has been tested in confirmatory clinical trials which have then been transported into the product label. The problem is that obese subjects are usually excluded from the drug industry's clinical development program and there is little incentive to obtain post marketing data. Dosing using TBW, assumes that the structural and functional aspects of the body are similar in the obese and non-obese population, which is not the case [30].

IBW was developed by Devine in 1974 as a metric to link weight to health risk based on life insurance tables that listed "desirable" weights for men and women over 25 years of age [33]. IBW aims to provide a measure of weight that is standardized by height. As this data was collected before the 1960s and reflects the demographics of the US population at the time of publication it has a conservative range of weights and heights that do not extrapolate to today's population. A formula by Robinson [34], based on the work by Devine is also used.

BMI is used as body size descriptor for mortality risk (section 1). It has not been used extensively to help understand PK over a range of body sizes and is therefore not used to calculate drug doses in clinical practice. BMI increases with TBW but cannot differentiate adipose tissue from muscle tissue.

BSA was derived almost a century ago [35] and has been re-defined to simplify its computation [36]. BSA seems a biologically plausible size descriptor as it considers height and weight in its derivation; however it does not consider sex. BSA is widely used in clinical practice to dose chemotherapeutic agents, and is probably considered the 'gold standard' metric for dosing such drugs.

PNWT is a relatively new body size descriptor which, unlike the other measures, was designed specifically for drug dosing in the obese population [37]. It characterizes an individual's fat mass into 'normal fat mass' and 'excess fat mass' and aims to describe the 'expected normal weight' of an obese individual by combining their lean mass with their normal fat mass. It is biologically more robust than some body size descriptors as it incorporates TBW, height and sex.

LBW is compromised of cellular mass and non-fatty intercellular connective tissue which includes bone, tendons and ligaments. It accounts for approximately 99% of the body's metabolic activity and is therefore an attractive size metric to use for dose adjustments in the obese population. There are various methods to determine LBW, such as dual-energy X-ray absorptiometry (DXA), and whole body densitometry measurements by underwater immersion. None of these methods can be used in clinical practice due to availability, cost, cooperation of the subject and need for technical expertise or equipment. Anthropometric measures (for example waist measurement) and bioelectrical impedance analysis (BIA) are other methods that can be used to predict LBW. These calculations can be easily performed in the clinical setting although their accuracy can depend on technical skill of the user. The most commonly cited equation to describe LBW was developed by Cheymol [26] who used data from a study by James [38].

The Limitations of Traditional Body Size Descriptors

What should we expect from a suitable body size descriptor? Firstly it should be based on sound biological principles and therefore include relevant covariates such as age, sex, weight and height which will limit any biological implausibility. Secondly, it should be transportable throughout the population with the ability to normalize PK parameters across a range of body compositions. Thirdly, there should be no mathematical inconsistencies when using the descriptor, especially at extremes of the covariate; for example it should be robust enough to use in both a 70kg and a 200kg subject. Finally, the descriptor should originate from a population representative of its use.

One overarching problem with the historic size descriptors, apart from PNWT, is that they were not specifically developed for scaling PK parameters and therefore drug doses across varying body compositions. Consequently, the extrapolation of their use to the obese remains questionable. Certainly body size descriptors, such as IBW, BMI and BSA, do not take into account the covariates required to describe biological variability between individuals. BSA and BMI do not consider sex and IBW is a function of height and sex only. These three metrics therefore fail to take into account the effect of changing body composition between normal weighted and obese subjects. IBW assumes that individuals of the same sex and height have exactly the same IBW, which does not seem biologically plausible. If used as a dosing scalar, all subjects of the same height would receive the same dose. Incorporating TBW into the IBW formula would add further information about the size of an individual over height alone. BMI contains TBW, however its use as a dosing scalar is limited as subjects of the same height with a large muscle mass would receive the same dose as subjects with a large fat mass. Due to the different compositions of these tissues, it is likely that obese subjects need dose individualization based on an alternative metric that accounts for varying proportions of muscle to fat.

The formula for LBW, despite incorporating TBW, was developed for reasons unrelated to PK [38]. It is also not transportable across weight ranges, primarily as the individuals used in the derivation of James' LBW equations in 1976 weighed considerably less than subjects commonly found in today's society (maximum BMI was 43 kg/m^2 and maximum TBW was

122 kg). This under-representation of obese subjects in James' population (only 9.2% of study subjects had a BMI ≥ 30 kg/m^2) leads to estimation of lower values of LBW at extremes of TBW and in some circumstances even lead to computation of negative values of LBW. This is shown in Figure 1, a three-dimensional plot of LBW, height (HT) and TBW demonstrating that, at extremes of TBW and HT, the calculation of LBW can be negative.

With none of these body size descriptors able to reliably be used as a dose scalar across a range of body sizes, what is the best body size descriptor to use to normalize PK parameters across a range of body compositions? Green et al [27] conducted a meta-analysis of studies that attempted to quantify the relationship between PK parameters and body size descriptors. The analysis found that few studies had explored the relationship adequately, with size descriptors that incorporate fat mass such as TBW preferred to describe V for lipophilic drugs. CL was best described by LBW with no single metric describing the influence of body size on both CL and V equally well. For drugs dosed chronically, where CL is of primary concern, dosing for obese subjects should not be based on their TBW. Instead, dosing the obese subject should be based on LBW. Recent research has focused on finding an optimal formula to describe LBW that does not have the limitations of traditional methods.

Development of a New Robust Body Size Descriptor

To overcome the limitations of the historic size descriptors above and given LBW seems the most scientifically justified body size metric to adjust drug doses, a semi-mechanistic model for LBW based on bioimpedance was developed in 2005 [32]. The model was developed from a population with a wide range of TBWs of which 71% of subjects were overweight or obese. The TBWs ranged from 40.7 to 216.5 kg and BMI values ranged from 17.1 to 69.9 kg/m^2.

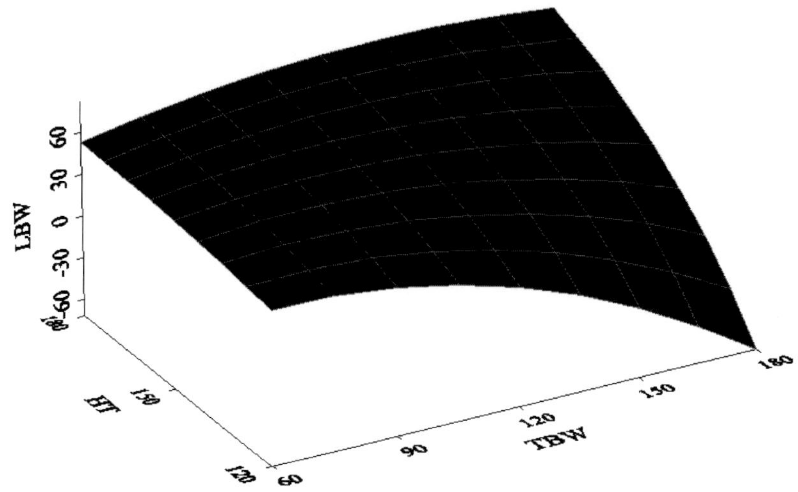

Figure 1. Estimated LBW for males of varying heights (HT) and TBW according to Cheymol [26] in which the x-axis is TBW (kg), the y-axis is HT (cm), and the z-axis is LBW (kg), (adapted from Green [65]). If this formula is used, LBW will become negative at extremes of HT and TBW.

The other key advantage of the new LBW model is that the estimate of LBW never declines as TBW increases and cannot therefore lead to negative values of LBW. Figure 2 graphically illustrates these properties by comparing the two formulae against increasing TBW (at a pre-defined subject HT of 1.7 meters). As seen, the new LBW (bold line) increases over the range of TBW while the old LBW (dotted line) decreases to a negative value.

The new equations for LBW are as follows:

$$\text{LBW (males), kg} = \frac{9270 \times TBW(kg)}{6680 + 216 \times BMI(kg/m^2)} \qquad \text{Eq. 2}$$

$$\text{LBW (females), kg} = \frac{9270 \times TBW(kg)}{8780 + 244 \times BMI(kg/m^2)} \qquad \text{Eq.3}$$

Renal Function and Body Size Descriptors

Renal function is a key covariate that affects the CL of many drugs. While not the focus of this chapter, some mention seems warranted as an appropriate body size descriptor should also be used when estimating an individual's renal clearance using equations such as the Cockcroft and Gault (C-G) formula [39]. The endogenous substance creatinine is predominantly eliminated by renal filtration and therefore incorporated into this equation.

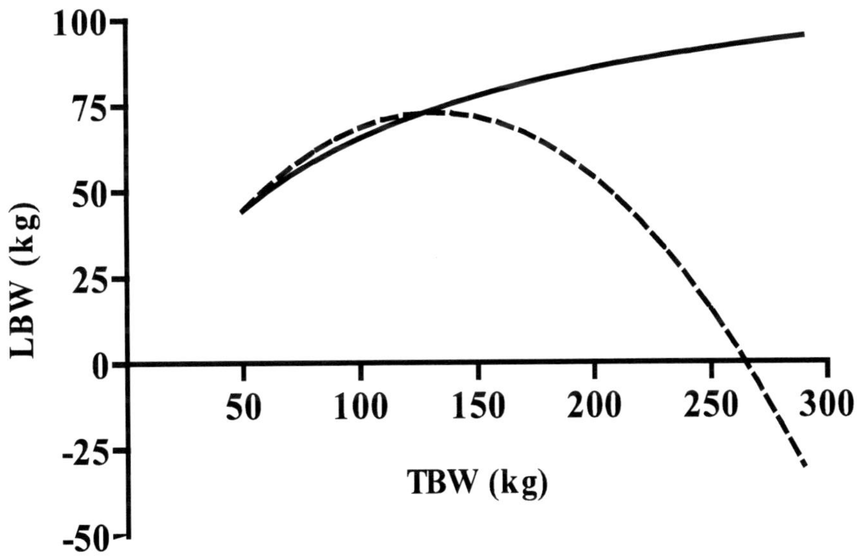

Figure 1. A comparison of estimated LBW for males of a height of 1.7 meters with increasing TBW, according to Cheymol [26] (dotted line) and Janmahasatian [32] (bold line), (adapted from Han [30]). LBW calculated using Cheymol's equation will decrease to a negative value while LBW calculated using Janmahasatian's equation with continue to increase with increasing TBW.

However, the C-G equation, like other predictive formulae furnish erroneously high estimates of glomerular filtration rate (GFR) in the obese subject, as excess body mass in the obese is mostly adipose tissue as opposed to muscle. Creatinine is a by-product of muscle metabolism, consequently, when no adjustment is made for the increase in total body mass, such as standardization with LBW, GFR will be routinely overestimated. As the C-G formula remains a predominant equation used clinically to estimate GFR, clinicians should be aware that it may be significantly biased when TBW is used to estimate GFR in obese subjects. A small study in 2008 confirmed this theory by demonstrating that GFR when normalized using LBW in the C-G formula, was not different between obese and normal weighted subjects [40].

5. Where Are the Clinical Trial Data to Support Drug Dosing in the Obese?

Currently, there is a substantial body of literature discussing the worldwide obesity health crisis, but few studies have quantified the influence of obesity on the PK (or PD) of drugs that are commonly administered to obese patients. Of the existing data available, the evaluation and interpretation is complicated by a number of factors usually related to study design and analysis. The complexities of trial design are beyond the scope of this chapter and we refer readers to Han et al [30] who provides an overview of this topic with an emphasis on studies in the obese population. We will briefly discuss two commonly encountered problems; recruitment and study analysis techniques.

Recruitment

The recruitment of subjects into a study that are representative of those likely to receive the drug is essential to allow unambiguous conclusions about the population in whom a drug will be used clinically i.e. the elderly, neonatal, renally impaired or obese populations. Unfortunately, obese subjects will often be excluded and therefore the ability to quantify any influence of obesity on PK parameters is difficult. Alternatively, studies evaluating the impact of obesity are often conducted in healthy subjects, restricting the potential influence of covariates, such as renal function on PK parameters. Finally, subjects are rarely recruited within a range of obesity. It is essential to assess parameters across a range of obesity, as a morbidly obese patient will influence a drug's PK in a distinctive way to a moderately obese patient [41].

Analysis

In PK studies that have involved obese subjects, the method of analysis is often unsatisfactory or uninformative. When conducting trials to evaluate the impact of obesity on PK, three primary methods can be used to interpret data [27]: method 1 is a statistical comparison of PK parameters between obese and non-obese populations; method 2 is a regression analysis of individual parameter values against a body size descriptor; and method 3 is the incorporation of a body size descriptor into a population analysis.

Method 1 cannot quantify the relationship between PK parameters and body size and should only be used in hypothesis ("yes-no") testing studies. If this method is used then the two study groups should not be matched for any body size descriptor that may correlate with a PK parameter, for example LBW if CL is the parameter of interest. Like any statistical analysis, no relationship will be found if the study groups are matched for the variable of interest.

Method 2 allows some quantification of the parameter-body size descriptor relationship and is therefore superior to method 1. In this method, individual subject parameters are determined which are then regressed against their respective body size descriptor. To ensure the individuals PK estimate is accurate, data sampling needs to be intensive and sampling times matched to maximize information about the PK parameters of interest. This can become complicated by subject specific drug dosing. In its simplest form, this method assumes a linear relationship between the parameter and the body size descriptor which may not be suitable for the obese population.

The third method is to incorporate the size descriptor into a population PK analysis. Population techniques accurately source and quantify both mean population parameter values, the variability of parameters between and within subjects and any remaining residual variability. Body size descriptors, or other patient characteristics, are then tested in the model to help explain the variability. The most influential characteristics can be statistically compared, using regression techniques, during the model building process. By characterizing parameters from a large number of patients, the resulting model can be used for the development of appropriate dosing guidelines and subsequent individualization of therapy. A major advantage of a population approach is that the nature of data can be highly variable. Data can be obtained using both sparse and intensively sampled designs that have been collected from uncontrolled conditions, such as clinical areas within hospitals. The sparse sampling methods will often reveal better estimates of the true inter-subject variability than the previous two methods that have been discussed. Most importantly the sources of variability are recognized, investigated and quantified [42, 43]. Interested readers are referred to excellent texts by Bonate [44] and Ette [45].

The scarcity of informative PK data in the obese is not surprising given the listed deficiencies in recruitment and analysis. As a result, clinicians usually have to assume that the results of PK studies in normal weighted subjects can be extrapolated to the obese population. This is an unsatisfactory method of dosing obese subjects who now constitute approximately 30% of today's population. A change in mind-set is required to eliminate arbitrary dosing methods and use methods based on scientific principles and mechanistic study design.

6. Is There a Scientifically Justified Method to Dose the Obese?

Optimal dosing regimens in the obese are often unknown with clinicians therefore having little confidence in doses they choose for the obese. They might also make arbitrary dose adjustments that may lead to therapeutic failure [46]. We now know that CL is more closely related to LBW than TBW and we also have a new LBW which is a robust body size descriptor capable of quantifying changes in CL for individuals of a wide range of body compositions. In a recent commentary [30], it has been proposed that clinicians shift the way they perceive the relationship between body composition and CL for all drugs and consider the following three hypotheses:

1. "Absolute CL Is Greater in Obese Individuals"

Obese individuals have a lower LBW:TBW ratio as compared to normal weighted individuals, although their total LBW is greater. This is represented in Figure 3 which illustrates how body composition changes with an increase in TBW. Normal weighted subjects, shown on the left-hand side, have a TBW consisting of normal LBW (LBWnorm) and fat body weight (FBWnorm) in an approximate ratio of 4:1. In contrast, an obese subject has an additional excess LBW (LBWexcess) and excess fat body weight (FBWexcess). The resulting LBW:TBW ratio is approximately 3:2, however there is a greater absolute LBW.

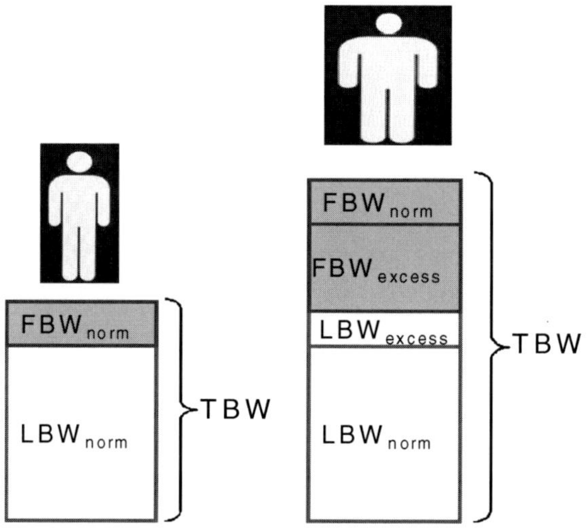

Figure 3. A pictorial comparison of a normal weighted subject (left-hand side) and an obese subject (right-hand side), depicting the approximate distribution of LBW and FBW. The obese patient has a lower LBW:TBW ratio but has a greater absolute LBW.

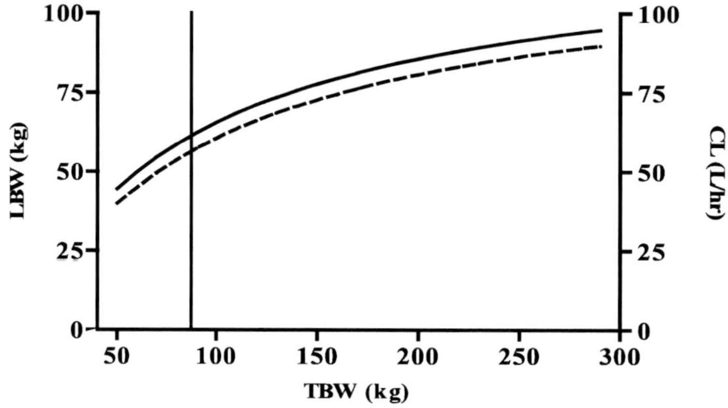

Figure 4. A plot of LBW and CL versus TBW in males of a standardized height of 1.7 meters. All individuals with a TBW greater than 87.5kg (vertical line) were considered obese (BMI > 30 kg/m2), (adapted from Han [30]). The plot illustrates the three hypotheses (section 6): CL (dashed line) is greater in the obese population; CL increases nonlinearly with TBW; CL increases linearly with LBW (solid line).

As metabolic processes such as CL are linked to LBW, it is not unreasonable to expect that the absolute CL of a drug is greater in the obese population. Consequently obese subjects require a greater dose than normal weighted patient and "dose capping" is not a scientifically justified method to use in the obese (refer to section 7). Figure 4 provides a graphical representation of this hypothesis. All individuals with a TBW greater than 87.5kg (vertical line) are considered obese (BMI $\geq$ 30) and a comparison of CL on both sides of this line indicates that absolute CL is greater in the obese population.

2. "CL Increases Non-Linearly with TBW"

As individuals become more obese their TBW will increase. Their ratio of LBW to TBW will however increase in a non-linear manner. Figure 4 demonstrates this hypothesis with CL (dashed line) increasing nonlinearly with TBW (x-axis). An individual with a TBW of 80kg for example has a CL of approximately 50 L/hr; however doubling TBW to 160kg only increases CL to approximately 70 L/hr. From a practical perspective, doubling the dose of a drug on the basis of TBW will not result in the doubling of CL with larger doses increasing the risk of an adverse event.

3. "CL Correlates Linearly with LBW"

The linear relationship between CL and LBW is also shown in Figure 4, where LBW (solid line) and CL (dashed line) run parallel to each other as TBW increases. It can be seen that CL does not increase linearly with TBW but does increase linearly with LBW. The subsequent effect on drug concentrations is pictorially represented in Figure 5. Dosing based on TBW (left hand boxes) will result in higher concentrations in the obese compared to normal weighted subjects, but concentrations will remain constant over all weight ranges when dosing is based on LBW (right hand boxes).

The hypotheses that link drug clearance to LBW instead of TBW have sparked interest in the development of novel individualized dose strategies in the field of cardiology. A relevant example is the LMWHs.

7. Motivating Example: *Enoxaparin*

The LMWHs are predominantly hydrophilic molecules with dose recommendations in approved labels based on TBW (mg/kg or units/kg). They are used to treat and prevent a variety of thromboembolic disorders and elicit their effect by potentiating the anti-thrombin 3 inhibition of factor Xa.

Enoxaparin is a LMWH that has been extensively researched with many purported advantages over UFH such as linear PK, an apparent predictable dose-concentration-response relationship with no need for TDM and improved outcomes in confirmatory clinical trials [47, 48]. Enoxaparin has proven to be at least as effective as UFH in phase 3 clinical trials [47, 48] and post-marketing studies for the treatment of acute coronary syndromes (ACS) [49, 50] together with other thromboembolic disorders [51, 52]. It is commonly recommended in contemporary clinical guidelines [53, 54] with an approved labelled dose in Australia [18],

Europe [55] and the United States [56] of 1mg/kg twice a day or 1.5mg/kg once a day, based on TBW. A dose reduction to 1mg/kg (TBW) once a day is recommended when the patient's creatinine clearance (CL_{CR}) is less than 30 ml/min (estimated using the C-G formula) [39].

The goals of LMWH therapy are to arrest the growth of a clot and prevent recurrence, while restricting adverse drug effects such as bleeding. Ideally, demonstrable relationships are sought between the dose and concentration and response (effectiveness or toxicity).

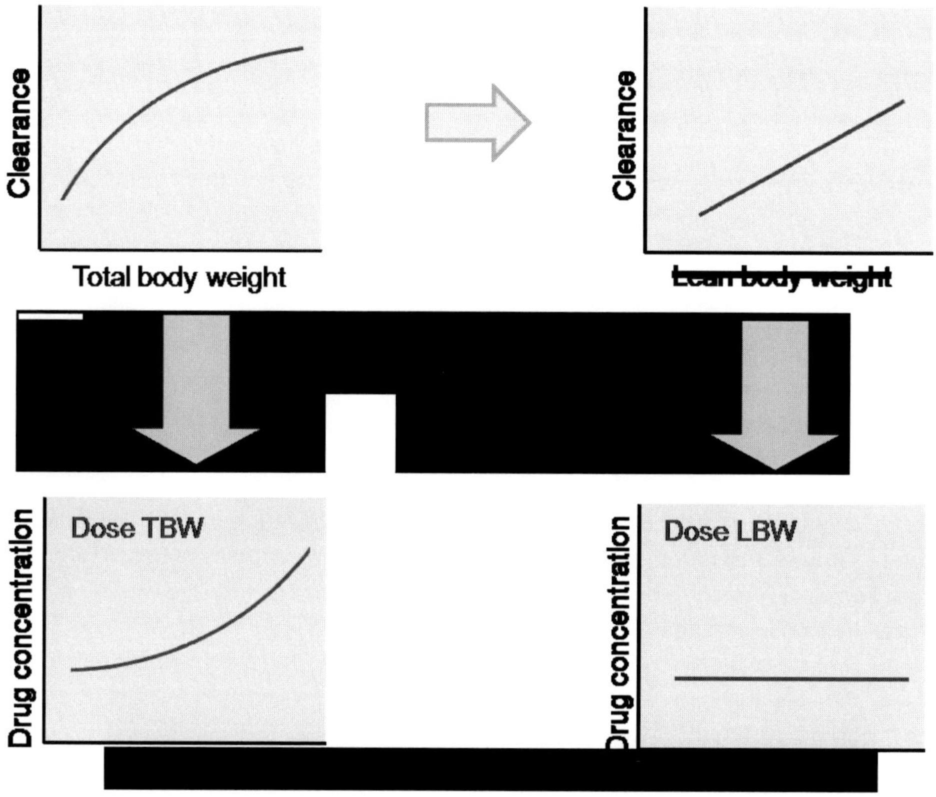

Figure 5. Pictorial representation of the effect on drug concentrations when TBW and LBW are used as dosing descriptors. Dosing based on TBW (left hand boxes) will result in higher concentrations in the obese compared to normal weighted subjects, but concentrations will remain constant over all weight ranges when dosing is based on LBW (right hand boxes).

However, for enoxaparin little information is known about this relationship in obesity as obese patients were generally excluded from drug development studies and only limited post marketing data exists. Consequently, the ideal dosing regimens in this patient population were unknown and outcomes were not predictable.

Many physicians recognize that dosing enoxaparin based on TBW increases the risk of adverse events and often introduce an arbitrary dose adjustment that has never been formally evaluated. One method is to dose 'cap' at 100 mg, regardless of the patients TBW. This was recently identified [57] and data is reproduced in Figure 6. In this study, non-adherence to the drug label (defined as ± 5mg) occurred in 58% of patients, with physicians primarily choosing to 'under-dose'. In addition, 79% of subjects whose TBWs were greater than 80 kg were under-dosed with all patients having a TBW >100kg dosed at or less than 100mg.

Capping is likely to result in sub-therapeutic concentrations of enoxaparin as CL does increase with the patient's size. This is of concern given that sub-therapeutic anti-Xa concentrations have been associated with an increase in mortality [46].

Two studies specifically sought to address this practical quandary and develop dosing guidelines for the obese [58] and renally impaired [59] (the other determinant on the CL of enoxaparin).

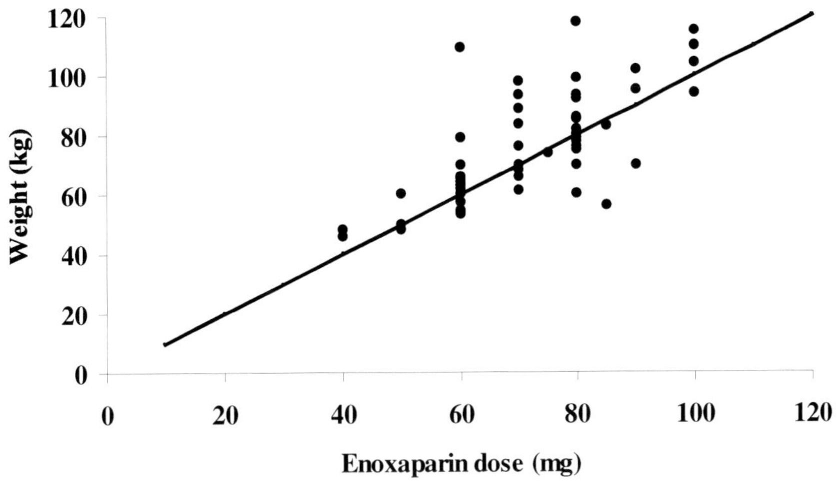

Figure 6. Plot of patient weight versus enoxaparin dose - line of identity is equal to a dose of 1mg/kg based on TBW, demonstrating the practice of "dose capping", (adapted from Barras [57]).

The dosing strategies developed from each study sought to increase the probability of achieving anti-Xa concentrations between 500-1000 International units (IU)/L (5-10 mg/L) which has been defined in the Thrombolysis in Myocardial Infarction (TIMI) 11A phase two study [60] as the range to maximize effectiveness and minimize bleeding events. The first study [58] demonstrated that enoxaparin dosing for patients with BMI values ranging from 15 to 45 kg/m^2, was best scaled by LBW. The second study [59], demonstrated that dosing was best scaled by CL_{CR}, using the C-G method, with 70% of the drug cleared renally and 30% metabolized as a function of LBW. As supported from the hypotheses described above, these studies showed that enoxaparin CL does not increase linearly with increasing TBW but increases linearly with LBW and CL_{CR}. Dose adjustments are therefore required in patients who are obese and unfortunately the current product label [18] does not have the flexibility to account for patients with obesity or renal impairment. The PK modeling used in this study also revealed that the best weight descriptor to use in the C-G formula (to determine CL_{CR}) was IBW and not TBW. More recent data suggests LBW should be used (section 4) [40].

A recent prospective study [57] evaluated the proposed individualized dosing guidelines and demonstrated that subjects who were dose individualized had fewer adverse events, with no apparent loss in effectiveness. In the study, individualized enoxaparin dosing based on LBW and CL_{CR} was compared to conventional dosing (product label). Patients in the individualized arm were initially dosed according to weight: non-obese TBW; obese using LBW. Doses were adjusted at 48 hours according to renal function. Patients in the conventional arm received enoxaparin according to current practice, as dictated by the prescriber. Dose individualized patients had fewer bleeding events (primary endpoint), (relative risk (RR) = 0.12, 95% CI = 0.01-0.89, P = 0.03) and composite bleeding and bruising events (secondary endpoint), (RR = 0.30, 95% CI = 0.12-0.71, P = 0.003) than those who received conventional dosing. In both arms of the study there were no recurrent thromboembolic events during treatment and no deaths had occurred at 30 days. Therefore there is now conclusive proof that dose individualization of enoxaparin in the obese populations will improve patient outcomes.

Other Drugs Used in Cardiology?

There are many other drugs used in cardiology that are currently dosed on TBW and have the potential to result in excessive drug exposure in the obese. Bivalirudin [20] has an approved drug label of 0.75 mg/kg (TBW) loading dose followed by a maintenance infusion also calculated using TBW. Eptifibatide [61], abciximab [21] and tirofiban [22] are other examples of drugs used in interventional cardiology that are dosed using TBW. UFH is often prescribed using an initial bolus (units/kg [TBW]) followed by a continuous infusion rate (units/kg/hour [TBW]) and subsequently adjusted on aPTT. Although nomograms have simplified UFH dose calculations, controversy exists as to which body size descriptor to use in obese patients. With the exception of case reports and retrospective studies that included small numbers of obese patients, there are few recommendations on how best use UFH to treat thromboembolic disorders such as ACS in the obese patient population [62]. Like enoxaparin, clinicians recognize the risk of excessive exposure and a dose cap is often implemented in dosing nomograms [19].

There are also drugs with a dichotomized dose structure based on TBW, for example carvedilol, a beta-receptor adrenergic blocking drug, used in the treatment of congestive heart failure (CHF) [63]. The dose-titration recommendation for carvedilol in the treatment of mild to moderate symptomatic CHF is to a maximum daily dose of 25mg twice daily in patients with a TBW < 85kg and 50mg twice daily for patients weighing ≥ 85kg. Consequently a patient weighing 85kg would receive twice the dose of a patient weighing 84 kg. Dichotomized dose strategies are simply another form of dose capping.

Other drugs that use wide dosing intervals based on TBW include fondaparinux, a pentasaccharide anti-thrombin used in the treatment of acute thromboembolic diseases [64]. The dose recommendation is this case is 2.5mg, subcutaneously, once daily for subjects with a TBW < 50kg, 5mg for patients ≥ 50kg and ≤ 100kg, and 10mg for patients > 100kg. Tenecteplase, a thrombolytic, also has a dose titration based on TBW. Sensibly, this dose increases with TBW between the weights of 60kg and 90kg (5mg per each 10kg increase in TBW); however there is a dose cap at 90kg.

In summary, many drugs used in the field of cardiology have dose strategies based on TBW without reference to obese patients in the product information; therefore clinicians will often be uncertain on how best to dose obese patients. Dose capping provides a "head in the sand" option for dosing obese patients and may restrict a subject from receiving the most effective dose. Dosing using LBW provides a superior alternative.

8. Future Research

With new evidence available to quantify and predict optimal drug doses in the obese using an appropriate metric such as LBW, future PK research for all drugs should focus on accurately describing the relationship between CL and LBW. The deficiencies of current study methods have been summarized in section 5, and we suggest a number of strategies when considering future research to accurately predict drug exposure in the obese population. Firstly, the appropriate recruitment of obese patients, in particular those with characteristics representative of the population in which the drug will be used; secondly, analyzing data using appropriate methods such as population PK modeling that will help accurately to quantify the CL-LBW relationship. Designing clinical trials that stratify across a range of TBWs can significantly improve the probability of finding this relationship [41]. Finally, future analyses in the obese population should avoid using body size descriptors such as IBW or BMI that do not accurately describe body composition and have no meaningful link to drug dosing in the clinical setting. If CL is expressed as a function of LBW, accurate quantification of CL across a broad range of body compositions will be possible.

9. Conclusion

In addition to renal function, TBW is the demographic variable that is often used to dose a medication. However, selecting a maintenance dose that is scaled according to TBW is unlikely to result in comparable exposures across the spectrum of body compositions. Identifying the optimal dose to use in obese patients is difficult and, in many cases, ill defined. Generally, drug dosing recommendations for many drugs are based on results from clinical trials where the obese subjects have been under-represented, or study design has been poor and the influence of obesity on the drug's PK not well defined. This results in the extrapolation of dosing recommendations from normal weighted subjects or arbitrary dose estimation. Drug dosing that is inappropriate for the patient's body composition may increase the risk of adverse events or alternatively reduce clinical effectiveness. In this chapter we have introduced the reader to new evidence that suggests that body composition should be measured as a function of LBW rather than TBW. We contend that using TBW to calculate maintenance doses for obese patients is scientifically unsound and that LBW takes into account changes in body composition that occur with obesity. Using LBW in dose calculations will help optimize pharmacological therapy in these patients.

References

[1] World Health Organisation. Obesity and overweight. What are overweight and obesity? [online]. 2007 [cited 2008 July 3]. Available from: http://www.who.int/topics/obesity/en/

[2] National Institutes of Health. Statistics related to overweight and obesity [online]. 2006 [cited 2008 6 July]. Available from: http://www.win.niddk.nih.gov/statistics/

[3] Centers for Disease Control and Prevention. Overweight and Obesity. [online]. [cited June 10, 2008]. Available from: http://www.cdc.gov/nccdphp/dnpa/obesity/

[4] Department of Health. Obesity [online]. 2007 [cited 2008 July 22]. Available from: http://www.dh.gov.uk/en/Publichealth/Healthimprovement/Obesity/index.htm

[5] Department of Health. Foresight - Tackling Obesities - Future Choices Project [online]. [cited July 22, 2008]. Available from: http://www.foresight.gov.uk/index.asp

[6] National Heart Foundation of Australia. Overweight and Obesity. Useful statistics and references-July 2007 [online]. 2007 [cited 2008 June 15]. Available from: http://www.heartfoundation.org.au/document/NHF/OWOB_StatsRefs_July2007.pdf

[7] National Heart Forum [online]. 2008 [cited July 23, 2008]. Available from: http://www.heartforum.org.uk/

[8] Hedley, A; Ogden, C; Johnson, C; Carroll, M; Curtain, L; Flegal, K. Prevalence of overweight and obesity among US children, adolescents, and adults, 1999-2002. *JAMA*. 2004; 291: 2847-50.

[9] Eckel, R; York, D; Rössner, S; Caterson, I; St. Jeor, S; Hayman, S, *et al.* Obesity, a Worldwide Epidemic Related to Heart Disease and Stroke: Executive Summary. *Circulation.* 2004; 110: 2968-75.

[10] Wannamethee, S; Shaper, A. Weight change and duration of overweight and obesity in the incidence of type 2 diabetes. *Diabetes Care.* 1999; 22: 1266-72.

[11] Haslam, D; James, W. Obesity. *Lancet*. 2005; 366: 1197-209.

[12] Kenchaiah, S; Evans, J; Levy, D; Wilson, P; Benjamin, E; Larson, M. Obesity and the risk of heart failure. *N. Engl. J. Med.* 2002; 347: 305-13.

[13] Poirier, P; Giles, T; Bray, G; Hong, Y; Stern, J; Pi-Sunyer, X, *et al.* Obesity and cardiovascular disease: Pathophysiology, Evaluation, and Effect of Weight Loss. *Circulation.* 2006; 113: 898-918.

[14] Yusuf, S; Hawken, S; Ounpuu, S. Effect of potentially modifiable risk factors associated with myocardial infarction in 52 countries (the INTERACT study): case-control study. *Lancet*. 2004; 364: 937-52.

[15] Yan, L; Daviglus, M; Liu, K; Stamler, J; Wang, R; Pirzada, A, *et al.* Midlife body mass index and hospitalization and mortality in older age. *JAMA*. 2006; 295: 190-8.

[16] Peeters, A; Barendregt, J; Willekens, F; Mackenbach, J; Al Mamun, A; Bonneux, L. Obesity in adulthood and its consequences for life expectancy: a life-table analysis. *Ann. Intern. Med.* 2003; 138: 24-32.

[17] Gibbs, H; Broom, J; Brown, J; Laws, R; Reckless, J; Noble, P, *et al.* The impact of obesity on drug prescribing in primary care. *Brit. J. Gen. Pract.* 2005; 55: 743-9.

[18] Clexane® Product Information [online]. 2007 [cited 2007 April 6]. Available from: http://www.sanofi-aventis.com.au/products/aus_pi_clexane.pdf

[19] Hirsh, J; Raschke, R. Heparin and low-molecular-weight heparin: the seventh ACCP conference on antithrombotic and thrombolytic therapy. *Chest.* 2004; 126: 188-204.

[20] Angiomax® product information [online]. 2007 [cited 2008 August 11]. Available from: http://secure.healthlinks.net.au/content/csl/pi.cfm?product=cspangio10106

[21] Reopro® Product Information [online]. 2008 [cited 2008 Sept 19]. Available from: http://www.reopro.com/about_reopro/product_information.jsp

[22] Aggrastat® Product Information [online]. 2006 [cited 2008 Sept 20]. Available from: http://www.aggrastat.com.sa/secure/resources/pi/pi.html

[23] Holford, N. Target concentration intervention: beyond Y2K. *Br J Clin Pharmacol.* 1999; 48: 9-13.

[24] Matthews, I; Kirkpatrick, C; Holford, N. Quantification justification for target concentration intervention - parameter variability and predictive performance using population pharmacokinetic models for aminoglycosides. *Br. J. Clin. Pharmacol.* 2004; 58 (1): 8-19.

[25] Evans, W; Relling, M; Rodman, J; Crom, W; Boyett, J; Pui, C. Conventional compared with individualized chemotherapy for childhood acute lymphoblastic leukemia. *New Engl. J. Med.* 1998; 338: 499-505.

[26] Cheymol, G. Effects of obesity on pharmacokinetics. Implications for drug therapy. *Clin. Pharmacokinet.* 2000; 39 (3): 215-31.

[27] Green, B; Duffull, S. What is the best size descriptor to use for pharmacokinetic studies in the obese? *Br. J. Clin. Pharmacol.* 2004; 58 (2): 119-33.

[28] Blouin, R; Warren, G. Pharmacokinetic considerations on obesity. *J. Pharm. Sciences.* 1999; 88: 1-7.

[29] Abernethy, D; Greenblatt, D. Drug disposition in obese humans. An update. *Clin Phamacokin.* 1986; 11: 199-213.

[30] Han, P; Duffull, S; Kirkpatrick, CMJ; Green, B. Dosing in obesity: A simple solution to a big problem. *Clin. Phamacol. Ther.* 2007; 82 (5): 505-8.

[31] Mayes, J; Watson, G. Direct effects of sex steroid hormones on adipose tissues and obesity. *Obesity Reviews.* 2004; 5: 197-216.

[32] Janmahasatian, S; Duffull, SB; Ash, S; Ward, LC; Byrne, NM; Green, B. Quantification of lean bodyweight. *Clin. Pharmacokinet.* 2005; 44 (10): 1051-65.

[33] Devine, B. Case study number 25 gentamicin therapy. Drug Intelligence and Clinical Pharmacy (cont'd as DICP- The Annals of Pharmacotherapy). 1974; 8: 650-5.

[34] Robinson, J; Lupkiewicz, S; Palenik, L. Determination of ideal body weight for drug dosage calculations. *Am. J. Hosp. Pharm.* 1983; 40: 1016-9.

[35] Du Bois, D; Du Bois, E. Clinical calorimetry. Tenth paper. A formula to estimate the approximate surface area if height and weight be known. *Arch. Intern. Med.* 1916; 17: 863.

[36] Mosteller, R. Simplified calculation of body surfaced area. *N. Engl. J. Med.* 1987; 317: 1098.

[37] Duffull, SB; Dooley, MJ; Green, B; Poole, SG; Kirkpatrick, CMJ. A standard weight descriptor for dose adjustment in the obese patient. *Clin. Pharmacokinet.* 2004; 43 (15): 1167-78.

[38] James, W. *Research on obesity*. London: Her Majesty's Stationary Office; 1976.

[39] Cockroft, DW; Gault, H. Prediction of creatinine clearance from serum creatinine. *Nephron.* 1976; 16: 31-41.

[40] Janmahasatian, S; Duffull, S; Chagnac, A; Kirkpatrick, C; Green, B. Lean body mass normalizes the effect of obesity on renal function. *Br. J. Clin. Pharmacol.* 2008; 65: 964-5

[41] Han, P; Kirkpatrick, C; Green, B. Informative study designs to identify true parameter-covariate relationships. PAGE (2008) Abstr 1253 [wwwpage-meetingorg/?abstract=1253]; Marseille

[42] Aarons, L. Population pharmacokinetics: theory and practice. *Br J Clin Pharmacol.* 1991; 32: 669-70.

[43] Holford, N; Sheiner, L. Understanding the dose-effect relationship: Clinical application of pharmacokinetic-pharacodynamic models. *Clin. Pharmacokinet.* 1981; 6: 429-53.

[44] Bonate, P. *Pharmacokinetic-pharmacodynamic modeling and simulation*. New York: Springer Science+Business Media; 2006.

[45] Ettte, E; Williams, P. Pharmacometrics. *The science of quantitative pharmacology*. Hoboken: John Wiley and Sons; 2007.

[46] Montalescot, G; Collet, J; Tanguy, ML; Ankri, A; Payot, L; Dumaine, R, *et al*. Anti-Xa activity relates to survival and efficacy in unselected acute coronary syndrome patients treated with enoxaparin. *Circulation*. 2004; 110 (4): 392-8.

[47] Cohen, M; Demers, C; Gurfinkel, E; Turpie, A; Fromell, G; Goodman, S, *et al*. A comparison of low molecular weight heparin with unfractionated heparin for unstable coronary artery disease. *New Engl. J. Med.* 1997; 337: 447-52.

[48] Antman, EM; McCabe, C; Gurfinkel, E; Turpie, A; Alexander, G; Bernink, P, *et al*. Enoxaparin prevents death and cardiac ischaemic events in unstable angina/non-Q-wave myocardial infarction. Results of the thrombolysis in myocardial infarction (TIMI) 11B trial. *Circulation*. 1999; 100: 1593-601.

[49] Antman, E; Morrow, D; McCabe, C; Murphy, S; Ruda, M; Sadowski, Z, *et al*. Enoxaparin versus unfractionated heparin with fibrinolysis for ST-Elevation Myocardial Infarction. *New. Engl. J. Med.* 2006; 354: 1477-88.

[50] The SYNERGY Trial Investigators. Enoxaparin vs unfractionated heparin in high-risk patients with non-ST-segment elevation acute coronary syndromes managed with an intended early invasive strategy. *JAMA*. 2004; 292 (1): 45-54.

[51] Merli, G; Spiro, T; Olsson, C; Abildgaard, U; Davidson, B; Eldor, A, *et al*. Subcutaneous enoxaparin once or twice daily compared with intravenous heparin for the treatment of venous thromboembolic disease. *Ann. Intern. Med.* 2001; 134: 191-202.

[52] Quinlan, DJ; McQuillan, A; Eikelboom, JW. Low-molecular-weight-heparin compared with intravenous heparin for treatment of pulmonary embolism. *Ann. Intern. Med.* 2004; 140 (3): 175-83.

[53] Aroney, CN; Aylward, P; Kelly, A-M; Chew, DP; Clune, E. Guidelines for the management of acute coronary syndromes 2006. *MJA*. 2006; 184 (Suppl) (8): S1-S32.

[54] Snow, V; Qaseem, A; Barry, P; Hornbake, ER; Rodnick, JE; Tobolic, T, *et al*. Management of venous thromboembolism: a clinical practice guideline from the American College of Physicians and the Academy of Family Physicians. *Ann. Intern. Med.* 2007; 146: 204-10.

[55] Product Information Clexane® [online]. 2006 [cited 2007 April 6]. Available from: http://www.sanofi-aventis.co.uk/prodcuts/Clexane_spc.pdf

[56] Lovenox® Prescribing Information [online]. 2006 [cited 2007 April 6]. Available from: http://www.sanofi-aventis.us/

[57] Barras, M; Duffull, S; Atherton, J; Green, B. Individualized compared to conventional dosing of enoxaparin. *Clin. Pharmacol. Ther.* 2008; 83 (6): 882-8.

[58] Green, B; Duffull, SB. Development of a dosing strategy for enoxaparin in obese patients. *Br. J. Clin. Pharmacol.* 2002; 54: 96-103.

[59] Green, B; Greenwood, M; Saltissi, D; Westhuyzen, J; Kluver, L; Rowell, J, *et al*. Dosing strategy for enoxaparin in patients with renal impairment presenting with acute coronary syndromes. *Br. J. Clin. Pharmacol.* 2004; 59 (3): 281-90.

[60] Antman, E. Dose-ranging trial of enoxaparin for unstable angina; results of TIMI 11A. *Journal of The American College of Cardiology*. 1997; 29 (7): 1474-82.

[61] Integrilin® Product Information [online]. 2007 [cited 2008 Sept 20]. Available from: http://www.integrilin.com/full_prescribing_information.html

[62] Schwiesow, S; Wessell, A; Steyer, T. Use of a modified dosing weight for heparin therapy in a morbidly obese patient. *Ann. Pharmacother.* 2005; 39: 753-6.

[63] Dilatrend® product information. [online]. [cited August 11, 2008]. Available from: http://www.roche-australia.com/downloads/dilatrend-pi.cfm?action=get

[64] Arixtra® product information [online]. 2006 [cited 2008 August 11]. Available from: http://www.gsk.com.au/products_prescription-medicined_detail.aspx?view=65

[65] Green, B; Duffull, SB. Caution when lean body weight is used as a size descriptor for obese subjects. *Clin. Phamacol. Ther.* 2002; 12: 743-4.

[66] Garrow, J; Webster, J. Quetelet's index (W/H^2) as a measure of fatness. *Int. J. Obes.* 1985; 9: 147-53.

In: Heart Disease in Men
Editors: A.B. Todd and M.H. Mosley, pp. 243-258
ISBN: 978-1-60692-297-2

Chapter 11

DIAGNOSTIC CLUES OF ETIOLOGICAL INVESTIGATIONS FOR CARDIOMYOPATHY

Yasuharu Tokuda*
Center for Clinical Epidemiology, St Luke's Life Science Institute, St Luke's International Hospital, 10-1 Akashi-cho, Chuo City, Tokyo 104-8560 Japan

Abstract

Cardiomyopathy is a disease of the myocardium that leads to impaired cardiac function and its common anatomical classifications include dilated, hypertrophic and restrictive cardiomyopathies. Many causes can precipitate a cardiomyopathy and the cause should be identified whenever possible since specific treatment, if available, can significantly improve the prognosis. In this chapter, we present the diagnostic clues and pitfalls for etiological investigations in patients with cardiomyopathy. The two major categories of the differential diagnosis are primary (idiopathic, familial and endomyocardial disease) and secondary myocardial involvement. Secondary causes include ischemic, valvular, hypertensive, infectious, inflammatory, metabolic, genetic, nutritional, toxic and peripartum cardiomyopathies. In this chapter, we focus on the non-cardiovascular causes of cardiomyopathy, i.e., etiologies other than ischemic, valvular, hypertensive, primary myocardial diseases, since physicians caring for patients with cardiomyopathy, mostly cardiologists, may find it difficult to determine these non-cardiovascular causes as part of the etiological diagnosis for cardiomyopathy. Since clinical examinations are simple and less expensive, but still can reveal many important clues for the crucial diagnosis, it is important to pay careful attention not only to laboratory, electrophysiological and imaging studies, but also to clinical examinations, such as history and physical examinations.

Clinical Classification of Cardiomyopathies

The cardiomyopathies are classified into one of three types on the basis of differences in their pathophysiology and clinical presentation, including dilated, restrictive, hypertrophic type [1].

* E-mail address: tokuyasu@orange.ocn.ne.jp. TEL& FAX 03-5550-2426

1) **Dilated cardiomyopathy (DCM):** This is characterized by left and/or right ventricular enlargement, impaired systolic function, congestive heart failure (CHF), various arrhythmias and embolic complications from ventricular thrombi.

2) **Hypertrophic cardiomyopathy (HCM):** Disproportionate left ventricular hypertrophy, also known as asymmetric septal hypertrophy (ASH), is the hallmark of HCM and typically involves the septum more than the free wall, usually of a non-dilated left ventricular cavity. Systolic anterior motion (SAM) of the mitral valve may be observed.

3) **Restrictive cardiomyopathy (RCM):** Endomyocardial scarring or myocardial infiltration, the main features of RCM, can result in restriction to left and/or right ventricular filling with diastolic dysfunction.

The cardiomyopathies are classified on an etiologic basis into two fundamental forms [2]: 1) a primary myocardial involvement, consisting of heart muscle disease of unknown cause; and 2) a secondary myocardial involvement, consisting of myocardial disease of known cause or associated with a disease involving other organ systems (Table). In the etiologic investigation of secondary cardiomyopathies, transvenous endomyocardial biopsy may be helpful but not always diagnostic. On the other hand, clinical examinations, such as history and physical examinations, are simple and less expensive but still can reveal many important clues for the crucial diagnosis. Thus, it is important to pay careful attention not only to laboratory studies, but also to clinical examinations.

Since we focus on the non-cardiovascular causes of a cardiomyopathy in this chapter, diseases of primary myocardial involvement (i.e., idiopathic, familial, endomyocardial fibrosis and eosinophilic endomyocardial disease) are not described here. Congenital myocardial involvement with infantile onset (e.g., mucopolysaccharidosis) is also not covered here. Thus, in this chapter, we review the diagnostic clues of the clinically important secondary causes (secondary myocardial involvement) of adult-onset cardiomyopathies.

Table. Etiologic Classification of Cardiomyopathies

PRIMARY MYOCARDIAL INVOLVEMENT
Idiopathic
Familial
Endomyocardial fibrosis
Eosinophilic endomyocardial disease
SECONDARY MYOCARDIAL INVOLVEMENT
Infective
Viral myocarditis
Bacterial myocarditis
Fungal myocarditis
Parasitic myocarditis
Spirochetal
Metabolic
Diabetic cardiomyopathy
Obesity-induced cardiomyopathy

Table. Continued

Familial storage diseases
Glycogen storage disease
Hereditary hemochromatosis
Fabry's disease
Nutritional Deficiency
Malnutrition heart disease
Thiamine deficiency
Connective tissue diseases
Systemic lupus erythematosus
Infiltrations and granulomas
Amyloidosis
Sarcoidosis
Neuromuscular diseases
Muscular dystrophy
Myotonic dystrophy
Friedreich's ataxia
Sensitivity and toxic reactions
Alcohol
Radiation
Drugs
Peripartum heart disease

*Modified from TABLE 221-1, Harrison's Principles of Internal Medicine [2]
This list is not comprehensive and includes only important causes.

Viral Myocarditis

Animal experiments suggest the pathogenesis of cardiomyopathy after viral myocarditis, particularly DCM-type cardiomyopathy [3]. Among infectious agents that can cause clinically significant acute myocarditis, viruses, especially Enteroviruses (e.g., Coxsackievirus B) and Adenoviruses, are the most common agents. Enteroviruses are considered the most prevalent, but Adenoviruses may be more prevalent in other series [4]. Although viral myocarditis is often self-limited and results in recovery without sequelae, some patients may progress to a chronic state of dilated cardiomyopathy. On the other hand, patients with fulminant viral myocarditis may require temporary mechanical cardiopulmonary support, but many of the survivors may exhibit good recovery of ventricular function.

The clinical manifestations range from an asymptomatic state, with the presence of transient electrocardiographic (ECG) ST-T-wave abnormalities and elevated serum levels of myocardial enzymes, to a fulminant condition, with various arrhythmias, CHF and death. In some patients, myocarditis mimics acute myocardial infarction, since they may present with chest pain, ECG changes and elevated serum levels of myocardial enzymes.

Patients with acute stage viral myocarditis often present with a history of a preceding upper respiratory tract infection or a flu-like syndrome. But myocarditis may occur up to several weeks after the acute viral infection. On physical examination, viral pharyngitis or tonsillitis may be evident clinically. Severe cases may show a muffled first heart sound, audible third heart sound and a murmur of mitral regurgitation. In patients with associated pericarditis, a pericardial friction rub may be audible.

Although testing for specific antibody titers is helpful in some cases, there are a number of viruses that can potentially cause myocarditis and testing for all classes of viruses is generally not feasible and thus it may not determine the specific classes of viruses in many cases. Some advocate viral isolation from pharyngeal swabs, stool, or other body fluids, but still the specific virus cannot be determined in a significant number of cases. Furthermore, there are no specific treatment modalities available for most viruses except for influenza viruses, Herpesviruses groups (herpes simplex, herpes zoster, Epstein-Barr virus and cytomegalovirus), human immunodeficiency virus (HIV) and hepatitis B (HBV) and C (HCV) virus. Therefore, it is advisable to not miss those cases that are infected with treatable viral agents. Endomyocardial biopsy, if conducted early in the course, may show lymphocyte infiltration and adjacent myocardial necrosis. There may be characteristic findings, such as inclusion bodies in giant cells, in patients infected with herpes virus groups. Polymerase chain reaction (PCR) used in conjunction with endomyocardial biopsy may enhance the likelihood of detecting viral genome in the myocardium of patients with clinical evidence of myocarditis [4].

HIV: HIV myocarditis is the most common cardiac complication in patients with HIV infection [5]. Subclinical cardiac involvement, including pericardial effusion, right ventricular dilatation and neoplastic infiltration, is frequently reported. Overt cardiac manifestation is reported in about 10% of HIV patients, but its diagnosis is occasionally missed, because of low clinical suspicion early in the illness. In patients with clinical AIDS, however, opportunistic infections may involve the myocardium, such as toxoplasmosis, as well as cardiac metastases of Kaposi's sarcoma.

HCV: A multi-center study of Japanese patients found that HCV antibody was present in about 10% of patients with hypertrophic cardiomyopathy and suggested that HCV infection may be a cause of hypertrophic cardiomyopathy [6]. The HCV-core protein may play an important role in the development of cardiomyopathy. Thus, HCV serology testing should be performed in patients with hypertrophic cardiomyopathy.

Bacterial Myocarditis

Infective endocarditis may lead to bacterial myocarditis with an involvement of abscess formation in valvular rings and the interventricular septum. In rare cases, septic patients may develop bacterial myocarditis, probably due to metastatic infection to the heart from bacteremia. For instance, myocarditis is being recognized as a rare consequence of Campylobacter infection [7].

Diphtheria: Patients with diphtheria (*Corynebacterium diphtheriae* infection) may develop myocarditis, which is a serious and potentially fatal complication [8]. Diphtheria toxin is a potent inhibitor of cellular protein synthesis and cause cardiac damage, leading to dilated cardiomyopathy along with conduction disturbances. Diphtheria should be considered in patients with fever, systemic toxicity, cervical lymphadenopathy, pharyngitis with white-grayish coalescent pseudomembranes, bloody discharge with scraping and palatal paralysis. Since rapidly-progressive CHF may occur after the first week of the illness and antitoxin therapy can be effective for the treatment, prompt diagnosis is crucial and can be achieved with culture of *C. diphtheriae* or positive toxin-production assay.

Fungal Myocarditis

Cardiac fungal infection is relatively uncommon, but its incidence is reported to be on the increase, especially fungal myocarditis [9]. Since fungal myocarditis is diagnosed infrequently before death, knowledge of the disease is largely derived from postmortem examinations. Cardiac surgery, malignancy, hematological disorders and excessive use of antibiotics and/or corticosteroids, are major underlying conditions. The most common organism causing fungal myocarditis is Candida, with Aspergillus and Mucor identified occasionally. Fungal myocarditis is commonly associated with multiple organ infections and exclusive cardiac involvement has been observed in only 10% of cases. As hematogenous spread is the main route to reach the heart, the presence of a systemic fungal infection should indicate the possibility of fungal myocarditis [9].

Parasitic Myocarditis

Chagas' disease: Among parasitic infections associated with myocarditis, Chagas' disease is the most important, particularly in many South American countries and it is due to infection of the protozoa, *Trypanosoma cruzi*. Indeed, Chagas' myocarditis is the most common form of cardiomyopathy in Latin-American countries. Chagas' disease consists of acute and chronic phases. In the acute phase, following an incubation period of 7 to 10 days after contact with the infected vector (triatomine insect or kissing bug), local skin swelling produces the typical portal of entry lesions known as chagomas. If the portal of entry of the vector's feces is the conjunctiva, unilateral periorbital edema with swelling of the eyelid is recognized (Romana's sign). Infection can also occur through blood transfusion and vertical transmission. The features of the acute phase include fever, myalgia, sweating, hepatosplenomegaly and signs of cardiac failure secondary to myocarditis, and, less frequently, meningoencephalitis. In the chronic phase, the pathophysiology is related to megaesophagus, megacolon and cardiac disease. Megaesophagus causes dysphagia and odynophagia, while megacolon typically causes constipation. Heart failure (particularly, right-side failure), arrhythmia and systemic/pulmonary thromboembolism from biventricular mural thrombi characterize chronic Chagas' heart disease. Echocardiography is useful to characterise and determine the prognosis of patients with chronic Chagas disease [10].

Trichinellosis: Trichinellosis is caused by the nematode, Trichinella and has been reported worldwide [11]. Human infections are acquired by eating meat containing cysts of Trichinella, including pig, walrus, bear, cougar, boar, cattle and horse [12]. Consumption of undercooked bear meat in wild game settings has emerged in recent years as a predominant source for Trichinellosis in US [13]. The incubation period is seven to 30 days but varies with the infectious dose, the host's immune status and the species of Trichinella involved [14]. Shorter incubation periods are generally related to a more severe disease.

First, during the intestinal stage about the 2-7th days after ingestion, larvae mature into adult worms, which burrow into the intestinal mucosa but patients may be asymptomatic or may be accompanied by abdominal pain, nausea/vomiting and diarrhea [14]. Second, during the muscle stage after the first week, adult-derived larvae in the intestines enter the bloodstream, disseminate hematogenously and enter the skeletal muscle, forming cysts within a host-derived cell (nurse cell). Various symptoms at this stage include high fever, subungual splinter hemorrhage, conjunctival hemorrhages and periorbital edema (chemosis), disturbed vision and ocular pain. Skeletal Myositis causes muscle pain, tenderness, swelling and weakness [14].

In serious infections, there may be cardiac (myocarditis), pulmonary (eosinophilic bronchitis, pneumonia and respiratory myositis), or central nervous system involvement (meningitis and encephalitis). In particular, cardiac complications are the most frequent cause of death in severe trichinellosis [15]. Although larvae do not encyst in cardiac muscle, larvae elicit an eosinophil-induced inflammatory myocarditis with occasional life-threatening arrhythmias [15]. Laboratory findings include eosinophilia and elevated serum muscle enzymes. The diagnosis of trichinellosis should be considered in cases of periorbital edema, myositis and eosinophilia in patients with a history of ingesting either inadequately cooked meat, particularly pork.

Spirochetal Myocarditis

Lyme disease: Lyme disease is a tick-borne spirochetal disease and is most common in the Northeast, upper Midwest and Pacific Coastal regions of the US during the summer. About 10% of patients develop cardiac involvement during the acute phase [16]. Conduction abnormalities (2nd- or 3rd-degree AV block) are the most common manifestations and may lead to syncope. Concomitant myocarditis can cause mild asymptomatic left ventricular dysfunction. However, chronic cardiac Lyme disease is uncommon [16].

Risk factors or possible evidence of *Borrelia burgdorferi* infection can be an indicator for the diagnosis and these include exposure (residence in or travel through an endemic area); tick bites; prior or current erythematous skin lesions (erythema migrans); coexistence of arthritis and neurologic diseases (meningoencephalitis, facial nerve palsy, or radiculoneuritis) compatible with Lyme disease. However, in some cases, heart block is the first and only manifestation of Lyme disease [17].

Cardiovascular syphilis: Late syphilis includes cardiovascular syphilis, gummas (skin and bone) and central nervous system syphilis (neurosyphilis) and can arise as early as one year after initial infection or up to 25 to 30 years later. Cardiovascular syphilis classically involves the ascending aorta resulting in aneurysm (calcified arch) and aortic regurgitation. The onset is typically insidious and clinical manifestations typically occur 15 to 30 years from initial infection in the untreated patients. Syphilitic aneurysms rarely lead to dissection. Syphilis may also involve the coronary arteries, resulting in coronary artery narrowing and thrombosis with myocardial infarction [18]. Serologic testing for syphilis is mandatory for patients with ascending aortic aneurysm.

Diabetic Cardiomyopathy

Patients with diabetes mellitus may develop myocardial dysfunction, independent of recognized causes, such as coronary artery disease and hypertension [19]. Diabetic cardiomyopathy contributes to excessive cardiovascular morbidity and mortality in patients with diabetes. The histological features include interstitial fibrosis with increased amounts of collagen, glycoprotein and lipids in the interstitial tissues of myocardium. In some patients, insulin therapy ameliorates myocardial dysfunction. Left ventricular dysfunction due to diabetic cardiomyopathy is manifested by systolic and/or diastolic dysfunction and some develop restrictive clinical cardiomyopathy. Multiple factors may contribute to ventricular dysfunction in such patients and these include autonomic neuropathy, microvascular dysfunction, impaired insulin responsiveness, calcium mishandling, upregulation of the renin-angiotensin system, increased reactive oxygen species and mitochondrial dysfunctions [20].

Obesity-induced Cardiomyopathy

Patients with morbid obesity may have cardiovascular system disturbances characterized by increases in total circulatory volume, cardiac output and left ventricular filling pressure [21]. The high cardiac output is likely to reflect a need for supporting the increased metabolic needs of the excessive adipose tissue. As a result of chronic volume overload, cardiac hypertrophy with ventricular dilatation, abnormal ventricular function, high-output heart failure and finally low-output heart failure may develop. The pathological findings are generalized cardiac dilatation with left ventricular hypertrophy in most patients and biventricular hypertrophy in some patients and are also involved with fatty infiltration of the myocardium [22]. Physical examination to evaluate cardiac failure in massively obese patients is sometimes difficult. Weight reduction is the therapy of choice, but rapid reduction may be dangerous since some develop cardiac arrhythmias and sudden death due to electrolyte imbalance.

Glycogen-storage Disease

Cardiomyopathy of glycogen storage disease is usually seen in infants or children. Glycogen storage disease II (Pompe disease), IV (Anderson disease) and VII (Tarui disease) can be a cause of child-onset cardiomyopathy associated with skeletal muscle and neurological diseases. However, some patients with glycogen storage disease may develop cardiomyopathy in adulthood.

Danon disease: Glycogen storage disease IIB (Danon disease) is a semi-dominant X-linked disorder that is caused by lysosome-associated membrane protein 2 (LAMP2) mutation and is characterized by cardiomyopathy, skeletal myopathy and variable mental retardation. This type of glycogen-storage cardiomyopathy leads to hypertrophic cardiomyopathy characterized by electrophysiological abnormalities, particularly ventricular preexcitation. Clinical features associated with defects in LAMP2 also include male gender, severe hypertrophy, early onset (at 8 to 17 years of age), ventricular preexcitation and asymptomatic elevations of two serum proteins [23].

Hereditary Hemochromatosis

The clinical manifestations of hereditary hemochromatosis are caused by systemic iron accumulation and include liver disease, skin hyperpigmentation, diabetes, arthropathy and impotence in males. In addition, hereditary hemochromatosis can cause excessive deposition of iron within the myocardium and lead to dilated cardiomyopathy characterized by heart failure and conduction disturbances, such as sick sinus syndrome [24]. Cardiac disease could be the presenting manifestation in some patients with hereditary hemochromatosis. To establish the diagnosis, in addition to serum iron studies (ferritin and transferrin saturation), various radiologic techniques, liver biopsy and/or HFE gene testing may be needed. Cardiac magnetic resonance imaging is characteristic for a very low signal intensity signal in the myocardium due to the effects of the iron deposits [25]. Treatment with phlebotomy or chelation therapy may reverse the left ventricular dysfunction.

Fabry's Disease

Fabry disease (angiokeratoma corporis diffusum or ceramide trihexosidosis) is an X-linked glycolipidosis caused by deficient activity of the lysosomal enzyme alpha-galactosidase A and tissue deposition of globotriaosylceramide [26]. Although Fabry disease was described as an X-linked recessive disorder, women with Fabry disease are increasingly recognized and it is now considered to exhibit an X-linked dominant transmission [27]. Clinical manifestations are evident by 10 years of age and typically include neuropathy and skin lesions. The neuropathy causes paroxysmal burning pains with hypohidrosis in the glove and stocking type distribution. Cutaneous angiokeratomas present as angioectatic papules that develop in the groin, hips and umbilical regions. Corneal dystrophy may also be identified. Renal involvement occurs in about 50 percent of patients and presents as progressive renal insufficiency with proteinuria. Polarized urine microscopy reveals oval fat bodies (tubular epithelial cells with lipid inclusions) with a lamellar structure and a Maltese cross pattern, while imaging studies may show multiple renal sinus cysts.

Cardiac involvement can lead to ventricular hypertrophy (HCM type), conduction defects, coronary artery disease, aortic and mitral valve regurgitation and aortic root dilation [28]. Echocardiography may show a characteristic binary appearance of the LV endocardial border. Since some mutations are associated with disease that is confined to the myocardium, there is a rationale for screening for Fabry disease by measurement of plasma alpha-galactosidase A in patients with unexplained concentric LVH [29]. Treatment with enzyme replacement therapy is available and has the potential to improve cardiac function.

Malnutrition Heart Disease

Severe protein-energy malnutrition is associated with one of two classical syndromes, marasmus (energy deficits) and kwashiorkor (protein deficits), or both [30]. Although profound states of malnutrition are most common in underdeveloped countries, significant nutritional heart disease may also occur in developed nations, particularly in patients with cancer or chronic debilitating diseases, in elderly bedridden patients with advanced dementia and in patients with advanced congestive cardiac failure (cardiac cachexia).

Common clinical findings include deficits in lean body mass and adipose tissue, low physical activity, mental apathy, anorexia and retarded psychomotor function. Additional physical findings in patients with marasmus include weak general appearance, hypothermia, atrophic, dry and redundant skin, and thin, sparse, easily plucked hair. Kwashiorkor is characterized by marked muscle atrophy with normal or increased body fat and physical examination findings include anasarca and pitting edema in the lower extremities and periorbital areas, dry, atrophic, peeling skin with confluent areas of hyperkeratosis and hyperpigmentation, dry and hypopigmented and easily plucked hair, hepatomegaly (from fatty liver), and distended abdomen with dilated intestinal loops and ascites. Subsequent protein intake restores hair color with resultant alternating loss of hair color interspersed between bands of normal pigmentation (flag sign).

These patients may develop a thin and flabby heart with myofibrillar atrophy and interstitial edema [31]. The systolic pressure, cardiac output and heart rate are low and the pulse pressure is minute. Generalized edema is common due to a combination of reduced plasma oncotic pressure (hypoalbuminemia) and myocardial dysfunction. These patients are more susceptible to infection, especially sepsis, pneumonia and enteritis. Clinical manifestations from deficiencies of electrolytes, vitamins and trace elements are also commonly recognized in these patients.

Thiamine Deficiency (beriberi heart)

Thiamine deficiency (beriberi or hypovitaminosis B1) may occur not only in people in the Far East (consumers of polished rice), alcoholics and food faddists, but also in a significant number of patients with chronic heart failure. Deficiency in such patients is likely to result from both reduced dietary intake and a diuretic-induced urinary excretion of thiamine [32]. Common clinical findings include generalized malnutrition, peripheral neuropathy, glossitis, unexplained lactic acidosis and anemia. The characteristic cardiovascular manifestation is high-output heart failure (wet beriberi), which is caused by the effects of vasomotor suppression and subsequent low systemic vascular resistance from deficiency in thiamine pyrophosphate coenzyme. The cardiac examination shows a wide pulse pressure, tachycardia and a third heart sound. The ECG may show low voltage, a prolonged QT interval and T-wave changes, while the chest x-ray generally shows a large heart with signs of congestive heart failure. Thiamine administration to these patients improves the left ventricular ejection fraction with the excretion of salt and water, often as quickly as within 12 to 48 hrs. However, delayed treatment may lead to eventual depression of myocardial function and the development of a low output state [33].

Systemic Lupus Erythematosus

Patients with systemic lupus erythematosus (SLE) frequently develop pericarditis with a benign course, although cardiac tamponade or constrictive pericarditis may rarely be recognised. In Libman-Sacks endocarditis, wart-like lesions are identified most often on the ventricular surface of the mitral valve, but hemodynamically important valvular regurgitation is rare. However, patients with antiphospholipid syndrome have an increased incidence of cardiovascular disturbances, including valvular regurgitant disease, venous and arterial thrombosis, pulmonary hypertension and cardiomyopathy. Although vasculitis of large coronary arteries may rarely result in myocardial ischemia, there is also an increased frequency of coronary atherosclerosis that may be related to hypertension or glucocorticoid therapy.

Myocarditis is an uncommon occurrence, which is often asymptomatic, or may accompany other cardiac manifestations, particularly pericarditis in SLE [1]. Clinical lupus myocarditis is seen in only a small percentage of patients with SLE. Myocarditis should be suspected if there are symptoms and signs of heart failure, electrocardiographic abnormalities and unexplained cardiomegaly in patients with SLE in the absence of other cardiac abnormalities (valvular, hypertensive, or coronary artery diseases). Echocardiography may show both systolic and diastolic dysfunction of the left ventricle. Myocarditis has been associated in some cases with antibodies to ribonucleoprotein [34].

Myocardial biopsy may be indicated to distinguish active myocarditis from fibrosis and other causes of cardiomyopathy (such as hydroxychloroquine cardiotoxicity) and may reveal active inflammation (lymphocyte infiltration of the myocardium) or cardiac fibrosis. Clinical lupus myocarditis should be treated using steroids and/or immunosuppressive treatment. However, cardiomyopathy with fibrosis is usually resistant to these treatments.

Amyloidosis

Cardiac involvement is the most frequent cause of death in primary amyloidosis (AL amyloidosis) and in transthyretin-associated amyloidosis, while clinically significant cardiac involvement is uncommon in the secondary form (AA amyloidosis) and in senile amyloidosis [35]. In patients with AL amyloidosis, the other major sites of clinically important amyloid deposition are the kidneys, liver, gastrointestinal tract, peripheral nervous system, musculoskeletal structure, lungs and skin. Cardiovascular complications include diastolic dysfunction (ultimately, restrictive cardiomyopathy), systolic dysfunction, arrhythmias and conduction disturbances, and orthostatic hypotension. The echocardiogram may show a thickened myocardium with a characteristic "speckled pattern" along with small pericardial effusion. The histological diagnosis is mandatory and can be performed by aspiration of abdominal fat or biopsy of the myocardium or other organs (rectal or duodenal mucosa or kidney). Cardiac transplantation may help selected patients and chemotherapy may improve survival in some cases, but the overall prognosis is poor, especially in AL amyloidosis with advanced cardiac involvement.

Sarcoidosis

A common cardiac manifestation of systemic sarcoidosis is right heart failure due to pulmonary hypertension as a result of pulmonary interstitial fibrosis. However, cardiac sarcoidosis can be associated with other systemic manifestations of sarcoidosis and may cause restrictive cardiomyopathy, mitral regurgitation, ventricular aneurysm and various arrhythmias, including high-grade AV block and ventricular tachycardia [36]. Both diastolic and systolic heart failure can be recognized, as cardiac infiltration by sarcoid granulomas causes increased stiffness of the myocardium as well as diminished systolic contractility. Thus, clinicians must be alert to the development of symptoms or signs suggestive of cardiac involvement among patients with known sarcoidosis. Diagnostic tests such as endomyocardial biopsy or imaging may be required, particularly in patients without other manifestations of the disease [37]. Treatment of cardiac sarcoidosis is aimed at controlling inflammation (corticosteroids) and preventing cardiac complications (pacemakers, implantable cardioverter defibrillators, cardiac surgery for mitral regurgitation or ventricular aneurysm, or cardiac transplantation).

Muscular Dystrophy

Duchenne's progressive muscular dystrophy (DPMD) is caused by mutations of the dystrophin gene and shows X-linked inheritance. Muscular weakness usually occurs between two and three years of age. When arising from the floor, affected boys use hand support to push themselves to an upright position (Gower's sign). An unusual waddling gait, lumbar lordosis and calf pseudohypertrophy are frequently observed. DPMD causes DCM-type cardiomyopathy with conduction defects and/or various supraventricular and ventricular arrhythmias [38]. Extensive fibrosis of the posterobasal left ventricular wall shows the characteristic electrocardiographic changes of tall right precordial R waves with an increased R/S ratio and deep Q waves in leads I, aVL and lateral chest leads. Involvement of the posterior papillary muscle can lead to massive mitral regurgitation. Symptomatic cardiomyopathy is evident in almost all patients older than 18 years [39]. Due to their inability to exercise, despite the high incidence of DCM, the majority of children with DPMD are relatively asymptomatic until they present with symptoms of acute CHF.

Myotonic Dystrophy

Myotonic dystrophy is the most common form of adult-onset muscular dystrophy and is an autosomal dominant disease. Initial clinical presentations may be cataracts, cardiac conduction abnormalities, infertility, alveolar hypoventilation syndrome, or insulin resistance, in addition to skeletal muscle weakness, pain and stiffness (myotonia). To examine myotonia, it is necessary to instruct the patient to firmly grip the examiner's fingers and to then rapidly let go. In this circumstance, the delayed relaxation (grip myotonia) can be recognized. In addition, by percussing the thenar muscles, the thumb will abduct but then relax slowly (percussion myotonia).

Myotonic dystrophy is associated with both cardiac conduction disturbances and structural heart abnormalities [40]. Atrial flutter and fibrillation are the most common arrhythmias and ventricular arrhythmias are less common. Clinical cardiomyopathy is uncommon, although echocardiography frequently shows left ventricular hypertrophy and dilatation, and occasionally left ventricular systolic dysfunction [41]. The diagnosis of myotonic dystrophy can usually be made clinically in a patient with the characteristic presentations and a positive family history. Electromyography for skeletal muscle and specific genetic testing may be useful adjuncts.

Friedreich's Ataxia

Friedreich's ataxia is an autosomal recessive disorder that affects the central nervous system, spinal cord, peripheral nerves, as well as the heart and pancreas. The major clinical manifestations include neurologic dysfunction, cardiomyopathy and diabetes mellitus. Many patients present with clinical onset under the age of 25, while about 10% have a later onset between 26 and 50 years of age. Common neurologic abnormalities include progressive ataxia of all four limbs and gait disturbance, optic atrophy, dysphagia, bladder dysfunction, as well as motor and sensory disturbances from involvement of the pyramidal and peripheral nerves.

Approximately 50% of patients with Friedreich's ataxia develop cardiac symptoms [42], while many more patients may have abnormal electrocardiographic (ST-segment and T-wave changes) or echocardiographic findings (left ventricular hypertrophy, with either symmetric or asymmetric hypertrophy of the left ventricular septum) [43]. The diagnosis of Friedreich ataxia is clinically made but can be confirmed by genetic testing.

Alcoholic Cardiomyopathy

Individuals with long-term alcohol dependence may develop a DCM-type cardiomyopathy and the risk of developing cardiomyopathy is partially genetically determined. Abstinence of alcohol consumption before developing clinical heart failure may halt disease progression or even reverse the clinical course. Although DCM in alcoholic patients may be related to beriberi heart, malnutrition or a combination of these factors, excessive alcohol use can also be an independent and sole cause of cardiomyopathy in some alcoholics [44]. Physical examination of the jugular venous pressure in patients with ascites is important in determining whether the ascites are due to alcoholic cardiomyopathy or cirrhosis (alcoholic liver disease). The jugular venous pressure is normal or low-normal in cirrhosis unless there are massive ascites which, via upward pressure on the diaphragm, can increase the intrathoracic and venous pressure [45].

However, the arrhythmogenic form of alcoholic cardiotoxicity is more prevalent among alcohol abusers, particularly alcoholic men [46]. A weekend of binge drinking is typically followed by atrial fibrillation, atrial flutter or ventricular premature contractions (holiday heart syndrome). Increased attention should be paid to the accompanying electrolyte abnormalities as contributing factors, such as hypomagnesemia and hypokalemia, which are frequently recognized in chronic alcoholics. Alcohol abstinence is the preventive treatment of choice rather than antiarrhythmic medications.

Radiation Cardiomyopathy

High dose irradiation of the heart can lead to cardiac damage, including the pericardium, myocardium, valves, coronary arteries, capillaries and conducting system [47]. Pericarditis is the typical acute manifestation of radiation injury, while some patients may develop chronic pericardial disease, coronary artery disease, cardiomyopathy (especially diastolic dysfunction), valvular disease and conduction abnormalities can manifest years or decades after the irradiation [48]. The typical histologic finding of radiation cardiotoxicity is diffuse interstitial fibrosis with a narrowing of capillary and arterial lumens. The risk is greater among patients whose coronary arteries receive >35 Gy of radiation exposure. Cardiac perfusion imaging and/or coronary calcium scoring by CT may reveal the abnormality. Since newer radiotherapy techniques reduce both dose of radiation and volume of the heart within the irradiation field, the risk of cardiac damage is likely to decrease in the future.

Drug-Induced Cardiomyopathy

A number of medications are associated with DCM-type cardiomyopathy. Among these, anthracycline (e.g., doxorubicin)-induced cardiomyopathy may lead to potentially fatal heart failure. The incidence of heart failure increases with the greater accumulated dose of the drug, as well as with several risk factors, including cardiac irradiation, higher age, underlying heart disease, hypertension, concomitant use of cyclophosphamide and genetic predisposition. Other drugs frequently related to cardiotoxicity include cyclophosphamide, trastuzumab, antiretroviral agents, tricyclic antidepressants, phenothiazines, lithium, chloroquine, clozapine and propofol. Further, cocaine abuse is associated with DCM-type cardiomyopathy as well as various cardiac complications, including sudden death, myocarditis and acute myocardial infarction (resulting from coronary spasm and/or thrombosis). Unexplained heart failure with DCM-type cardiomyopathy in a young person should raise the possibility of cocaine abuse, since abstinence can restore myocardial dysfunction.

Peripartum Cardiomyopathy

Unexplained myocardial dilatation and dysfunction related to pregnancy, or peripartum cardiomyopathy (PPCM), may develop during the last trimester of pregnancy or within 6 months after delivery. Most patients develop symptoms of CHF in the month before or during the first four to five months after delivery. In contrast, pregnant women with underlying cardiac disease (e.g., valvular heart disease) tend to develop symptoms of CHF during the second trimester of gestation due to the hemodynamic burden. Risk factors for PPCM include age greater than 30 years, multiparity, African descent, multiple pregnancy, history of preeclampsia or eclampsia, maternal cocaine abuse and long-term (more than four weeks) use of tocolytic therapy with beta adrenergic agonists.

Common symptoms include fatigue, cough, chest discomfort, dyspnea, orthopnea, paroxysmal nocturnal dyspnea or hemoptysis. Abdominal pain from acute congestive liver (rapid stretch of the hepatic capsule) may mimic the conditions of acute abdomen. Systemic and pulmonary emboli are common in patients with PPCM, likely because of the hypercoagulable state associated with pregnancy. The diagnosis of PPCM is based upon four clinical criteria: peripartum development of heart failure; absence of an identifiable cause for the heart failure; absence of recognizable heart disease prior to the last month of pregnancy; and left ventricular systolic dysfunction. The prognosis in these patients is related to whether the heart size returns to normal after the first episode of CHF. If cardiomegaly persists, further pregnancies frequently produce refractory and fatal CHF.

References

[1] Richardson P, McKenna W, Bristow M, Maisch B, Mautner B, O'Connell J, et al. Report of the 1995 World Health Organization/International Society and Federation of Cardiology Task Force on the Definition and Classification of cardiomyopathies. *Circulation*. 1996 Mar 1;93(5):841-2.

[2] Harrison TR, Braunwald E. Harrison's principles of internal medicine. 15th ed. New York: McGraw-Hill 2001.

[3] Sole MJ, Liu P. Viral myocarditis: a paradigm for understanding the pathogenesis and treatment of dilated cardiomyopathy. *J Am Coll Cardiol*. 1993 Oct;22(4 Suppl A):99A-105A.

[4] Martin AB, Webber S, Fricker FJ, Jaffe R, Demmler G, Kearney D, et al. Acute myocarditis. Rapid diagnosis by PCR in children. *Circulation*. 1994 Jul;90(1):330-9.

[5] Barbaro G, Di Lorenzo G, Grisorio B, Barbarini G, The Gruppo Italiano per lo Studio Cardiologico dei Pazienti Affetti da A. Incidence of Dilated Cardiomyopathy and Detection of HIV in Myocardial Cells of HIV-Positive Patients. *New England Journal of Medicine*. 1998 October 15, 1998;339(16):1093-9.

[6] Matsumori A, Matoba Y, Sasayama S. Dilated cardiomyopathy associated with hepatitis C virus infection. Circulation. 1995 Nov 1;92(9):2519-25.

[7] Wanby P, auml, Olsen B, ouml, rn. Myocarditis in a Patient with Salmonella and Campylobacter enteritis. *Scandinavian Journal of Infectious Diseases*. 2001;33(11): 860 - 2.

[8] Brady WJ, Ferguson JD, Ullman EA, Perron AD. Myocarditis: emergency department recognition and management. *Emergency Medicine Clinics of North America*. 2004;22(4):865-85.

[9] Chinen K, Tokuda Y, Sakamoto A, Fujioka Y. Fungal infections of the heart: A clinicopathologic study of 50 autopsy cases. *Pathology - Research and Practice*. 2007; 203 (10): 705-15.

[10] Viotti RJ, Vigliano C, Laucella S, Lococo B, Petti M, Bertocchi G, et al. Value of echocardiography for diagnosis and prognosis of chronic Chagas disease cardiomyopathy without heart failure. *BMJ*. 2004 June 1, 2004;90(6):655-60.

[11] Murrell KD, Pozio E. Trichinellosis: the zoonosis that won't go quietly. *Int J Parasitol*. 2000 Nov;30(12-13):1339-49.

[12] Ancelle T, Dupouy-Camet J, Desenclos JC, Maillot E, Savage-Houze S, Charlet F, et al. A multifocal outbreak of trichinellosis linked to horse meat imported from North America to France in 1993. *Am J Trop Med Hyg*. 1998 Oct;59(4):615-9.

[13] Trichinellosis associated with bear meat--New York and Tennessee, 2003. *MMWR Morb Mortal Wkly Rep*. 2004 Jul 16;53(27):606-10.

[14] Kociecka W. Trichinellosis: human disease, diagnosis and treatment. *Vet Parasitol*. 2000 Dec 1;93(3-4):365-83.

[15] Compton SJ, Celum CL, Lee C, Thompson D, Sumi SM, Fritsche TR, et al. Trichinosis with ventilatory failure and persistent myocarditis. *Clin Infect Dis*. 1993 Apr;16(4):500-4.

[16] Steere AC, Batsford WP, Weinberg M, Alexander J, Berger HJ, Wolfson S, et al. Lyme carditis: cardiac abnormalities of Lyme disease. *Ann Intern Med*. 1980 Jul;93(1):8-16.

[17] Kimball SA, Janson PA, LaRaia PJ. Complete heart block as the sole presentation of Lyme disease. *Arch Intern Med*. 1989 Aug;149(8):1897-8.

[18] Kennedy JL, Barnard JJ, Prahlow JA. Syphilitic coronary artery ostial stenosis resulting in acute myocardial infarction and death. *Cardiology*. 2006;105(1):25-9.

[19] Zarich SW, Nesto RW. Diabetic cardiomyopathy. *Am Heart J*. 1989 Nov;118(5 Pt 1):1000-12.

[20] Boudina S, Abel ED. Diabetic cardiomyopathy revisited. *Circulation*. 2007 Jun 26;115(25):3213-23.

[21] Kenchaiah S, Evans JC, Levy D, Wilson PW, Benjamin EJ, Larson MG, et al. Obesity and the risk of heart failure. *N Engl J Med*. 2002 Aug 1;347(5):305-13.

[22] McGavock JM, Victor RG, Unger RH, Szczepaniak LS. Adiposity of the heart, revisited. Ann Intern Med. 2006 Apr 4;144(7):517-24.

[23] Arad M, Maron BJ, Gorham JM, Johnson WH, Jr., Saul JP, Perez-Atayde AR, et al. Glycogen storage diseases presenting as hypertrophic cardiomyopathy. *N Engl J Med*. 2005 Jan 27;352(4):362-72.

[24] Olson LJ, Edwards WD, McCall JT, Ilstrup DM, Gersh BJ. Cardiac iron deposition in idiopathic hemochromatosis: histologic and analytic assessment of 14 hearts from autopsy. *J Am Coll Cardiol*. 1987 Dec;10(6):1239-43.

[25] Anderson LJ, Holden S, Davis B, Prescott E, Charrier CC, Bunce NH, et al. Cardiovascular T2-star (T2*) magnetic resonance for the early diagnosis of myocardial iron overload. *Eur Heart J*. 2001 Dec;22(23):2171-9.

[26] Desnick RJ, Brady R, Barranger J, Collins AJ, Germain DP, Goldman M, et al. Fabry disease, an under-recognized multisystemic disorder: expert recommendations for diagnosis, management and enzyme replacement therapy. *Ann Intern Med*. 2003 Feb 18;138(4):338-46.

[27] Kampmann C, Baehner F, Whybra C, Martin C, Wiethoff CM, Ries M, et al. Cardiac manifestations of Anderson-Fabry disease in heterozygous females. *J Am Coll Cardiol*. 2002 Nov 6;40(9):1668-74.

[28] Kampmann C, Baehner F, Ries M, Beck M. Cardiac involvement in Anderson-Fabry disease. *J Am Soc Nephrol*. 2002 Jun;13 Suppl 2:S147-9.

[29] Nakao S, Takenaka T, Maeda M, Kodama C, Tanaka A, Tahara M, et al. An atypical variant of Fabry's disease in men with left ventricular hypertrophy. *N Engl J Med*. 1995 Aug 3;333(5):288-93.

[30] Castiglia PT. Protein-energy malnutrition (Kwashiorkor and Marasmus). *Journal of Pediatric Health Care*. 1996;10(1):28-30.
[31] Webb JG, Kiess MC, Chan-Yan CC. Malnutrition and the heart. *CMAJ*. 1986 Oct 1;135(7):753-8.
[32] Sica DA. Loop diuretic therapy, thiamine balance and heart failure. *Congest Heart Fail*. 2007 Jul-Aug;13(4):244-7.
[33] Abelmann WH, Lorell BH. The challenge of cardiomyopathy. *J Am Coll Cardiol*. 1989 May;13(6):1219-39.
[34] Borenstein DG, Fye WB, Arnett FC, Stevens MB. The myocarditis of systemic lupus erythematosus: association with myositis. Ann Intern Med. 1978 Nov;89(5 Pt 1):619-24.
[35] Dubrey SW, Cha K, Anderson J, Chamarthi B, Reisinger J, Skinner M, et al. The clinical features of immunoglobulin light-chain (AL) amyloidosis with heart involvement. *QJM*. 1998 Feb;91(2):141-57.
[36] Smedema JP, Snoep G, van Kroonenburgh MP, van Geuns RJ, Dassen WR, Gorgels AP, et al. Cardiac involvement in patients with pulmonary sarcoidosis assessed at two university medical centers in the Netherlands. *Chest*. 2005 Jul;128(1):30-5.
[37] Chapelon-Abric C, de Zuttere D, Duhaut P, Veyssier P, Wechsler B, Huong DL, et al. Cardiac sarcoidosis: a retrospective study of 41 cases. *Medicine (Baltimore)*. 2004 Nov;83(6):315-34.
[38] Perloff JK. Cardiac rhythm and conduction in Duchenne's muscular dystrophy: a prospective study of 20 patients. *J Am Coll Cardiol*. 1984 May;3(5):1263-8.
[39] Nigro G, Comi LI, Politano L, Bain RJ. The incidence and evolution of cardiomyopathy in Duchenne muscular dystrophy. *Int J Cardiol*. 1990 Mar;26(3):271-7.
[40] Phillips MF, Harper PS. Cardiac disease in myotonic dystrophy. *Cardiovasc Res*. 1997 Jan;33(1):13-22.
[41] Bhakta D, Lowe MR, Groh WJ. Prevalence of structural cardiac abnormalities in patients with myotonic dystrophy type I. *Am Heart J*. 2004 Feb;147(2):224-7.
[42] Child JS, Perloff JK, Bach PM, Wolfe AD, Perlman S, Kark RA. Cardiac involvement in Friedreich's ataxia: a clinical study of 75 patients. *J Am Coll Cardiol*. 1986 Jun;7(6):1370-8.
[43] Gunal N, Saraclar M, Ozkutlu S, Senocak F, Topaloglu H, Karaaslan S. Heart disease in Friedreich's ataxia: a clinical and echocardiographic study. *Acta Paediatr Jpn*. 1996 Aug;38(4):308-11.
[44] McKenna CJ, Codd MB, McCann HA, Sugrue DD. Alcohol consumption and idiopathic dilated cardiomyopathy: a case control study. *Am Heart J*. 1998 May;135(5 Pt 1):833-7.
[45] Guazzi M, Polese A, Magrini F, Fiorentini C, Olivari MT. Negative influences of ascites on the cardiac function of cirrhotic patients. *Am J Med*. 1975 Aug;59(2):165-70.
[46] Mukamal KJ, Tolstrup JS, Friberg J, Jensen G, Gronbaek M. Alcohol consumption and risk of atrial fibrillation in men and women: the Copenhagen City Heart Study. *Circulation*. 2005 Sep 20;112(12):1736-42.
[47] Adams MJ, Lipsitz SR, Colan SD, Tarbell NJ, Treves ST, Diller L, et al. Cardiovascular status in long-term survivors of Hodgkin's disease treated with chest radiotherapy. *J Clin Oncol*. 2004 Aug 1;22(15):3139-48.
[48] Heidenreich PA, Hancock SL, Vagelos RH, Lee BK, Schnittger I. Diastolic dysfunction after mediastinal irradiation. *Am Heart J*. 2005 Nov;150(5):977-82.

In: Heart Disease in Men
Editors: A.B. Todd and M.H. Mosley, pp. 259-274
ISBN: 978-1-60692-297-2

Chapter 12

THE ROLE OF NATRIURETIC PEPTIDES IN INVESTIGATION OF VARIOUS CARDIOVASCULAR DISEASES

K. Kotaška and R. Průša
Department of Clinical Biochemistry and Pathobiochemistry, 2nd Faculty of Medicine, Charles University, University Hospital Motol, Prague, Czech Republic

Abstract

The natriuretic peptides are well established serum biomarkers for acute and chronic heart failures. The prevalence of heart diseases increases markedly with age. Among all investigated neurohormones and natriuretic peptides, BNP and NT-proBNP are the best markers to rule out left ventricular dysfunction. The levels of BNP and NT-proBNP increase with the severity of the left ventricular impairment. Natriuretic peptides show good ability to discriminate patients with mild and severe left ventricular dysfunction. Brain natriuretic peptides are due to their higher sensitivity, specificity and negative predictive values well approved in diagnosis of severe and moderate left ventricular dysfunction. Various studies have pointed out the role of brain natriuretic peptides as markers of myocardial dysfunction. Natriuretic peptides play significant role as prognostic factors and long term clinical outcome predictors after acute myocardial infarction. Levels of natriuretic peptides A and B increase significantly in patiens with congenital and valvular heart diseases including transposition of great arteries and ventricular septal defect, thus, natriuretic peptides are clinicaly useful markers for monitoring various types of heart diseases of different etiology.

1. Introduction

During the past 100 years, cardiovascular disease (CVD) has become a leading cause of morbidity and mortality worldwide. At the beginning of the 21st century CVD now accounts for nearly one half of all deaths in the developed world and 25% in developing world due to the significant increase in CVD risk factors (obesity, diabetes). Heart failure is characterized with myocardial injury, usually secondary to myocardial infarction, ischemia, hypertension or other etiologies (Bhalla et al., 2004)

Acute coronary syndrome (ACS) is a complex syndrome with heterogeneous etiology. The most common cause is atherosclerotic coronary artery disease with erosion or rupture of atherosclerotic plaque resulting in formation of partially obstructive or only transiently occlusive intracoronary thrombus. Principal causes of ACS are: 1) plaque rupture with acute thrombosis, 2) progressive mechanical obstruction, 3) inflammation, 4) secondary unstable angina due to severe anaemia or hypothyreoidism and dynamic obstruction resulting in coronary vasoconstriction (Alpert et al., 2000)

Valvular heart disease is any disease process involving one or more of the valves of the heart (the aortic and mitral valves on the left and the pulmonary and tricuspid valves on the right). Valve problems may be congenital (inborn) or acquired (due to another cause later in life). Treatment may be with medication but often (depending on the severity) involves valve repair or replacement (insertion of an artificial heart valve). Congenital heart disease refers to a problem with the heart's structure and function due to abnormal heart development before birth.

1.1. Physiology and Biochemistry of Cardiovascular Diseases

The physiologic compensatory mechanisms of heart disease included activation of renin-angiotensin-aldosterone system (RAAS), natriuretic peptide system, sympathetic nervous system, endothelins and other neurohormonal factors. Activation of these mechanisms leads to the progressive worsening of left ventricular systolic function and increasing remodelling and overall work of the heart. Left ventricular systolic dysfunction is defined in terms of ejection fraction. Left ventricular ejection fraction (LVEF) is a good clinical indicator of left ventricular systolic function. Normal ejection fraction is 0.50 or more ($\geq$50%), nevertheless, in many studies presented below, the normal left ventricular ejection fraction is set at 0.60 ($\geq$60%). The effect of natriuresis, diuresis and vasodilatory mechanisms leads to the progressive deterioration of heart function with worsened symptoms of heart failure (dyspnoea, peripheral oedema, tachycardia and volume overload). Natriuretic peptides are released from cardiac myocytes in response to increases in cardiovascular stress. BNP is released from the atria and ventricles of the heart in response to volume overload, increased filling pressures and myocardial wall stretching. BNP causes vasodilatation, reduces blood pressure and stimulates sodium and water excretion. (Bhalla et al., 2004)

The BNP gene is located on chromosome 1 (1p36.2) (Seilhamer et al., 1989). The hormone originates from the precursor peptides preproBNP (134 amino acid) and proBNP (108 amino acids; 12 kDa). ProBNP is the *in situ* precursor of both the biologically active BNP hormone (32 amino acids; 4 kDa), and its inactive metabolite, NT-proBNP (76 amino acids; 8 kDa). Both forms circulate in the blood of normal subjects and in those with heart failure. ProBNP also circulates in blood in monomeric and trimeric (approximately 36 kDa) forms (Shimizu et al., 2002). The estimated *in vivo* half-life of BNP in blood is 20 minutes and between 1 and 2 hours for NT-proBNP and its related forms. BNP is cleared by a combination of receptors, neutral endopeptidases, proteolytic enzymes and renal clearance. Atrial natriuretic peptide (ANP) is present in the ventricular tissue of fetuses and neonates in hypertrophied ventricles as well as in low concentrations in normal ventricles. C-type natriuretic peptide (CNP) is expressed primarily in the central nervous system and vascular tissues, and unlike ANP and BNP is nearly non-existent in cardiac tissue. Nevertheless, CNP does play an important role in cardiovascular physiology as a potent vasorelaxant, as well as an inhibitor of vascular smooth muscle proliferation and endothelial cell migration. (Vanderheyden et al., 2004)

The structure of natriuretic peptides is listed in figure 1.

Mechanism of biological activity of natriuretic peptides is listed in figure 2.

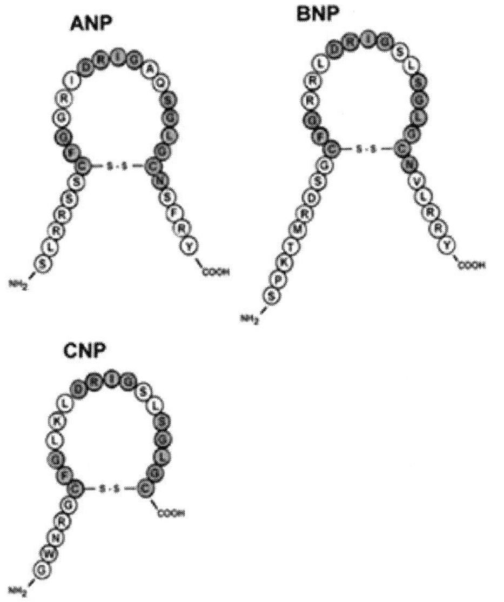

Figure 1. The structure of the natriuretic peptides.

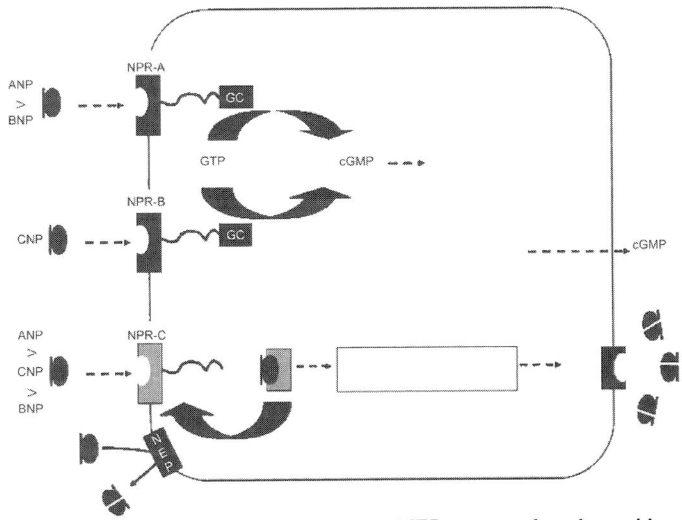

NPR –A,B,C – natriuretic peptide receptors A, B and C, NEP – neutral endopeptidase, GC – guanylate cyclase RAAS – Renin-angiotensin aldosterone system

Figure 2. Mechanism of biological activity of natriuretic peptides adapted from (Vanderheyden et al., 2004).

Wall stress in chamber is directly related to the diameter of the chamber and the transmural pressure and inversely related to the thickness of the wall. Increases both in the diameter and pressure within the left ventricle during remodeling after transmural infarction or as a consequence of prior ischemic damage may contribute to elevation of natriuretic peptides observed in patients with acute myocardial infarction. Chronic heart failure is characterized by an impaired pump function with reduced cardiac output and subsequent venous congestion. Neurohormonal system including natriuretic peptides play important role in disease progression (Bhalla et al., 2004). In the first stage of heart failure (NYHA I) during which is cardiac function minimally diminished, atrial natriuretic peptide (ANP), which is stored in atria and released predominantly in response to distension of the atrial walls and BNP, which mainly reflect the ventricular overload, and is released from the cardiomyocytes primarily in response to the elevation of the end diastolic ventricular pressure or the ventricular stretching, have compensatory effect. If the cardiac output is reduced in the initial stage of heart failure (NYHA I) the sympathetic nervous system and renin-angiotensin aldosterone system are stimulated and blood pressure and cardiac output increase. During the progression of heart failure (NYHA II) the impairment of neurohormonal regulation leads to the peripheral vasoconstriction and natriuretic peptides are not able to compensate for the constricting effect and water retention occurs. (Puschendorf and Mair, 2003)

With increasing cardiac failure (NYHA III) renal perfusion becomes disturbed and sympathetic nervous system and RAAS are more stimulated, resulting in peripheral vascular resistence and brain natriuretic peptides lose their peripheral effect on kidney. The NYHA stage IV represent decompensated heart failure during which moderately and greatly elevated concentration of natriuretic peptides are measured and their vasodilatatory and natriuretic effect is not present. The summary of the severity of the heart diseases according to the NYHA classification is listed in table 1 (Puschendorf and Mair, 2003). Increased plasma concentrations of natriuretic peptides are not strictly specific for heart diseases and also lack sensitivity in the chronic compensated state. Diuretics, angiotensin-converting enzyme (ACE) inhibitors, angiotensin receptor antagonists, and spironolactone have been shown to decrease BNP and NT-proBNP in parallel with clinical and hemodynamic improvement (Angermann and Ertl, 2004).

Table 1. NYHA classification

Class	Patient Symptoms
Class I (Mild)	No limitation of physical activity. Ordinary physical activity does not cause undue fatigue, palpitation, or dyspnea (shortness of breath).
Class II (Mild)	Slight limitation of physical activity. Comfortable at rest, but ordinary physical activity results in fatigue, palpitation, or dyspnea.
Class III (Moderate)	Marked limitation of physical activity. Comfortable at rest, but less than ordinary activity causes fatigue, palpitation, or dyspnea.
Class IV (Severe)	Unable to carry out any physical activity without discomfort. Symptoms of cardiac insufficiency at rest. If any physical activity is undertaken, discomfort is increased.

2. Role of Natriuretic Peptides in Heart Diseases

2.1. Natriuretic Peptides in Acute Coronary Syndromes

Many studies show strong association between BNP and NT-proBNP and outcomes in patients with acute coronary syndrome (ACS). After presentation of transmural infarction, the plasma concentrations of BNP rise rapidly and peaks at 24 hours with the peak concentration proportional to the size of myocardial infarction. In patients with severe heart failure, second peak at 5 days could occur, resulting in development of adverse ventricular remodelling. Elevated values of NT-proBNP and BNP have been shown to predict cardiovascular mortality independently to other prognostic factors and variables including left ventricular ejection fraction. The plasma concentrations of natriuretic peptides are directly associated with older age, female sex, renal insufficiency, left ventricular dysfunction, clinical evidence of heart failure, presence of myocardial necrosis. Nevertheless, prognostic relationship between the natriuretic peptides and mortality is independent of the other clinical risk factors. Natriuretic peptides clearly identified patients without systolic dysfunction or sign of heart failure who are at higher risk of death and heart failure and provide similar prognostic efficiency as the cardiac troponin I did. It is well shown, that elevated serum concentrations of NT-proBNP and BNP have strong relationship with risk of short- and long-term mortality. Elevated B-type natriuretic peptide (BNP) levels are associated with increased risk for mortality in patients with non-ST-segment-elevation (NSTE) acute coronary syndromes (ACS) (Atwater et al., 2007; Jernberg et al., 2005)

2.2. Natriuretic Peptides in Left Ventricular Dysfunction

Echocardiography is the method of choice to detect left ventricular systolic dysfunction. Nevertheless, there are some limitations especially in primary care. However, access to echocardiography in a primary care setting is limited. To date, general practitioners have to identify patients in need of a referral to echocardiography by clinical information, which is routinely obtained from medical history and physical examination. Therefore, a screening test (such as blood natriuretic peptide concentrations) which could easily be administered in primary care and reliably rule out left ventricular systolic dysfunction would reduce referral rates for echocardiography and lower health care costs. A retrospective analysis of cost-effectiveness showed that brain natriuretic peptide (BNP) testing could have reduced the costs per detected case by 26% compared to echocardiography (Nielsen et al., 2003).

Among all investigated neurohormones and natriuretic peptides, BNP and NT-proBNP are the best markers to rule out left ventricular dysfunction (de Lemos et al., 2003; Hammerer-Lercher et al., 2001; Yamamoto et al., 1996). In many studies, severe ventricular dysfunction was defined as LVEF $\leq$ 25%, moderate LVSD was defined as a LVEF of 26-40%, mild systolic ventricular dysfunction was defined as LVEF 41-59%, values of LVEF$\geq$ 60% were considered as normal. (Kotaska et al., 2006a; Pfister et al., 2004; Seino et al., 2004) Population-based studies (de Lemos et al., 2003; Hunt et al., 1997; McDonagh et al., 1998) as well as studies in patients with acute dyspnoea in emergency department (Lainchbury et al., 2003; Maisel, 2001; Palladini et al., 2003) have shown that low levels of natriuretic peptides effectively rule out left ventricular systolic dysfunction. (Del Ry et al., 2007) show, that CNP is specifically increased in patients with idiopathic left ventricular systolic dysfunction.

2.3. Natriuretic Peptides in Congenital and Valvular Heart Diseases

Patients with congenital and valvular heart diseses had significantly elevated levels of natriuretic peptides. (Taniguchi et al., 2006; Kotaska et al., 2006a; Kotaska et al., 2006b; Flezzani et al., 1988; Yasumura, 2004) Plasma NT-proBNP levels were significantly elevated in patients with rheumatic mitral stenosis (Selcuk et al., 2007) and with Senning/Mustard corrected transposition, congenitally corrected transposition and Fontan/total cavopulmonary connection.(Larsson et al., 2007) Circulating levels of atrial natriuretic peptide and brain natriuretic peptide (BNP) are elevated in patients with cyanotic congenital heart disease and associated with the severity of ventricular dysfunction.(Khan et al., 2008). The differences between various types of congenital heart diseases are mentioned in many studies. (Koch et al., 2008). Pro-ANP levels show very good diagnostic efficiency in patients with transposition of great arteries and ventricular septal defect (Kotaska et al.,unpublished data).

2.4. Natriuretic Peptides as Prognostic Factors in Various Heart Diseases

The determination of B-type natriuretic peptides (BNP) provides powerful and independent prognostic information in patients at all stages of the evolution of chronic heart failure (HF), in a variety of clinical settings. The best evidence of the prognostic value of amino-terminal pro-BNP (NT-proBNP) in chronic HF comes from statistically robust controlled clinical trials that include a large number of clinically well-characterized patients from different sites. A single determination of NT-proBNP at any time during the progression of chronic HF provides a clinically useful tool for risk stratification. As with acute HF, the hypothesis that repeated measurements could carry prognostic information beyond that of a single measure has been confirmed in different settings. The value of repeated determinations of NT-proBNP levels is of special interest for monitoring progression of disease and may help in evaluating the clinical effects of medical therapy. For instance, as noted, changes in NT-proBNP levels during hospitalization were independent predictors of 6-month hospital readmission and death of patients hospitalized for decompensated HF (Bettencourt et al., 2004). In another study, patients who experienced a reduction of NT-proBNP levels less than 50% after cardiac resynchronization therapy had a more favorable outcome than the rest of the population, and this was associated with positive changes in left ventricular remodeling and exercise capacity. (Yu et al., 2005). Omland et al., (2007) describe the strong association between natriuretic peptide concentrations and the incidence of cardiovascular mortality, fatal or nonfatal myocardial infarction, heart failure, and stroke. The prognostic value of NT-proBNP is generally superior to that of other circulating biomarkers used in chronic HF (endothelin peptides, adrenomedullin, tumor necrosis factor, C-reactive protein, norepinephrine, and erythropoietine (Gardner et al., 2005), markers of cardiac injury (cardiac troponin T,troponin I) (Taniguchi et al., 2004) or imaging techniques (echocardiography) (Bruch et al., 2006b).

Decision limits based on cut off values have graded relationship with risk for short- and long-term mortality (James et al., 2003; Morrow et al., 2003). If the cut off value for the NT-proBNP is four times higher than the upper limit of the reference interval, the probability of survival in patients with various types of heart impairment decrease significantly (Long term survival rate is less than 70%). On the contrary, in patients, where the serum levels of BNP and NT-proBNP are below the cut off value, is the probability of long term survival more than 90%. (Heeschen et al., 2004) shows, that baseline NT-proBNP levels >250 ng/l were associated with death after MI during 30 days follow up.

2.5. Natriuretic Peptides as Tools for Therapeutic Decision Making in Heart Failure

The diagnostic utility of blood natriuretic peptide levels in the acute heart failure setting has interest in evaluation of these biomarkers as screening tools for patients with underlying cardiac dysfunction, but no overt signs and symptoms – asymptomatic left ventricular dysfunction due to structural cardiac abnormalities. Higher NT-proBNP levels have also been associated with greater likelihood of detecting incident heart failure in population with stable coronary artery disease (Bibbins-Domingo et al., 2007). Many studies pointed out the role of natriuretic peptides as the therapy guides in patients with mild-to-moderate chronic heart failure (Jourdain et al., 2007; Troughton and Richards, 2008). These studies found significant decrease of severe cardiovascular events (death, decompensated heart failure). Natriuretic peptides play significant role in the assessment of decompensated heart failure (Cheng et al., 2001; O'Brien et al., 2003). Diagnostic use of natriuretic peptides in other heart impairment is summarized in table 1 adapted from (Phua et al., 2005)

Table 1. Diagnostic use of natriuretic peptides in other heart impairment

Concentration	Type of heart impairment	Remarks
Significantly elevated concentrations (BNP > 500 ng/l, NTproBNP > 1000 ng/l)	Decompensated heart failure	
Gray zone (BNP 100 – 500 ng/l, NT-proBNP 250 – 1000 ng/l)	Ventricular dysfunction	
	Acute coronary syndrome	High risk of cardiovascular mortality if the level is elevated
	Unstable angina pectoris	
Mild elevation or normal values (BNP less than 100 ng/l, NT-proBNP less than 250 ng/l)	Hearth fibrosis	Elevated BNP secretion
	Cardiac arythmia	
	Myocardial hypoxia	Elevated BNP levels due to the paracrine vascular regulation (protection against other ischemic processes)
	Endotelial dysfunction	Elevated secretion of natriuretic peptides by the humoral factors (endothelin, TNF alpha, TGF beta)
	Stable angina pectoris	
	Increased atrial and ventricular volume	

Other potential diagnostic uses of natriuretic peptides are: diagnosing diastolic dysfunction, monitoring cardiotoxic drugs (doxorubicin, trastuzumab), timing of surgery for valve disease (aortic, mitral), Cardiovascular complications could also occur in other pathological states including diabetes, transplantation, renal failure. Natriuretic peptides are appropriate in following patients with diabetes (Hildebrandt and Richards, 2008), monitoring transplant rejection (Martinez-Dolz et al., 2007; Sun et al., 2008), rule out acute respiratory distress syndrome (Maisel and DiSomma, 2007; Phua et al., 2005), screening for hypertrophic cardiomyopathy (Tigen et al., 2007), BNP act as significant predictor in patients with renal failure and in hemodialyzed patients (Biasioli et al., 2007; Bruch et al., 2006a; Hildebrandt and Richards, 2008; Sommerer et al., 2007). Variety of noncardiac causes may also lead to moderate elevations of the markers (BNP plasma concentrations of 100–400 pg/ml). In addition, normal marker levels may be observed in > 20% of patients with long-term stable heart failure. (Morrison et al., 2002)

2.6. Biochemical and Analytical Issues for Natriuretic Peptides

Concentration of natriuretic peptides is determined by various immunoassays using antibodies directed to the different epitopes. All natriuretic peptides are derived from preprohormones (preproANP and and preproBNP) containing signal sequence at the N-terminal end. The prohormones (proANP and proBNP) are produced by cleavage of signal peptide and then are further split into inactive longer N-terminal fragments (NT-proANP or NT-proBNP) and biologically active shorter C-terminal peptide (ANP and BNP). Both N- and C-terminal fragments are released in blood in equimolar amounts. However, ANP and BNP have shorter plasma half-lives and lower plasma concentration than NT-proBNP and NT-proANP. Thus, setting up an immunoassay for N-terminal fragments should be easier because their plasma concentrations are higher than those BNP and ANP. NT-proBNP may be affected by the several analytical problems concerning specifities and various linearities (Clerico and Emdin, 2004). Summary of relative advantages of active peptide assays and inactive propeptide assays is listed in table 2 (adapted from Clerico and Emdin, 2004)

Table 2. Relative advantages of ANP/BNP and NT-proANP/NTproBNP assays

ANP/BNP	NT-proANP/BNP
Close correlation between hormonal and immunologic activities	Higher and more stable circulating concentrations
	Lower degradation *in vivo* and *in vitro*
Better correlation with physiologic or clinical conditions after acute changes of hemodynamics	Longer half-life

2.6.1. Specimen Collection

For NT-proBNP, serum, or heparin plasma is the specimen of choice on the larger instruments in clinical laboratories. EDTA plasma gives a consistent negative bias (8-10%) compared with serum samples of NT-proBNP. For ANP and proANPx, EDTA plasma is preferred.

For BNP, EDTA anticoagulated whole blood or plasma appears to be only acceptable specimen of choice. The influence of stabilizing and anticoagulant additives has been mentioned (Lubien et al., 2002; Morrison et al., 2002).

2.6.2. Diagnostic Accuracy of Natriuretic Peptide Assays

Various studies evaluated the diagnostic efficiency of natriuretic peptides as screening method in general population (Nakamura et al., 2002; Vasan et al., 2002) and in patients with suspected heart failures in low-risk and high risk populations (Apple et al., 2003; Cowie et al., 1997; Hobbs et al., 2002; Maisel et al., 2002; Richards et al., 1998). Some studies mentioned the similar diagnostic efficiency in patients with congenital, valvular or chronic ischemic heart diseases and left ventricular impairment (Kotaska et al., 2006b; Vanderheyden et al., 2006). Significant importance show also studies in elderly people suspected to have heart failure (Hutcheon et al., 2002). Summary of selected studies is listed in table 3.

Table 3. Study protocols and diagnostic accuracy of natriuretic peptide assay in patients with various heart diseases

Reference	No. of patients, Diagnosis	Peptide, Cut off (Assay)	AUC	Sensitivity (%)	Specificity (%)	PPV (%)	NPV (%)
Cowie et al., 1997	122 patients, HF	ANP (RIA) NT-proANP (RIA) BNP (RIA)	0.93 0.89 0.96	97 97 97	72 66 84	55 54 70	98 98 98
Vasan et al., 2002	3177, LVH	BNP (IRMA)	0.75		95	38 Men 30 Women	92 Men 93 Women
Nakamura et al., 2002	1098, low prevalence CHD	BNP(IRMA), 50 ng/l	0.97	90	95	44	100
Apple et al., 2003	334, HF, 8 month monitoring	BNP (ILMA), 28.9 pmol/l	0.92	95	77	85	91
Hobbs et al., 2002	591, risk of HF	NT-proBNP (ELISA), 36 pmol/l	0.92	100	70	7	100
Richards et al., 1998	121, AMI	NT-proBNP (RIA), 160 pmol/l		91	72	39	97
Kotaska et al., 2006b	42, CD,CHD,VD	NT-proBNP (ECLIA), 130 ng/l	0.93	98	79	-	-
Vanderheyden et al., 2006	72, ventricular dysfunction	NT-proBNP (ECLIA), 358 ng/l BNP (Biosite), 139 ng/l	0.8 0.85	100 84	61 71	66 68	100 85
Hutcheon et al., 2002	299, old patients, abnormal ECG	BNP (RIA), 35 ng/l		94	69	24	97

LVH- left ventricular hypertrophy
CHD – chronic heart disease
HF- heart failure
CD – congenital heart disease
VD – valvular heart disease
ECG - echocardiogram

AUC – Area under the curve
NPV – negative predictive value
PPV – positive predictive value

On the contrary, some studies are less convincing regarding the ability of natriuretic peptide assays to identify patients with significant ventricular damage after acute myocardial infarction (Omland et al., 1996; Panteghini et al., 2003)

2.6.3. Reference Values of Natriuretic Peptides

The influence of age, gender, ethnicity has been shown to influence what may be considered as a physiological concentration (Alehagen et al., 2007; Clerico et al., 2002; Clerico and Emdin, 2004; Hess et al., 2005; Jensen et al., 1997; Redfield et al., 2002). Paediatric reference values are mentioned in many studies (Ationu and Carter, 1993; Mir et al., 2006; Yoshibayashi et al., 1995) Reference values are related also to the type of the immunoassay (Puschendorf and Mair, 2003). The summary of selected reference values in various age groups is listed in table 4.

Table 4. Reference values of natriuretic peptides in various age groups

Study	Method/number of individuals	Reference values
Ationu and Carter, 1993	RIA/ 40 individuals	Children: BNP: 31± 4 pg/ml ANP: 27± 3 pg/ml Adults: BNP: 12± 2 pg/ml ANP: 36± 2 pg/ml
Yoshibayashi et al., 1995	IRMA/ 58 individuals	Newborn: BNP: 56.7±49.6 pg/ml Umbilical cord: BNP:2.7±1.4 pg/ml
Jensen et al., 1997	RIA/124 individuals	BNP: 1.8± 1 pg/ml
Clerico et al., 2002	IRMA/216 adult individuals	ANP: Men: 16.7±10 pg/ml Women: 18.8± 11.7 pg/ml BNP: Men: 7.7±7.1 pg/ml Women: 12.2±10.2 pg/ml
Clerico and Emdin, 2004	IRMA/292 adult individuals	BNP: Men 20 – 50 years: 5.9±6.0 ng/l Men > 50 years: 10.1±7.8 ng/l Women 20 – 50 years: 10.0±8.3 ng/l Women > 50 years: 15.6±11.8 ng/l
Hess et al., 2005	ECLIA/1980 blood donors	NT-proBNP: Males: cut off value 84 pg/ml Females: cut off value 146 pg/ml
Mir et al., 2006	434 individuals	NT-proBNP: 0-9 years: cut off 12.6 fmol/ml 10-14 years: cut off 9.4 fmol/ml 15-19 years: cut off 4.1 fmol/ml >19 years: cut off 4,1 fmol/ml
Alehagen et al., 2007	218 individuals, elder, mean age 73 years	NT-proBNP: cut off 540 pg/ml BNP: cut off 97 pg/ml
Puschendorf and Mair, 2003	RIA	ANP: 0.11-0.60 nmol/l (plasma without extraction) BNP: 1.5-9 pmol/l
Roche NT-proBNP	ECLIA	NT-proBNP: Men < 50 years: 5 – 84 ng/l Men 50 - 75 years: 5 - 94 ng/l Men > 75 years: 5 – 450 ng/l Women < 50 years: 5 – 155 ng/l Women 50-75 years: 5 – 222 ng/l Women > 75 years 5 – 450 ng/l

Conversion factors: ANP: 1 pg/ml = 0.325 pmol/l, BNP: 1 pg/ml = 0.289 pmol/l, NT-proBNP: 1 pg/ml=0.118pmol/l

Conclusion

Nariuretic peptides are clinicaly useful markers for monitoring various types of heart diseases of different etiology as well as prognostic factors and tools for therapeutic decision making in various types of heart impairment.

References

Alehagen, U., Goetze, J. P., and Dahlstrom, U. (2007): Reference intervals and decision limits for B-type natriuretic peptide (BNP) and its precursor (Nt-proBNP) in the elderly. *Clin Chim Acta* **382**, 8-14.

Alpert, J. S., Thygesen, K., Antman, E., and Bassand, J. P. (2000): Myocardial infarction redefined--a consensus document of The Joint European Society of Cardiology/American College of Cardiology Committee for the redefinition of myocardial infarction. *J Am Coll Cardiol* **36**, 959-69.

Angermann, C. E., and Ertl, G. (2004): [Natriuretic peptides--new diagnostic markers in heart disease]. *Herz* **29**, 609-17.

Apple, F. S., Trinity, E., Steen, J., Prawer, S., and Wu, A. H. (2003): BNP test utilization for CHF in community hospital practice. *Clin Chim Acta* **328**, 191-3.

Ationu, A., and Carter, N. D. (1993): Brain and atrial natriuretic peptide plasma concentrations in normal healthy children. *Br J Biomed Sci* **50**, 92-5.

Atwater, B. D., Milford-Beland, S., Newby, L. K., Hernandez, A. F., Peacock, W. F., Gibler, W. B., Christenson, R. H., Ohman, E. M., Peterson, E. D., and Roe, M. T. (2007): Patterns and implications of B-type natriuretic peptide measurement in patients with non-ST-segment elevation acute coronary syndromes. *Am J Cardiol* **100**, 1727-33.

Bettencourt, P., Azevedo, A., Pimenta, J., Frioes, F., Ferreira, S., and Ferreira, A. (2004): N-terminal-pro-brain natriuretic peptide predicts outcome after hospital discharge in heart failure patients. *Circulation* **110**, 2168-74.

Bhalla, V., Willis, S., and Maisel, A. S. (2004): B-type natriuretic peptide: the level and the drug--partners in the diagnosis of congestive heart failure. *Congest Heart Fail* **10**, 3-27.

Biasioli, S., Zamperetti, M., Borin, D., Guidi, G., De Fanti, E., and Schiavon, R. (2007): Significance of plasma B-type natriuretic peptide in hemodialysis patients: blood sample timing and comorbidity burden. *Asaio J* **53**, 587-91.

Bibbins-Domingo, K., Gupta, R., Na, B., Wu, A. H., Schiller, N. B., and Whooley, M. A. (2007): N-terminal fragment of the prohormone brain-type natriuretic peptide (NT-proBNP), cardiovascular events, and mortality in patients with stable coronary heart disease. *Jama* **297**, 169-76.

Bruch, C., Reinecke, H., Stypmann, J., Rothenburger, M., Schmid, C., Breithardt, G., Wichter, T., and Gradaus, R. (2006a): N-terminal pro-brain natriuretic peptide, kidney disease and outcome in patients with chronic heart failure. *J Heart Lung Transplant* **25**, 1135-41.

Bruch, C., Rothenburger, M., Gotzmann, M., Sindermann, J., Scheld, H. H., Breithardt, G., and Wichter, T. (2006b): Risk stratification in chronic heart failure: independent and incremental prognostic value of echocardiography and brain natriuretic peptide and its N-terminal fragment. *J Am Soc Echocardiogr* **19**, 522-8.

Clerico, A., Del Ry, S., Maffei, S., Prontera, C., Emdin, M., and Giannessi, D. (2002): The circulating levels of cardiac natriuretic hormones in healthy adults: effects of age and sex. *Clin Chem Lab Med* **40**, 371-7.

Clerico, A., and Emdin, M. (2004): Diagnostic accuracy and prognostic relevance of the measurement of cardiac natriuretic peptides: a review. *Clin Chem* **50**, 33-50.

Cowie, M. R., Struthers, A. D., Wood, D. A., Coats, A. J., Thompson, S. G., Poole-Wilson, P. A., and Sutton, G. C. (1997): Value of natriuretic peptides in assessment of patients with possible new heart failure in primary care. *Lancet* **350**, 1349-53.

de Lemos, J. A., McGuire, D. K., and Drazner, M. H. (2003): B-type natriuretic peptide in cardiovascular disease. *Lancet* **362**, 316-22.

Del Ry, S., Giannessi, D., Maltinti, M., Prontera, C., Iervasi, A., Colotti, C., Emdin, M., L'Abbate, A., and Neglia, D. (2007): Increased levels of C-type natriuretic peptide in patients with idiopathic left ventricular dysfunction. *Peptides* **28**, 1068-73.

Flezzani, P., McIntyre, R. W., Xuan, Y. T., Su, Y. F., Leslie, J. B., and Watkins, W. D. (1988): Atrial natriuretic peptide plasma levels during cardiac surgery. *J Cardiothorac Anesth* **2**, 274-80.

Gardner, R. S., Chong, V., Morton, I., and McDonagh, T. A. (2005): N-terminal brain natriuretic peptide is a more powerful predictor of mortality than endothelin-1, adrenomedullin and tumour necrosis factor-alpha in patients referred for consideration of cardiac transplantation. *Eur J Heart Fail* **7**, 253-60.

Hammerer-Lercher, A., Neubauer, E., Muller, S., Pachinger, O., Puschendorf, B., and Mair, J. (2001): Head-to-head comparison of N-terminal pro-brain natriuretic peptide, brain natriuretic peptide and N-terminal pro-atrial natriuretic peptide in diagnosing left ventricular dysfunction. *Clin Chim Acta* **310**, 193-7.

Heeschen, C., Hamm, C. W., Mitrovic, V., Lantelme, N. H., and White, H. D. (2004): N-terminal pro-B-type natriuretic peptide levels for dynamic risk stratification of patients with acute coronary syndromes. *Circulation* **110**, 3206-12.

Hess, G., Runkel, S., Zdunek, D., and Hitzler, W. E. (2005): Reference interval determination for N-terminal-B-type natriuretic peptide (NT-proBNP): a study in blood donors. *Clin Chim Acta* **360**, 187-93.

Hildebrandt, P., and Richards, A. M. (2008): Amino-terminal pro-B-type natriuretic peptide testing in patients with diabetes mellitus and with systemic hypertension. *Am J Cardiol* **101**, 21-4.

Hobbs, F. D., Davis, R. C., Roalfe, A. K., Hare, R., Davies, M. K., and Kenkre, J. E. (2002): Reliability of N-terminal pro-brain natriuretic peptide assay in diagnosis of heart failure: cohort study in representative and high risk community populations. *Bmj* **324**, 1498.

Hunt, P. J., Espiner, E. A., Nicholls, M. G., Richards, A. M., and Yandle, T. G. (1997): The role of the circulation in processing pro-brain natriuretic peptide (proBNP) to amino-terminal BNP and BNP-32. *Peptides* **18**, 1475-81.

Hutcheon, S. D., Gillespie, N. D., Struthers, A. D., and McMurdo, M. E. (2002): B-type natriuretic peptide in the diagnosis of cardiac disease in elderly day hospital patients. *Age Ageing* **31**, 295-301.

Cheng, V., Kazanagra, R., Garcia, A., Lenert, L., Krishnaswamy, P., Gardetto, N., Clopton, P., and Maisel, A. (2001): A rapid bedside test for B-type peptide predicts treatment outcomes in patients admitted for decompensated heart failure: a pilot study. *J Am Coll Cardiol* **37**, 386-91.

James, S. K., Lindahl, B., Siegbahn, A., Stridsberg, M., Venge, P., Armstrong, P., Barnathan, E. S., Califf, R., Topol, E. J., Simoons, M. L., and Wallentin, L. (2003): N-terminal pro-brain natriuretic peptide and other risk markers for the separate prediction of mortality and subsequent myocardial infarction in patients with unstable coronary artery disease: a Global Utilization of Strategies To Open occluded arteries (GUSTO)-IV substudy. *Circulation* **108**, 275-81.

Jensen, K. T., Carstens, J., Ivarsen, P., and Pedersen, E. B. (1997): A new, fast and reliable radioimmunoassay of brain natriuretic peptide in human plasma. Reference values in healthy subjects and in patients with different diseases. *Scand J Clin Lab Invest* **57**, 529-40.

Jernberg, T., James, S., Lindahl, B., Stridsberg, M., Venge, P., and Wallentin, L. (2005): NT-ProBNP in non-ST-elevation acute coronary syndrome. *J Card Fail* **11**, S54-8.

Jourdain, P., Jondeau, G., Funck, F., Gueffet, P., Le Helloco, A., Donal, E., Aupetit, J. F., Aumont, M. C., Galinier, M., Eicher, J. C., Cohen-Solal, A., and Juilliere, Y. (2007): Plasma brain natriuretic peptide-guided therapy to improve outcome in heart failure: the STARS-BNP Multicenter Study. *J Am Coll Cardiol* **49**, 1733-9.

Khan, A. R., Birbach, M., Cohen, M. S., Ittenbach, R. F., Spray, T. L., Levy, R. J., and Gaynor, J. W. (2008): Chronic hypoxemia increases ventricular brain natriuretic peptide precursors in neonatal swine. *Ann Thorac Surg* **85**, 618-23.

Koch, A. M., Zink, S., and Singer, H. (2008): B-type natriuretic peptide in patients with systemic right ventricle. *Cardiology* **110**, 1-7.

Kotaska, K., Popelova, J., Tiserova, M., Telekes, P., Vrzanova, M., Bronsky, J., Halacova, M., Kukacka, J., and Prusa, R. (2006a): NT-proBNP and BNP values in cardiac patients with different degree of left ventricular systolic dysfunction. *Biomed Pap Med Fac Univ Palacky Olomouc Czech Repub* **150**, 125-30.

Kotaska, K., Popelova, J., Tiserova, M., Telekes, P., Vrzanova, M., Bronsky, J., Halacova, M., Kukacka, J., and Prusa, R. (2006b): The relevance of brain natriuretic peptides investigation in various cardiovascular diseases. *Biomed Pap Med Fac Univ Palacky Olomouc Czech Repub* **150**, 285-8.

Lainchbury, J. G., Campbell, E., Frampton, C. M., Yandle, T. G., Nicholls, M. G., and Richards, A. M. (2003): Brain natriuretic peptide and n-terminal brain natriuretic peptide in the diagnosis of heart failure in patients with acute shortness of breath. *J Am Coll Cardiol* **42**, 728-35.

Larsson, D. A., Meurling, C. J., Holmqvist, F., Waktare, J. E., and Thilen, U. J. (2007): The diagnostic and prognostic value of brain natriuretic peptides in adults with a systemic morphologically right ventricle or Fontan-type circulation. *Int J Cardiol* **114**, 345-51.

Lubien, E., DeMaria, A., Krishnaswamy, P., Clopton, P., Koon, J., Kazanegra, R., Gardetto, N., Wanner, E., and Maisel, A. S. (2002): Utility of B-natriuretic peptide in detecting diastolic dysfunction: comparison with Doppler velocity recordings. *Circulation* **105**, 595-601.

Maisel, A. S. (2001): Practical approaches to treating patients with acute decompensated heart failure. *J Card Fail* **7**, 13-7.

Maisel, A. S., and DiSomma, S. (2007): B-type natriuretic peptide-guided therapy and prognosis in acutely ill patients with pulmonary disease. *Crit Care Med* **35**, 301-3.

Maisel, A. S., Krishnaswamy, P., Nowak, R. M., McCord, J., Hollander, J. E., Duc, P., Omland, T., Storrow, A. B., Abraham, W. T., Wu, A. H., Clopton, P., Steg, P. G.,

Westheim, A., Knudsen, C. W., Perez, A., Kazanegra, R., Herrmann, H. C., and McCullough, P. A. (2002): Rapid measurement of B-type natriuretic peptide in the emergency diagnosis of heart failure. *N Engl J Med* **347**, 161-7.

Martinez-Dolz, L., Almenar, L., Moro, J., Aguero, J., Hervas, I., Rueda, J., Rivera, M., Arnau, M. A., Mateo, A., and Salvador, A. (2007): Prognostic value of brain natriuretic peptide in heart transplant patients. *J Heart Lung Transplant* **26**, 986-91.

McDonagh, T. A., Robb, S. D., Murdoch, D. R., Morton, J. J., Ford, I., Morrison, C. E., Tunstall-Pedoe, H., McMurray, J. J., and Dargie, H. J. (1998): Biochemical detection of left-ventricular systolic dysfunction. *Lancet* **351**, 9-13.

Mir, T. S., Flato, M., Falkenberg, J., Haddad, M., Budden, R., Weil, J., Albers, S., and Laer, S. (2006): Plasma concentrations of N-terminal brain natriuretic peptide in healthy children, adolescents, and young adults: effect of age and gender. *Pediatr Cardiol* **27**, 73-7.

Morrison, L. K., Harrison, A., Krishnaswamy, P., Kazanegra, R., Clopton, P., and Maisel, A. (2002): Utility of a rapid B-natriuretic peptide assay in differentiating congestive heart failure from lung disease in patients presenting with dyspnea. *J Am Coll Cardiol* **39**, 202-9.

Morrow, D. A., de Lemos, J. A., Sabatine, M. S., Murphy, S. A., Demopoulos, L. A., DiBattiste, P. M., McCabe, C. H., Gibson, C. M., Cannon, C. P., and Braunwald, E. (2003): Evaluation of B-type natriuretic peptide for risk assessment in unstable angina/non-ST-elevation myocardial infarction: B-type natriuretic peptide and prognosis in TACTICS-TIMI 18. *J Am Coll Cardiol* **41**, 1264-72.

Nakamura, M., Endo, H., Nasu, M., Arakawa, N., Segawa, T., and Hiramori, K. (2002): Value of plasma B type natriuretic peptide measurement for heart disease screening in a Japanese population. *Heart* **87**, 131-5.

Nielsen, O. W., McDonagh, T. A., Robb, S. D., and Dargie, H. J. (2003): Retrospective analysis of the cost-effectiveness of using plasma brain natriuretic peptide in screening for left ventricular systolic dysfunction in the general population. *J Am Coll Cardiol* **41**, 113-20.

O'Brien, R. J., Squire, I. B., Demme, B., Davies, J. E., and Ng, L. L. (2003): Pre-discharge, but not admission, levels of NT-proBNP predict adverse prognosis following acute LVF. *Eur J Heart Fail* **5**, 499-506.

Omland, T., Aakvaag, A., Bonarjee, V. V., Caidahl, K., Lie, R. T., Nilsen, D. W., Sundsfjord, J. A., and Dickstein, K. (1996): Plasma brain natriuretic peptide as an indicator of left ventricular systolic function and long-term survival after acute myocardial infarction. Comparison with plasma atrial natriuretic peptide and N-terminal proatrial natriuretic peptide. *Circulation* **93**, 1963-9.

Omland, T., Sabatine, M. S., Jablonski, K. A., Rice, M. M., Hsia, J., Wergeland, R., Landaas, S., Rouleau, J. L., Domanski, M. J., Hall, C., Pfeffer, M. A., and Braunwald, E. (2007): Prognostic value of B-Type natriuretic peptides in patients with stable coronary artery disease: the PEACE Trial. *J Am Coll Cardiol* **50**, 205-14.

Palladini, G., Campana, C., Klersy, C., Balduini, A., Vadacca, G., Perfetti, V., Perlini, S., Obici, L., Ascari, E., d'Eril, G. M., Moratti, R., and Merlini, G. (2003): Serum N-terminal pro-brain natriuretic peptide is a sensitive marker of myocardial dysfunction in AL amyloidosis. *Circulation* **107**, 2440-5.

Panteghini, M., Cuccia, C., Bonetti, G., Pagani, F., Giubbini, R., and Bonini, E. (2003): Rapid determination of brain natriuretic peptide in patients with acute myocardial infarction. *Clin Chem Lab Med* **41**, 164-8.

Pfister, R., Scholz, M., Wielckens, K., Erdmann, E., and Schneider, C. A. (2004): Use of NT-proBNP in routine testing and comparison to BNP. *Eur J Heart Fail* **6**, 289-93.

Phua, J., Lim, T. K., and Lee, K. H. (2005): B-type natriuretic peptide: issues for the intensivist and pulmonologist. *Crit Care Med* **33**, 2094-13.

Puschendorf, B and Mair, J: Cardiac Diseases, In: Thomas, L, Clinical laboratory diagnostics, 1st Edition, TH Books, Frankfurt, pages 101-120.

Redfield, M. M., Rodeheffer, R. J., Jacobsen, S. J., Mahoney, D. W., Bailey, K. R., and Burnett, J. C., Jr. (2002): Plasma brain natriuretic peptide concentration: impact of age and gender. *J Am Coll Cardiol* **40**, 976-82.

Richards, A. M., Nicholls, M. G., Yandle, T. G., Frampton, C., Espiner, E. A., Turner, J. G., Buttimore, R. C., Lainchbury, J. G., Elliott, J. M., Ikram, H., Crozier, I. G., and Smyth, D. W. (1998): Plasma N-terminal pro-brain natriuretic peptide and adrenomedullin: new neurohormonal predictors of left ventricular function and prognosis after myocardial infarction. *Circulation* **97**, 1921-9.

Seilhamer, J. J., Arfsten, A., Miller, J. A., Lundquist, P., Scarborough, R. M., Lewicki, J. A., and Porter, J. G. (1989): Human and canine gene homologs of porcine brain natriuretic peptide. *Biochem Biophys Res Commun* **165**, 650-8.

Seino, Y., Ogawa, A., Yamashita, T., Fukushima, M., Ogata, K., Fukumoto, H., and Takano, T. (2004): Application of NT-proBNP and BNP measurements in cardiac care: a more discerning marker for the detection and evaluation of heart failure. *Eur J Heart Fail* **6**, 295-300.

Selcuk, M. T., Selcuk, H., Maden, O., Erbay, A. R., Temizhan, A., Aksu, T., Saydam, G. S., and Korkmaz, S. (2007): The effect of percutaneous balloon mitral valvuloplasty on N-terminal- pro B- type natriuretic peptide plasma levels in mitral stenosis. *Int Heart J* **48**, 579-90.

Shimizu, H., Masuta, K., Aono, K., Asada, H., Sasakura, K., Tamaki, M., Sugita, K., and Yamada, K. (2002): Molecular forms of human brain natriuretic peptide in plasma. *Clin Chim Acta* **316**, 129-35.

Sommerer, C., Beimler, J., Schwenger, V., Heckele, N., Katus, H. A., Giannitsis, E., and Zeier, M. (2007): Cardiac biomarkers and survival in haemodialysis patients. *Eur J Clin Invest* **37**, 350-6.

Sun, T. W., Zhang, S. Y., and Wang, L. X. (2008): Plasma B-type natriuretic peptide for early diagnosis of allograft rejection after renal transplantation. *Med Hypotheses* **70**, 1160-2.

Taniguchi, R., Sato, Y., Nishio, Y., Kimura, T., and Kita, T. (2006): Measurements of baseline and follow-up concentrations of cardiac troponin-T and brain natriuretic peptide in patients with heart failure from various etiologies. *Heart Vessels* **21**, 344-9.

Taniguchi, R., Sato, Y., Yamada, T., Ooba, M., Higuchi, H., Matsumori, A., Kimura, T., and Kita, T. (2004): Combined measurements of cardiac troponin T and N-terminal pro-brain natriuretic peptide in patients with heart failure. *Circ J* **68**, 1160-4.

Tigen, K., Karaahmet, T., Kahveci, G., Tanalp, A. C., Bitigen, A., Fotbolcu, H., Bayrak, F., Mutlu, B., and Basaran, Y. (2007): N-terminal pro brain natriuretic peptide to predict prognosis in dilated cardiomyopathy with sinus rhythm. *Heart Lung Circ* **16**, 290-4.

Troughton, R. W., and Richards, A. M. (2008): Outpatient monitoring and treatment of chronic heart failure guided by amino-terminal pro-B-type natriuretic peptide measurement. *Am J Cardiol* **101**, 72-5.

Vanderheyden, M., Bartunek, Claeys, G., Manoharan, G., Beckers, J. F., and Ide, L. (2006): Head to head comparison of N-terminal pro-B-type natriuretic peptide and B-type natriuretic peptide in patients with/without left ventricular systolic dysfunction. *Clin Biochem* **39**, 640-5.

Vanderheyden, M., Bartunek, J., and Goethals, M. (2004): Brain and other natriuretic peptides: molecular aspects. *Eur J Heart Fail* **6,** 261-8.

Vasan, R. S., Benjamin, E. J., Larson, M. G., Leip, E. P., Wang, T. J., Wilson, P. W., and Levy, D. (2002): Plasma natriuretic peptides for community screening for left ventricular hypertrophy and systolic dysfunction: the Framingham heart study. *Jama* **288**, 1252-9.

Yamamoto, K., Burnett, J. C., Jr., Jougasaki, M., Nishimura, R. A., Bailey, K. R., Saito, Y., Nakao, K., and Redfield, M. M. (1996): Superiority of brain natriuretic peptide as a hormonal marker of ventricular systolic and diastolic dysfunction and ventricular hypertrophy. *Hypertension* **28**, 988-94.

Yasumura, Y. (2004): [Natriuretic peptides and valvular heart disease]. *Nippon Rinsho* **62** Suppl 9, 93-4.

Yoshibayashi, M., Kamiya, T., Saito, Y., Nakao, K., Nishioka, K., Temma, S., Itoh, H., Shirakami, G., and Matsuo, H. (1995): Plasma brain natriuretic peptide concentrations in healthy children from birth to adolescence: marked and rapid increase after birth. *Eur J Endocrinol* **133**, 207-9.

Yu, C. M., Fung, J. W., Zhang, Q., Chan, C. K., Chan, I., Chan, Y. S., Kong, S. L., Sanderson, J. E., and Lam, C. W. (2005): Improvement of serum NT-ProBNP predicts improvement in cardiac function and favorable prognosis after cardiac resynchronization therapy for heart failure. *J Card Fail* **11**, S42-6.

In: Heart Disease in Men
Editors: A.B. Todd and M.H. Mosley, pp. 275-291
ISBN 978-1-60692-297-2

Chapter 13

SEX-RELATED DIFFERENCES IN TIME TO SURGICAL REVASCULARIZATION AND POSTOPERATIVE MORTALITY*

***B. Sobolev*[1]*, G. Fradet*[2]*, L. Kuramoto*[3] *and A. Levy*[1]**
[1]The University of British Columbia, Vancouver, BC, Canada
[2]St. Paul's Hospital, Vancouver, BC, Canada
[3]Centre for Clinical Epidemiology and Evaluation, Vancouver, BC, Canada

Abstract

In this chapter, we compare the risk of postoperative in-hospital death between men and women undergoing coronary artery bypass grafting. Using data from a population-based registry, we examine whether postoperative mortality during admission for the procedure differed between the sexes and whether any such differences were related to the time that patients waited for surgery, independent of other risk factors. We found a significant difference in the risk of death: 1.4% for men and 2.4% for women. Post-operative death was more likely among patients who were older, had higher operative risk, and had more coexisting medical conditions. After adjustment for clinical risk factors, the rate of postoperative mortality was similar for men and women in the high-risk group but differed for the lower risk groups. In terms of other aspects of care, we also found differences between the sexes in time to surgical revascularization, but only among those with lower operative risk. However, the time that patients waited for surgery after diagnostic catheterization did not influence the difference in the risk of postoperative death between men and women.

1. Introduction

Coronary artery bypass grafting (CABG) is indicated to alleviate symptoms and to reduce the risk of death among patients who have limiting angina that persists despite optimal medical treatment and suitable coronary anatomy [1]. Randomized trials and observational

*This chapter has been peer reviewed.

studies have demonstrated survival benefits associated with CABG. The intervention has been shown to improve long-term survival in symptomatic patients with left main coronary disease, triple-vessel disease, or two-vessel disease with significant stenosis of the proximal left anterior descending coronary artery whose condition is stable [2]. In practice, postoperative morbidity and mortality may be higher among patients who are older, or sicker, those with multiple comorbidities, and those for whom percutaneous coronary intervention has failed or who do not qualify for such treatment [3, 4, 5].

The proportion of patients who die after surgery before they can be discharged from hospital (i.e., during the same hospital admission) is an important indicator of the quality of surgical care [6, 7]. It also reflects the impact of differences in clinical factors among patients treated at different sites [8]. A number of observational studies comparing rates of postoperative death between men and women have provided evidence of greater in-hospital and 30-day mortality among women [9, 10, 11, 12, 13, 14], with several studies reporting no difference after adjustment for clinical characteristics [15, 16, 17, 18]. For example, a recent report based on the Society of Thoracic Surgeons National Cardiac Surgery Database showed a postoperative mortality rate of 2.2% for men and 3.5% for women [19].

Reasons offered for the higher rates among women include older age, more urgent need for revascularization, and greater burden of coexisting diseases, all of which would augment their operative risk. To investigate this issue, Edwards et al. [10] analyzed records from the Society of Thoracic Surgeons database on the postoperative survival of more than 300,000 patients who underwent CABG between 1994 and 1997. After adjustment for other risk factors, sex remained an independent factor associated with postoperative mortality for all patients except those with very high risk.

Studies from the Cleveland Clinic and the Northern New England Study Group have shown the impact of body size on postoperative mortality after CABG [20]. Women's smaller coronary arteries are thought to present greater technical challenges and thus to increase the potential for incomplete revascularization [21, 22]. Other proposed explanations for sex-related differences in postoperative mortality include variation in time to surgical treatment after cardiac catheterization, a test in which dye is injected into the patient's circulatory system to show blockages in the heart's blood vessels; this variation is thought to occur because of gender bias in decision-making related to cardiac care [23]. King et al. [24] have extended our current understanding of sex-related differences in the outcomes of surgical revascularization by identifying a close link between coronary anatomy and the treatment modality after cardiac catheterization such as medication or procedures to open the vessels or bypass the blockages.

Surprisingly, few studies have correlated the in-hospital mortality rate with the timing of surgery, yet this relation is important in deciding how much capacity is required to avoid unacceptable delays that put patients at greater risk [25]. In addition, it has been argued that cardiologists, when referring a patient for consultation with a cardiac surgeon, have a duty to inform those patients of the likely extent of treatment delay and the associated risks [26]. To date, however, there have been no direct estimates of the reduction in postoperative mortality afforded by performing CABG within the time deemed acceptable to consultant surgeons. Therefore, the impact of time between cardiac catheterization and surgical revascularization on sex-related differences in postoperative mortality is not known.

In this chapter, we report the results of a study examining whether postoperative mortality during admission for CABG differed between men and women and whether any such differences were related to the time that patients waited for surgery, independent of other risk factors. We determined the survival after surgical revascularization, using data from a population-based registry of all adults for whom a cardiac surgeon booked an operating room for coronary artery bypass surgery in one of the participating hospitals between 2000 and 2005. We focused only on the first revascularization procedure within a year of catheterization because that is the surgical procedure most likely indicated by the results of coronary angiography.

2. Evidence from a Population-Based Registry

2.1. Methods

Data Sources

We obtained data for this study from the British Columbia Cardiac Registries (BCCR). This prospective database stores dates of catheterization and surgical procedure, along with disease severity and other risk factors, for all patients who have undergone revascularization since 1991 in any of the 4 tertiary care hospitals providing cardiac care to adult residents of British Columbia, Canada [27]. To identify hospital admission and discharge dates, mode of admission for surgery, coexisting conditions, and in-hospital deaths, we used patients' Provincial Health Numbers to link deterministically BCCR records to the British Columbia Linked Health Database Hospital Separations File [28]. Emergency admissions were identified by the emergency or urgent code for admission from the emergency department or the emergency code for admission from the admitting department after registration on a surgical wait list. Coexisting conditions were identified on the basis of diagnoses reported in discharge abstracts created during the calendar year before the treatment [29].

Patients

The inception cohort consisted of all adult residents of British Columbia with established coronary artery disease and a record of surgery for isolated CABG in one of the participating hospitals between January 1, 2000, and December 31, 2005. We identified 11,521 patients meeting the initial inclusion criteria, but we excluded 475 records that contained either invalid data (date of surgery was not between the date of admission and the discharge date; n = 212) or insufficient information (date of catheterization in the year preceding surgery was not reported; n = 263). We excluded an additional 40 records for which urgency of treatment was unknown. The final study cohort therefore consisted of 11,006 patients who had undergone isolated CABG during the study period.

Operative Risk

We compared mortality rates for women and men, with patients categorized, on the basis of mode of admission, urgency of treatment, and extent of disease, into four groups emergency, high risk, medium risk and low risk (Table 1). When accepting patients for CABG, the cardiac surgeons used a common algorithm to set the urgency of treatment, taking account of the severity of patients' condition and considerations of expected benefit, such that the operation could be performed within a clinically appropriate time (shown in Table 1), as previously described [30].

Table 1. Definition of levels of operative risk

Operative risk	Target time for surgery	Description
Emergency		Emergency admission
High	3 days	Patients with left-main stenosis more than 70%
Medium	6 weeks	Patients with stable angina and extensive coronary artery disease (left-main stenosis more than 50%, triple-vessel disease, or double-vessel disease with significant proximal left anterior descending stenosis and impaired left ventricular function)
Low	12 weeks	Stable symptomatic patients with limited coronary artery disease (double-vessel disease with no lesion in the proximal left anterior descending artery and normal left ventricular function or single-vessel disease with significant stenosis of the proximal left anterior descending artery)

Time to Surgery

Upon consultation with a cardiac surgeon after diagnostic catheterization, access to CABG in British Columbia is managed either through direct admission to hospital or admission from a priority wait list. The number of patients undergoing surgery through direct admission and through wait lists is approximately the same. Because scheduling of surgery is done weekly, time to surgery for each patient was computed as the number of calendar weeks from catheterization to surgery. In this chapter, the phrases "time since catheterization" and "time to surgery" are used interchangeably.

Statistical Analysis

The primary outcome was death occurring after surgery but before discharge from hospital (i.e., during the same hospital admission) [8]. We used proportions to characterize the probability that a postoperative death occurred during the hospital admission and chi-square testing to compare the proportions between men and women. The effect of sex on the odds of in-hospital death was estimated by means of logistic regression, which yielded the odds ratio (OR) [31]. An OR less than 1 indicated that the odds of in-hospital death were lower for men than for women. Time to surgery was compared across study factors using the log–rank test [31].

In multivariate analysis, the effect of sex was adjusted for age, operative risk, known comorbidity during the year before the time of surgery, 2-year calendar period, institution where surgery was performed, method of managing access to surgery (i.e., direct admission or registration on a wait list), and time to surgery, because the existing literature suggests that these factors may be potential confounders for measuring the difference in mortality between the sexes. Specifically, elderly patients are more likely to undergo revascularization as an urgent procedure [32], and coexisting medical conditions may delay open heart surgery [33]. To control for coexisting conditions, each patient was classified as (1) presenting with no coexisting conditions; (2) presenting with congestive heart failure, diabetes mellitus, chronic obstructive pulmonary disease, rheumatoid arthritis, or cancer; or (3) presenting with other coexisting chronic conditions, specifically peripheral vascular disease, cerebrovascular disease, dementia, peptic ulcer disease, hemiplegia, renal disease, or liver disease [34]. The first set of coexisting conditions was used in a previous study on the appropriateness of coronary revascularization [35]. Because we were concerned that other illnesses might also delay surgery, we added the second set, which included conditions from the Charlson comorbidity index [36]. We entered two indicator variables in the models to represent three comorbidity categories, whereby patients without coexisting conditions formed the referent category.

Initially, the multivariate analysis adjusted for age, operative risk, comorbidity, 2-year calendar period, institution, and method of access management yielded partially adjusted ORs. Further adjustment for time to surgery yielded fully adjusted ORs. For emergency and high risk patients, time to surgery was entered as a continuous variable. For medium and low operative risk patients, time to surgery was entered as an indicator variable, with a value of 1 denoting a wait time beyond the recommended time for surgery. Patients who waited for CABG longer than the recommended time (6 or 12 weeks, depending on urgency) were classified as having undergone late surgery. Those who waited less than the recommended time were classified as having undergone early surgery.

The results in this chapter have been reported according to guidelines [37]. The University of British Columbia Ethics Board approved the study.

2.2. Results

Relation between Sex and Other Factors

We analyzed data for 11,006 patients who underwent CABG in British Columbia between 2000 and 2005, of whom 8,973 (81.5%) were men and 2,033 (18.5%) were women. The distribution of age, operative risk, extent of disease, comorbidity, and method of access management differed by sex (Table 2). Among patients who underwent CABG, men tended to be younger than women, with the largest age groups being 60 to 69 years for men (34.3%) and 70 to 79 years for women (40.7%) ($\chi^2 = 137.9$, df = 4, $p < 0.001$). Higher operative risks were less prevalent among men than among women (33.4% versus 38.7% for emergency and high-risk group combined) ($\chi^2 = 21.5$, df = 3, $p < 0.001$). The extent of disease differed by sex, with the percentage of patients with limited coronary artery disease being lower for men than for women (6.6% versus 9.3%) ($\chi^2 = 18.9$, df = 2, $p < 0.001$).

With a lower rate of major coexisting medical conditions among men than among women (42.7% versus 54.4%), sicker patients were less likely to be men ($\chi^2 = 105.1$, df = 2, $p < 0.001$). The number of procedures was similar across 2-year calendar periods for each sex ($\chi^2 = 2.6$, df = 2, $p = 0.28$). There was little variation by sex in the distribution of institutions, with the smallest percentage of men (22.5%) treated at institution 1 and the

Table 2. Characteristics of 11,006 patients who underwent isolated coronary artery bypass grafting in British Columbia in 2000–2005, by sex

	Sex; no. (%) of patients			
Characteristic	All ($n = 11,006$)	Men ($n = 8,973$)	Women ($n = 2,033$)	*p* value*
Age group (years)				
<50	728 (6.6)	626 (7.0)	102 (5.0)	< 0.001
50–59	2,412 (21.9)	2,093 (23.3)	319 (15.7)	
60–69	3,705 (33.7)	3,074 (34.3)	631 (31.0)	
70–79	3,604 (32.7)	2,777 (30.9)	827 (40.7)	
≥80	557 (5.1)	403 (4.5)	154 (7.6)	
Operative risk				
Emergency	1,568 (14.2)	1,245 (13.9)	323 (15.9)	< 0.001
High	2,215 (20.1)	1,752 (19.5)	463 (22.8)	
Medium	6,691 (60.8)	5,545 (61.8)	1,146 (56.4)	
Low	532 (4.8)	431 (4.8)	101 (5.0)	
Extent of disease				
Left main	2,529 (23.0)	2,062 (23.0)	467 (23.0)	< 0.001
Multivessel†	7,697 (69.9)	6,320 (70.4)	1,377 (67.7)	
Limited‡	780 (7.1)	591 (6.6)	189 (9.3)	
Comorbidity				
Major conditions§	4,936 (44.8)	3,831 (42.7)	1,105 (54.4)	< 0.001
Other conditions‖	3,930 (35.7)	3,275 (36.5)	655 (32.2)	
None	2,140 (19.4)	1,867 (20.8)	273 (13.4)	
Calendar period				
2000–2001	3,569 (32.4)	2,895 (32.3)	674 (33.2)	0.28
2002–2003	3,669 (33.3)	2,975 (33.2)	694 (34.1)	
2004–2005	3,768 (34.2)	3,103 (34.6)	665 (32.7)	
Institution				
1	2,511 (22.8)	2,018 (22.5)	493 (24.2)	0.08
2	2,616 (23.8)	2,171 (24.2)	445 (21.9)	
3	3,211 (29.2)	2,601 (29.0)	610 (30.0)	
4	2,668 (24.2)	2,183 (24.3)	485 (23.9)	
Access management				
Direct admission	5,261 (47.8)	4,177 (46.6)	1,084 (53.3)	< 0.001
Admission from a wait list	5,745 (52.2)	4,796 (53.4)	949 (46.7)	

*Chi-square test of association

†Two- or three-vessel disease with proximal left anterior descending coronary artery (PLAD)

‡Two-vessel disease with no PLAD or one-vessel disease with PLAD

§Congestive heart failure, diabetes mellitus, chronic obstructive pulmonary disease, rheumatoid arthritis, or cancer

‖Peripheral vascular disease, cerebrovascular disease, dementia, peptic ulcer disease, hemiplegia, renal disease, or liver disease

smallest percentage of women (21.9%) at institution 2 ($\chi^2 = 6.7$, df = 3, $p = 0.08$). A lower percentage of men than women accessed surgery via direct admission (46.6% versus 53.3%) ($\chi^2 = 30.4$, df = 1, $p < 0.001$).

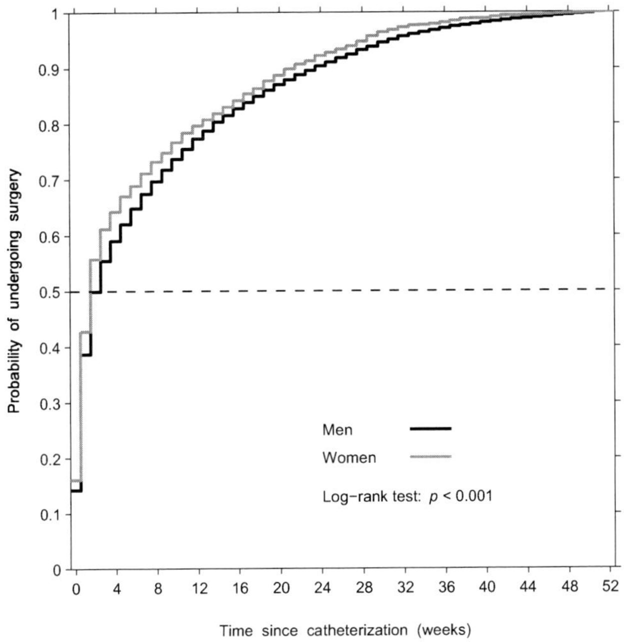

Figure 1. Probability of undergoing coronary artery bypass grafting according to time since catheterization, by sex, for all patients.

Distribution of Times from Catheterization to Surgery

The distribution of times from catheterization to surgery differed across all factors examined (Table 3). Men had longer waiting times to surgery than women (log–rank test statistic = 17.9, df = 1, $p < 0.001$) (Figure 1). Specifically, waiting times for men were such that 25%, 50%, and 75% underwent surgery within 1, 3, and 11 weeks after catheterization, respectively, whereas 50% and 75% of women underwent surgery within 2 and 10 weeks, respectively.

As expected, operative risk had a substantial influence on time to surgery, with shorter times for higher risk groups (log–rank test statistic = 2516.7, df = 3, $p < 0.001$). Men had longer waiting times (1 week) in the medium and low risk groups (log–rank test statistic = 9.9, df = 1, $p = 0.002$), but there was no difference in the emergency and high risk groups (log–rank test statistic = 0.28, df = 1, $p = 0.60$) (Figure 2).

Access to surgery differed by age group, with shorter waiting times for older patients (log–rank test statistic = 46.2, df = 4, $p < 0.001$). Extent of coronary artery disease also influenced waiting times, with shorter times among patients with left main coronary artery stenosis and longer times among patients with multivessel disease (log–rank test statistic = 373.3, df = 2, $p < 0.001$). In terms of comorbidities, waiting times tended to be longest for patients with no comorbidities, were shorter for those with major comorbidities, and were shortest for those with other coexisting medical conditions (log–rank test statistic = 630.3, df = 2, $p < 0.001$).

Calendar period was also associated time to surgery which were longest for the period

Table 3. Distribution of waiting times for isolated coronary artery bypass grafting, by various patient characteristics

Characteristic	No. of patients	Mean (SD)	Median (IQR)
Sex			
Men	8,973	8 (11)	3 (1–11)
Women	2,033	7 (10)	2 (1–10)
Age group (years)			
<50	728	7 (10)	2 (1–10)
50–59	2,412	8 (11)	2 (1–12)
60–69	3,705	8 (11)	3 (1–12)
70–79	3,604	7 (10)	2 (1–10)
≥80	557	6 (9)	2 (1–7)
Operative risk			
Emergency	1,568	2 (5)	1 (0–2)
High	2,215	3 (6)	1 (0–2)
Medium	6,691	10 (11)	5 (1–14)
Low	532	19 (13)	16 (8–29)
Extent of disease			
Left main	2,529	5 (8)	1 (1–6)
Multivessel*	7,697	9 (11)	3 (1–13)
Limited†	780	5 (10)	1 (0–5)
Comorbidity			
Major conditions‡	4,936	8 (11)	2 (1–11)
Other conditions§	3,930	5 (8)	1 (1–5)
None	2,140	12 (11)	9 (3–18)
Calendar period			
2000–2001	3,569	7 (10)	2 (1–11)
2002–2003	3,669	9 (12)	3 (1–14)
2004–2005	3,768	6 (9)	2 (1–8)
Institution			
1	2,511	9 (11)	3 (1–13)
2	2,616	5 (7)	2 (1–8)
3	3,211	8 (11)	2 (1–11)
4	2,668	9 (11)	2 (1–14)
Access management			
Direct admission	5,261	3 (6)	1 (1–2)
Admission from a wait list	5,745	12 (12)	8 (2–18)

Abbreviations: SD = standard deviation, IQR = interquartile range

*Two- or three-vessel disease with proximal left anterior descending coronary artery (PLAD)

†Two-vessel disease with no PLAD or one-vessel disease with PLAD

‡Congestive heart failure, diabetes mellitus, chronic obstructive pulmonary disease, rheumatoid arthritis, or cancer

§Peripheral vascular disease, cerebrovascular disease, dementia, peptic ulcer disease, hemiplegia, renal disease, or liver disease

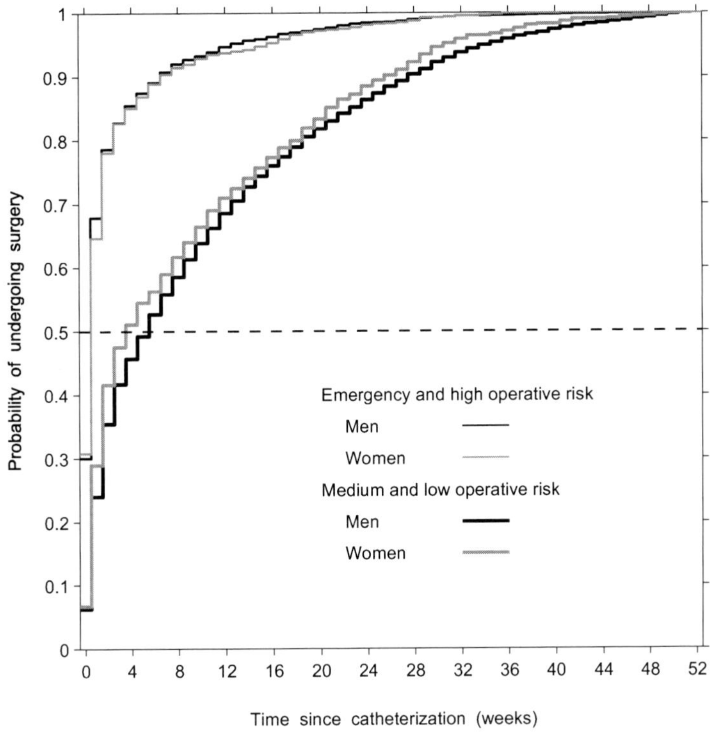

Figure 2. Probability of undergoing coronary artery bypass grafting according to time since catheterization, by sex and operative risk, for all patients.

2002–2003 (log–rank test statistic = 149.2, df = 2, $p < 0.001$). Three of the institutions had similar waiting times, but institution 2 had much shorter times (log–rank test statistic = 165.7, df = 3, $p < 0.001$). There was a strong association between method of access management and time to surgery, with shorter times experienced by patients who were admitted for surgery directly (log–rank test statistic = 2870.6, df = 1, $p < 0.001$).

Effect of Sex on Postoperative Mortality Rate

Of the 11,006 patients in this study, 177 (1.6%) died during the same hospital admission; more specifically, 1.4% of the men (129/8,973) and 2.4% of the women (48/2,033) died (Table 4). Among men who underwent the operation, in-hospital death was three-fifths as likely as among women (unadjusted OR = 0.60, 95% confidence interval [CI] 0.43–0.84) (Figure 3).

The risk of death was constant, at 1.6%, across the three 2-year calendar periods. The percentage of in-hospital deaths across institutions varied from 1.4% (37/2,668) at institution 4 to 1.9% (60/3,211) at institution 3. The risk of death was more than 2 times higher for patients who were admitted directly than for those who were admitted from a wait list (2.3% versus 1.0%) (unadjusted OR = 2.33, 95% CI 1.70–3.20).

The percentage of patients who died before discharge increased with age, from 0.5%

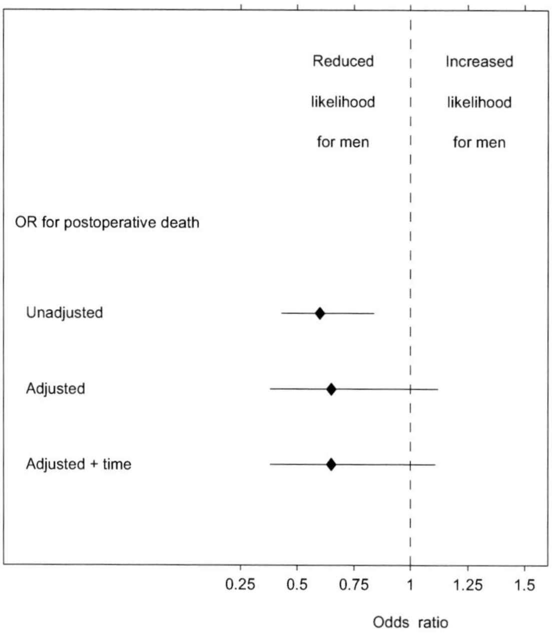

Figure 3. The odds ratios for postoperative death among medium and low operative risk patients.

(4/728) for patients less than 50 years of age to 1.1% (41/3,705) for patients 60 to 69 years of age to 5.0% (28/557) for patients 80 years of age or older (Table 4). There was an approximately linear relation between the logarithm of odds of in-hospital death and age (Figure 4), with an 0.56 increase, on average, for each decade in age. Therefore, in the multivariate models, age was entered as a continuous variable and the odds ratio for a decade increase in age was reported. Emergency patients were almost 5 times as likely as medium-risk patients to die in hospital (unadjusted OR = 4.92, 95% CI 3.48–6.97), and patients with high operative risk were 2 times as likely as medium risk patients to die in hospital (unadjusted OR = 2.02, 95% CI 1.36–3.00). Compared with patients with no comorbidities, patients with major coexisting medical conditions were 9 times as likely to die during the same admission (unadjusted OR = 9.08, 95% CI 4.00–20.63), and patients with other comorbidities were 4 times as likely to die (unadjusted OR = 4.39, 95% CI 1.88–10.28).

Among emergency and high operative risk patients, men were equally likely as women to experience in-hospital death, after adjustment for age, operative risk, comorbidity at surgery, calendar period, institution, and method of access management (adjusted OR = 0.96, 95% CI 0.61–1.50). The effect remained the same after additional adjustment for time since catheterization (fully adjusted OR = 0.97, 95% CI 0.62–1.51).

Among 7,223 patients with medium and low operative risk combined, 3,950 (54.7%) and 3,273 (45.3%) underwent surgery within and beyond the recommended time, respectively; men were two-thirds as likely as women to experience in-hospital death, after adjustment for age, operative risk, comorbidity at surgery, calendar period, institution, and method of access management (adjusted OR = 0.65, 95% CI 0.38–1.12) (Table 5, Figure 3).

Table 4. Percentage of patients who died in hospital and unadjusted odds ratios for in-hospital death among patients who underwent isolated coronary artery bypass grafting, derived from logistic regression models

Factor	No. of patients	Deaths No.	Deaths % (95% CI)	Unadjusted OR (95% CI)
Sex				
Men	8,973	129	1.4 (1.2–1.7)	0.60 (0.43–0.84)
Women	2,033	48	2.4 (1.7–3.0)	1.00
Age group (years)				
<50	728	4	0.5 (0.0–1.1)	0.49 (0.18–1.38)
50–59	2,412	19	0.8 (0.4–1.1)	0.71 (0.41–1.23)
60–69	3,705	41	1.1 (0.8–1.4)	1.00
70–79	3,604	85	2.4 (1.9–2.9)	2.16 (1.48–3.14)
≥80	557	28	5.0 (3.2–6.8)	4.73 (2.90–7.71)
Operative risk				
Emergency	1,568	69	4.4 (3.4–5.4)	4.92 (3.48–6.97)
High	2,215	41	1.9 (1.3–2.4)	2.02 (1.36–3.00)
Medium	6,691	62	0.9 (0.7–1.2)	1.00
Low	532	5	0.9 (0.1–1.8)	1.01 (0.41–2.53)
Comorbidity				
Major conditions*	4,936	123	2.5 (2.1–2.9)	9.08 (4.00–20.63)
Other conditions†	3,930	48	1.2 (0.9–1.6)	4.39 (1.88–10.28)
None	2,140	6	0.3 (0.1–0.5)	1.00
Calendar period				
2000–2001	3,569	58	1.6 (1.2–2.0)	1.00
2002–2003	3,669	59	1.6 (1.2–2.0)	0.99 (0.69–1.43)
2004–2005	3,768	60	1.6 (1.2–2.0)	0.98 (0.68–1.41)
Institution				
1	2,511	38	1.5 (1.0–2.0)	1.00
2	2,616	42	1.6 (1.1–2.1)	0.92 (0.58–1.44)
3	3,211	60	1.9 (1.4–2.3)	1.24 (0.82–1.87)
4	2,668	37	1.4 (0.9–1.8)	1.06 (0.68–1.65)
Access management				
Direct admission	5,261	120	2.3 (1.9–2.7)	2.33 (1.70–3.20)
Admission from a wait list	5,745	57	1.0 (0.7–1.2)	1.00

Abbreviations: OR = odds ratio, CI = confidence interval

*Congestive heart failure, diabetes mellitus, chronic obstructive pulmonary disease, rheumatoid arthritis, or cancer

†Peripheral vascular disease, cerebrovascular disease, dementia, peptic ulcer disease, hemiplegia, renal disease, or liver disease

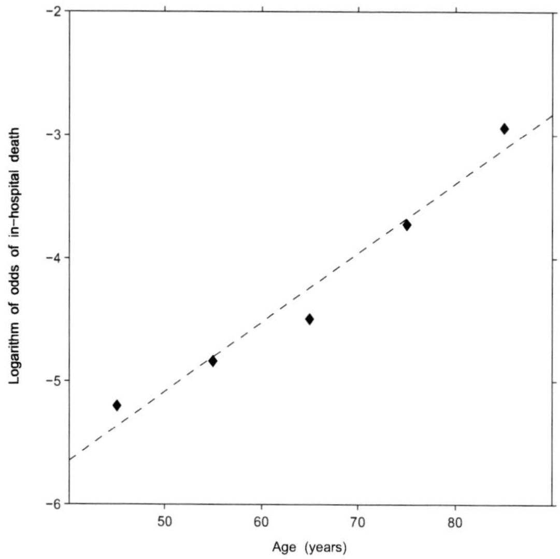

Figure 4. Linear relation between age groups and logarithm of odds for postopeartive death.

Additional adjustment for time since catheterization did not alter this effect (fully adjusted OR = 0.65, 95% CI 0.38–1.11) (Table 5, Figure 3). Treating time since catheterization as a continuous variable, rather than as a dichotomized variable, yielded similar results.

3. Conclusion

In previously reported comparisons of men and women who are to undergo surgical coronary revascularization, the women have been older, have had a greater extent of coronary artery disease, and have been more likely to have comorbid medical conditions such as diabetes, renal disease, or hypertension [10, 12, 17, 18]. Sex-related differences in outcomes after CABG appear sensitive to time after surgery, such that short-term outcomes tend to show greater differences than longer-term outcomes [24].

The purpose of our study was to investigate if time to surgery influences sex-related differences in postoperative in-hospital mortality, independent of clinical characteristics. Although there is considerable literature on the risk of adverse events while waiting for CABG, only a few studies have reported on the effect of delays in undergoing the procedure on postoperative mortality, an important measure of performance [31]. For this study, we used a data set representing all British Columbia patients who underwent first-time isolated CABG over a 6-year period.

In this cohort of 11,006 patients with angiographically proven coronary artery disease and complete records of surgical revascularization, who underwent CABG, the sex distribution was 81.5% men and 18.5% women, which is similar to other published reports. We found that the risk of death was 1.4% among men and 2.4% among women, a difference that we then tested in the context of several sex-related differences in clinical factors and time to surgery. Men tended to be younger than women (34.3% versus 31.0% between 60

Table 5. Adjusted odds ratios for in-hospital death among medium and low operative risk patients who underwent isolated coronary artery bypass grafting, derived from logistic regression models

	OR (95% CI)	
Factor	**Partially adjusted**	**Fully adjusted**
Sex		
Men	0.65 (0.38–1.12)*	0.65 (0.38–1.11)†
Women	1.00	1.00
Age (per decade)	2.00 (1.48–2.71)	2.01 (1.49–2.73)
Operative risk		
Medium	1.00	1.00
Low	1.18 (0.45–3.09)	1.16 (0.44–3.03)
Comorbidity		
Major conditions‡	4.24 (1.65–10.88)	4.38 (1.70–11.28)
Other conditions§	1.71 (0.60–4.84)	1.80 (0.63–5.16)
None	1.00	1.00
Calendar period		
2000–2001	1.00	1.00
2002–2003	1.24 (0.70–2.18)	1.23 (0.70–2.18)
2004–2005	0.71 (0.36–1.40)	0.74 (0.38–1.46)
Institution		
1	1.00	1.00
2	1.30 (0.61–2.76)	1.31 (0.62–2.79)
3	1.24 (0.62–2.48)	1.26 (0.63–2.52)
4	1.24 (0.57–2.66)	1.27 (0.59–2.74)
Access management		
Direct admission	1.44 (0.85–2.44)	1.61 (0.88–2.94)
Admission from a wait list	1.00	1.00
Time since catheterization		
Early surgery	NA	1.00
Late surgery	NA	1.24 (0.69–2.23)

Abbreviations: OR = odds ratio, CI = confidence interval, NA = not applicable

*With adjustment for age, operative risk, cormorbidity, 2-year calendar period, institution, and method of access management

†With adjustment for age, operative risk, cormorbidity, 2-year calendar period, institution, method of access management, and time between catheterization and surgery

‡Congestive heart failure, diabetes mellitus, chronic obstructive pulmonary disease, rheumatoid arthritis, or cancer

§Peripheral vascular disease, cerebrovascular disease, dementia, peptic ulcer disease, hemiplegia, renal disease, or liver disease and 69 years of age and 30.9% versus 40.7% between 70 and 79 years of age), men had lower operative risk (19.5% versus 22.8% in the high-risk category) and fewer coexisting medical conditions (42.7% versus 54.4% with major conditions), and fewer men accessed surgery by direct admission (46.6% versus 53.3%).

In examining the difference in risk of death in relation to these clinical factors, we first found differences between the sexes in times to CABG among those with lower operative risk, but not among high-risk patients. Second, after adjustment for clinical risk factors, the rate of postoperative in-hospital mortality was similar for men and women in the higher risk group but was 35% less likely for men in the medium- and low-risk groups combined. More generally, in-hospital death was more likely among patients who were older, had higher operative risk, had more coexisting medical conditions, and had access to CABG through direct admission. Third, the time that patients waited for surgery after catheterization did not influence the difference in the risk of postoperative death between men and women.

Our study was observational and therefore required risk adjustment for potential differences among the treated patients. The existing literature suggests that elderly patients are more likely to undergo revascularization as an urgent procedure [32], that a smaller coronary vessel diameter may account for the higher risk of adverse cardiovascular events among women [22], that coexisting medical conditions may delay open heart surgery [33], that postoperative survival depends on institutional constraints and individual care providers [38], and that changes in practice or supplementary funds may reduce time until surgery [30]. All of these factors were entered into multivariate regressions in our study directly or through the proxy variable of institution. Another factor that might have affected time to surgery was change in urgency status during the preoperative period. Because an increase in urgency would reduce the time to surgery, those who underwent CABG after their urgency status was upgraded might have been more ill, which might have resulted in a downward bias in the survival effect. However, there was no record of the timing of such changes between catheterization and surgery and we were therefore unable to adjust for such upgrades.

Although the data in the current study have been validated locally at each hospital, no external audit was performed to evaluate the quality of the registry records. Misclassification of the recorded urgency for treatment is a potential concern in this analysis, because surgeons may select patients from wait lists on the basis of other considerations, such as best use of operating time or availability of hospital resources.

The data set did not have enough events to allow adjustment for the surgical operator, and outcomes might have been influenced by the individual surgeon's threshold for accepting a patient for nonurgent treatment. Similarly, we were unable to adjust for a possible imbalance in urban versus rural referrals between the study groups. Nevertheless, our findings suggest that time between cardiac catheterization and surgical revascularization had no independent effect on sex-related differences in postoperative in-hospital mortality.

References

[1] Rihal CS, Raco DL, Gersh BJ, Yusuf S. Indications for coronary artery bypass surgery and percutaneous coronary intervention in chronic stable angina: review of the evidence and methodological considerations. *Circulation* 2003;108:2439–2445.

[2] Yusuf S, Zucker D, Peduzzi P, Fisher LD, Takaro T, Kennedy JW, et al. Effect of coronary artery bypass graft surgery on survival: overview of 10-year results from randomised trials by the Coronary Artery Bypass Graft Surgery Trialists Collaboration. *Lancet* 1994;344:563–570.

[3] Eagle KA, Guyton RA, Davidoff R, Ewy GA, Fonger J, Gardner TJ, et al. ACC/AHA guidelines for coronary artery bypass graft surgery: executive summary and recommendations : A report of the American College of Cardiology/American Heart Association Task Force on Practice Guidelines. *Circulation* 1999;100:1464–1480.

[4] Ivanov J, Weisel RD, David TE, Naylor CD. Fifteen-year trends in risk severity and operative mortality in elderly patients undergoing coronary artery bypass graft surgery. *Circulation* 1998;97:673–680.

[5] Trachiotis GD, Weintraub WS, Johnston TS, Jones EL, Guyton RA, Craver JM. Coronary artery bypass grafting in patients with advanced left ventricular dysfunction. *Annals of Thoracic Surgery* 1998;66:1632–1639.

[6] Guru V, Anderson GM, Fremes SE, O'Connor GT, Grover FL, Tu JV. The identification and development of Canadian coronary artery bypass graft surgery quality indicators. *Journal of Thoracic and Cardiovascular Surgery* 2005;130:1257.e1–1257.e11.

[7] Tekkis PP, McCulloch P, Steger AC, Benjamin IS, Poloniecki JD. Mortality control charts for comparing performance of surgical units: validation study using hospital mortality data. *British Medical Journal* 2003;326:786–788.

[8] Bridgewater B. Mortality data in adult cardiac surgery for named surgeons: retrospective examination of prospectively collected data on coronary artery surgery and aortic valve replacement. *British Medical Journal* 2005;330:506–510.

[9] Fisher LD, Kennedy JW, Davis KB, Maynard C, Fritz JK, Kaiser G, et al. Association of sex, physical size, and operative mortality after coronary artery bypass in the Coronary Artery Surgery Study (CASS). *Journal of Thoracic and Cardiovascular Surgery* 1982;84:334–341.

[10] Edwards FH, Carey JS, Grover FL, Bero JW, Hartz RS. Impact of gender on coronary bypass operative mortality. *Annals of Thoracic Surgery* 1998;66:125–131.

[11] Aldea GS, Gaudiani JM, Shapira OM, Jacobs AK, Weinberg J, Cupples AL, et al. Effect of gender on postoperative outcomes and hospital stays after coronary artery bypass grafting. *Annals of Thoracic Surgery* 1999;67:1097–1103.

[12] Vaccarino V, Abramson JL, Veledar E, Weintraub WS. Sex differences in hospital mortality after coronary artery bypass surgery: evidence for a higher mortality in younger women. *Circulation* 2002;105:1176–1181.

[13] Ghali WA, Quan H, Shrive FM, Hirsch GM. Outcomes after coronary artery bypass graft surgery in Canada: 1992/93 to 2000/01. *Canadian Journal of Cardiology* 2003;19:774–781.

[14] Guru V, Fremes SE, Tu JV. Time-related mortality for women after coronary artery bypass graft surgery: a population-based study. *Journal of Thoracic and Cardiovascular Surgery* 2004;127:1158–1165.

[15] Carey JS, Cukingnan RA, Singer LK. Health status after myocardial revascularization: inferior results in women. *Annals of Thoracic Surgery* 1995;59:112–117.

[16] Hammar N, Sandberg E, Larsen FF, Ivert T. Comparison of early and late mortality in men and women after isolated coronary artery bypass graft surgery in Stockholm, Sweden, 1980 to 1989. *Journal of the American College of Cardiology* 1997;29:659–664.

[17] Abramov D, Tamariz MG, Sever JY, Christakis GT, Bhatnagar G, Heenan AL, et al. The influence of gender on the outcome of coronary artery bypass surgery. *Annals of Thoracic Surgery* 2000;70:800–805.

[18] Koch CG, Khandwala F, Nussmeier N, Blackstone EH. Gender and outcomes after coronary artery bypass grafting: a propensity-matched comparison. *Journal of Thoracic and Cardiovascular Surgery* 2003;126:2032–2043.

[19] Edwards FH, Ferraris VA, Shahian DM, Peterson E, Furnary AP, Haan CK, et al. Gender-specific practice guidelines for coronary artery bypass surgery: perioperative management. *Annals of Thoracic Surgery* 2005;79:2189–2194.

[20] O'Connor GT, Morton JR, Diehl MJ, Olmstead EM, Coffin LH, Levy DG, et al. Differences between men and women in hospital mortality associated with coronary artery bypass graft surgery. The Northern New England Cardiovascular Disease Study Group. *Circulation* 1993;88:2104–2110.

[21] Christakis GT, Weisel RD, Buth KJ, Fremes SE, Rao V, Panagiotopoulos KP, et al. Is body size the cause for poor outcomes of coronary artery bypass operations in women? *Journal of Thoracic and Cardiovascular Surgery* 1995;110:1344–1356.

[22] O'Connor NJ, Morton JR, Birkmeyer JD, Olmstead EM, O'Connor GT. Effect of coronary artery diameter in patients undergoing coronary bypass surgery. Northern New England Cardiovascular Disease Study Group. *Circulation* 1996;93:652–655.

[23] Ghali WA, Faris PD, Galbraith PD, Norris CM, Curtis MJ, Saunders LD, et al. Sex differences in access to coronary revascularization after cardiac catheterization: importance of detailed clinical data. *Annals of Internal Medicine* 2002;136:723–732.

[24] King KM, Ghali WA, Faris PD, Curtis MJ, Galbraith PD, Graham MM, et al. Sex differences in outcomes after cardiac catheterization: effect modification by treatment strategy and time. *Journal of the American Medical Association* 2004;291:1220–1225.

[25] Rexius H, Brandrup-Wognsen G, Oden A, Jeppsson A. Waiting time and mortality after elective coronary artery bypass grafting. *Annals of Thoracic Surgery* 2005;79:538–543.

[26] O'Neill BJ, Brophy JM, Simpson CS, Sholdice MM, Knudtson M, Ross DB, et al. General commentary on access to cardiovascular care in Canada: universal access, but when? Treating the right patient at the right time. *Canadian Journal of Cardiology* 2005;21:1272–1276.

[27] Sobolev B, Levy A, Hayden R, Kuramoto L. Does wait-list size at registration influence time to surgery? Analysis of a population-based cardiac surgery registry. *Health Services Research* 2006;41:23–39.

[28] Chamberlayne R, Green B, Barer ML, Hertzman C, Lawrence WJ, Sheps SB. Creating a population-based linked health database: a new resource for health services research. *Canadian Journal of Public Health* 1998;89:270–273.

[29] Humphries KH, Rankin JM, Carere RG, Buller CE, Kiely FM, Spinelli JJ. Comorbidity data in outcomes research: are clinical data derived from administrative databases a reliable alternative to chart review? *Journal of Clinical Epidemiology* 2000;53:343–349.

[30] Levy A, Sobolev B, Hayden R, Kiely M, FitzGerald M, Schechter M. Time on wait lists for coronary bypass surgery in British Columbia, Canada, 1991 - 2000. *BMC Health Services Research* 2005;5:22.

[31] Sobolev B, Kuramoto L. *Analysis of Waiting-Time Data in Health Services Research.* 1st ed. Springer; 2008.

[32] Christenson JT, Simonet F, Schmuziger M. The influence of age on the outcome of primary coronary artery bypass grafting. *Journal of Cardiovascular Surgery (Torino)* 1999;40:333–338.

[33] Naylor CD, Baigrie RS, Goldman BS, Basinski A. Assessment of priority for coronary revascularisation procedures. *Lancet* 1990;335:1070–1073.

[34] Romano PS, Roos LL, Jollis JG. Adapting a clinical comorbidity index for use with ICD-9-CM administrative data: differing perspectives. *Journal of Clinical Epidemiology* 1993;46:1075–1079.

[35] Naylor CD, Levinton CM, Baigrie RS. Adapting to waiting lists for coronary revascularization. Do Canadian specialists agree on which patients come first? *Chest* 1992;101:715–722.

[36] Charlson ME, Pompei P, Ales KL, MacKenzie CR. A new method of classifying prognostic comorbidity in longitudinal studies: development and validation. *Journal of Chronic Diseases* 1987;40:373–383.

[37] Lang TA, Secic M. *How to report statistics in medicine.* 2nd ed. American College of Physicians; 2006.

[38] DeLong ER, Nelson CL, Wong JB, Pryor DB, Peterson ED, Lee KL, et al. Using observational data to estimate prognosis: an example using a coronary artery disease registry. *Statistics in Medicine* 2001;20:2505–2532.

In: Heart Disease in Men
Editors: A.B. Todd and M.H. Mosley, pp. 293-316
ISBN: 978-1-60692-297-2

Chapter 14

Cardiovascular Disease and Erectile Dysfunction The Evolving Role of Phosphodiesterase-5-Inhibitors

Ujjaini Khanderia and Randolph E. Regal
University of Michigan Hospitals and Health Centers,
Ann Arbor, Michigan 48109, USA

Introduction

The exact prevalence of erectile dysfunction (ED) is difficult to determine due to under-reporting of this condition. This is because of patient reluctance to talk about personal problems related to sexual functioning. One of the most frequently cited studies on the epidemiology of ED is the Massachusetts Male Aging Study.[1] This landmark study interviewed 1,290 men with a self-administered questionnaire regarding sexual activity. The findings showed that 52% of men age 40 to 70 years had some degree of ED, and that about 10% of these men experienced a total absence of erectile function. With increased age, the prevalence of ED also increased, such that 68% of men aged 60 to 70 years experienced ED of some magnitude. After adjusting for age, ED directly correlated with the presence of coronary artery disease (CAD), hypertension, diabetes mellitus, low serum levels of high-density lipoprotein cholesterol (HDL-C), depression, and cigarette smoking.

There is compelling evidence that ED precedes the formation of atherosclerotic plaques and may serve as an early marker of coronary atherosclerosis. The manifestation of ED may therefore serve as a useful clinical tool for identifying men at high risk for cardiovascular disease (CVD).[2,3] ED and CVD share many conventional risk factors including hypertension,[1,4] dyslipidemia,[5,6] type 2 diabetes mellitus[7,8], cigarette smoking.[1,9] and obesity.[10] The severity of ED appears to correlate with the presence of an increasing number of risk factors, all of which are associated with endothelial dysfunction. It is now well established that the endothelium plays a key role in the pathogenesis of all systemic vascular diseases, including ED.[11]

In this chapter, we review the association between ED and underlying CVD. The pharmacology, clinical efficacy and safety of the available phosphodiesterase -5 inhibitors (PDEIs) will be discussed. Clinical trials that have investigated the use of PDEIs in men with ED and concomitant cardiovascular conditions such as heart failure (HF), hypertension, pulmonary hypertension, diabetes mellitus, and coronary artery disease will be addressed.

Endothelial Dysfunction

The link between ED and atherosclerosis is endothelial dysfunction. The endothelium is present throughout the arterial vasculature, and consequently, symptoms of endothelial dysfunction manifested as ED may also indicate problems in the coronary arteries. Indeed, the pathogenesis of ED is closely related to the atherosclerotic process,[12-14] with both conditions being characterized by disturbed endothelial function.[2,15] Endothelial dysfunction results from the inability of arterial smooth muscle to relax in a process regulated by the nitric oxide-cyclic guanosine-3’5’-monophosphate (NO-cGMP) system.[14,16,17,18] Nitric oxide (NO), synthesized by nitric oxide synthase (NOS) from the amino acid L-arginine, regulates vasomotor tone and plays a major role in mediating smooth muscle relaxation in normal penile erection. Oxidative stress, which interferes with the NO pathway and is directly toxic to the endothelium, causes vascular damage associated with both preclinical as well as clinically evident CVD. A deficiency in NO, brought about by impaired production or increased degradation by reactive oxidant species (i.e., superoxides), prevents normal vasodilation in the penile arteries.[19,20]

ED resulting from insufficient NO-mediated dilatation of relatively small penile arteries may occur at a stage when atherosclerosis in the larger coronary, carotid or femoral arteries is not yet clinically manifested.[21] In one study using flow mediated brachial artery vasodilation, systemic endothelial function was examined in 30 men with ED compared with 27 age-matched controls.[17] Men with ED had impaired endothelium-dependent flow-mediated vasodilation ($p \leq 0.05$) as well as endothelium-independent vasodilation, defined as a blunted response to sublingual nitroglycerin, compared with the control group ($p=0.02$).[17] The abnormalities preceded any evidence of coronary or vascular disease.

Erectile Dysfunction as a Surrogate Marker for Cardiovascular Disease

The prevalence of ED in patients with CVD is higher than that seen in the general population, ranging from 60% in men with previous myocardial infarction (MI) or who had undergone coronary artery bypass surgery[22] to 75% of men with chronic CAD.[23] In fact, one study found that men with ED had a twofold increased risk for acute MI compared to their cohorts without ED.[24]

Until recently, ED was generally regarded as a late consequence of generalized atherosclerosis. This view has been contradicted in recent times, and questions have arisen as to whether ED could be a marker predating the development of future cardiac events. The

Prostate Cancer Prevention Trial[25] was a landmark study that used data from 9457 men to determine whether ED was associated with the subsequent development of CVD. Around 15% of the men (1394 of 9457) had CVD at study entry. All patients were evaluated every three months over a 9-year period for evidence of ED and CVD. Of the 4247 men who did not have ED at study entry, 2420 (57%) developed ED (incident ED) in the subsequent 5 years. After adjusting for other CVD risk factors, incident ED was associated with a hazard ratio of 1.25 for the development of new CV events (p=0.04). Thus, ED had significant prognostic value for the subsequent development of CVD. For men who either had ED at the start of the study or developed it during the course of the study, the hazard ratio for developing CVD during the course of the study was 1.45 (p<0.001).

ED may already be present prior to the clinical manifestations of coronary artery or peripheral vascular disease.[3,26,27] A large study of 25, 650 men found a 75% increased risk of peripheral vascular disease in men with pre-existing ED.[28] Pritzker[29] studied 50 men who had ED but no history or symptoms of CVD, yet 80% of these men had multiple risk factors for CAD as assessed by questionnaire analysis. Furthermore, 56% failed a treadmill stress test and had an abnormal exercise electrocardiogram (ECG). When 20 of these 28 men had coronary angiography, all were found to have one- to three- vessel disease. Vlachopoulos et al.[30] documented that up to 19% of patients with ED have documented silent CAD.

ED is now considered to be a surrogate marker for occult vascular or coronary artery disease (CAD). The diameter of penile arteries is around 1-2 mm, which is a much smaller compared with that of the coronary artery (3-4 mm) or carotid artery (5-7 mm). Consequently, the amount of plaque sufficient to block blood flow through the penile artery, and therefore cause ED, produces only a 30-40% stenosis and no apparent symptoms in arteries with a larger diameter.[21] Thus, compared to penile arteries, the larger coronary arteries can better tolerate the same amount of atherosclerotic plaque without inducing obstructive flow-limiting stenosis. It follows then that damage to the penile vascular bed precedes the development of atherosclerotic lesions, and may serve as an early marker of systemic atherosclerosis. Thus, ED may be the first clinical manifestation of coronary atherosclerosis, and patients presenting with ED should be investigated for CVD. Early detection could facilitate prompt intervention and aggressive management of CV risk factors to prevent future cardiovascular events.

Phosphodiesterase Inhibitors

At the time of this writing, three phosphodiesterase inhibitors (PDEIs), sildenafil (Viagra®), vardenafil (Levitra®), and tadalafil (Cialis®) are available in the US market for treating ED of organic, psychogenic, or mixed etiology. Sildenafil has also been recently labeled under a different strength and trade name (Revatio®) for treating pulmonary hypertension. Ironically, before these agents became widely marketed and aggressively publicized as the drugs of choice for ED, the PDEIs were studied as a potential pharmaceutical panacea for a gamut of cardiovascular-related diseases such as chronic heart failure, essential hypertension, and diabetes mellitus. However, further long-term studies are necessary to measure their true overall utility for these conditions.

Mechanism of Action: Thus far, eleven discrete phosphodiesterase (PDE) families have been identified within the human body, and at least 40 different isoforms have been described. The enzyme families are similar in structure, but differ in terms of tissue distribution, selectivity for cyclic nucleotides, and sensitivity for inhibitors and activators. Because of these differences, each family occupies a unique niche in terms of its ultimate physiological role. As will be further addressed in this section, the currently marketed PDEIs are relatively specific to the family known as PDE 5.[31-33]

PDE enzymes catalyze the degradation of both cyclic adenosine monophosphate (cAMP) and cyclic guanosine monophosphate (cGMP). It is established that cAMP and cGMP play pivotal roles in a plethora of intracellular signaling pathways. In the case of cGMP, this compound acts as a vital messenger that initiates complex signaling cascades which regulate such diverse functions as vascular smooth muscle tone , homeostasis of interstitial fluid and electrolytes, and induction of phototransduction within the retina. In terms of its function on vascular smooth muscle within the penis specifically, cGMP is the second messenger in the enzymatic cascade that elicits relaxation of the smooth muscle in the penile vascular spaces and penile vessels, including the corpus cavernosa. Of course, potentiation of these processes then facilitates the effect of penile erection.[32] Once introduced into the systemic circulation, PDEIs penetrate into smooth muscle cells to inhibit tissue-local PDE. Obviously, when PDEIs prevent the degradation of cGMP, they subsequently induce vasodilation leading to an increase in penile blood flow; and ultimately potentiate the achievement of penile erection.[31-34]

It is important to understand the synergistic physiologic process which PDEIs exact with nitric oxide (NO). NO is a potent activator of guanylate cyclases, a group of enzymes which catalyze the synthesis from guanosine triphosphate to cGMP. One can recall that these compounds make up part of the NO-cGMP system which was alluded to earlier in the article. As a result of their ability to activate guanylate cyclases, NO and related nitrates directly elevate cGMP levels. This NO effect of elevating cGMP levels acts in consort with PDEIs, since PDEIs prevent cGMP degradation. Understanding the synergy between PDEIs and NO/nitrates helps to practically explain two important clinical pearls that clinicians must remember about PDEI therapy. First, this helps explain why the concomitant use of nitrates and PDEIs can cause a profound and prolonged drop in blood pressure; the hypotension results from vasodilation caused by excessive cGMP buildup. Second, this helps explain why in order to facilitate optimal erectile responses, PDEIs still need the concomitant presence of endogenous nitric oxide from neuronal or endothelial cells, a process initiated by normal sexual stimulation, in order to be optimally effective.[31,33,35,36]

History of Pharmaceutical Development: Of the eleven PDE families, much research initially focused on the subtype known as PDE5. This is because in the mid -1980s, the PDE5 family was found to be present in high concentrations in vascular smooth muscle as well as within platelets. Of course, both of these effects were already recognized as being of benefit in treating various cardiovascular conditions, such as angina.[31] Thus, in hopes of synthesizing an agent that elicited vasodilator effects as well as platelet anti-aggregation, a selective PDE5 inhibitor was sought after for research and development. Although the PDE5 enzyme is especially plentiful in the corpus cavernosum of the penis, it was recognized earlier that the PDE5 family was ubiquitous, and could be found in vascular smooth muscles throughout the body.[31,32]

In 1989, sildenafil citrate was synthesized as a potent and selective inhibitor of PDE5. Though initially studied for angina, this aspiration was countermanded by the emergence of self-limiting and transient visual side effects. Vision changes were observed at high doses of

150mg and 200mg daily. It was later realized that these side effects were due to sildenafil's weak inhibitory effect on PDE6, an enzyme concentrated in the photoreceptor cells within the retina. Serendipitously, another side effect reported in clinical trials was penile erections. Shortly thereafter, the somewhat parallel and complementary role of NO in sexual stimulation and erectile production was also discovered. With the added knowledge of PDE5's presence in the smooth muscle of the corpus cavernosum, sildenafil's first pilot study in men with ED was started in 1993.[31] The drug was eventually approved for the treatment of ED in 1998. Since then, two more PDE inhibitors under the generic names of vardenafil and tadalafil, were approved in or around 2004.

In terms of PDE5 potency, sildenafil and tadalafil appear to have equal potency, whereas vardenafil has greater potency.[32] Vardenafil appears to share the same cross-affinity for PDE6 receptors as does sildenafil, whereas tadalafil apparently cross-reacts with PDE 11 enzymes, which happen to be located in cardiac tissue, the pituitary gland, and the testes.[32] In addition, sildenafil, but not vardenafil or tadalafil, shows relatively high affinity for PDE1c, a subtype PDE enzyme which has been found to distribute in high concentrations in lung tissue. This last observation regarding sildenafil's PDE1c selectivity may explain its emergence as the first PDEI to be studied and approved to treat pulmonary hypertension.[37]

Pharmacokinetics and Dosing: The pharmacokinetics of PDEIs is summarized in Table 1.[38] The most clinically important difference between the three agents is that tadalafil possesses a much longer half-life than either sildenafil or vardenafil.[39-41] In this class of drugs, the durations of action appear commensurate with the elimination half-lives, thus owing tadalafil to nicknames such as "*Le weekender*" in France.

The PDEIs share many similarities. All are primarily hepatically eliminated, with CYP 3A4 as the major CYP pathway for metabolism. Thus, caveats exist for use and dosing of PDEIs in patients with liver disease, as well at those taking concomitant drugs which have been identified as potent CYP 3A4 inhibitors (Table 2). Conversely, drugs that may induce the CYP 3A4 system could reduce PDEI effectiveness.[33,37] Both sildenafil and vardenafil have 2C isozymes listed as secondary pathways, but no warnings exist as to drug interactions with important 2C inhibitor drugs for either one of these drugs.[38-41]

In addition to hepatic elimination, the PDE inhibitors also have sufficient renal elimination such that dose reductions are recommended for patients with creatinine clearances between 30 and 50 ml/min and below, depending on the drug.[39-41] For example, in the case of tadalafil's active catechol metabolite, its half-life increases from 36 hours in healthy individuals to 54-77 hours in patients with end stage renal disease.[37]

In terms of systemic oral absorption, bioavailability tends to be low for the PDEIs, at 40, 36, and 15% for sildenafil, tadalafil, and vardenafil, respectively.[37] In the case of at least sildenafil, the low systemic bioavailability is attributed to a high first pass effect.[37] All three agents bypass absorption in the stomach, and are rapidly absorbed in the small intestine. Thus, delays in drug onset can result from conditions or activities that delay gastric emptying.[32] The absorption of both sildenafil and vardenafil are slowed by high fat meals, such that the time to peak is increased and maximum drug concentration in the serum is decreased, but the area under the curve (AUC) is apparently not changed.[33] Tadalafil's absorption is not affected significantly by food consumption, but the concomitant use of antacids may reduce its absorption.[38-41]

Table 1. PDE5 -Inhibitor Comparison: Dosing and Pharmacokinetics

Parameter	Sildenafil(Viagra)	Vardenafil(Levitra)	Tadalafil(Cialis)
Dosage Availability (mg)	25, 50, 100	2.5, 5, 10, 20	5, 10, 20
Dosing	50mg orally 1hr (usally 0.5-4hr) prior to sexual intercourse (may decrease to 25mg or increase to 100mg per day as tolerated)	10mg orally 1hr prior to sexual intercourse (max 20mg/day)	10mg orally prior to sexual intercourse (may decrease to 5mg or increase to 20mg per day as tolerated)
Onset of Action (min)	30-60	30-120	16-30
Duration of Action (hr)	3-5	4-5	24-36
Half-life (hr)	4	4-5	17.5
Metabolism	Hepatic	Hepatic	Hepatic
P-450 Isozyme Pathways	3A4 (major) 2C9 (minor)	3A4 3A5, 2C	3A4
Plasma Protein Binding	96%	95%	94%
Mean Volume of Distribution (L)	105	208	63
Absorption	F= 0.40 Time to peak prolonged and Cmax reduced with high-fat foods. No change in AUC	F=0.15 Time to peak prolonged and Cmax reduced with high-fat foods. No change in AUC.	F=0.36 Unchanged with food; decreased with antacids
Dose Adjustments for Renal or Hepatic Impairment	Dose reduction for patients > 65yr, hepatic impairment, severe renal impairment (CrCl < 30ml/min)	Dose reduction for patients > 65yr, hepatic impairment, moderate to severe renal impairment (CrCl < 50ml/min)	No dosage adjustment for age; not recommended for use with severe hepatic impairment; decrease dose for moderate to severe renal impairment (CrCl < 50ml/min)

All three agents are highly lipophilic and highly protein bound at approximately 95%.[32,38-41] High protein binding may limit the dialyzability of PDEIs, as reported with sildenafil.[39]

Clinical Efficacy for ED: Sildenafil, the prototype PDEI, appears to be effective in about 50-80% of men with ED. Response rates in men with primarily psychogenic disease is reported to be as high as 84% compared to 68% in those thought to have primarily organic disease.[33] Response rates to sildenafil appear to be slightly lower (about 59%) in men who have diabetes mellitus, and even lower (around 31%) in those who have undergone radical retropubic prostectomy, especially when the local nerve fibers were not spared. In patients with ED secondary to radiotherapy, response rates to sildenafil have been around 70%.[36]

Table 2. PDE5 Inhibitor Comparison of Side Effects, Drug Interactions

Parameter	Sildenafil(Viagra)	Vardenafil(Levitra)	Tadalafil(Cialis)
Side Effects	Headache, flushing, dyspepsia, nasal congestion, abnormal vision, priapism	Headache, flushing, dyspepsia, rhinitis, abnormal color vision, priapism	Headache, flushing, nasal congestion, dyspepsia, back pain, myalgia 12-24hr after dose, rare color vision changes, priapism
Collateral PDE Family Inhibition	PDE 6, PDE 1c	PDE 6	PDE 11
Precautions/ Contraindications	Hypersensitivity; concurrent use of nitrates; not for use in children	Hypersensitivity; concurrent use of nitrates; not for use in children	Hypersensitivity; concurrent use of nitrates; not for use in children
Drug Interactions	Non-specific interactions w/ strong CYP3A4 inhibitors (e.g., ritonavir, indinavir, ketoconazole, itraconazole) & moderate CYP3A4 inhibitors (e.g., erythromycin); increased plasma levels w/ CYP450 inhibitor cimetidine; potential hypotension w/ nitrates and α-adrenergic blockers	Increased plasma levels w/ strong CYP3A4 inhibitors (e.g., ritonavir, indinavir, ketoconazole, itraconazole); potential hypotension w/ nitrates and α-adrenergic blockers	Increased plasma levels w/ strong CYP3A4 inhibitors (e.g., ritonavir, indinavir, ketoconazole, itraconazole); potential hypotension w/ nitrates and α-adrenergic blockers
Additional Information	None	May prolong QT interval	Nitrates given no sooner than 48hr after dose; substantial consumption of EtOH increases orthostatic hypotension; no BP drop w/ tamsulosin

Nitric oxide deficiency has been identified as one of the underlying causes of ED.[32] PDEIs have been less effective in various disease states associated with deficiencies in neuronal or endothelial nitric oxide synthetase, leading to low local levels of NO. As previously discussed in the "Mechanism of Action" section earlier in this text, both stimulation of cGMP production from endogenous NO and inhibition of cGMP breakdown from PDEIs are important features in inducing cGMP mediated vasodilation in the corpus cavernosum and surrounding tissues. The presence of endogenous nitric oxide is necessary for PDEIs to work effectively, and men with underlying organic disorders appear to be relatively deficient in endogenous NO production and/or secretion.[36]

There is a paucity of head-to-head clinical trials comparing response rates to sildenafil with that of the two newer agents, vardenafil and tadafadil. Despite differences in terms of pharmacokinetics, the clinical efficacy for treating ED appears to be comparable between the three agents.[31,32,36] Response rates of 80% have been reported with vardenafil.[36,42] One study with tadalafil showed an 81% improvement rate compared to 17% in the placebo group.[43]

Tolerability and Side Effects: Table 2 provides a summary of the various side effects reported with each of the three agents. The preponderance of side effects attributed to the PDEIs are usually related to either their PDE5-mediated vasodilatory effects or "collateral damage" from affected PDE enzymes outside of the PDE5 isozyme.

Headache, a classic vasodilator-related effect, is the most common side effect reported with all three PDE inhibitors (11-16%).[39-41] Other side effects include flushing, reported in 11% of patients on vardenafil, 4-14% on sildenafil, and only 2-3% with tadalafil. Direct comparison data are lacking, however. It is possible that the longer half-life and more gradual time-to-peak effect of tadalafil might somewhat ameliorate the flushing. Nasal congestion has been reported with sildenafil (4%) as well as vardenafil (3-9%) and tadalafil (2-3%); and dizziness may occur with all three agents (around 2%).[39-41]

Gastrointesinal (GI) side effects including indigestion and diarrhea have been reported with all three PDEIs, with an incidence of around 4%.[39-41] The "dyspeptic" GI side effects are of interest, because they are though to be primarily due to relaxation of the lower esophageal sphincter muscle. In other words, PDEIs may cause or potentiate gastroesphageal reflux disease (GERD), a malady that already afflicts a large percentage of the male population taking these medications.[33] In one study with sildenafil that used a direct question and answer design to assess each side effect associated with the medication, patient response to "heartburn" was positive 10.5% of the time. When side effects are specifically elicited in this manner, the reported numbers are generally higher than open-end volunteering of complaints. For instance, in the same study using self-referred males in a university-based practice, all side effects, including flushing (30.8%), headache (25.4%), nasal congestion (18.7%), and visual changes (5.8%) were higher than the rates reported in clinical trials.[33,44]

For reasons related to the aforementioned collateral PDEI inhibition of PDE6 which subsequently leads to an effect on retinal transduction, visual changes have been reported with all three agents.[39-41] However, the incidence has been lowest with tadalafil, probably because, unlike sildenafil and vardenafil, tadalafil has very little affinity for PDE 6 receptors.[32] While the visual changes are often mild and transient, PDEIs have been associated with non-arteritic anterior ischemic optic neuropathies (NAAION) with attendant permanent vision loss.[45] More study is currently underway to gain a better understanding of the relationship between PDEIs and ophthalmologic side effects.

A recently identified side effect of PDEIs is sudden hearing loss.[46] In some incidences, the loss was associated with vestibular symptoms such as tinnitus, vertigo, and dizziness. In almost all cases, the malady was unilateral. The hearing loss reported was temporary in about 1/3 of those affected, with uncertainty regarding the duration to resolution.[46] As with the ophthalmologic side effects, more study is currently underway to better characterize the relationship between PDEI use and hearing loss.

As previously mentioned, tadalafil selectively inhibits PDE-11. This has been concerning because high levels of PDE-11 are present in cardiac myocytes, pituitary gland, and the testes. Consequently, the possibility of adversely affecting cardiac function as well as reproductive and sexual-hormone axes cannot be dismissed. However, no data from clinical trials has suggested that tadalafil causes an increased risk of cardiac toxicity, and the clinical ramifications of PDE-11 inhibition are not clear at this time.[32,47,48]

Contraindications and Warnings: All three agents are contraindicated if there is a known hypersensitivity. There is no indication for the use of PDEIs in children. The vasodilating effects of PDEIs may result in a small drop in arterial pressure. In healthy individuals this is rarely a problem, but in patients with cardiovascular disease who have low blood pressure at baseline, this could be concerning. PDEIs potentiate the hypotensive effects of organic nitrates. If used concurrently, the result may be a synergistic drop in blood pressure leading to profound hypotension. To avoid the possibility of prolonged hypotension, nitrates should be held for at least 24 hours before a PDE inhibitor can be given.[32] Further, nitrates should not be given within 24 hours of sildenafil or vardenafil, and 48 hours after tadalafil.[32,39-41] There is also a precaution for PDEI use with α-adrenergic blockers. It is well known that α-adrenergic blockers can cause orthostatic hypotension; consequently PDEIs can potentiate the hypotention.[49-50] The drug labeling for tadalafil, however, allows for concomitant use of the α-adrenergic blocker, tamsulosin, upto a dose of 0.4 mg once daily.[41] Despite contraindications and warnings, the concomitant use of PDEIs with various antihypertensive drugs has been reported to be reasonably safe.[33,39,41]

An additional warning on the package label that is unique to vardenifil states: "Patients with congenital QT prolongation and those taking Class 1A (quinidine, procainamide) or Class III (amiodarone, sotalol) antiarrhythmics should avoid using Levitra."[40] Unlike vardenafil, tadalafil and sildenafil do not carry this warning.[39,41] Although there have been no documented cases of Torsades de Pointes, small increases in QTc were observed in one study with vardenafil.[50] In a premarketing study of 59 healthy males, vardenafil 10mg resulted in mean QT corrected change of 4 msec. Consequently, vardenafil should be avoided in patients with congenital QT prolongation and patients taking class IA or class III antiarrythmic medications.[40] At recommended therapeutic doses, sildenafil has not shown significant electrophysiologic effects on the myocardium.[39]

Drug Interactions: As previously mentioned, all three PDEIs are hepatically removed as cytochrome 3A4 (CYP 3A4) substrates.[39-41] Therefore, warnings exist for the use and the dosing of PDEIs in patients taking a plethora of agents known to be potent CYP 3A4 inhibitors (Table 2). Studies have shown that drugs such as ketoconazole, erythromycin, and sequinavir significantly increase the plasma levels of PDE inhibitor agents. In the case of sildenafil, these drugs increase the area under the curve (AUC) without affecting the half-life, which points to an inhibition of first pass metabolism leading to increased bioavailability. In one study with tadalafil, therapeutic doses of ketoconazole increased the tadafadil AUC by 4.1 fold, while increasing the peak plasma concentration slightly by 1.2-fold. Thus, PDEI potentiation by 3A4 inhibitors can result from either increased PDEI bioavailability, reduced PDEI elimination, or a combination of both mechanisms.[33,37] Conversely, drugs that induce the CYP 3A4 system can reduce the effectiveness of PDEIs. Bosentan, a potent CYP 3A4 inducer, reduces plasma sildenafil levels by about 50% when used concomitantly with sildenafil.[37]

Both sildenafil and vardenafil have 2C isozymes listed as secondary pathways, but no warnings exist as to drug interactions with important 2C inhibitor drugs. More research is needed to better characterize the possibility of PDEI potentiation through medications known to inhibit the 2C9 and 2C19 pathways.

Use of PDEIs in Patients with CVD

Heart Failure

Lack of exercise tolerance, a prevailing symptom of heart failure (HF), has been identified as a major predictor of patient prognosis.[51,52] Several studies have shown that PDEIs improve exercise capacity in patients with HF.[53-55] The benefits may be attributable to multiple mechanisms, including the alleviation of pulmonary hypertension and improvement of vascular endothelial function. Pulmonary hypertension, secondarily identified in 68-78% of patients with severe left ventricular systolic dysfunction, is often associated with concomitant right ventricular dysfunction.[54] In chronic left ventricular dysfunction, dysregulation of vascular smooth muscle tone frequently results in an elevation of pulmonary vascular resistance (PVR). Not surprisingly, PVR and right ventricular function are major predictors of both exercise tolerance and global prognosis in HF populations.[54]

In one study, Lewis and colleagues[56] investigated the acute effects of a single 50 mg dose of sildenafil on cardiopulmonary exercise parameters and hemodynamic effects in 13 patients with stable New York Heart Association Class III HF. One hour after sildenafil administration, pulmonary arterial pressure was reduced by 14%; systemic and pulmonary vascular resistance was reduced by 19% and 21%, respectively. Resting and exercise cardiac index were increased by 20% and 12%, respectively ($p < 0.05$ for all parameters). However, there was no significant change in terms of arterial pressure, heart rate, or pulmonary capillary wedge pressure.

The same authors investigated the chronic effects of PDEIs.[54] Thirty-four patients with symptomatic HF and pulmonary hypertension received 12 weeks of treatment with sildenafil at doses of 25 to 75mg given orally three times daily. Again, at peak exercise, sildenafil significantly decreased pulmonary vascular resistance (PVR) by 23% ($p=0.008$) and increased cardiac output (CO) by 38%($p=0.004$). Conversely, there was no effect on pulmonary capillary wedge pressure (PCWP), heart rate, arterial pressure, or systemic vascular reisistance(SVR) with longer term use. Commensurate with these findings, a four week study with sildenafil 50 mg given orally three times daily, conducted by Behling,[55] and a 6 month study using a 50mg twice daily regimen, conducted by Guazzi,[53] found significantly decreased systolic pulmonary artery pressure from baseline ($p=0.004$ for Behling, $p <0.01$ for Guazzi).

Patients with left ventricular assist devices (LVADs) have also benefited from sildenafil's ability to reduce pulmonary artery and systemic arterial pressures. The findings from a retrospective review of 10 consecutive LVAD patients concluded that sildenfil decreased pulmonary artery pressure and facilitated weaning from inhaled nitric oxide and inotropes without causing adverse hemodynamic effects.[57]

PDEIs are also thought to improve endothelial dysfunction, a hallmark of hemostasis-gone-wrong in HF patients. The endothelium is involved in a number of physiologic processes, including growth of smooth muscle cells, regulation of vascular tone and permeability, and maintenance of the balance between coagulation and fibrinolysis. The development of endothelial dysfunction in HF is related to increased SVR and other adversely altered pulmonary hemodynamics.[55] Disruption in endothelial function causes reduced vascular nitric oxide release, impairs skeletal blood flow during exercise, and is associated with decreased functional capacity.[58,59]

Katz and colleagues[60] investigated the possibility that PDE5 inhibition could have beneficial effects on endothelial function in HF patients. Using brachial artery ultrasound imaging to measure flow-mediated, endothelium-dependent vasodilation in response to transient arterial occlusion, the investigators found that, compared to placebo, the administration of sildenafil 25 and 50 mg resulted in a significant increase in brachial artery diameter after the release of 1, 3 and 5 min occlusions ($p < 0.05$). A study by Hryniewicz and colleagues[61] also utilized brachial artery ultrasound imaging and found that the concomitant doses of sildenafil and ACE-inhibitor ramipril had additive effects on brachial artery diameter at four hours after co-administration in HF patients.

The chronic effects of PDE5 inhibition on endothelial dysfunction have also been studied. In a four week trial, Behling and associates[55] assigned 11 patients to receive sildenafil 50 mg three times daily added to their current heart failure regimens. Patients in the placebo group showed a trend toward decreased forearm blood flow (FBF) (30% reduction, $P = 0.07$) after reactive hyperemia, while patients receiving the sildenafil regimen did not demonstrate any significant changes in FBF after reactive hyperemia from baseline. The investigators were unable to definitively state that there had been an improvement in endothelial function.

Guazzi and colleagues[53] found that HF patients receiving the same regimen for six months, again in addition to their current heart failure regimens, experienced significant increases in brachial artery flow-mediated dilatation (FMD) at 3 and 6 months compared to baseline (13.4% and 14.2% respectively, $P < 0.01$ for both). The findings suggest that chronic sildenafil administration is associated with improved long term endothelial function. Since there is thought to be a link between endothelial function and ergoreflex activity, the authors also sought to investigate the role of sildenafil in relief of abnormal skeletal muscle signaling due to muscle metabolic byproducts, a phenomenon known as ergoreflex. The study found that the ergoreflex effect on ventilation decreased significantly from baseline after 3 and 6 months of sildenafil treatment (67 and 72% respectively, $P < 0.01$ for both) suggesting that PDE5 inhibitors may have endothelium-mediated effects on muscle over-signaling that results in undesirable vasoconstriction.[53]

Regardless of the underlying mechanism, patients with HF treated chronically with sildenafil have shown increased exercise capacity and improvement in quality of life.[54] Clinical trials have shown a significant increase in peak oxygen uptake, ventilator efficiency, Minnesota Living with Heart Failure Score, and fewer hospitalizations for HF.[53-55] However, there is reason for caution. For example, in patients with predominant right ventricular heart failure, cardiac output increases with sildenafil, suggesting that the drug has an inotropic effect.[62] Nagendran and colleagues[63] found that although PDE5 is not normally present in the right ventricular myocardium, in patients with a hypertrophied right ventricular myocardium, it is present.[63] If PDE5 is also present in diseased, hypertrophied left ventricular tissue, there is concern about the safety of long-term administration of PDEIs in patients with systolic heart failure. Indeed, the long-term use of milrinone, an inotropic

PDE3 inhibitor, was found to increase morbidity and mortality in patients with severe chronic heart failure, and this could be a caveat regarding the use of PDEIs in this population.[64,65]

Hypertension

PDEIs produce mild systemic vasodilator effects without causing sympathomimetic-mediated increases in heart rate. Thus, they have the potential to lower blood pressure (BP) without inducing an increase in cardiac oxygen demand.[66] This desirable pharmacologic profile presents the opportunity for a new class of antihypertensive drugs. However, the acute effects of currently studied PDEIs, at least in terms of decreasing blood pressure, have thus far appeared relatively modest.

In a single-blind, four-way crossover trial by Jackson and colleagues,[67] eight healthy men aged 18-45 years received single doses of 100, 150, and 200 mg of sildenafil. BP was monitored at -1, 1, 3, 6, 9, and 12 hours after sildenafil administration. The result was a mean maximum reduction of 10 mm Hg systolic and 7 mm Hg diastolic BP. The BP reduction reached a peak at 3 hours post administration, and returned to baseline for most subjects 6 hours post-dose. In another study involving healthy volunteers receiving tadalafil 10 or 20 mg daily for 10 days, the drug did not significantly reduce systolic BP or have much of an effect on other BP parameters, but it did reduce diastolic pressure in the standing position by about 5 mm Hg compared to placebo by day 10 of therapy ($p < 0.05$).[68]

A study of the chronic effects of PDEIs on BP was conducted by Oliver and colleagues.[69] In a randomized, double-blind, two-way crossover study, 22 previously untreated hypertensive patients received either sildenafil 50 mg three times daily or placebo for 16 days. Both clinic and ambulatory BPs were measured. In the clinic, BPs decreased 5/4 mm Hg from baseline, similar to responses observed with other antihypertensive medications given as monotherapy. Meanwhile, ambulatory daytime BPs were reduced 8 /6 mm Hg, and nighttime pressures were reduced 5/4 mm Hg, compared to baseline ($p < 0.05$ for both parameters). Although sildenafil treatment decreased 24-hour, daytime, and nighttime pressures significantly, the magnitude of the BP-lowering effect was lower at nighttime. The findings suggest that the overnight dosing interval may be too long. This is an important observation because early morning surges in blood pressure are associated with increased cardiovascular morbidity and mortality, due in part to resultant silent ischemic events and cerebrovascular infarcts. Finally, patients with substantially elevated systolic BPs at baseline had greater decreases in BP than those with lower baseline BP, suggesting that sildenafil may be more useful in treating patients with more severe hypertension than those with milder disease.[70,71]

In the aforementioned study, Oliver and colleagues [69] also investigated mechanisms other than systemic vasodilation through which PDEIs may exert beneficial effects in hypertension. By measuring carotid-femoral pulse wave velocity (CF-PWV), the authors assessed sildenafil's effects on arterial stiffness. They found no significant changes from baseline. However, there was a trend toward progressive reductions in CF-PWV, suggesting that sildenafil reduced arterial stiffness. The same authors also assessed sildenafil's effect on endothelial function through flow-mediated vasodilation (FMD) and did not find any significant changes in this parameter after 16 days. This study indicated that, contrary to findings reported in healthy and chronic heart failure subjects, sildenafil did not improve endothelial dysfunction in this particular venue. The authors hypothesized that hypertensive patients, unlike non-hypertensive patients, may rely on a vasodilatory pathway other than that involving nitric oxide. However, FMD is not significantly improved with a variety of other BP-lowering drugs, so sildenafil's potential as an antihypertensive drug should not be dismissed simply based upon this observation.[69]

Interestingly, PDEIs may be useful as antihypertensive agents due to psychological as well as physiological effects. A retrospective cohort study by Scranton and colleagues[72] found that treating ED with PDEIs for two years in 3,384 hypertensive men had a beneficial effect on BP. Consistent with Oliver's aforementioned speculation, men with BP ≥ 160 mm Hg experienced the greatest BP reduction, with a mean decrease in systolic pressure of 17.8 mm Hg from baseline in the two year interval. The authors concluded that the beneficial benefits of starting a PDEI inhibitor therapy are likely multifactorial. For one, the benefits appear to be related to the intensification of an antihypertensive regimen, which involves an increase in the frequency of BP monitoring after a PDEI is prescribed.[72] Other theories are that patients are more likely to embark in more measures of good self-care, such as losing weight and exercising, when sexual activity is restored.[73]

It has been observed that PDEIs have an additive effect with other BP-lowering medications. Webb and colleagues[74] reported that sildenafil, when administered to hypertensive patients taking amlodipine for one month, appreciated a modest maximal reduction of 8/7 and 10/8 mm Hg in sitting and standing BP, respectively. On the other hand a study by Zusman et al.[75] concluded that the additive effects of sildenafil, in combination with beta-blockers, diuretics, and ACE-inhibitors, was smaller than the effects found with amlodipine, and that the BP-lowering changes were unlikely to be clinically significant.

PDEIs have potential in treating patients with essential hypertension. However, further studies are needed. For example, an extended-release version of sildenafil, or the use of one of the longer acting drugs in its class, may result in a less fluctuant steady-state plasma concentration profile. The less fluctuant concentration-time curves would, of course, ameliorate or even eradicate nighttime or early morning decreases in BP-lowering.[69]

Pulmonary Hypertension

The previous section on PDEIs in HF addressed many studies that looked at the use of these agents in treating pulmonary hypertension (PH) secondary to HF. Outside of this disease state, the majority of studies with PDEIs have involved patients with idiopathic PH, or PH associated with connective tissue diseases.

The empiric use of PDEIs for PH seems to be logical. As discussed earlier, sildenafil, unlike vardenafil or tadalafil, shows a relatively high affinity for PDE 1c, a subtype PDE enzyme found in high concentrations in lung tissue.[37] Sildenafil has long been known to reduce pulmonary vascular resistance in a dose-dependent manner. In fact, the vasodilator effects appeared to be greater in the pulmonary circulation than in any other vascular bed within the human body. In addition, sildenafil has typically shown synergy with other commonly used agents, such as the inhaled prostacyclin analogue, iloprost. Sildenafil augmented and prolonged the therapeutic effect of iloprost.[37]

In one study, all three PDEIs were assessed and compared for their hemodynamic influences over a two hour period in 60 consecutive patients with PH. All three agents induced significant pulmonary vasodilation, with peak effects occurring at 40-45 minutes for vardenafil, 60 minutes for sildenafil, and 75-90 minutes for tadalafil. Sildenafil and tadalafil caused a significant reduction in pulmonary SVR, whereas vardenafil did not. Significant improvement in arterial oxygenation only occurred with sildenafil. Thus, it is important to note that the three agents differ in terms of their pharmacokinetic properties, their selectivity for the pulmonary vascular beds, and their impact on arterial oxygenation. Of the three PDEIs, sidenafil exhibited the most desirable hemodynamic profile in this study.[76]

In terms of chronic management, several small single center studies have reported beneficial effects of sildenafil for the long term treatment of PH.[37] However, the sentinel study that catapulted sildenafil into its new FDA indication was the SUPER-1 study.[77] This study involved 278 patients with symptomatic PH who were treated with either placebo or sildenafil at 20, 40, or 80 mg three times daily for 12 weeks. The primary endpoint was measurement of hemodynamic changes and total walking distance after a 6 minute walk distance test. The test was performed at baseline and at 12 weeks into treatment. All three sildenafil doses improved exercise capacity ($p < 0.001$ for all three doses) and WHO functional class rankings ($p=0.003$ for 20 mg, $p< 0.001$ for 40 and 80mg doses), as well as various hemodynamic markers, including mean arterial pulmonary pressure ($p=0.04$ for 20mg, $p=0.01$ for 40mg, and $p< 0.01$ for 80mg) over the placebo arm. However, despite apparent trends towards a dose-response relationship, there were no statistical differences found between the three dose regimens. In addition, the increase in the 6 minute walk distance achieved in the placebo controlled trial phase was sustained for up to 3 months when these patients were maintained on open label drug at the 80mg dose.

Because the dose-response curve appeared statistically flat in the SUPER-1 trial, the FDA decision was to license the drug at a fixed dose of 20mg administered three times daily. However, this single dose labeling has created a conundrum for clinicians treating PH with sidenafil.[37] If used with the known sildenafil inducer bosentan, the sildenafil dose is ostensibly only equivalent to about half, or 10mg three times daily, due to the metabolic induction elicited by bosentan.[78,79] Also, many clinicians feel that over time, as the disease progresses, larger doses may be needed. At least in one aspect, the Super-1 study supported a dose-response relationship, where 80mg given three times daily had a greater effect on PVR than did the lower doses.[79]

Combination therapy with sildenafil has been studied, but currently there are only unblinded trials. Despite the aforementioned pharmacokinetic interaction, sildenafil with the endothelin-receptor antagonist bosentan has been found to arrest clinical deterioration.[78,79] Combination therapy with sildenafil and sitaxentan or ambrisentan, two newer endothelin receptor antagonists not known to be CYP-inducers, lacks the pharmacokinetic interaction, but pharmacodynamic data is currently lacking.[37] Finally, beneficial short and long term effects have been observed when sildenafil was combined with inhaled iloprost.[80,81]

Sildenafil has also been effective in treating PH associated with HIV,[82,83] PH related to high altitude exposure,[84] PH in patients with non-operable chronic thromboembolism,[85,86] and hypoxia-associated PH.[87] If sildenafil can improve parameters for hypoxia-associated PH, it may provide a modicum of hope for patients suffering from COPD, interstitial lung disease, and obstructive sleep apnea.[37,88]

Continued interest in studying PDEIs for various types of PH prevails. For one, these agents are the only ones available that reduce PVR without compromising V'/Q'matching and subsequent oxygenation, which makes them more desirable in the treatment of patients who already have underlying lung disease. Secondly, these drugs may help improve right ventricular function by inhibiting PDE 5 found in the cardiac tissues of patients with right ventricular hypertrophy. The local PDE 5 inhibiting effect would enhance contractility and bolster CO, favorably changing two parameters that have already been linked to better outcomes in determining patient prognosis in those who have clinically succumbed to the adverse effects of PH.[37]

Diabetes

ED and diabetes mellitus share many risk factors such as endothelial dysfunction, autonomic neuropathy, and vascular and hormonal abnormalities. Using a national managed care claims database Sun et al.[89] conducted a retrospective study to compare the prevalence rates of diabetes between men with ED (285,436) and men without ED (1,584,230). The findings showed that men with ED were more than twice as likely to have diabetes as men without ED (20.0% vs 7.5%). After adjusting for age and concurrent diseases, men with ED were still more likely to have diabetes than men without ED (odds ratio 1.60, $p < 0.001$). In the Massachusetts Male Aging Study (MMAS),[1] the prevalence of any degree of ED in diabetic men aged 40 to 70 years was estimated to be around 52%, and men with diabetes were three to four times more likely to have ED compared with those without diabetes.

ED may predate the clinical diagnosis of type 2 diabetes by years, and in fact, may be the first symptom of yet undiagnosed diabetes.[90] The United Kingdom Prevention of Diabetes Study (UKPDS) revealed that 20% of patients had ED at the time their diabetes was diagnosed.[91] Based on these findings, it has been suggested that ED can be used as an early, observable marker to detect diabetes earlier.

In men with silent ischemia and angiographic evidence of CHD, Gazzaruso et al.[92] reported that ED was significantly more prevalent than in men without silent ischemia (33.8% vs. 4.75, $p=0.001$). In fact, after adjustment for confounding variables, ED appeared to be the most efficient independent predictor of silent CAD. This suggests that ED in patients with diabetes can provide a rationale for screening for silent coronary artery disease.

The etiology of ED in the setting of diabetes is often complex and related to poor glycemic control, dyslipidemia, microvascular and macrovascular disease, autonomic neuropathy, and endothelial dysfunction. ED is often related to the duration and severity of diabetes and correlates with glycemic control.[93] It has been demonstrated that controlling blood sugar levels does improve erectile function.[93]

Treatment with PDEIs is now considered first-line therapy because of convenience, effectiveness, and generally good tolerance to the drugs. Sildenafil, vardenafil, and tadalafil have not been directly compared in a head-to-head trial, but all three drugs significantly improve erectile function in patients with diabetes and ED.

In a 16-week randomized, double-blind, placebo-controlled, and fixed-dose study, 282 men (mean age, 46.4 years) with ED (mean duration, 3.6 years) and diabetes (mean duration, 11 years) were randomly assigned to receive 100 mg sildenafil or placebo approximately 1 hour before planned sexual activity.[94] The efficacy of the two treatments was assessed using responses to the International Index of Erectile Function (IIEF) questionnaire.[95] Positive clinical results were obtained in 68 (51%) of 134 patients in the sildenafil group compared with 14 (11%) of 128 patients in the placebo group ($p<0.003$). Boulton et al.[96] in a 12-week double blind, placebo-controlled randomized clinical trial, evaluated the effectiveness of sildenafil in 219 men with ED and type 2 diabetes. Primary criteria for efficacy included questions 3 (achieving an erection) and 4 (maintaining an erection) from the International Index of Erectile Function (IIEF, score range, 0-5). After 12 weeks, the mean scores for questions 3 and 4 had improved significantly in patients receiving sildenafil compared with placebo ($p < 0.0001$). In this study sildenafil was well tolerated and improved ED in men with type 2 diabetes independent of the degree of glycemic control or the presence of neuropathic and vascular complications. In a similar study, Rendel et al.[97] randomized 268 diabetic men with ED to receive either sildenafil or placebo for 12 weeks. In the sildenafil arm, 56% of the patients reported improved erections, compared to 10% in the placebo group ($p< 0.001$). A meta-analysis of 11 randomized, double-blind, placebo-controlled trials of sildenafil in patients with diabetes reported improved erections in 59% of patients with type 1 diabetes and 63% with type 2 diabetes.[98] Improvement has been noted regardless of age, race, severity and duration of ED.[99] However, the response rate in men with diabetes was less than the 83% improvement observed in men with ED who did not have diabetes. Randomized trials have also documented the effectiveness of tadalafil[100, 101] and vardenafil[42] in men with diabetes and ED. A multicenter, double-blind, placebo-controlled study assessed the effectiveness of tadalafil (10 or 20 mg) in 216 men with diabetes and severe ED.[100] Improved erectile function was reported in 22.2% and 22.6% of men receiving 10 and 20 mg respectively of tadalafil as compared with a decline of 4.1% for those patients receiving placebo.

Studies comparing response rates to PDEIs in diabetic versus non-diabetic men with ED have reported variable findings. In a multi-center study of 1,511 patients with ED, the response rates to sildenafil was lower for patients with diabetes (77.9%), as compared to those without diabetes (86.5%) ($p<0.01$).[102] Patients with diabetes also required a higher dose of sildenafil as compared to those without diabetes. In another study with tadalafil, 76% of men with diabetes had improved erections, although only 58% of those receiving tadalafil (20 mg) reported erections sufficient for satisfactory intercourse.[101] In men without diabetes, the comparable rates were 81% and 75%, respectively. Similar findings have been observed with verdenafil.[42] The poorer efficacy of PDEIs in the diabetic population is thought to be related to poor vascular supply to the penile arteries resulting from macrovascular disease,[103] reduced production of nitric oxide as a result of advanced glycosylation product accumulation,[104] and impaired neurogenic and endothelium-dependent relaxation in penile arteries.[105] Many men with diabetes have subclinical neuropathy that may decrease the effectiveness of PDEIs.

Coronary Artery Disease

The relationship between CV disease and ED is well documented. In one study, 49% of patients who had acute chest pain and had angiographically documented CAD also had ED.[27] Others have demonstrated a correlation between ED, the number of affected coronary vessels, and the severity of ischemic coronary disease. Recent findings from clinical trials suggest that ED may be an early marker of atherosclerosis, subclinical or undiagnosed CVD, and systemic vascular disease. The presence and recognition of ED, therefore provides a clinical tool to identify men at an early stage prior to the development of atherosclerosis or an adverse vascular event.

The PDEIs have been shown to be effective in men with known coronary artery disease.[106,107] Conti et al.[108] showed that sildenafil improved erections in 70% of men with known coronary artery disease compared with 20% in patients who received placebo. A recent analysis by DeBusk et al.[106] confirmed these results. Patients with ED and clinically stable coronary artery disease were randomized to sildenafil or placebo for 12 weeks. By 12 weeks, patients receiving sildenafil had significantly better improvements on question 3 and 4 of the International Index of Erectile Function than did patients receiving placebo ($n=72$; $p < 0.01$). Patients taking sildenafil were more likely to report improved erections (64%) and improved intercourse (65%) vs patients receiving placebo (21% and 19%).

Sildenafil, vardenafil, and tadalafil have not been associated with serious adverse cardiovascular events. Results from clinical trials do not indicate an increase in cardiac ischemia, MI, or mortality in patients taking PDEIs.[106-108] It has been shown that when given to patients with stable CAD during exercise stress testing, PDEIs do not exacerbate ischemia compared with placebo.[109,110]

In a double-blind placebo-controlled crossover study of 105 men at high risk for CAD, the effects of sildenafil 50 mg and 100 mg were compared with placebo, using exercise echocardiography.[109] The findings showed no adverse effects on the left ventricular wall motion score with a similar hemodynamic response regarding heart rate, blood pressure, and exercise capacity. Fox et al.[111] tested sildenafil 100 mg in a study that included 108 men with stable angina. The primary end point was time to limiting angina, and secondary end points included time to angina, time to ST-segment depression, and exercise duration. All patients had ischemia at baseline and underwent exertion on a treadmill 1 hour after receiving sildenafil or placebo. In this study, sildenafil increased primary and secondary end points ($p<0.05$) and was generally well tolerated.

Mittleman et al.[112] pooled data from 124 double-blind clinical trials involving 5054 placebo-treated and 6896 sildenafil-treated patients and found that the overall incidence of MI and CV death were low and comparable between sildenafil and placebo treatments, $p = 0.801$. Studies that have extensively evaluated the use of tadalafil in patients with CVD have shown a similar safety profile compared to sildenafil with no adverse effects on cardiac function or ischemic threshold.[49,113] Because safety has not been established in patients with recent serious CV events, the use of PDEIs is not recommended in patients with unstable CAD, a recent history of MI and stroke (in the past 6 to 8 weeks or earlier), moderate to severe HF, cardiomyopathy and severe valvular heart disease.

The vasodilating effects of PDE inhibitors can be concerning, particularly in patients with CV disease, left ventricular outflow obstruction or aortic stenosis.[114,115] In the setting of angina, alternatives to nitrates should be considered after PDE inhibitor therapy. If a patient has taken sildenafil or vardenafil (half-life of 4 hours) and then develops angina, the recommendation from the American College of Cardiology/American Heart Association Consensus Committee is to withhold nitrates for 24 hours.[114] However, if a patient takes tadalafil (half-life of 17.5 hours) and then has angina, nitrates should be withheld for about 48 hours.[115] During the period of time in which nitrates should not be administered, other antianginal and anti-ischemic drugs may be used such as beta-blockers, calcium-channel blockers, aspirin, and others. Although nitrates are antianginal agents, they have not been shown to reduce adverse CV events or reduce cardiac mortality in the setting of an acute coronary syndrome.

Summary

ED is now considered both an early manifestation and an independent predictor of cardiovascular disease. In men presenting with ED, cardiovascular risk factors should be evaluated and managed in order to prevent future cardiac events. PDEIs provide a promising clinical therapeutic modality for improving not only the symptoms of ED, but also treating the underlying endothelial dysfunction that initially caused the ED. The PDEIs are now established as first- line therapy in the treatment for ED. All three agents appear equally effective in treating ED, but some differences in pharmacokinetics and side effect profiles may drive physician and patient preferences towards one specific agent. Overall, PDEIs are well tolerated, and have been found safe in a wide array of patients, including those with comorbidities such as diabetes, hypertension, coronary artery disease, and heart failure.

References

[1] Feldman HA, Goldstein I, Hatzichristou DG, et al. Impotence and it medical psychosocial correlates: results of the Massachusetts Male Aging Study. *J Urol* 1994;151:54-61.

[2] KL, Bank AJ, Padma-Nathan H, et al. Erectile dysfunction is a marker for cardiovascular disease: results of the Minority Health Institute expert advisory panel. *J Sex med* 2005;2:40-52.

[3] Speel TG, van Langen H, Meuleman EJ. The risk of coronary heart disease in men with erectile dysfunction. *Eur Urol* 2003;44:366-370.

[4] Jensen J, Lendorf A, Stimpel H et al. The prevalence and etiology of impotence in 101 male hypertensive outpatients. *Am J hypertens* 1999;12:271-275.

[5] Wei M, Macera CA, Davis DR et al. Total cholesterol and high density lipoprotein cholesterol as important predictors of erectile dysfunction. *Am J Epidemiol* 1994;140:930-937.

[6] Roumeguere T, Wespes E, Carpentier Y et al. Erectile dysfunction is associated with a high prevalence of hyperlipidemia and coronary heart disease risk. *Eur Urol* 2003;44:355-359.

[7] Bacon CG, Hu FB, Biovannucci E et al. Association of type and duration of diabetes with erectile dysfunction in a large cohort of men. *Diabetes Care* 2002;25:1458-63.

[8] Moulik PK, Hardy KJ. Hypertension, antihypertensive drug therapy and erectile dysfunction in diabetes. *Diabet Med* 2003;20:290-293.

[9] Rosen MP, Greenfield AJ, Walker TG et al. Cigarette smoking: an independent risk factor for atherosclerosis in the hypogastric-cavernous arterial bed of men with arteriogenic impotence. *J Urol* 1991;145:759-63.

[10] Fung MM, Bettencourt R, Barrett-Connor E. Heart disease risk factors predict erectile dysfunction 25 years later: the Rancho Bernardo study. *J Am Coll Cardiol* 2004;43;1405-1411.

[11] Esposito K, Giugliano F, Martedi E et al. High proportions of erectile dysfunction in men with erectile dysfunction. *Diabetes Care* 2005;28:1201-1203.
[12] Solomon H, Man JW, Jackson G. Erectile dysfunction and the cardiovascular patient: endothelial dysfunction is the common denominator. *Heart* 2003;89:251-253.
[13] Virag R, Bouilly P, Frydman D. Is impotence an arterial disorder? A study of arterial risk factors in 440 impotent men. Lancet 1985;1:181-184.
[14] Jackson G. Erectile dysfunction and cardiovascular disease. *Int J Clin Pract* 1999;53:363-368.
[15] Guay AT. ED2: erectile dysfunction = endothelial dysfunction. *Endocrinol Metab Clin North Am* 2007;36:453-463.
[16] Sullivan ME, Thompson CS, Dashwood MR et al. Nitric oxide and penile erection: Is erectile dysfunction another manifestation of vascular disease? *Cardiovasc Res* 1999;43:658-665.
[17] Kaiser DR, Billups K, Mason C, et al. Impaired brachial artery endothelium-dependent and –independent vasodilation in men with erectile dysfunction and no other clinical cardiovascular disease. *J Am Coll Cardiol* 2004;43:179-184.
[18] Tikkanen MJ, Jackson G, Tammela T, et al. Erectile dysfunction as a risk factor for coronary heart disease: implications for prevention. *Int J Clin Pract* 2007;61(2):265-268.
[19] Miner M, Billups KL. Erectile dysfunction and dyslipidemia: relevance and role of phosphodiesterase type-5 inhibitors and statins. *J Sex Med* 2008;5:1066-1078.
[20] Kawashima S, Yokoyama M. Dysfunction of endothelial nitric oxide synthase and atherosclerosis. *Arterioscler Thromb Vasc Biol* 2004;24:998-1005.
[21] Kirby M, Jackson G, Simonsen U. Endothelial dysfunction links erectile dysfunctiont to heart disease. *Int J Clin Pract* 2005;59:225-229.
[22] Dhabuwala CB, Kumar A, Pierce JM. Myocardial infarction and its influence on male sexual function. *Arch Sexual Behav* 1986;15:499-504.
[23] Kloner RA, Mullin SH, Shook T, et al. Erectile dysfunction in the cardiac patient: how common and should we treat? *J Urol* 2003;170 (suppl):S46-S50.
[24] Blumentals WA, Gomez-Caminero A, Joo S, et al. Should erectile dysfunction be considered as a marker for acute myocardial infarction? Results from a retrospective cohort study. *Int J Impot Res* 2004;16:350-353.
[25] Thompson IM, Tangen CM, Goodman PJ, et al. Erectile dysfunction and subsequent cardiovascular disease. *JAMA* 2005;294:2996-3002.
[26] Billups KL. Erectile dysfunction as an early sign of cardiovascular disease. *Int J Impot Res* 2005;17 (suppl):S19-S24.
[27] Montorsi F, Briganti A, Salonia A et al. Erectile dysfunction prevalence, time of onset and association with risk factors in 300 consecutive patients with acute chest pain and angiographically documented coronary artery disease. *Eur Urol* 2003;44:360-5.
[28] Blumentals WA, Gomez-Caminero A, Joo S et al. Is erectile dysfunction predictive of peripheral vascular disease? *Aging Male* 2003;6:217-221.
[29] Pritzker MR. The penile stress tests: a window to the hearts of Man? *Circulation* 1999;100(suppl 1):350-353.
[30] Vlachopoulos C, Rokkas K, Iokeimides N, et al. Prevalence of asymptomatic coronary artery disease in men with vasculogenic erectile dysfunction: a prospective angiographic study. *Eur Urol* 2005;48:996-1003.

[31] Kloner RA. *Heart Disease and Erectile Dysfunction*. Humana Press Inc. Totowa, New Jersey. 2004.

[32] McCullough AR. An update on the PDE-5 inhibitors. *J Androl* 2003;24 (suppl):S52-S58.

[33] Salonia A, Rigatti P, Montorsi F. Sildenafil in erectile disfunction: A critical review. *Curr Med Res Opin* 2003;19:241-262.

[34] Jackson G. Hemodynamic and exercise effects of phosphodiesterase 5 inhibitors. *Am J Cardiol* 2005; 96 (suppl): 32M- 35M.

[35] Hellstrom WJG, Kendirci M. Type 5 phosphodiesterase inhibitors: curing erectile dysfunction. *Eur Urol* 2006;49:942-945.

[36] Seftel AD. Challenges in oral therapy for erectile dysfunction. J Androl 2002;23:729-736.

[37] Wilkins MR, Wharton J, Grimminger F, Ghofrani HA. Phosphodiesterase inhibitors for the treatment of pulmonary hypertension. *Eur Respir J* 2008;32:198-209.

[38] Rakel: Textbook of Family Medicine on MD Consult, 7th Ed. Male Sexual Disorders. (2007). URL: http://www.mdconsult.com/das/book/body/93087398-3/698678431/1481/608.html Accessed: April 24, 2008.

[39] *Sildenafil prescribing information*. New York, NY:Pfizer;2007.

[40] *Vardenafil prescribing information*. Kenilworth, NJ:Schering-Plough;2007.

[41] *Tadalafil prescribing information*. Indianapolis, IN: Eli Lilly and Company; 2008.

[42] Porst H, Rosen R, Padma-Nathan H Golstein I, et al. The efficacy and tolerability of vardenafil, a new oral selective phosphodiesterasetype 5 inhibitor in patients with erectile dysfunction: the first at home clinical trial. *Int J Impot Res* 2001;13:192-199.

[43] Padma-Nathan H, McMurral JG, Pullman WE, et al. On-demand IC351(Cialis) enhances erectile function in patients with erectile dysfunction. *Int J Impot Res* 2001;13:2-9.

[44] Moreira SG, Brannigan RE, Sitz A, et al. Side effect profile of sildenafil citrate (Viagra) in clinical practice. *Urology* 2000;56:474-6.

[45] Sowka J, Neiberg L, Vollmer L. Optic atrophy after sildenafil use. *J Am Optometry Assoc* 2003;78:122-128.

[46] Waknine Y. Erectile dysfunction drugs linked to risk for hearing loss. Medscape Medical News 2007 http://www.medscape.com/viewarticle/564533.

[47] Baxendale RW, et al. Selectivity of sildenafil and other phosphodiesterase type 5 (PDE5) inhibitors against phosphodiesterase types 7-11. *J Clin Pharmacol* 2001;41:1015.

[48] Montorsi F, Nathan HP, McCullough A, et al. Tadalfil in the treatment of erectile dysfunction following nerve sparing radical retropubic prostectomy: a randomized, double blind placebo controlled trial. *J Urol* 2004;172:1036-41.

[49] Jackson G, Rosen RC, Kloner RA, et al. The second princeton consensus on sexual dysfunction and cardiac risk: new guidelines for sexual medicine. *J Sex Med* 2006;3:28-36.

[50] Kloner RA. Medscape: Erectile dysfunction and the cardiovascular disease connection: An update for clinicians. Accessed online: http://www.medscape.com/viewprogram/5895_pnt.

[51] De Groote P, Dagorn J, Soudan B, et al. B-type natriuretic peptide and peak exercise oxygen consumption provide independent information for risk stratification in patients with stable congestive heart failure. *J Am Coll Cardiol* 2004;43:584-1589.

[52] Bittner V, Weiner DH, Yusuf S. Prediction of mortality and morbidity with a 6-minute walk test in patients with left ventricular dysfunction. SOLVD investigators. *JAMA* 1993;270 1702-1707.

[53] Guazzi M, Samata M, Arena R. Long-term use of sildenafil in the therapeutic management of heart failure. *J Am Coll Cardiol* 2007;50:2136-2144.

[54] Lewis GD, Shah R, Shahzad K. Sildenafil improves exercise capacity and quality of life in patients with systolic heart failure and secondary pulmonary hypertension. *Circulation* 2007;116:1555-1561.

[55] Behling A, Rohde LE, Colombo FC. Effects of 5'-phosphodiesterase four-week long inhibition with sildenafil in patients with chronic heart failure: A double-blind, placebo-controlled clinical trial. *J Cardiac Failure* 2008;14:189-196.

[56] Lewis GD, Lachmann J, Camuso J. Sildenafil improves exercise hemodynamics and oxygen uptake in patients with systolic heart failure. *Circulation* 2007;115:59-65.

[57] Klodell CT, Morey TE, Lobato ED. Effect of sildenafil on pulmonary artery pressure, systemic pressure, and nitric oxide utilization in patients with left ventricular assist devices. *Ann of Thorac Surg* 2007;83: 68-71.

[58] Katz SD, Krum H, Khan T. Exercise-induced vasodilation in forearm circulation of normal subjects and patients with congestive heart failure: Role of endothelium-derived nitric oxide. *J Am Coll Cardiol.*1996; 28:585-590.

[59] Nakamura M, Ishikawa M, Funakoshi T, et al.. Attenuated endothelium-dependent peripheral vasodilation and clinical characteristics in patients with chronic heart failure. *Am Heart J* 1994;128:11641169.

[60] Katz SD, Balidemaj K, Homma S. Acute type 5 phosphodiesterase inhibition with sildenafil enhances flow-mediated vasodilation in patients with chronic heart failure. *J Am Coll Cardiol* 2000;36:845-851.

[61] Hryniewicz K, Dimayuga C, Hudaihed A. Inhibition of angiotensin-converting enzyme and phosphodiesterase type 5 improves endothelial function in heart failure. *Clinical Science*. 2005;108:331-337.

[62] Michelakis E, Tymchak W, Lien D. Oral sildenafil is an effective and specific pulmonary vasodilator in patients with pulmonary arterial hypertension: Comparison with inhaled nitric oxide. *Circulation* 2002;105:2398-2403.

[63] Nagendran J, Archer SL, Soliman D. Phosphodiesterase type 5 is highly expressed in the hypertrophied human right ventricle, and acute inhibition of phosphodiesterase type 5 improves contractility. *Circulation* 2007;116:238-248.

[64] Goldsmith SR. Type 5 phosphodiesterase inhibition in heart failure: The next step. *J Am Coll Cardiol* 2007;50:2136-44.

[65] Packer M, Carver JR, Rodeheffer RJ. Effect of oral milrinone on mortality in severe chronic heart failure. The PROMISE study research group. *N Engl J Med* 1991;325:1468-1475.

[66] Ghiadoni L. Phosphodiesterase 5 inhibition in essential hypertension. *Current Hypertension Reports* 2008;10:52-57.

[67] Jackson G, Benjamin N, Jackson N, et al. Effects of sildenafil citrate on human hemodynamics. *Am Cardiol* 1999;83:13-19.

[68] Kloner RA, Mitchell M, Emmick JT. Cardiovascular effects of tadalafil. *Am J Cardiol* 2003;92 (suppl):37M-46M.
[69] Oliver JJ, Melville VP, Webb DJ, et al. Effect of regular phosphodiesterase type 5 inhibition in hypertension. *Hypertension* 2006;48:622-627.
[70] Mancia G, De Backer G, Dominiczak A. 2007 guidelines for the management of arterial hypertension: The task force for the management of arterial hypertension of the European Society of Hypertension (ESH) and of the European Society of Cardiology (ESC) *Eur Heart J* 2007;28:1462.
[71] Giles TD. Circadian rhythm of blood pressure and the relation to cardiovascular events. *J Hypertension* 2006;24 (suppl):S11-S16.
[72] Scranton RE, Lawler E, Botteman M, et al. Effect of treating erectile dysfunction on management of systolic hypertension. *Am J Cardiol* 2007;100:459-463.
[73] Yao S, Messerle FH. Blood pressure control and sildenafil-carrot stick or sword of damocles? *Am J Cardiol* 2007;100:552-553.
[74] Webb DJ, Freestone S, Allen MT. Sildenafil citrate and blood-pressure-lowering drugs: Results of drug interaction studies with an organic nitrate and a calcium antagonist. *Am J Cardiol* 1999;83:21-28.
[75] Zusman RM, Prisant LM, Brown MJ. Effect of sildenafil citrate on blood pressure and heart rate in men with erectile dysfunction taking concomitant antihypertensive medication. Sildenafil study group. *J Hypertension* 2000;18:1865-1869.
[76] Ghofrani HA Voswininckel E Reichenberger F, et al. Differences in hemodynamic and oxygenation responses to three different phosphodiesterse-5 inhibitors in patients with pulmonary arterial hypertension: a randomized prospective study. *J Am Coll Cardiol* 2004;44:1488-1496.
[77] Galie N, Ghofrani HA, Torbicki A, et al. Sildenafil citrate therapy for pulmonary arterial hypertension. *N Engl J Med* 2005;353:2148-2153.
[78] Hoeper MM, Faulenbach C Golpon H, et al. Combination therapy with bosentan and sildenafil in idiopathic pulmonary hypertension. *Eur Respir J* 2004;24:1007-1010.
[79] Mathai SC, Girgis RE, Fisher MR, et al. Addition of sidenafil to bosentan monotherapy in pulmonary arterial hypertension. *Eur Respir J* 2007;29:469-475.
[80] Ghofrani HA, Wiedeman R, Rose F, et al. Combination therapy with oral sidenafil and inhaled iloprost for severe pulmonary hypertension. *Ann Intern Med* 2002;136:515-522.
[81] Ghofrani HA, Rose F, Schermuly RT, et al. Oral sildenafil as long-term adjunct therapy to inhaled iloprost in severe pulmonary arterial hypertension. *J Am Coll Cardiol* 2003;42:158-164.
[82] Carlsen J, Kjeldsen K, Gerstoft j. Sildenfil as a successful treatment of otherwise fatal HIV-related pulmonary hypertension. *AIDS* 2002;16:1568-1569.
[83] Schumacher YO, Zdebik A, Huonker M, et al. Sildenafil in HIV-related pulmonary hypertension. *AIDS* 2001;15:1747-1748.
[84] Ghofrani HA, Reichenberger F, Kohstall MG, et al. Sidenafil increases exercise capacity during hypoxia at low altitudes and at Mount-Everest base camp: a randomized, double-blind, placebo-controlled crossover trial. *Ann Intern Med* 2004;141:169-177.
[85] Ghofrani HA, Schermuly RT, Rose F., et al. Sildenafil for long term treatment of non-operable chronic thromboembolic pulmonary hypertension. *Am J Resp Crit Care Med* 2003;167:1139-1141.

[86] Reichenberger F, Voswinckel R, Enke B, et al. .Long-term treatment with sidenafil in chronic thromboembolic pulmonary hypertension. *Eur Respir J* 2007;30:922-927.
[87] Richalet JP, Gratadour P, Robach P, et al. Sildenafil inhibits altitude-induced hypoxemia and pulmonary hypertension. *Am J Respir Crit Care Med* 2005;171:275-281.
[88] Higginbottam T. Pulmonary hypertension and chronic obstructive pulmonary disease: a case for treatment. *Proc Am Thorac Soc* 2005;2:12-19.
[89] Sun P, Cameron A, Seftel A, et al. Erectile dysfunction-An observable marker of diabetes mellitus? A Large national epidemiological study. *J Urol* 2006;176:1081-1085.
[90] Deutsh S, Sherman L. Previously unrecognized diabetes mellitus in sexually impotent men. *JAMA* 1980;244:2430-2.
[91] Manley SM, Meyer LC, Neil HAW et al. Complications in newly diagnosed type 2 diabetic patients and their association with different clinical and biochemical risk factors. *Diabetes Res* 1990;13:1-11.
[92] Gazzaruso C, Giordanetti S, De Amici E, et al. Relationship between erectile dysfunction and silent myocardial ischemia in apparently uncomplicated type 2 diabetic patients. *Circulation* 2004; 110:22-26.
[93] Romeo JH, Seftel AD, Madhun ZT, et al. Sexual function in men with diabetes type 2: association with glycemic control. *J Urol* 2000;163:788-791.
[94] Safarinejad MR. Oral sildenafil in the treatment of erectile dysfunction in diabetic men: a randomized double-blind and placebo-controlled study. *J Diabetes and Its Complications* 2004;18:205-210.
[95] Rosen RC, Riley A, Wagner G, et al. The International Index of Erectile Function (IIEF): A multidimensional scale for assessment of erectile dysfunction. *Urology* 1997;49:822-830.
[96] Boulton AJM, Selam JL, Sweeney M, et al. Sildenafil citrate for the treatment of erectile dysfunction in men with type 2 diabetes mellitus. *Diabetologia* 2001;44:1296-1301.
[97] Rendell MS, Rajfer J, Wicker PA, et al. Sildenafil for treatment of erectile dysfunction in men with diabetes: a randomized controlled trial. *JAMA* 1999;281:421-426.
[98] Fink HA, Mac DR, Rutks IR, et al. Sildenafil for male erectile dysfunction: a systematic review and meta-analysis. *Arch Intern Med* 2002;162:1349-60.
[99] Carson CC, Burnett AL, Levine LA, et al. The efficacy of sildenafil citrate (Viagra) in clinical populations: an update. *Urology* 2002;60 (suppl 2):12-27.
[100] Saenz de Tejada I, Anglin G, Knight JR, et al. Effects of tadalafil on erectile dysfunction in men with diabetes. *Diabetes Care* 2002;25:2159-64.
[101] Brock GB, Mcmahon CG, Chen KK et al. Efficacy and safety of tadalafil for the treatment of erectile dysfunction: results of integrated analyses. *J Urol* 2002;168:1332-1336.
[102] Ng KK, Lim HCP, Ng FC, et al. The use of sildenafil in patients with erectile dysfunction in relation to diabetes mellitus – A study of 1,511 patients. *Singapore Med J* 2002; 43(8):387-390.
[103] Kadioglu A, Erdogru T, Karsidag K et al. Evaluation of penile arterial system with color Doppler ultrasonography in nondiabetic and diabetic males. *Eur Urol* 1995; 27:311-314.

[104] Seftel AD, Vaziri ND, Ni Z et al. Advanced glycation end products in human penis: elevation in diabetic tissue, site of deposition, and possible effect through iNOS or eNOS. *Urology* 1997;50:1016-1026.

[105] Saenz de Tejada I, Goldstein I, Azadzoi K, et al. Impaired neurogenic and endothelium-mediated relaxation of enile smooth muscle from diabetic men with impotence. *N Engl J Med* 1989;320:1025-1030.

[106] DeBusk RF, Pepine CJ, Glasser DB, et al. Efficacy and safety of sildenafil citrate in men with erectile dysfunction and stable coronary artery disease. *Am J Cardiol* 2004;93:147-153.

[107] Olsson AM, Persson CA. Efficacy and safety of sildenafil citrate for the treatment of erectile dysfunction in men with cardiovascular disease. *Int J Clin Pract* 2001;55:171-176.

[108] Conti CR, Peine CJ, Sweeney M. Efficacy and safety of sildenafil citrate in the treatment of erectile dysfunction in patients with ischemic heart disease. *Am J Cardiol* 1999;83:29C-34C.

[109] Arruda-Olson AM, Mahoney DW, Nehra A, et al. Cardiovascular effects of sildenafil during exercise in men with known or probable coronary artery disease: a randomized crossover trial. *JAMA* 2002;287:719-725.

[110] Thadani U, Smith W, Nash S, et al. The effect of vardenafil, a potent and highly selective phosphodiesterase-5 inhibitor for the treatment of erectile dysfunction on the cardiovascular response to exercise in patients with coronary artery disease. *J Am Coll Cardiol* 2002;40:2006-2012.

[111] Fox KM, Thadani U, Ma PT, et al. Sildenafil citrate does not reduce exercise tolerance in men with erectile dysfunction and chronic stable angina. *Eur Heart J* 2003;24:2206-2212.

[112] Mitttleman MA, Glasser DB, Orazem J. Clinical trials of sildenafil citrate (Viagra) demonstrate no increase in risk of myocardial infarction and cardiovascular death compared with placebo. *Int J Clin Pract* 2003;57;597-600.

[113] Kloner RA, et al. Cardiovascular safety of vardenafil, a potent, highly selective PDE5 inhibitor in patients with erectile dysfunction: An analysis of five placebo-controlled trials. *Pharmacotherapy* 2002;22:1371.

[114] Cheitlin MD, Hutter AM, Brindis RG, et al. ACC/AHA expert consensus document use of sildenafil (Viagra) in patients with cardiovascular disease. *J Am Coll Cardiol* 1999;33:272-281.

[115] DeBusk R, Drory Y, Goldstein I, et al. Management of sexual dysfunction in patients with cardiovascular disease: recommendations of the Princeton Consensus Panel. *J Am Coll Cardiol* 2000;86:175-181.

[116] Kloner RA, Hutter AM, Emmick JT, et al. Time course of the interaction between tadalafil and nitrates. *J Am Coll Cardiol* 2003;42:1855-1860.

In: Heart Disease in Men
Editors: A.B. Todd and M.H. Mosley, pp. 317-332
ISBN: 978-1-60692-297-2

Chapter 15

Congenital Heart Disease in Adults- Challenges and Management Issues

Rajesh Vijayvergiya** and Puspendra Garg
Department of Cardiology, Post Graduate Institute of Medical Education & Research, Chandigarh- 160 012, INDIA

Abstract

Advances in diagnostic, percutaneous and surgical interventions in pediatric patients suffering from congenital heart disease (CHD) has resulted in increased number of adults with partial or totally corrected CHD. In developed countries, the burden of adult congenital heart disease (ACHD) constitute more of intervened patients, while in developing countries there is more number of un-intervened complicated ACHD patients. It has resulted into a significant number of ACHD populations world-wide. They present the challenging and complicated problems like atrial and ventricular arrhythmias, sudden cardiac death, infective endocarditis, congestive heart failure, right heart failure, pulmonary hypertension and Eisenmenger syndrome, hyperviscosity syndrome, and issues related with exercise and pregnancy. There are technical problems in management of CHD patients once they develop ventricular systolic dysfunction, pulmonary hypertension, atrial or ventricular tachy-arrhythmias and associated co-morbid illnesses. Post intervention patients have problems like graft infection, malfunction, valvular regurgitation and under-sizing in a growing child. There is also a need for heart and heart lung transplantation in few of the un-operable CHD patients during adulthood, which requires the technical expertise for surgery and intensive post-operative and follow-up management; which is available at limited centers in the world. To deal with these unusual problems of adult CHD patients, there is a need for multi-disciplinary, comprehensive approach involving pediatrician, cardiologist, electro-physiologist, pediatric cardiac surgeon, anesthesiologist, internist, psychiatrist and social worker. There is a need to setup adult CHD clinics with trained specialists, who can deal and coordinate different problems of this emerging sub-specialty of the cardiology. As the trained specialists are very limited, there is an urgent need for comprehensive training of health manpower in this field. There is also a

* E-mail address: rajeshvijay999@hotmail.com. Tel No +91-172-2756512. Fax No +91-172-2744401. Address for Correspondence: Dr Rajesh Vijayvergiya, MD, DM, Assistant Professor, Department of Cardiology, Post Graduate Institute of Medical Education & Research (PGIMER), Chandigarh – 160 012, INDIA.

need for development of cheap, easy and innovative therapies for management of these patients, so that poor patients can also be benefited.

Key Words: Congenital heart disease (CHD), Adult congenital heart disease (ACHD), Implantable cardioverter defibrillator (ICD), Tetralogy of Fallot (TOF), atrial septal defect (ASD), Ventricular septal defect (VSD), patent ductus arteriosus (PDA), infective endocarditis (IE).

1. Introduction

Congenital heart disease (CHD) is most common birth defect and affects large number of children throughout the world. Its incidence varies from 4-12/1000 live births in various community and hospital based studies [1]. The number of CHD cases recognized in the first year of life is about 75% of the total number of cases recognized in a population of children followed up till their teens[2]. A substantial number of adult congenital heart disease (ACHD) patients are there in both developed and developing countries. In developed countries, the ACHD patients following palliative or corrective surgeries are in significant number, even the total number of ACHD patients has become equal to the number of children with CHD[3]. In developing countries, the burden of uncorrected ACHD patients is more than intervened CHD patients because of limited health resources & manpower, poverty, lack of health awareness and insurance policies[1]. The burden of ACHD patients results in greater long term expenditures for care and loss of productivity for this ever growing population.

The complex patho-physiology of corrected or uncorrected CHD in adulthood poses a challenge to pediatric and adult cardiologists. Both have a limited expertise in management of these patients and require interaction in a comprehensive and coordinated manner under the adult CHD programs. Though in recent years, ACHD referral centers has been introduced in various countries, the patients attended are mostly those who needs surgical and catheter interventions, ignoring rest of the patients requiring long term monitoring and follow-up. This is due to lack of organized effort to monitor these patients either because of lack of health care delivery which falls far short of that for adults with acquired heart disease like coronary heart disease & heart failure or children with CHD & rheumatic heart disease. Reluctance of relatively asymptomatic ACHD patients to attend these clinics may also be contributory.

2. Burden of Disease

Advancement in management of CHD has lead to a marked increased in number of ACHD patients in most of the developed countries. In the United States itself, there are about a million adults with CHD and the number of patients with >20 years is greater than those with <20 years of age[3]. The exact data regarding total burden of ACHD patient is lacking because different criteria for structural defect's inclusion or exclusion have been used in various epidemiological studies. For example exclusion of bicuspid aortic valve which is present in 1% of live birth or inclusion of atrial septal defect (ASD), ventricular septal defect (VSD) and patent ductus arteriosus (PDA), which have the high spontaneous closure rate by the age of adulthood, changes the burden of ACHD patients. Similarly, different criteria for diagnosis like physical examination, echocardiography, and registry data from community or hospital based setup yield varying prevalence of CHD. It is estimated that about 80% of infants born with CHD survive till adulthood[2]. And the additional diagnosis like ASD, Ebstein's anomaly, corrected transposition (L-TGA) etc. are diagnosed later in the life. The number of CHD cases recognized in the first year of life is about 75% of the cases at >15 years age[2]. Among the ACHD patients, about 65% patients who have moderate to complex CHD needs regular long term follow-up in ACHD clinics[2]. In contrast to developed countries, ACHD burden is different in developing countries because of lack of health awareness and health care facilities/manpower. This has resulted into higher number of uncorrected adult CHD patients, comparatively high morbidity and mortality for moderate and complex CHD during early childhood and substantial number of cases presents late in the course of disease, when it has already become inoperable or have high risk for surgery.

4. Disease Pattern

The increasing number of patients with palliative or corrective surgery is reaching the adulthood. The post intervention unnatural history of CHD is different in term of hemodynamics and cardiac problems, for example osteal coronary artery stenosis following arterial switch operation or systemic ventricle dysfunction following Mustard or Senning procedure, graft stenosis or thrombosis following Fontan procedure, ventricular or atrial tachy-arrhythmias following surgical scar formation, etc. There is a need for periodic review of post-operative patients with atresia, single ventricle, transpositions variants, Ebstein's anomaly, Tetralogy of Fallot (TOF), pulmonary vascular disease, and complex septal defects. This is required for general cardiac evaluation, assessment for type and timing of further intervention and post intervention follow-up strategy. The postoperative adult not only confronts with surgically modified congenital malformation and its residua/sequelae, but also acquires other cardiovascular diseases like hypertension, obesity, atherosclerotic coronary artery disease and diabetes mellitus[4]. A complex combination of these diseases makes the management difficult and challenging.

A. Improved Diagnostic Modality

Echocardiography is an important diagnostic tool for structural and hemodynamic evaluation of CHD. Its ready availability, portability and familiarity to most of the cardiologists make it a superior and practical investigational tool for CHD. Trans-esophageal and more recently, intra-cardiac echocardiography are very helpful during percutaneous or surgical interventions in these patients. In the developing countries where health resources and manpower is limited, echocardiography is the best investigational tool for all purposes. Nevertheless, interpretation and exact diagnosis of complex CHD and those with surgical shunt requires experienced echocardiographer /pediatric cardiologist which is lacking in most of the centers.

The latest generation of non-invasive imaging modalities likes 3-D echocardiography and trans-esophageal echo, computed tomography (CT) and magnetic resonance imaging (MRI) have made a great impact on defining the subtle anatomy and hemodynamics of most of ACHD without causing significant discomfort to the patients. The information regarding hemodynamic data, coronary anatomy, aorto-pulmonary collaterals status; for which catheterization was the only answer in the past, can now be non-invasively defined with these imaging modalities. The multi-slice CT has advantages of superior visualization around metallic implants and defining coronary arteries. However, it has the limitation of radiation exposure, needs slow heart rate and breath holding during image acquisition. MRI can provide the detailed structural and functional information like gradient across stenotic segment or valve, planimetry of valve areas, relative pulmonary blood flow, collateral vessel flow, leak across the baffle etc. It has limitations like non-availability, non-portable, required lengthy time for image reconstruction and interpretation, high cost, inadequate operator's experience in the CHD field, and non-feasibility in patients with pacing devices, cerebral aneurysm clips, foreign bodies in eye, MRI non-compatible stents and other devices. More important than the newer technology and costliest equipment is the availability of imaging specialists to conduct the study, interpret it expertly, report it insightfully, and caution if there are limitations that should be known about. There is a need for collaborative and integrated approach among radiologist, echocardiographer, interventional cardiologist and cardiac surgeon for proper and optimal utilization of these imaging modalities.

With the advancement in non-invasive diagnostic modalities, cardiac catheterization is mostly performed for preoperative evaluation of coronary arteries, assessment of pulmonary vascular resistance and its response to vasodilator therapy, and for morphologic and hemodynamic evaluation of complex CHD. In the recent decades, interventional catheterization has become common for lesions like valvular pulmonic stenosis, pulmonary artery stenosis, residual or recurrent coarctation of aorta, arteriovenous fistula, device closure of ASD, VSD, PDA and ruptured sinus of Valsalva, aorto-pulmonary window, dilatation of stenotic or thrombotic palliative shunts, and coil embolization of aorto-pulmonary collaterals.

B. Impact of Cardiac Surgery

Though there are improved surgical results for most of the CHD, it is not similar all over the world as outcome varies depending on the centers, their annual volume and operator's expertise. High volume centers operating upon CHD patients have the lower mortality as compared to low volume centers[5]. The work load for coronary artery bypass surgery or valvular heart disease is much higher compared to CHD in most of the centers; hence priority and expertise are utilized in these patients instead for managing CHD patients. The scenario is different in developing countries where there is limited number of expert cardiac surgeons for CHD surgery. The co-morbid conditions associated with ACHD patients like hypertension, coronary artery disease, ventricular systolic dysfunctions, and pulmonary artery hypertension also adversely affect the result of surgery. In addition, expertise for cardiac transplantation or heart lung transplantation as needed in some of complex CHD is available at only few CHD centers throughout the world. There should be a close collaboration between cardiac surgeons, cardiologists, echocardiographers, interventional cardiologist, anesthesiologist and intensive care unit paramedical staff for improvement in surgical outcomes in these patients.

In addition, the advancement in percutaneous valve replacement for pulmonic, aortic and mitral valve; minimal invasive off pump surgery with hybrid approach, magnetic navigation system and robotic assistance during catheterization and intervention are likely to change the clinical practice in coming years.

In contrast to developed countries, where so much stress is given upon setting up the ACHD clinics, developing countries are facing the problems of lack of diagnostic & treatment facility and unaffordable cost of medical care, which add to huge burden of un-intervened CHD patients. The cost of surgery is forbidding and most of the patients have to live without it. There is also a gross mismatch in demand and supply for cardiac surgery in developing countries. It is estimated that about 1222 cardiac surgeries being done in North America, which is far more than 25 surgeries in Asia and 18 surgeries in Africa, per million population annually[6]. It is estimated that only 7% of needy patients undergo cardiac surgery in Asia, Africa, South America and Russia[6]. This is because of non-availability of infrastructure, expertise, non-affordable cost and lack of medical insurance policy. Even following corrective or palliative surgery, there is a need of long term care and monitoring for infective endocarditis, heart failure, arrhythmias, post intervention sequelae/residue, pregnancy and contraception, which is lacking in developing countries because of limited health resources and manpower. There is a need for developing effective inter-country, inter-regional and global networks for concerted global action to enhance the capacity of underprivileged countries to meet the health care needs. The developed countries can help in building infrastructure, providing the expertise, training the local physicians/surgeons and facilitating the availability of low cost surgeries to these countries. With the advancement in information technology, there should be more live demonstration or video conferencing among experts in the cardiac field with those sitting in other under privileged countries/community, to help them to become independents, and also to improve the standard and quality care in this field.

5. Specific Medical Issues

a. Transition & Transfer to Adulthood

The transition from childhood to adulthood is associated with multiple problems like cognitive and physical disability, social adjustment, lack of employment and public insurance, discontinuation of medical care because of various social or financial factors. Adequate physical and mental capability for most of the professional work and belief of cure of CHD following childhood surgery makes them unwilling to attend the ACHD services. There is a need for comprehensive and individualized education regarding their cardiac conditions and health care needs. It includes specific information on diagnosis and future operations, medications and their side effects, infective endocarditis prophylaxis, contraception and family planning, pregnancy related risk, arrhythmias, frequency of medical follow-up, dental care and other hygiene related instruction.

b. Infective Endocarditis

Infected endocarditis (IE) is a life long risk for many of the operated and un-operated CHD patients. About 4% CHD patients with infective endocarditis being admitted in ACHD clinics[7]. The risk factors for IE are previous cardiac surgery and dental, surgical and cardiac interventional procedures without proper antibiotic prophylaxis. However, about 60% of patients do not have the recognizable risk factor[7]. The most common CHD cases with IE are of VSD, aortic stenosis, and mitral valve disease, while operated cases includes TOF and Atrio-ventricular septal defects. Though the IE is uncommon in cyanotic CHD, post operative patients have higher risk of IE for example those with residual lesions or shunts, prosthetic valves/conduits and palliative aorto-pulmonary shunts. It is rare in ASD, repaired VSD or ductus, pulmonic valve stenosis, anomalous pulmonary venous drainage, Ebstein's, post-Fontan, post-Mustard/Senning patients. The usual organisms are Staphylococcus and Streptococcus, but unusual organism including fungi can also be involved[7]. As IE is associated with significant morbidity and about 10% mortality[8], it is essential to diagnose it early and start the antibiotics on time. Surgical intervention should be done well within time in patients with appropriate indications.

c. Pregnancy & Contraception in Women

The most common structural heart disease during pregnancy is CHD in developed nations, while it is the second common following rheumatic heart disease in developing countries. These pregnant CHD patients need a multi-specialty care by obstetrician, cardiologist, neonatologist and anesthesiologist for improvement of maternal and fetal outcomes. The risk associated with pregnancy in CHD patients can be categorized in 3 types:-

a. Maternal Risk.
b. Fetal Risk.
c. Risk of CHD recurrence in offspring.

a. Maternal Risk during Pregnancy

The hemodynamic stress of pregnancy which peaks during late second, early third trimester period and also during labor can adversely affect the outcome in certain CHD. The potential risk factors for adverse outcome are poor maternal functional class, significant pulmonary artery hypertension, Eisenmenger syndrome, significant obstructive lesion, heart failure, cyanosis, uncontrolled arrhythmias and left ventricular systolic dysfunction[9]. Patient with left to right shunt lesions like ASD, VSD and those with valvular regurgitation generally tolerate increased blood volume and cardiac output very well during pregnancy, unless there is precipitating factor for congestive heart failure like arrhythmias, anemia, infection, pulmonary thrombo-embolism, thyrotoxicosis, pre-eclampsia or hypertension. Congenital heart disease like mitral stenosis, aortic stenosis, coarctation of aorta, and TOF are associated with moderate maternal risk, while Eisenmenger and Marfan syndrome with aortic root dimension of >4 cm is associated with high maternal risk[10]. Those with cyanotic CHD have worsening of hypoxemia following increase in right to left shunt secondary to decrease systemic vascular resistance. The physiological increase in procoagulant activity during pregnancy can be deleterious in cyanotic patients having haemostatic disorder and hyperviscosity syndrome. Patient with Marfan syndrome, bicuspid aortic valve with stenosis, coarctation of aorta and those with post aortic valve replacement having aortic root dilatation have high risk of aortic dissection during pregnancy[11]. There is a need of thorough knowledge about course and management of individual CHD and its complication with special reference to pregnancy. The risk can be appreciably reduced by meticulous attention to fetal lung maturity assessment by amniocentesis, controlled induced vaginal delivery, lumbar epidural anesthesia, and meticulous post partum care. The medical termination of pregnancy is an option in unplanned pregnancy and in patients of moderate to high risk groups. It should be done at earliest preferably in first trimester only, as advancing gestational age is associated with higher maternal complication rate.

b. Fetal Risk

There is a greater risk of prematurity, intrauterine growth retardation, fetal and neonatal death in CHD patients during pregnancy. The risk factors for adverse outcomes are NYHA functional class greater than II, cyanosis, obstructive structural heart disease, congestive heart failure and Eisenmenger syndrome[10]. The management of fetus includes serial Ultrasonography for growth assessment, fetal echocardiography to rule out CHD, and selective amniocentesis for fetal lung maturation.

c. Risk of CHD Recurrence in Offspring

Genetic counseling regarding etiology, inheritance, recurrence risk, and prenatal diagnosis should be explained to ACHD patients. The proper counseling regarding discontinuation of cardiac drugs like Angiotensin converting enzyme inhibitors, Angiotensin II receptor antagonists, oral anticoagulants, Amiodarone and other anti-arrhythmic drugs should be done prior to conception. Preconception consumption of multivitamins including folic acid decreases the incidence of CHD[12]. The recurrence rate of CHD in offspring varies from 3-50%, maximum with Marfan, Noonan and Holt–Oram syndrome[13]. The recurrence with one previously affected sibling is 2.3% and with two previously affected siblings is 7.3%. If mother is having CHD, the recurrence risk to her offspring is 6.7%, and if the father is affected, the risk is 2.1%[14]. A fetal echocardiographic screening at 16-18 weeks is recommended in all CHD patients. In patients with high suspicion of fetal malformation, the chorionic villus sampling or amniocentesis may be useful for prenatal diagnosis of chromosomal disorders. With improved management of CHD including the complex one, the CHD in fetus needs a detail discussion with parents regarding the outcome during post natal life of individual heart defect. The parents may be benefited in such situation from additional counseling by a psychiatrist.

Contraception

The proper and timely counseling regarding choice of contraceptive method in female ACHD patients to avoid unplanned pregnancy should be done by gynecologist in consultation with cardiologist, as none of the present contraceptive method is ideal. The barrier and natural methods have high failure rates and can not be recommended in women whom pregnancy carries a significant risk. Combined contraceptives (estrogen and progesterone) have the risk of thrombo-embolism and can result into worsening of pulmonary hypertension, paradoxical embolism, post-Fontan shunt thrombosis and valvular prosthesis malfunction. Progesterone-only oral contraceptive though have the minimal risk of thrombo-embolism, it has the higher failure rate than combined oral contraceptives. Depot injections of progesterone is an alternative to oral preparation, when compliance is poor and pregnancy carries a high risk. An intra-uterine contraceptive device is highly effective and relatively safe with minimal risk of infection and infective endocarditis. Tubectomy in women with high risk CHD has the surgery related procedural complications[10].

d. Cardiac Arrhythmias & Its Management

The late onset arrhythmias during adulthood in CHD patients are associated with significant morbidity and mortality, which requires a special attention by both adult cardiologist and electro-physiologist. It is estimated that about 50% of ACHD patients experiences some arrhythmogenic problem during long term follow-up. The supra-ventricular arrhythmias are more common than the ventricular arrhythmias. The arrhythmias occurs as a consequence of underlying structural abnormality, chamber dilatation and fibrosis, ventricular systolic dysfunction, previous operative myocardial scar and adverse hemodynamics. There is paucity of evidence based management protocol; therefore the usual clinical practice is based upon experience of large ACHD centers and individual experiences. Pharmacologic management may be limited in a given situation because of concomitant sinus node disease, ventricular systolic dysfunction, or female patients willing for the pregnancy. The non-pharmacologic options like percutaneous catheter ablation, surgical ablation during heart surgery, and devices like implantable cardioverter defibrillators (ICD) and pacemaker with special algorithm for management of atrial tachy-arrhythmias are effective in a significant number of patients. Both diagnostic and therapeutic electrophysiological procedures may be challenging because of difficult vascular access and complex post-surgical anatomy as in cases of Fontan, Mustard and Senning operations. There is a need for integrated collaborative approach of surgeon, electrophysiologist, and cardiologist for effective management of these patients.

The risk of ventricular tachycardia and sudden cardiac death is increased in specific subset of ACHD patients like those with post ventriculotomy scar or patients with long standing hemodynamic stress like aortic valve disease, corrected transposition (L-TGA) with systemic right ventricular dysfunction, severe Ebstein's anomaly, Eisenmenger syndrome, and TOF[15]. The risk stratification for primary prevention of VT in this population remains unclear and literature data are still limited. Patient with TOF have significant arrhythmia burden as one third of operated cases have symptomatic atrial tachycardia by adulthood[16], 10% develops high grade ventricular arrhythmias[17], 5% requires pacemaker for surgically acquired AV block or sinus node dysfunction[18] and increasing number of patients are requiring ICD for both primary and secondary prevention of SCD[19]. The clinical variables like high grade ventricular ectopics, abnormal right or left ventricular systolic functions, more than 180msecs QRS duration, inducible VT on electro-physiological study and surgery at older age can be considered for further risk stratification and management of ventricular tachy-arrhythmias in these patients[15]. There is also an upcoming trend in implantation of cardiac resynchronization therapy (CRT) and CRT plus ICD in selected CHD patients with ventricular systolic dysfunction, dysynchrony and risk of sudden cardiac death[20,21].

Patients with Ebstein's anomaly and corrected transposition (L-TGA) are typically associated with multiple accessory pathways across the abnormal tricuspid valve. A significant number of adult patients have AV reentrant tachycardia and also atrial tachy-arrhythmias with fast conduction through accessory pathways, which needs radiofrequency catheter ablation. However, this therapy has lower success rate in these patients because of challenges associated with distorted anatomical landmarks, difficulty in identifying the true

AV groove, extremely fractionated electrogram, and high incidence of multiple accessory pathways[22,23].

Another tachycardia specific to CHD is intra-atrial reentrant tachycardia or incisional tachycardia, which occurs following atrial scar formation subsequent to surgery. This tachycardia is problematic in patients requiring atrial support for cardiac output like Mustard or Senning atrial switch surgery and Fontan surgery. Though the acute episode of IART can be controlled with class I or class III anti-arrhythmic drugs, electrical cardioversion or overdrive pacing maneuvers; the prevention of recurrence is difficult with various anti-arrhythmic drugs. Patients with frequent, symptomatic and hemodynamically unstable episodes or with atrial thrombus formation need aggressive treatment, for which the various therapeutic options should be tailored depending on individual patient. The options are like anti-arrhythmic drugs, pacemaker for bradycardia and anti-tachycardia pacing, catheter ablation, and surgically modified atrial maze operation[24].

Sino-atrial nodal dysfunction and atrial fibrillation is associated with heterotaxy, sinus venosus ASD, secondum ASD and secondary to surgical trauma cased during Mustard, Senning, and Fontan surgery. The issues related with venous assess, intracardiac shunts, associated venous anomalies, and risk of thrombo-embolism preclude transvenous lead placement for device mediated therapy in few of these patients. A combined surgical approach for both structural defect and surgical ablation is successful in patients with Ebstein's anomaly, Fontan revision, and TOF. There has been surgical refinement following experience of adverse long term electrophysiological outcomes with standard procedures for example atrial switch is replaced by arterial switch in complete transposition (D-TGA), Fontan being replaced by modified cavo-pulmonary shunt in single ventricle and right ventricle approach being replaced by right atrial and or pulmonary artery approach in TOF.

Technical Aspects of Pacemaker and ICD

The standard transvenous endocardial pacing lead placement may be difficult or contraindicated in many CHD patients because of complex venous drainage from upper limbs, cavo-pulmonary shunt surgery and atrial switch surgery, or presence of intra-cardiac shunt resulting in significant risk of systemic thrombo-embolism. Epicardial lead implantation is an alternative but it also have the problems like associated morbidity of sternotomy /thoracotomy for lead implantation, poor long term performance of lead including frequent lead fracture, difficulty in achieving good pacing parameters and optimal site of pacing and difficult surgical resection in patients with prior cardiac surgery[25].

As indication of ICD for primary prevention is not very clear, electrophysiologists are not very aggressive in device implantation in this subset of patients, considering the technical difficulty of implantation and short and long term troubles associated with generators and leads. The rate of appropriate discharge for ventricular tachy-arrhythmias is about 35% over 5 years of follow-up, and inappropriate shocks are around 25% due to lead malfunction and atrial tachycardia[26]. Overall, the rate of device utilization is satisfactory and life saving, therefore present individualized case selection criteria seems to be appropriate. Another problem with ICD is lead fracture, which is reported in about 20% patients over 5 years[26]. The possible mechanism is high level of activity and the physical growth in children. These cases of lead fracture are challenging because of difficulty in lead extraction, venous thrombosis or occlusion, and repeat thoracotomy for epicardial lead placement.

e. Eisenmenger Syndrome

In CHD with shunt lesions, the severe pulmonary artery hypertension develops over the period of time because of irreversible pathological pulmonary vascular changes resulting into "Eisenmenger" syndrome. Though in developed nations, its incidence has decreased because of timely management of CHD during childhood, the prevalence is still high in developing countries. The spectrum of patients is also different like complex CHD with palliative shunt repair during childhood having Eisenmenger syndrome is more frequent in developed countries while the simple cardiac lesions like ASD, VSD and PDA is more frequent with Eisenmenger syndrome in underdeveloped countries. In addition to cyanosis, hypoxemia and pulmonary artery hypertension, these patients also suffer from multi-system disorder manifesting as bleeding or thrombotic diathesis, ischemic complication, infective endocarditis, cerebral abscess, congestive heart failure, sudden cardiac death, hepatic and renal involvement, and pregnancy related adverse fetal and maternal outcomes[27].

The survival of Eisenmenger syndrome is better than idiopathic pulmonary artery hypertension, and most of the patients survive till 3rd-4th decade, if managed appropriately. The risk factor for poor survival includes poor functional class, right ventricular dysfunction, complex underlying cardiac defect, increased serum creatinine and uric acid, associated Down syndrome and pregnancy[27].

The treatment option in these patients is limited to palliative measures only, which includes adequate hydration, correction of iron deficiency anemia and hyperviscosity syndrome, avoidance of pregnancy and appropriate use of contraceptives, oral anticoagulants, and prompt treatment of cardiac arrhythmias, avoidance of strenuous exercise and competitive sports and infective endocarditis prophylaxis. Recently, drugs like Sildenafil and Bosentan has shown encouraging results in improvement of functional class and pulmonary artery hypertension in this subset of patients[28,29], however their long term efficacy is not proven and required further studies. The lung or heart lung transplantation can be a definitive treatment in selected cases, however the non-availability of dual donor organ, lack of expertise for complex surgical procedure, difficult post operative immuno-suppression and lack of experienced cardiologist for post-operative care are few of the reasons, because of which the surgery is limited to only few centers throughout the world.

f. Exercise and Physical Activity

ACHD patients have the subnormal exercise tolerance, whether it is simple defects like ASD, VDS; stenotic lesions like pulmonic or aortic stenosis or complex lesions like single ventricle, Ebstein's Anomaly, transposition of great arteries. They should be cautioned about participation in competitive athletic activities. The detailed recommendation of individual CHD regarding exercise training and competitive sport's participation is described under 26th Bethesda Conference- task force report[30]. There is a need for safe and efficacious structured exercise rehabilitation strategy for these patients to improve fitness and aerobic capacity.

g. Psychological Issues

With increasing number of ACHD patients in the community, there is a concern about quality of life, social integration/ support, and achievement of professional or educational goals in these patients. These psychological issues are affected by lesion severity and need for repeated hospital admission and intervention, physician consultation, functional disability, phenotypic appearance, and mental capabilities. Patients needs regular counseling for enhancing their knowledge of CHD, its course and further management issues, and also in dealing with acute stress and transition period associated psychological problems during adolescence. For this purpose, trained cardiac psychologists can be integrated in the multi-disciplinary ACHD care teams, who can provide the clinical service, coordinate research with other team members, and provide the professional education to trainees in cardiology, nursing and psychology[31].

h. Anesthesia

These patients need special attention during non-cardiac and cardiac surgeries. Issues pertaining to IE prophylaxis, peri-operative anticoagulation management, and adverse effect of anesthetic drugs or stress should be discussed among anesthesiologist, surgeon and cardiologist. The risk assessment for non-cardiac surgery is required in setting of poor functional class, ventricular dysfunction, congestive heart failure, persistent shunt and risk of systemic air embolism, arrhythmias, pulmonary disease and pulmonary hypertension including Eisenmenger syndrome, erythrocytosis and hyperviscosity syndrome. Regional or general anesthesia for cardiac or non-cardiac surgeries in CHD patients is challenging as one needs to understand the hemodynamic of CHD and effects of various anesthetic agents on it. A tilt in the balance between systemic and pulmonary vascular resistance ratio, decrease cardiac output, hypotension and fall in systemic saturation which are the common side effect of most of the anesthetic agents can deteriorate the hemodynamic and clinical condition of the patient. Therefore, a dedicated cardiac anesthesiologist is required who can coordinate and share the knowledge with cardiologist and cardiac surgeon for better outcome of these patients. Various factors like polycythemia and hyperviscosity syndrome, hydration, deficient coagulation factors and platelet dysfunction, risk of paradoxical air embolism from intravenous lines, ventilatory effects of positioning during surgery, one lung ventilation, pregnancy, presence and type of pacemaker, risk of supra-ventricular and ventricular tachy-arrhythmias should be evaluated and managed properly during peri-operative period[32].

i. Residua & Sequelae Following Intervention

The residua following reparative surgery for CHD can be electrophysiological or structural. The electrophysiological residua are like prolongation of AV node conduction and complete heart block in operated case of corrected transposition (L-TGA), atrial tachy- and brady–arrhythmias in patients with sinus venosus and secondum ASD and persistence of supraventricular tachycardia, atrial flutter & fibrillation in operated cases of ASD and Ebstein's anomaly. The structural residua are like morphologic right ventricle in systemic position following atrial switch operation in transposition of great arteries and bicuspid aortic valve. The peripheral vascular residua are like aneurysm of circle of Willis, ascending aorta dilatation and hypertension following coarctation of aorta repair[33].

Sequelae are as a result of corrective surgery for CHD and can again be of two types-electrophysiological or structural. Electrophysiological sequelae are like ectopic atrial bradycardia following damage to SA node during sinus venosus ASD repair, atrial tachyarrhythmias and sinus bradycardia following secondum ASD repair, atrial switch operation, Fontan operation; impaired atrio-ventricular conduction following peri-membranous VSD or primum ASD repair. Post ventriculotomy incision site monomorphic ventricular tachyarrhythmias and sudden cardiac death is a concern following CHD repair. An electrophysiological study and scar site ablation is the indicated in these patients especially in subgroup with baseline QRS duration of >180msecs. The structural sequelae are like significant pulmonary valve regurgitation following right ventricular outflow repair in TOF, degeneration of autologous aortic valve in Ross procedure; prosthetic valve or conduits malfunction, stenosis, thrombosis and infective endocarditis. The structural sequelae of percutaneous intervention also exist for example structurally abnormal bicuspid aortic valve following balloon aortic dilatation may pose the risk of infective endocarditis and ascending aorta dilatation secondary to associated medial abnormality and aneurysm formation following coarctation segment dilatation[33].

6. Special Health Care Needs

With the growing number of ACHD population, there is urgent need for specially trained physicians who can provide comprehensive and effective outpatient and in-patient care. Presently, these patients are looked by either pediatric or adult cardiologists, and both of them have lack of training/ professional expertise in managing them. On the one hand the pediatric cardiologist has little or no experience in comprehensive adult care, the adult cardiologist lacks the training in diagnosis and management of CHD. This discrepancy can be corrected by collaborative approach from different sub-specialty of cardiology and cardiac surgery under ACHD program. For the effective ACHD program in the community, the main requirements are[34]:-

1. Education of a modest number of ACHD specialists who can lead highly specialized teams and serve as a referral and continuing educational resource for the greater number of providers with training in either adult or pediatric cardiology.
2. Integration of highly specialized centers with community based providers and with each other in order to provide a high level of care for all patients and to provide an informational base for continual improvement in care; and
3. Free access to an appropriately trained provider for all adults with CHD.

There is a need for basic and advanced professional training to physicians, nurses, interventionist, intensive care providers, cardiac surgeons, electro-physiologist, obstetricians and anesthesiologists for running the effective ACHD programs. As described by Core Cardiology Training Symposium 2 (COCATS II)[35], the level for training for cardiology services can be defined from basic level 1 to advanced level 3 as follows:-

Level 1—requires basic training of all adult (medical) cardiology trainees so they may become competent consulting cardiologists.

Level 2 requires additional training in a specialized area to enable the cardiologist to perform or interpret, or both, specific procedures or skills at an intermediate skill level.

Level 3—requires additional training in a specialized area to enable the cardiologist to perform, interpret, and train others to perform and interpret specific procedures or acquire skills and knowledge at a high level.

The ultimate goal of ascending level of training is to make the experts and teachers in the field of ACHD[36]. The competence to be achieved by them is as follows:-

1. Medical and surgical management of ACHD.
2. Technical expertise for diagnosis and percutaneous interventions by invasive and non-invasive cardiac procedures.
3. Expertise in the management of cardiac arrhythmias. A fully equipped and properly staffed service with a full range of ablative and pacing therapies should be available at ACHD tertiary care centre.
4. Recognition and management of acquired cardiovascular and cardiopulmonary disease.
5. Cardiac management of pregnant females.
6. Direct and meaningful experience of clinical and epidemiological research in CHD.
7. Principles of health promotion and management of psychosocial disorders in adults.

In addition, there is a need for training the professionals from other specialties like cardiac anesthesiologist for peri-operative care including training in trans-thoracic and trans-esophageal echocardiography; cardiac perfusionists with expertise in ventricular assist device (VAD) and extra-corporeal membrane oxygenator (ECMO) setup, delivery and maintenance; cardiac surgeons having expertise and appropriate annual volume of CHD surgeries and also affiliated with cardiac transplant unit; Intensive care unit staff and fellows trained for advanced and critical care support including capability of open chest resuscitation, implementing and monitoring VAD and ECMO, and management of acquired cardiovascular and other diseases.

7. Conclusion

In conclusion, the emerging new sub-specialty of adult CHD population, which is steadily growing needs a proper attention and management by health providers. Presently, these patients are treated by both pediatric and adult cardiologist individually, who have limited education and expertise in managing them. These patients have challenging and complicated problems which needs a multi-disciplinary, comprehensive approach involving pediatrician, cardiologist, electro-physiologist, pediatric cardiac surgeon, anesthesiologist, internist, psychiatrist and social worker under ACHD program. At present, the trained specialist and setup for the ACHD clinics is limited to few centers, which needs to be expanded to other tertiary care centers throughout the world, both in developed and developing countries. This will help in improving clinical care, advance the knowledge, open the new frontiers for further research and patient management, and provide ongoing professional education for the larger population of adult and pediatric cardiologists. With the limited manpower and health resources, especially in developing countries, the concept of ACHD program can be integrated with available health resources, which will be more practical and cost effective.

Acknowledgment

We are thankful to Drs. Ashish Jha & Anupam Vijayvergia for correction of the manuscript. There is no conflict of interest of any of the authors of the manuscript.

References

[1] Grover A, Vijayvergiya R, Thingam ST. Burden of rheumatic and congenital heart disease in India: lowest estimate based on the 2001 census. *Indian Heart J.* 2002; 54(1):104-7.

[2] Wren C, O'Sullivan JJ. Survival with congenital heart disease and need for follow up in adult life. *Heart.* 2001; 85(4):438-43.

[3] Marelli AJ, Mackie AS, Ionescu-Ittu R, Rahme E, Pilote L. Congenital heart disease in the general population: changing prevalence and age distribution. *Circulation.* 2007; 115(2):163-72.

[4] Billett J, Cowie MR, Gatzoulis MA, Vonder Muhll IF, Majeed A. Comorbidity, health care utilisation and process of care measures in patients with congenital heart disease in the UK: cross-sectional population-based study with case control analysis. *Heart.* 2008; 94(9):1194-9.

[5] Spiegelhalter DJ. Mortality and volume of cases in paediatric cardiac surgery: retrospective study based on routinely collected data. *BMJ.* 2002; 324(7332):261-3.

[6] Cox JL. Presidential address: changing boundaries. *J Thorac Cardiovasc Surg.* 2001;122(3):413-8.

[7] Li W, Somerville J. Infective endocarditis in the grown-up congenital heart (GUCH) population. *Eur Heart J.* 1998;19(1):166-73.

[8] Niwa K, Nakazawa M, Tateno S, Yoshinaga M, Terai M. Infective endocarditis in congenital heart disease: Japanese national collaboration study. *Heart.* 2005;91(6):795-800.

[9] Siu SC, Sermer M, Colman JM, et al. Cardiac Disease in Pregnancy (CARPREG) Investigators. Prospective multicenter study of pregnancy outcomes in women with heart disease. *Circulation.* 2001;104(5):515-21

[10] Uebing A, Steer PJ, Yentis SM, Gatzoulis MA. Pregnancy and congenital heart disease. *BMJ.* 2006;332(7538):401-6.

[11] Immer FF, Bansi AG, Immer-Bansi AS, et al. Aortic dissection in pregnancy: analysis of risk factors and outcome. *Ann Thorac Surg.* 2003;76(1):309-14.

[12] Wilson RD, Johnson JA, Wyatt P, et al. Genetics Committee of the Society of Obstetricians and Gynaecologists of Canada and The Mother risk Program. Pre-conceptional vitamin/folic acid supplementation 2007: the use of folic acid in combination with a multivitamin supplement for the prevention of neural tube defects and other congenital anomalies. *J Obstet Gynaecol Can.* 2007; 29(12):1003-26.

[13] Kafka H, Johnson MR, Gatzoulis MA. The team approach to pregnancy and congenital heart disease. *Cardiol Clin.* 2006; 24(4):587-605.

[14] Perloff JK, Koos B. Pregnancy and congenital heart disease. In: Perloff JK, Child JS, eds. *Congenital Heart Disease in Adults.* 2nd ed. Philadelphia: Saunders; 1998.

[15] Walsh EP, Cecchin F. Arrhythmias in adult patients with congenital heart disease. *Circulation*. 2007; 115(4):534-45.

[16] Roos-Hesselink J, Perlroth MG, McGhie J, Spitaels S. Atrial arrhythmias in adults after repair of tetralogy of Fallot: correlations with clinical, exercise, and echocardiographic findings. *Circulation*. 1995; 91:2214–2219.

[17] Harrison DA, Harris L, Siu SC, MacLoghlin CJ, Connelly MS, Webb GD, Downer E, McLaughlin PR, Williams WG. Sustained ventricular tachycardia in adult patients late after repair of tetralogy of Fallot. *J Am Coll Cardiol*. 1997; 30:1368 –1373.

[18] Weindling SN, Gamble WJ, Mayer JE, Walsh EP. Duration of complete atrioventricular block after congenital heart disease surgery. *Am J Cardiol*. 1998; 82:525–527.

[19] Berul CI, Van Hare GF, Kertesz NJ, et al. Results of a multicenter retrospective implantable cardioverter-defibrillator registry of pediatric and congenital heart disease patients. *J Am Coll Cardiol*. 2008; 51(17):1685-91.

[20] Janousek J, Gebauer RA. Cardiac resynchronization therapy in pediatric and congenital heart disease. *Pacing Clin Electrophysiol*. 2008; 31 Suppl-1:S21-3.

[21] Khairy P. Defibrillators and cardiac resynchronization therapy in congenital heart disease: evolving indications. *Expert Rev Med Devices*. 2008; 5(3):267-71.

[22] Rudnick AG, Deger FT, Greenberg RM. Ablation of atrioventricular conduction in corrected transposition of the great arteries. *Heart Rhythm*. 2006; 3(5):598-600.

[23] Chetaille P, Walsh EP, Triedman JK. Outcomes of radiofrequency catheter ablation of atrioventricular reciprocating tachycardia in patients with congenital heart disease. *Heart Rhythm*. 2004; 1(2):168-73.

[24] Kannankeril PJ, Fish FA. Management of intra-atrial reentrant tachycardia. *Curr Opin Cardiol*. 2005; 20(2):89-93

[25] Karpawich PP. Technical aspects of pacing in adult and pediatric congenital heart disease. *Pacing Clin Electrophysiol*. 2008; 31 Suppl-1:S28-31.

[26] Walsh EP. Practical aspects of implantable defibrillator therapy in patients with congenital heart disease. *Pacing Clin Electrophysiol*. 2008; 31 Suppl-1:S38-40.

[27] Diller GP, Gatzoulis MA. Pulmonary vascular disease in adults with congenital heart disease. *Circulation*. 2007; 115(8):1039-50.

[28] Singh TP, Rohit M, Grover A, Malhotra S, Vijayvergiya R. A randomized, placebo-controlled, double-blind, crossover study to evaluate the efficacy of oral sildenafil therapy in severe pulmonary artery hypertension. *Am Heart J*. 2006;151(4): 851.e1-5.

[29] Gatzoulis MA, Beghetti M, Galiè N, et al. BREATHE-5 Investigators. Longer-term bosentan therapy improves functional capacity in Eisenmenger syndrome: results of the BREATHE-5 open-label extension study. *Int J Cardiol*. 2008; 127(1):27-32.

[30] Graham TP Jr, Driscoll DJ, Gersony WM, Newburger JW, Rocchini A, Towbin JA. Task Force 2: congenital heart disease. *J Am Coll Cardiol*. 2005; 45(8):1326-33.

[31] Kovacs AH, Silversides C, Saidi A, Sears SF. The role of the psychologist in adult congenital heart disease. *Cardiol Clin*. 2006; 24(4):607-18.

[32] Heggie J, Karski J. The anesthesiologist's role in adults with congenital heart disease. *Cardiol Clin*. 2006; 24(4):571-85.

[33] Perloff JK, Warnes CA. Challenges posed by adults with repaired congenital heart disease. *Circulation*. 2001; 103(21):2637-43.

[34] Webb GD, Williams RG. Care of the adult with congenital heart disease: introduction. *J Am Coll Cardiol.* 2001; 37(5):1166.
[35] Beller GA, Bonow RO, Fuster V; Core Cardiology Training Symposium (COCATS). ACC revised recommendations for training in adult cardiovascular medicine. Core Cardiology Training II (COCATS 2).*J Am Coll Cardiol.* 2002; 39(7):1242-6.
[36] Child JS, Collins-Nakai RL, Alpert JS, et al. Task force 3: workforce description and educational requirements for the care of adults with congenital heart disease. *J Am Coll Cardiol.* 2001; 37(5):1183-7.

Additional Educational Resources for Professionals and Patients Related with Adult Congenital Heart Disease

http://www.guch.org.uk/ - Grown Up Congenital Heart Patients Association
http://www.cachnet.org/ - Canadian Adult Congenital Heart Network
http://www.isaccd.org/ - International Society for Adult Congenital Cardiac Disease.
http://www.cchaforlife.org/ - The Canadian Congenital Heart Alliance.
http://www.achaheart.org/ - The Adult Congenital Heart Association.
http://tchin.org/ - Congenital heart information network.

In: Heart Disease in Men
Editors: A.B. Todd and M.H. Mosley, pp. 333-346
ISBN: 978-1-60692-297-2

Chapter 15

CORONARY ARTERY SURGERY IN MEN: RISKS AND OUTCOMES

Justin D. Blasberg and Sandhya K. Balaram *

Division of Cardiothoracic Surgery, St. Luke's-Roosevelt Hospital Center,
Columbia University College of Physicians and Surgeons

Abstract

Over the past fifteen years, gender studies in coronary artery bypass graft (CABG) surgery outcomes have focused on women, although the majority of patients diagnosed with coronary artery disease and those who undergo intervention are predominantly male. A marked increase in public interest in women's health accompanied by new scientific research has produced increasing evidence that women carry a higher operative mortality after CABG surgery. The fact that this data remains somewhat controversial emphasizes the complexity of the issue. It has become clear that differences in profiles between men and women contribute to variation in outcomes after CABG. Biologic differences play a role in etiology, progression, and treatment outcomes. Furthermore, some risk factors have been shown to be unique to each gender. Ultimately, determination of specific independent predictors for long-term mortality after CABG may be helpful in improving surgical results. The purpose of this chapter is to summarize and analyze the current body of knowledge of male gender as an independent variable in coronary artery bypass surgery.

Introduction

Coronary artery bypass surgery has been shown in numerous trials to be a safe and effective treatment for coronary artery disease [1-4]. The role of gender differences in outcomes has been studied extensively over the past several years. Data from large retrospective studies have resulted in specific recommendations being made for women undergoing surgical revascularization [5]. These include the use of internal mammary artery grafts and the appropriate management of hyperglycemia and anemia [5].

* Phone: (212) 523-2798. Fax (212) 523- 5344. Address for Correspondence: 1111 Amsterdam Avenue, New York, NY 10025

Less attention has focused directly on men who undergo coronary surgery. It has been shown that risk profiles of men and women who undergo CABG vary widely [6-10]. Furthermore, the impact of a given risk factor has been variable between these two groups. Although definitive conclusions regarding causation, risk factors, and modifiable predictors have not been completely clarified by available data, a number of evidence-based differences have been described. A review of these differences in terms of the biologic manifestations of disease, risk factors, and surgical outcomes, reveals that male gender in itself is a specific variable that must be considered in patients undergoing coronary bypass surgery.

Differences in Biology

One important issue in surgical outcomes is the difference in the biologic manifestation of a given disease. A difference in underlying substrate is partially responsible for the severity of a disease state. In cardiac surgery, this includes age at presentation, patient size, and the location and nature of coronary disease. In addition, studies performed in animal models highlight the hormonal and metabolic differences that influence formation of coronary artery disease and focus on estrogen, androgens, and cholesterol levels.

Age at presentation with coronary disease is a clear and reproducible difference between men and women. Although male surgical patients outnumber women by a wide margin, an increasing percentage of older patients presenting for CABG are female [8]. Overall, men with coronary artery disease present at a younger age compared to their female counterparts [11, 12]. Interestingly, younger women with coronary disease appear to carry a more virulent form of the disease as compared to older women; both percutaneous intervention and surgery carry a significantly higher mortality in this group [13, 14]. At present, the majority of patients over the age of 70 undergoing surgery are female and those below 70 are predominantly male [8].

In terms of biology, estrogen is known to play a key role as a protective cardiovascular factor, and in men, estrogen absence reduces or even eliminates that effect over time. Atheroma and atheroscleorosis formation are partially mediated through estrogen receptors that regulate vasodilatory and vasoconstrictor proteins [15]. Villablanca et al studied estrogen receptors in male mice as they relate to the formation of atherosclerosis. With the knowledge that a specific estrogen receptor (ER-α) is important in the development of arterial disease, they devised a rat model which showed that male mice without these receptors fed cholesterol diets were unable to effectively process and eliminate their cholesterol load. These mice developed early, larger, and more advanced atheromatous lesions [15]. Removal of testosterone decreased the rate of these lesions. This supports the role of atherosclerosis formation as mediated thru estrogen receptors, and testosterone in the male counterpart has physiologic effects on atheroma formation thru known pathways converting testosterone to estrogen [15].

Other studies support this link. Chronic treatment of male mice with 17β-estradiol lead to decreased serum glucose and triglyceride levels and decreased the size of existing atheromatous lesions [16]. This showed a clear benefit that long term estrogen supplementation would have on the formation of atherosclerotic lesions [16]. In a related study, 17β-estradiol had a gender-independent effect on atheroma formation in a rabbit model subjected to intimal injury [17]. This supplementation was also associated with a reduced serum cholesterol level. In rabbits with elevated cholesterol profiles, 17β estradiol supplementation was associated with a gender independent decrease in atheroma development in the face of neo-intimal injury [17].

Androgens are important in determining the onset of coronary artery disease in men [18]. Macrophages, which play a critical role in atherosclerosis formation, are known to replicate in the presence of androgens. In addition, they exhibit a large up-regulation of specific genes in response to androgen exposure. These include genes related to lipoprotein processing, cell-surface adhesion, extracellular signaling, coagulation, fibrinolysis, and transport proteins. These findings were not observed in the absence of androgens [18]. Androgens may thus provide a direct stimulatory effect at sites of atherosclerosis formation.

A difference in the processing of cholesterol may also play an important role in coronary disease in men. Male hamsters fed a hypercholesterolemic diet were found to have higher LDL and total cholesterol levels, lower HDL levels, and larger atherosclerotic lesion size. Their female counterparts had larger LDL particle size, percentage of LDL in the particles assessed, and increased rate of LDL oxidation; all parameters associated with smaller atherosclerotic plaque size. Female estradiol levels were noted to be significantly higher than in their male counterpart, which was postulated to be a common factor to explain this difference [19]. These findings have not, however, been substantiated across models. For instance, in a mouse model, no difference was found between male and female mice fed cholesterol-rich diets in terms of the formation of aortic atheromatous lesions [20].

In addition to metabolic and hormonal factors, another manifestation of the biological difference between men and women is in the location and nature of the coronary disease. Although the location of the disease most frequently involves the left anterior descending artery in both sexes, men have a clearly higher incidence of diffuse three vessel disease [21]. Furthermore, men have been shown to have significant increase in severity and location of coronary stenoses when compared to women [21]. Women have been shown to have smaller left anterior descending and left main coronary arteries as measured by intravascular ultrasound, suggesting an effect of gender on coronary dimensions. [22]. Other studies claim that both sexes have similar plaque burden, and that differences in body surface area (BSA) may account for this discrepancy in coronary size and lesions [23].

In summary, studies show that men do not enjoy potential benefits of estrogen, perhaps accounting for the presence of coronary disease at a younger age. Estrogen receptors in men likely play an important role in atherogenesis [17, 19]. Androgens may also promote the formation of disease [18]. The diffuse nature of atherosclerotic changes among men may be a result of a combination of both hormonal and metabolic factors.

Risk Factors for Men

Male and female risk profiles are markedly different and have been implicated as the main reason for differences in surgical outcomes [5,8,9,11,13,24]. In direct examination of high-risk patients, risk factors appear to be more important than gender in terms of outcomes. Once expected mortality approaches 30%, some studies show no obvious differences in gender comparisons [6]. In this setting, any differences in gender are perhaps overshadowed by the potential of a given risk factor to influence outcome.

In general, men present with less severe medical co-morbidities at the time of surgery when compared to women. The exact reason for this is not known. Women present with unstable angina for more urgent procedures and carry a diagnosis of diabetes, hypercholesteremia, hypertension, and cerebrovascular disease, more often than men [25,26]. One crucial factor is age: women tend to be older, and with that age also carry a number of age-related co-morbidities. It may follow that coronary disease in women is more a direct result of these associated co-morbid conditions. This difference in age of presentation may have to do with an intrinsic biological factor as discussed above that puts males at more risk for heart disease at a younger age. In fact, younger women who present with coronary disease may have an unknown risk factor or lack of a protective mechanism unlike other women their age [27]. The previous rarity of this condition in young women may account for observed increased surgical risk and subsequent referral bias for these often very ill patients [13].

Studies of patients undergoing CABG have demonstrated that the risk profile for men and women are not similar. Men have presented with significantly higher creatinine, previous myocardial infarction (MI), and left ventricular hypertrophy (LVH) [25]. In addition, poor cardiac function, multiple cardiac operations, and a current or recent history of smoking are more common in men [8, 25]. This differs from those risk factors commonly attributed to women: age above 70, a history of congestive heart failure (CHF), the need for an urgent or emergent operation, diabetes mellitus, Class 3 or 4 angina, hypertension (HTN), and peripheral vascular disease (PVD) [8]. Despite this list of significant systemic diseases, men have been shown to consistently have more three-vessel disease than women. i.e. more diffuse disease [28]. The prevalence of diabetes and hypertension as a specific co-morbidity in women is reproducible across studies [13, 26, 28-31] and signifies a more secondary nature of coronary disease in women. [See Figure 1]

Men	Women
Diffuse Disease	Smaller Size/BSA
Smoking	Older Age
Decreased LV Function	Diabetes
Previous MI	HTN

Figure 1. Common Preoperative Risk Factors By Gender.

Multivariate analysis shows that in gender comparisons, some of the risk factors may be similar, but the weight of the risk factors is different. Comparison of operative mortality for certain groups of risk factors shows a difference in outcome between men and women, i.e. risk factors affect each gender differently [29]. There are likely gender-specific responses to cardiovascular disease. One of the most important factors related to late survival by univariate analysis is peripheral vascular disease or stroke, which decreases men's survival overall to approximately 50% at 10 years. Poor cardiac function (EF< 20%) decreases 10-year survival for men to 54% [28]. Other predictors of decreased survival include poor LV function, CHF, PVD, advanced age, small body size, and class IV New York Heart Association (NYHA) symptoms [28].

Variable	CABG in men	CABG in women
BMI >29	1.97 (1.18-3.29), $P = .010$	—
Emergency operation	1.72 (1.29-2.29), $P < .001$	—
Previous cardiac operation	1.44 (1.11-1.88), $P = .007$	—
PVD	1.47 (1.22-1.78), $P < .001$	—
LV hypertrophy	1.32 (1.09-1.59), $P = .004$	—
Current CHF	1.30 (1.03-1.64), $P = .025$	—
Past CHF	1.48 (1.16-1.88), $P = .002$	—
COPD	1.26 (1.02-1.54), $P = .028$	—
Preoperative renal failure on dialysis	2.01 (1.18-3.42), $P = .010$	—
Preoperative thrombolysis	0.49 (0.32-0.76), $P = .001$	—
Intraoperative stroke	1.91 (1.31-2.77), $P = .001$	—
Postoperative renal failure	2.95 (1.59-5.45), $P - .001$	—
Malignant ventricular arrhythmia	—	2.37 (1.33-4.22), $P = .003$
Calcified aorta	—	1.70 (1.19-2.42), $P = .003$
Preoperative renal failure	—	4.10 (2.45-6.88), $P < .001$
Age	1.059 (1.049-1.070), $P < .001$	1.063 (1.048-1.079), $P < .001$
Ejection fraction category (1: <30%, 2: 30%-50%, 3: >50%)	0.79 (0.68-0.91), $P = .001$	0.62 (0.51-0.76), $P < .001$
Diabetes mellitus	1.49 (1.24-1.80), $P < .001$	1.37 (1.06-1.76), $P = .016$
>2 Arterial grafts	0.75 (0.63-0.90), $P = .002$	0.74 (0.56-0.98), $P = .035$
Postoperative MI	2.16 (1.01-4.60), $P = .046$	3.62 (1.46-8.96), $P = .005$
Deep sternal wound infection	2.16 (1.18-3.97), $P = .001$	3.62 (1.71-7.67), $P = .001$
Sepsis, endocarditis, or both	2.44 (1.44-4.14), $P = .001$	2.72 (1.20-6.15), $P = .017$
Gastrointestinal complications	1.73 (1.06-2.82), $P = .029$	3.59 (1.64-7.88), $P = .001$
Respiratory failure	2.09 (1.46-2.97), $P < .001$	2.51 (1.63-3.86), $P < .001$

>*CABG*, Coronary artery bypass grafting; *BMI*, body mass index; *PVD*, peripheral vascular disease; *LV*, left ventricular; *CHF*, congestive heart failure; *COPD*, chronic obstructive pulmonary disease; *MI*, myocardial infarction.

Toumpoulis, IK; Anagnostopoulos, CE; Ioannidis, JP; Toumpoulis, SK; Chamogeorgakis, T; Swistel, DG; Derose JJ. The importance of independent risk-factors for long-term mortality prediction after cardiac surgery. *European Journal of Clinical Investigation,* September 2006, Volume 9, Pages 599-607.

Figure 2. Independent predictors for long-term mortality (hazard ratios and 95% confidence intervals) in men and women

Lists of preoperative risk factors overall favor men, but emphasize that despite a younger age of presentation, men also carry significant co-morbidities. In fact, one study found men carry 21 independent predictors of long-term mortality whereas women had only 12 [29]. [See Figure 2]. Other preoperative characteristics found to be more prevalent in men included their rate of transmural MI and poor EF. The presence of COPD, renal failure, and emergency operations between men and women were similar as was their presentation with hemodynamic instability or shock [29].

While some research agrees that certain predictors are statistically significant in respect to gender comparison, a recent analysis attempted to stratify and analyze data comparing men to women matched by propensity scores. These scores can be compared as equalizing risk factors for mortality but a true matching was only possible for a very small percentage of patients [30]. While men and women can be compared based on presenting comorbidities, for the most part their profiles are so different that extrapolating data from that comparison may not be truly representative of surgical outcomes. This may account for the discrepancy found between studies of gender outcomes.

Surgical Outcomes for Men

Multiple retrospective studies show the specifics of gender outcome data in respect to CABG surgery. Although some have found no difference and have attributed mortality rates strictly to differences in risk [8, 31], others have shown that gender does make a difference. Many studies have demonstrated that women carry significantly higher postoperative mortality and complication rates [6-8, 13, 25,32-34].

One issue discussed repeatedly in gender studies is in regards to body surface area (BSA) and differences in anatomy. BSA and coronary artery luminal diameter are shown to be a powerful determinant of mortality for both men and women [10]. Females have a smaller BSA and smaller coronary arteries, which may be a cause of reduced graft patency. In addition, women have been found to suffer post-operative angina more frequently than men, possibly due operative difficulties with particularly small coronary vessel diameters [35-37]. Smaller BSA and coronary artery size have been associated with an increased risk of hospital mortality [10, 36]. Men generally have a larger BSA which has been correlated directly with decreased hospital mortality. In one study, the presence of a BSA < 1.6 was associated with a 5x higher mortality than for a patient with a BSA > 2.0, man or woman [10].

Others have found that both men and women equally were at risk for coronary vessels to be less than 1.5mm [28]. This size makes a distal coronary anastomosis more challenging; placing the patient at increased risk for post-operative myocardial infarction or recurrent angina. Men in fact have more diffuse disease, which can increase operative mortality and perhaps neutralize any benefit that they carry for an increased BSA [31].

The association between body size and outcomes has been also studied with respect to blood transfusion rates. Transfusions are known to be an independent predictor of both increased mortality and intensive care unit length of stay [38]. Smaller body surface area is associated with intraoperative hemodilution necessitated by cardiopulmonary bypass, and may subsequently prompt transfusion. Men with smaller body surface area were more likely to receive transfusions, and thus at higher risk for postoperative mortality and complications [38]. Others disagree, finding that smaller body size does not increase operative mortality, but may contribute to low-output syndrome in the postoperative period [39].

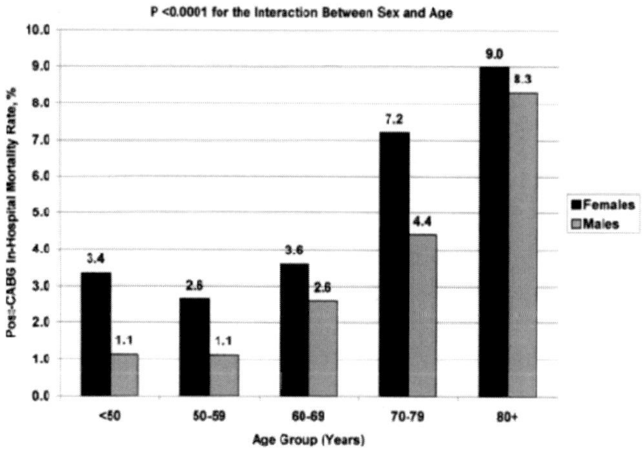

Comparison of crude post-CABG in-hospital mortality rates between men and women according to age group.

Guru, V; Fremes, SE; Austin, PC; Blackstone, EH; Tu, JV. Gender Differences in Outcomes After Hospital Discharge From Coronary Artery Bypass Grafting. *Circulation*, January 2006, Volume 113, Pages 507 - 516.

Figure 3.

An important distinction is made between short and long-term mortality after CABG. Co-morbidities for women indicate they are more at risk for short-term mortality

[6,8,10,13,40,41] [See Figure 3]. Men endure an earlier onset of coronary disease, but most studies show that they have better long-term survival [28, 41]. When attributing a gender role to CABG outcome, the more common co-morbidities which are specific to gender are a better predictor of outcome than attributing outcome to gender alone [8].

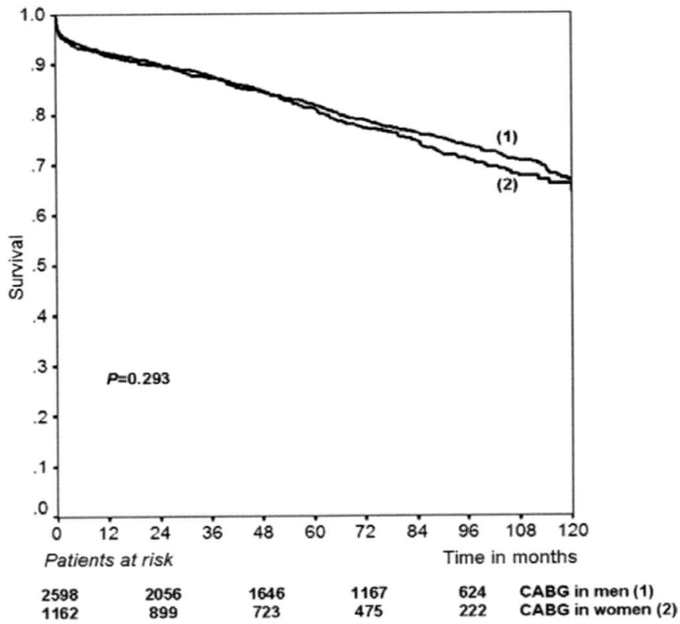

Toumpoulis, IK; Anagnostopoulos, CE; Ioannidis, JP; Toumpoulis, SK; Chamogeorgakis, T; Swistel, DG; Derose JJ. The importance of independent risk-factors for long-term mortality prediction after cardiac surgery. *European Journal of Clinical Investigation,* September 2006, Volume 9, Pages 599-607.

Figure 4. Kaplan-Meier survival plots if men and women undergoing coronary artery bypass grafting (CABG).

Other studies suggest that specific predictors of outcome exist between genders that directly effect survival [Figures 4 and 5]. At our institution, Toumpoulis et al assessed 3760 patients over a 10-year period to assess predictors of outcome. While there was no difference between genders in hospital mortality or 5-year survival, they did discover female sex to be an independent predictor of survival with adjustment for specific risk factors and mortality [29]. This contradicts prior claims that women suffer from a higher 30-day mortality. The assessment was based on a model using the EuroSCORE algorithm, which has been shown to be an independent predictor of long-term mortality after CABG [2, 42, 43]. Risk factors unique to men which were identified as causative for mortality included the necessity for an emergency operation, previous cardiac operation, the presence of peripheral vascular disease, left ventricular hypertrophy, current and past congestive heart failure, history of a previous MI, chronic obstructive pulmonary disease, a body mass index of greater than 29, preoperative dialysis, thrombolysis within 7 days before coronary artery bypass grafting, intraoperative stroke, and postoperative renal failure.

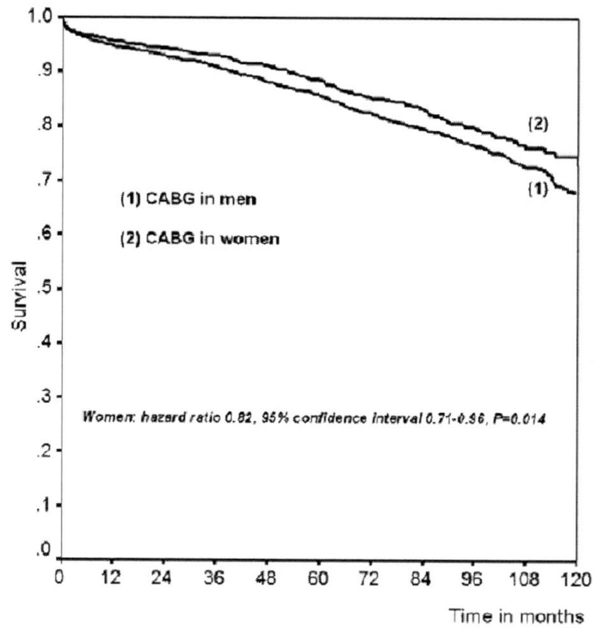

Toumpoulis, IK; Anagnostopoulos, CE; Ioannidis, JP; Toumpoulis, SK; Chamogeorgakis, T; Swistel, DG; Derose JJ. The importance of independent risk-factors for long-term mortality prediction after cardiac surgery. *European Journal of Clinical Investigation,* September 2006, Volume 9, Pages 599-607.

Figure 5. Risk-adjusted Kaplan-Meier survival plots of men and women undergoing coronary artery bypass grafting (CABG) adjusted for all independent preoperative, interoperative, and post-operative predictors for long-term mortality (age, race, emergency operation, ejection fraction previous cardiac operation, peripheral vascular disease, ≥ 1 previous myocardial infractions, intravenous nitroglycerin, congestive heart failure, malignant ventricular arrhythmia, chronic obstructive pulmonary disease, diabetes mellitus, preoperative renal failure, preoperative renal failure on dialysis, thrombolysis, off-pump coronary artery bypass, ≥ 2 arterial grafts, interoperative stroke, postoperative myocardial infarction, deep sternal wound infection, sepsis and/or endocarditis, gastrointestinal complications, and respiratory failure).

Postoperative complications were not different between genders in this study, and except for a longer postoperative inpatient stay for females, 30-day characteristics of mortality were evenly matched [29]. Had the patients been evenly matched, a difference in 30-day and 5-year mortality may have been uncovered. However, as shown in other studies, matching males to females evenly for preoperative characteristics is difficult as those features are inherently different across gender lines. This study also subdivided its data into 5-year blocks to assess whether changes in surgical technique might have affected the data; they found no such relationship [29].

Although some risk factors were found to be common between sexes, women generally present with a greater increase in mortality due to their presence [See Figure 6] [28]. Men in this study were more likely to have a lower EuroSCORE, and were younger upon presentation for surgery. This is consistent with other studies which have shown that males undergo surgery at a younger age due to earlier development of arterial disease, but in this study while the need for urgent or emergency surgery was greater in females, the immediate post-operative mortality and 5-year outcomes were not necessarily worse [28].

	Survival of men at			Survival of women at		
	5 y	10 y	*P* value	5 y	10 y	*P* value
Age						
<60	96	83	<.001	93	87	.053
>60	89	70		91	74	
Left ventricular ejection fraction						
>60%	97	87	<.001	94	83	.028
20%-60%	92	74		91	78	
<20%	75	54		85	38	
CHF	78	37	<.001	79	69	.135
None	94	81		93	79	
PVD	82	52	<.001	78	54	<.001
None	94	80		95	84	
Diabetes	89	58	<.001	87	64	.009
None	93	80		93	83	
Stroke/TIA	84	49	.001	72	54	.001
None	93	78		94	82	
MI 30 days preop	88	66	.178	83	62	.013
BSA						
<1.8 m^2	90	67	.008	92	80	.862
>1.8 m^2	93	79		91	75	
LITA	94	79	<.001	93	83	.039
None	85	64		90	70	
Ischemic MR	81	66	<.001	89	78	.232
None	93	77		93	78	
Timing						
Elective	94	79	.001	92	79	.232
Urgent	88	65		91	77	
Poorly visualized	91	73	.004	89	78	.403
Well visualized	93	78		93	79	
Left main stenosis	92	78	.330	90	72	.092
None	93	76		92	80	

MR, Mitral regurgitation.

Mickleborough, LL; Carson, S; Ivanov, J. Gender differences in quality of distal vessels: effect on results of coronary artery bypass grafting. *Journal of Thoracic and Cardiovascular Surgery*, October 2003, Volume 126, Issue 4, Pages 950-958.

Figure 6. Factors related to late survival by univariate analysis.

Other studies have found that men have better five-year survival when compared to women [44]. This can be partially attributed to the increased early mortality in women in addition to their advanced age at presentation. After the initial period, one study the adjusted mortality rates are equal between men and women [44]. Other studies support 5-year mortality with equal survival for both genders [29,45,46].

Studies that support that gender plays *no* role in mortality consistently find that mortality was increased in both men and women in the face of poor ventricular performance, congestive heart failure, and peripheral vascular disease. Men specifically had worse outcome in the presence of increased age, NYHA class IV symptoms, small vessel size, small body size (BSA < 1.8m^2) and lack of a left internal thoracic artery graft. Men were more likely to be smokers at presentation, present with worse left ventricular function, and more extensive angiographic evidence of coronary disease. However, these qualities were not found to be statistically significant predictors of increased mortality [7].

In matched samples, unadjusted analysis uncovers predictors of poor outcome, which can be applied to both genders. Factors independently associated with worse outcome include advanced age, history of peripheral vascular disease and heart failure, previous bypass grafts, major perioperative blood transfusion, and abnormal left ventricular function [30].

Thus far the largest gender-based CABG study was published using 344,913 patients in the Society of Thoracic Surgery (STS) database [6]. Operative mortality was significantly reduced in men as compared to women (2.6 % vs 4.5 %). Low and medium risk male subsets had a lower mortality compared to their female counterparts. However, in high risk patients, mortality was not statistically associated with gender. As a group, men were more likely to have tobacco use, cardiomegaly, COPD, previous MI, a higher NYHA classification, elective procedures, triple vessel disease, and an ejection fraction of less than 30% [6].

Men can expect to have good outcomes from coronary bypass surgery. They carry a low operative mortality and excellent long-term survival. Particularly when compared to women, men have shown greater relief of angina and higher graft patency rates [37]. They have improved post-operative ability to carry out activities of daily living, and fewer symptoms related to congestive heart failure, despite having decreased left ventricular function and the presence of more diffuse disease [37, 41, 47].

Conclusion

The purpose of coronary bypass surgery is to improve both quality of life and long-term survival. Assessment of early and long-term mortality in CABG patients has been an arena of significant interest, especially in an age where angioplasty and percutaneous therapies have become more prevalent. Outcomes data for CABG in terms of gender differences has been the focus of much research over the past several years, and its analysis has allowed clinicians to observe specific differences in risk assessment and outcome. Further research in the field of gender outcomes will assist in providing improved results for all patients.

References

[1] Peduzzi, P; Kamina, A; Detre, K. Twenty-two year follow-up in the VA Cooperative Study of Coronary Artery Bypass Surgery for Stable Angina. *American Journal of Cardiology,* June 1998, Volume 81, Issue 12, 1393-1399.

[2] European Coronary Surgery Study Group: long-term results of prospective randomized study of coronary artery bypass surgery in stable angina pectoris. *Lancet,* 1982, Volume ii, 1173-1180.

[3] Seung, KB; Park, DW; Kim, YH; Lee, SW; Lee, CW; Hong, MK; Park, SW; Yun, SC; Gwon, HC; Jeong, MH; Jang, Y; Kim, HS; Kim, PJ; Seong, IW; Park, HS; Ahn, T; Chase, IH; Tahk, SJ; Chung, WS; Park, SJ. Stents versus Coronary-Artery Bypass Grafting for Left Main Coronary Artery Disease. *New England Journal of Medicine,* April 2008, Volume 358, Issue 17, 1781-1792.

[4] Malenka, DJ; Leavitt, BJ; Hearne, MJ; Robb, JF; Baribeau, YR; Ryan, TJ; Helm, RE; Kellett, MA; Dauerman, HL; Dacey, LJ; Silver, MT; VerLee, PN; Weldner, PW; Hettleman, BD; Olmstead, EM; Piper, WD; O'Connor, GT. Comparing Long-Term

Survival Of Patients With Multivessel Coronary Disease After CABG or PCI: Analysis Of BARI-like Patients in Northern New England. *Circulation,* August 2005, Volume 112, I371-376.

[5] Edwards, FH; Ferraris, VA; Shahian, DM; Peterson, E; Furnary, AP; Haan, CK; Bridges, CR. Gender-Specific Practice Guidelines for Coronary Artery Bypass Surgery: Perioperative Management. *The Annals of Thoracic Surgery*, June 2005, Volume 79, Issue 6, 2189-2194.

[6] Edwards, FH; Carey, JS; Grover, FL; Bero, JW; Hartz, RS. Impact of gender on coronary bypass operative mortality. *The Annals of Thoracic Surgery*, July 1998, Volume 66, Issue 1, 125-131.

[7] Mickleborough, LL; Takagi, Y; Maruyama, H; Sun, Z; Mohamed, S. Is Sex a Factor in Determining Operative Risk for Aortocoronary Bypass Graft Surgery? *Circulation*, November 1995, Volume 92. 80-84.

[8] Abramov, D; Tamariz, MG; Sever, JY; Christakis, GT; Bhatnagar, G; Heenan, AL; Goldman, BS; Fremes, SE. The influence of gender on the outcome of coronary artery bypass surgery. *The Annals of Thoracic Surgery*, September 2000, Volume 70, Issue 3, 800-805.

[9] Edwards, FH; Grover, FL; Shroyer, LW; Schwartz, M; Bero, J. The Society of Thoracic Surgeons National Cardiac Surgery Database: Current Risk Assessment. *The Annals of Thoracic Surgery,* March 1997, Volume 63, Issue 3, 903-908.

[10] O'Connor, GT; Morton, JR; Diehl, MJ; Olmstead, EM; Coffin, LH; Levy, DG; Maloney, CT; Plume, SK; Nugent, W; Malenka, DJ. Differences between men and women in hospital mortality associated with coronary artery bypass graft surgery. The Northern New England Cardiovascular Disease Study Group. *Circulation,* November 1993, Volume 88, 2104-2110.

[11] Haskell, WL; Alderman, EL; Fair, JM; Maron, DJ; Mackey, SF; Superko, HR; Williams, PT; Johnstone, IM; Champagne, MA; Krauss, RM. Effects of intensive multiple risk factor reduction on coronary atherosclerosis and clinical cardiac events in men and women with coronary artery disease. The Stanford Coronary Risk Intervention Project (SCRIP). *Circulation*, March 1994, Volume 89, 975-990.

[12] Gottlieb, S; Harpaz, D; Shotan, A; Boyko, V; Leor, J; Cohen, M; Mandelzweig, L; Mazouz, B; Stern, S; Behar, S. Sex Differences in Management and Outcome After Acute Myocardial Infarction in the 1990s: A Prospective Observational Community-Based Study. *Circulation*, November 2000, Volume 102, 2484-2490.

[13] Vaccarino, V; Abramson, JL, Veledar, W; Weintraub, WS. Sex Differences in Hospital Mortality After Coronary Artery Bypass Surgery: Evidence for a Higher Mortality in Younger Women. *Circulation*, March 2002, Volume 105, 1176–1181.

[14] Bell, MR; Grill, DE; Garratt, KN; Berger, PB; Gersh, BJ; Holmes, DR Jr. Long-Term Outcome of Women Compared With Men After Successful Coronary Angioplasty. *Circulation*, June 1995, Volume 91, Issue 12, 2876-2881.

[15] Villablanca, A; Lubahn, D; Shelby, L; Lloyd, K; Barthold, S. Susceptibility to Early Atherosclerosis in Male Mice is Mediated by Estrogen Receptor Alpha. *Arteriosclerosis, Thrombosis, and Vascular Biology,* June 2004, Volume 24, 995-997.

[16] Tse, J; Martin-McNaulty, B; Halks-Miller, M; Kauser, K; DelVecchio, V; Vergona, R; Sullivan, ME; Rubanyi, GM. Accelerated Atherosclerosis and Premature Calcified Cartilaginous Metaplasia in the Aorta of Diabetic Male Apo E Knockout Mice Can Be

Prevented by Chronic Treatment with 17β-estradiol. *Atherosclerosis*, June 1999, Volume 144, Issue 2, 303-313.

[17] Finking, G; Krauss, N; Römer, S; Eckert, S; Lenz, C; Kamenz, J; Menke, A; Brehme, U; Hombach, V; Hanke, H. 17β-estradiol, Gender Independently, Reduces Atheroma Development But Not Neointimal Proliferation After Balloon Injury in the Rabbit Aorta. *Atherosclerosis,* January 2001, Volume 154, Issue 1, 39-49.

[18] Ng, MK; Quinn, CM; McCrohon, JA; Nakhla, S; Jessup, W; Handelsman, DJ; Celermajer, DS; Death, AK. Androgens Up-Regulate Atherosclerosis-Related Genes in Macrophages From Males But Not Females. *Journal American College of Cardiology*, October 2003, Volume 42, 1306-1313.

[19] Wilson, TA; Nicolosi, RJ; Lawton, CW; Babiak, J. Gender Differences in Response to a Hypercholesterolemic Diet in Hamsters: Effects on Plasma Lipoprotein Cholesterol Concentrations and Early Aortic Atherosclerosis. *Atherosclerosis*, September 1999, Volume 146, Issue 1, 83-91.

[20] Johnston, TP; Coker, JW; Paigen, BJ; Tawfik, O. Sex Does Not Seem To Influence The Formation Of Aortic Lesions In The P-407-Induced Mouse Model Of Hyperlipidemia and Atherosclerosis. *Journal of Cardiovascular Pharmacology,* March 2002, Volume 39, Issue 3, 404-411.

[21] Kyriakidis, M; Petropoulakis, P; Androulakis, A; Antonopoulos, A; Apostolopoulous, T; Barbetseas, J; Vyssoulis, G; Toutouzas, P. Sex Differences In The Anatomy Of Coronary Artery Disease. *Journal of Clinical Epidemiology*, June 1995, Volume 48, Issue 6, 723-730.

[22] Sheifer, SE; Canos, MR; Winfurt, KP; Arora, UK; Mendelsohn, FO; Gersh, BJ; Weissman, NJ. Sex Differences In Coronary Artery Size Assessed By Intravascular Ultrasound. *American Heart Journal*, April 2000, Volume 139, Issue 4, 649-653.

[23] Kornowski, R; Lansky, AJ; Mintz, GS; Kent, KM; Pichard, AD; Satler, LF; Bucher, TA; Popma, JJ; Leon, MB. Comparison of Men Versus Women In Cross-Sectional Area Luminal Narrowing, Quantity of Plaque, Presence Of Calcium In Plaque, And Lumen Location In Coronary Arteries By Intravascular Ultrasound In Patients With Stable Angina Pectoris. *American Journal Cardiology,* June 1997, Volume 79, Issue 12, 1601-1605.

[24] Murabito, JM; Evans, JC; Larson, MG; Levy, D. Prognosis after the onset of coronary heart disease. An investigation of differences in outcome between the sexes according to initial coronary disease presentation. *Circulation*, December 1993, Volume 88, 2548-2555.

[25] Woods, SE; Noble, G; Smith, JM; Hasselfeld, K. The influence of gender in patients undergoing coronary artery bypass graft surgery: an eight-year prospective hospitalized cohort study. *Journal of the American College of Surgeons,* March 2003, Volume 196, Issue 3, 428-434.

[26] Vaccarino, V; Lin, ZQ; Kasl, SV; Mattera, JA; Roumanis, SA; Abramson, JL; Krumholz, HM. Sex Differences in Health Status After Coronary Artery Bypass Surgery. *Circulation*, November 2003, Volume 108, 2642 - 2647.

[27] Wexler LF. Studies of acute coronary syndromes in women: lessons for everyone. *N Engl J. Med.* 1999; 341:275-276.

[28] Mickleborough, LL; Carson, S; Ivanov, J. Gender differences in quality of distal vessels: effect on results of coronary artery bypass grafting. *Journal of Thoracic and Cardiovascular Surgery*, October 2003, Volume 126, Issue 4, 950-958.
[29] Toumpoulis, IK; Anagnostopoulos, CE; Balaram, SK, Rokkas, CK; Swistel, DG, Ashton, RC; DeRose, JJ. Assessment of independent predictors for long-term mortality between women and men after coronary artery bypass grafting: Are women different from men?. *The Journal of Thoracic and Cardiovascular Surgery*, February 2006, Volume 131, Issue 2, Pages 343-351.
[30] Koch, CG; Khandwala, F; Nussmeier, N; Blackstone, EH. Gender and outcomes after coronary artery bypass grafting: a propensity-matched comparison. *Journal of Thoracic and Cardiovascular Surgery*, December 2003, Volume 126, Issue 6, 2032-2043.
[31] Aldea, GS; Gaudiani, JM; Shapira, OM; Jacobs, AK; Weinberg, J; Cupples, AL; Lazar, HL; Shemin, RJ. Effect of gender on postoperative outcomes and hospital stays after coronary artery bypass grafting. *The Annals of Thoracic Surgery*, April 1999, Volume 67, Issue 4, 1097-1103.
[32] Ibrahim JF, Paparella D, Ivanov J, Buchanan MR, Brister SJ. Gender-related differences in morbidity and mortality during combined valve and coronary surgery. *J Thorac Cardiovasc Surg*. 2003; 126 (4) : 959-964.
[33] Rahimtoola Sh, Bennet AJ, Grunkemeier GL, Block P, and Starr A. Survival at 15-18 years after coronary bypass surgery for angina in women. *Circulation* 1993 nov ;88 II71-8.
[34] Carey JS, Cukingnan RA, and Singer L.K.M. Health Status after Myocardial Revascularization: Inferior Results in Women. *Ann Thor Surg* 1995; 59:112-7.
[35] O'Connor, NJ; Morton, JR; Birkmeyer, JD; Olmstead, EM; O'Connor, GT. Effects of Coronary Artery Diameter in Patients Undergoing Coronary Bypass Surgery. *Circulation*, February 1996, Volume 93, Pages 652-655.
[36] Fisher, LD; Kennedy, JW; Davis, KB; Maynard, C; Fritz, JK; Kaiser, G; Myers, WO. Association of sex, physical size and operative mortality after coronary artery bypass in the Coronary Artery Surgery Study (CASS). *Journal of Thoracic Cardiovascular Surgery*, September 1982, Volume 84, 334-341.
[37] Johnson WE, Kayser KL, Pedraza PM. Angina pectoris and coronary bypass surgery: patterns of prevention and recurrences in 3105 consecutive patients followed up to 11 years. *Am Heart J* 1984;108:1190-7.
[38] Ranucci, M; Pazzaglia, A; Bianchini, C; Bozzetti, G; Isgrò, G. Body Size, Gender, and Transfusions as Determinants of Outcome After Coronary Operations. *The Annals of Thoracic Surgery*, February 2008, Volume 85, Issue 2, Pages 481-486.
[39] Christakis GT, Weisel RD, Buth KJ, Fremes SE, Rao V, Panagiotopoulos KP, Ivanov J, Goldman BS, and David TE. Is body size the cause for poor outcomes of coronary artery bypass operations in women? *J Thorac Cardiovasc Surg*. 1995 nov 110(5) 1344-56.
[40] Jacobs AK, Kelsey SF, Brooks MM, Faxon DP, Chaitman BR, Bittner V, Mock MB, Weiner BH, Dean L, Winston C, Drew L, Sopko G. Better outcome for women compared with men undergoing coronary revascularization : a report from the Bypass Angioplasty Revascularization Investigation (BARI) *Circulation* 1998;98:1279-1285.
[41] Guru, V; Fremes, SE; Austin, PC; Blackstone, EH; Tu, JV. Gender Differences in Outcomes After Hospital Discharge From Coronary Artery Bypass Grafting. *Circulation*, January 2006, Volume 113, 507 - 516.

[42] Nashef, SA; Roques, F; Michel, P; Gauducheau, E; Lemeshow, S; Salamon, R. European system for cardiac operative risk evaluation (EuroSCORE). *European Journal of Cardiothoracic Surgery,* July 1999, Volume 16, 9–13.

[43] Nashef, SA; Roques, F; Hammill, BG; Peterson, ED; Michel, P; Grover, FL; Wyse, RK; Ferguson, TB. EuroSCORE Project Group. Validation of European System for Cardiac Operative Risk Evaluation (EuroSCORE) in North American cardiac surgery. *European Journal of Cardiothoracic Surgery,* July 2002, Volume 22, 101–105.

[44] Herlitz, J; Brandrup-Wognsen, G; Karlson, BW; Sjöland, H; Karlsson, T; Caidahl, K; Hartford, M; Haglid, M. Mortality, risk indicators of death, mode of death and symptoms of angina pectoris during 5 years after coronary artery bypass grafting in men and women. *Journal of Internal Medicine*, April 2000, Volume 247, Issue 4, 500-506.

[45] Loop, FD; Golding, LR; Macmillian, JP. Coronary artery surgery in women compared with men: analysis of risks and long-term results. *Journal of the American College of Cardiology,* 1983, Volume 1, 383-90.

[46] Davis, KB; Chaitman, B; Ryan, T; Bittner, V; Kennedy, JW. Comparison of 15-year survival for men and women after initial medical or surgical treatment for coronary artery disease: a CASS registry study. *Journal of the American College of Cardiology,* April 1995, Volume 25, 1000-1009.

[47] Jessup M, Pina IL. Is it important to examine gender differences in the epidemiology and outcome of severe heart failure? *J Thorac Cardiovasc Surg*. 2004; 127;1247-1252.

In: Heart Disease in Men
Editors: A.B. Todd and M.H. Mosley, pp. 347-364
ISBN: 978-1-60692-297-2

Chapter 17

EVALUATION OF CORONARY ARTERY DISEASE BY EXERCISE ECHOCARDIOGRAPHY

Jesus Peteiro **[*]** ***and Beatriz Bouzas***

Laboratory of Echocardiography, Service of Cardiology,
Juan Canalejo Hospital, University of A Coruña,
A Coruña, Spain

Abstract

Stress echocardiography is an established tool for clinical decision making, with and average sensitivity of 80% and specificity of 86%. Among available stress techniques, exercise is safer and more physiologic, therefore represents the first choice for the patient able to exercise. Peak exercise imaging, although challenged in treadmill, has greater sensitivity than post-exercise imaging. Apical images are as good as those acquired during the post-exercise period. Some tips may increase the successfulness of peak treadmill exercise imaging.

The role of new technology is promising for exercise echo. Doppler tissue and speckle imaging can assess myocardial velocities and deformation. Doppler tissue imaging increases the agreement and accuracy among novel readers, although it is not better than visual assessment performed by experienced observers. The role of speckle imaging is hopeful, as it can easily measure myocardial torsion, which has been found to be diminished under ischemic conditions. Finally, 3-dimensional echocardiography can also be used during exercise since a full volume of the entire myocardium can be acquired in only a few cardiac cycles.

Detection of myocardial ischemia is a must for cardiologists attending patients with confirmed or suspected coronary artery disease (CAD). Ischemia detection allows the diagnosis of CAD. Besides, ischemia is associated to poor quality of life, its magnitude is related to the extension of CAD, and produces left ventricular (LV) dysfunction and

---

[*] E-mail address: pete@canalejo.org. Fax 34-81-178001. Address for correspondence: Jesus C Peteiro, P/Ronda 5-4º izda.15011-A Coruña, Spain

ventricular arrhythmias. Furthermore, for a long time it has been well known that the outcome of CAD patients is more related to the extension of the myocardial ischemia during stress than to the number of diseased vessels on coronary angiography (1-3). Therefore, the decisions related to revascularization procedures should be based not only on the coronary anatomy, but also in the evidence that a particular coronary stenosis has an objective functional significance.

Several non-invasive techniques allow for the detection of myocardial ischemia and the stratification of patients with more severe or extensive CAD that should go to coronary angiography and eventually to revascularization, namely ECG exercise testing, stress echo, nuclear techniques and magnetic resonance (MR). Besides, coronary computed axial tomography (CAT) offers anatomical assessment with high accuracy.

The advantages of stress echo over these other techniques include: low cost (if 1 is the cost of an ECG exercise testing, 2 would be that of an exercise echo, but 5.7 would be the cost of a nuclear technique) (4); safety (approximately 1 event/7000 exercise echo, 1/700 pharmacological stress echo) (5-6); relatively high sensitivity (80%) and specificity (86%) (7), comparable to the rest of the non-invasive methods but ECG exercise testing (lower sensitivity and specificity), nuclear techniques (lower specificity), and coronary CAT (higher sensitivity); solid prognostic data (less that 1% events/year in those with a negative stress echo) (8-10); and the fact that it is a green technology (other methods as those based on nuclear medicine or CAT, even with optimized protocols, radiate the same or more than a coronary angiography, an equivalent to more than 300 single chest-X-ray) (11). As stress echo is usually performed and interpreted by cardiology staff in a quick fashion, the results are commonly available in a short-term.

Exercise Echocardiography

Within the stress echo modalities (exercise, pharmacological stress), exercise is safer, more physiological and more accurate (12), therefore it represents the first choice for the patient able to exercise. Exercise echo consists simply on the addition of echocardiography to a conventional exercise testing. Thus, besides the clinical information (symptoms during exercise) and ECG information (ST segment changes), we will obtain resting echo data (resting wall motion abnormalities suggesting necrosis, valvular or myocardial disease,...etc), and exercise echo data (new wall motion abnormalities indicating ischemia). This is the reason for its superior sensitivity and specificity when compared to conventional exercise testing. As it can be inferred from above, its major advantage dwells on the evaluation of patients with resting ECG abnormalities and in the evaluation of those with an inconclusive or doubtful ECG exercise testing. Table 1 shows the up-to-date recommendations for the performance of stress echo on the management of chest pain according to recent ESC guidelines (13). The recommendation stating that exercise echo should be considered as a diagnostic and/or prognostic alternative to ECG exercise testing in the centers with wide availability will likely spread the method.

Table 1. Recommendations for the use of exercise stress in the initial diagnostic assessment of angina *.

Class I

Diagnostic and/or prognostic evaluation in patients with resting ECG abnormalities, LBBB, >1 mm ST-depression, paced rhythm, or WPW.

Diagnostic and/or prognostic evaluation in patients with a non-conclusive exercise ECG.

Class IIa

Diagnostic evaluation in patients with prior revascularization and/or coronary lesions in angiography in whom localization of ischaemia is important.

As an alternative to exercise ECG in patients where facilities, costs, and personnel resources allow.

As an alternative to exercise ECG in patients with a low pre-test probability of disease such as women with atypical chest pain˙

Prognostic evaluation in symptomatic patients after revascularization.

*pharmacological stress with imaging techniques is recommended if the patient is unable to exercise adequately.

Modified from: ESC Guidelines on the management of stable angina pectoris: executive summary. *Eur Heart J 2006.*

Abbreviations: EE, stress echocardiography; WPW, Wolf-Parkinson-White; LBBB, left bundle brand block; CAD, coronary artery disease.

Class I: Is commonly accepted that benefits are greater than risks, therefore the procedure should be performed;

Class IIa: Benefits are greater than risks, although additional studies are required. It is reasonable to perform the procedure.

How to Perform an Exercise Echo

Treadmill and bicycle are the most commonly used exercise modalities, although treadmill is more likely performed worldwide. Treadmill exercise produces more oxygen consumption, and patients able to walk are usually able to do it in a treadmill but are not always able to cycle. ECG and blood pressure are monitorized all through the test as they are in a conventional exercise testing. Protocols adjusted to the clinical patient characteristics should be used, although Bruce protocol (change in speed and step every 3 min) is the most commonly used. We occasionally ask the patients to walk out of the treadmill, previously to the exercise testing, to decide about the more adequate protocol for each particular patient.

We acquire resting images on the table, and peak exercise in the treadmill with the patient walking or running (apical and parasternal views). In case of non-conclusive peak images (bad quality or doubtful), images during the immediate post-exercise time are also acquired. Our group has demonstrated that peak treadmill imaging is more sensitive than post-exercise imaging for the diagnosis of CAD, and that the quality of peak images are similar to those

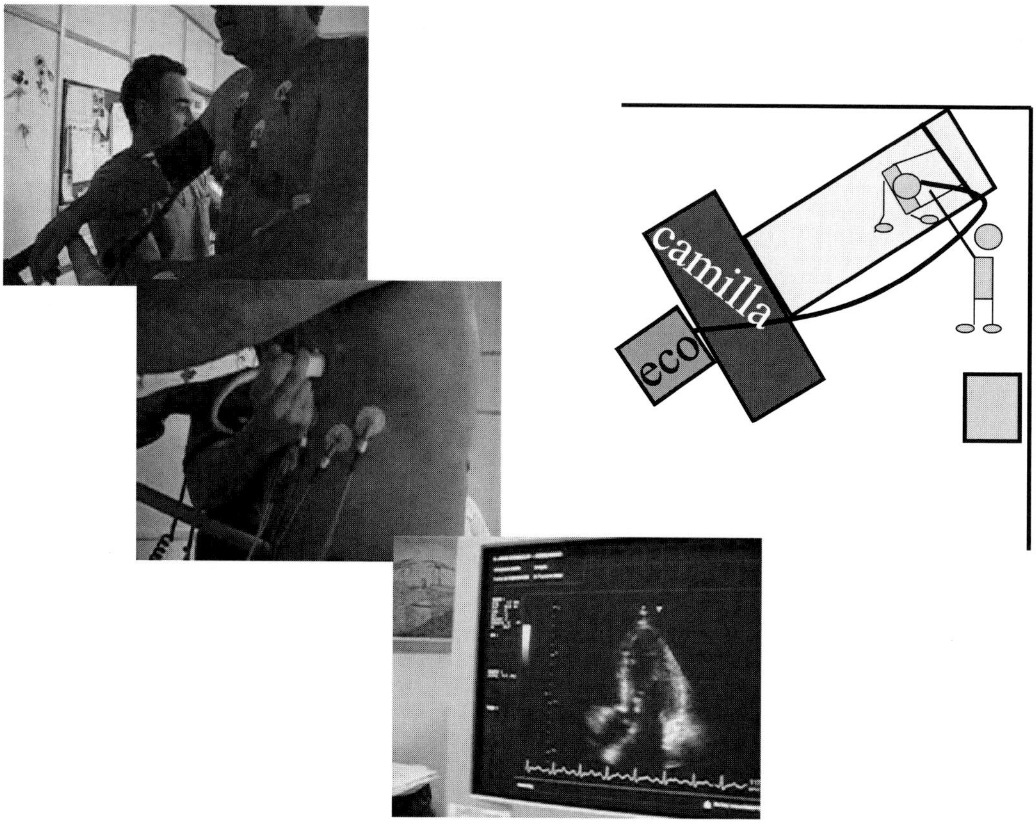

Figure 1. Exercise echo. When the patient is exhausted or some termination criteria is achieved (symptoms, significative ST changes, decrease or increase in blood pressure..etc), the observer acquires images by placing the transducer in the cardiac apex, then in the parasternal region. Note the placement of the table, the treadmill and the echo machine for feasible imaging evaluation at peak and post-exercise.

acquired at post-exercise (14-15). Others have also demonstrated higher sensitivity with peak instead of post-exercise during bicycle exercise echo (16). A proper training in peak exercise imaging has other several advantages: 1) patient scanning during different phases of the exercise testing is feasible, and it can be performed in case of concern about the appropriateness of stopping the test, for example in case of symptoms or ECG changes that can be doubtful; 2) the narrow window time we have for post-exercise imaging does not exist; in this last case imaging acquisition should be no longer than 45 s, otherwise wall motion abnormalities can rapidly recover. To scan the patient both during peak exercise and quickly during post-exercise requires a particular spatial disposition of the treadmill, the table and the echo machine, being each one next to the others. In the Fig 1, we show their disposition in our laboratory. The length of the probe should be as long as possible, considering it is not the same for all the manufacturers.

Nevertheless, 3 technical requirements are mandatory to achieve effectiveness in peak and/or post-exercise imaging acquisition and interpretation: 1) direct ECG wire connexion between the echo machine and the ergometer to optimize the ECG signal, unavoidable to obtain well registered RR cycles; 2) a continuous imaging acquisition system. This system allows the acquisition of a continuous loop containing multiple cardiac cycles during several minutes. After the test, the interpreter has only to choose the more appropriate cycles corresponding to the different views to compare them with the resting ones; and 3) a quad-format screen to compare resting and exercise images. Almost all the manufacturers offer these requirements. The cost-effectiveness of a stress laboratory may be optimized if an off-line computer is available to read the studies, as the echo machine may be used meanwhile.

Imaging Interpretation

With stress echo, CAD is considered when there are resting or stress-induced wall motion abnormalities (WMA) (hypokinesia, akinesia, dyskinesia). When the same WMA are present at rest and stress the condition is defined as fixed WMA or necrosis. When the WMA appear only at stress the condition is defined as induced-WMA or ischemia. When there are WMA at rest that increase with stress the condition is defined as mixed necrosis and ischemia (see Figs 2 to 10). In this latter situation the WMA can develop in the same territory or in another one (ischemia at a distance). A semi-quantitative system is used to calculate a score by dividing the LV in 16 or 17 segments (17) and assigning 1 to each normal segment, 2 hypokinesia, 3 akinesia, and 4 diskinesia. The sum of all the segments divided by the number of segments is the WMA score (if=1, normal case; if >1, abnormal). Most laboratories also calculate resting and exercise LV ejection fraction.

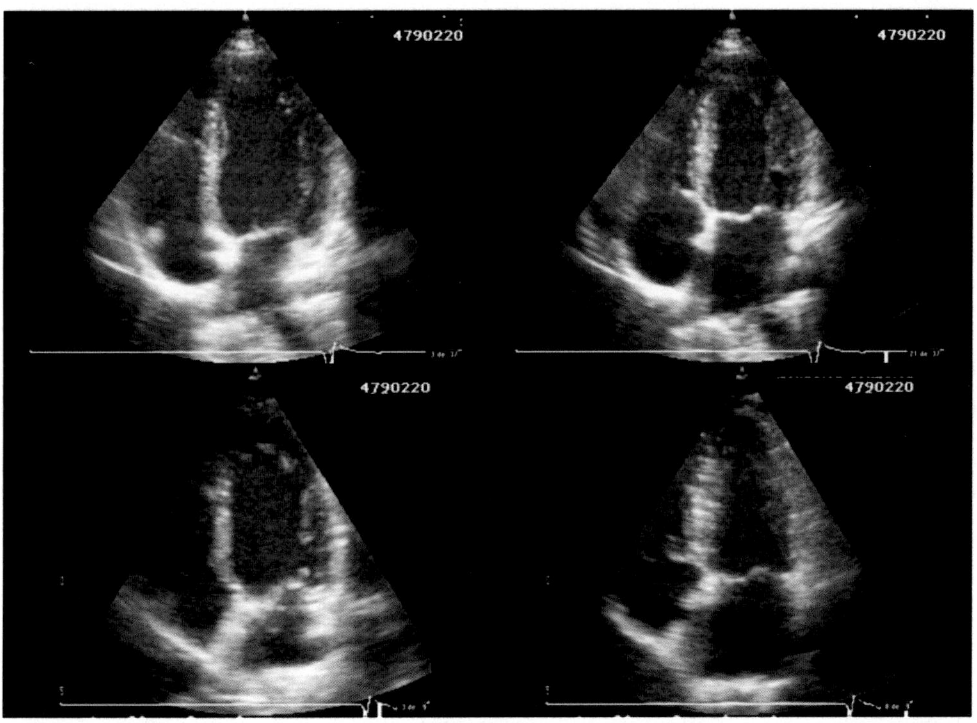

Figure 2. Resting echo (top) and peak exercise echo (bottom) in the 4-Ch apical view (diastolic frames on the left, systolic frames on the right) in a patient with normal results. Note the LV cavity dimensions decrease with exercise and the increase in LV ejection fraction.

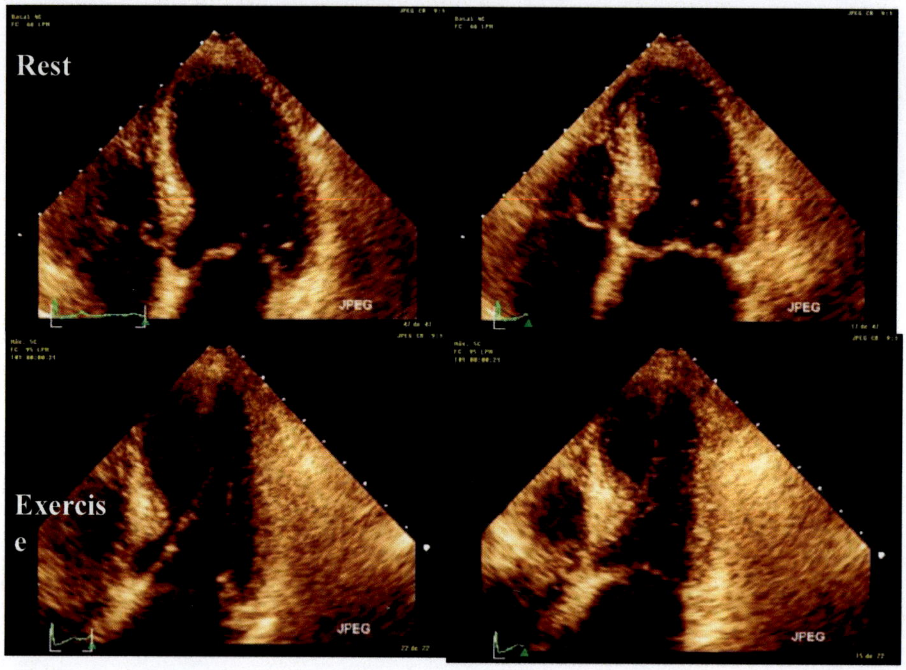

Figure 3. Resting echo (top) and peak exercise echo (bottom) in the 4-Ch apical view (diastolic frames on the left, systolic frames on the right) in a patient with significant coronary stenoses in the left anterior descending artery (99%) and right coronary artery (70%). At rest, wall motion is normal, whereas at exercise a septoapical dyssinergia is observed with the typical 8-shaped LV.

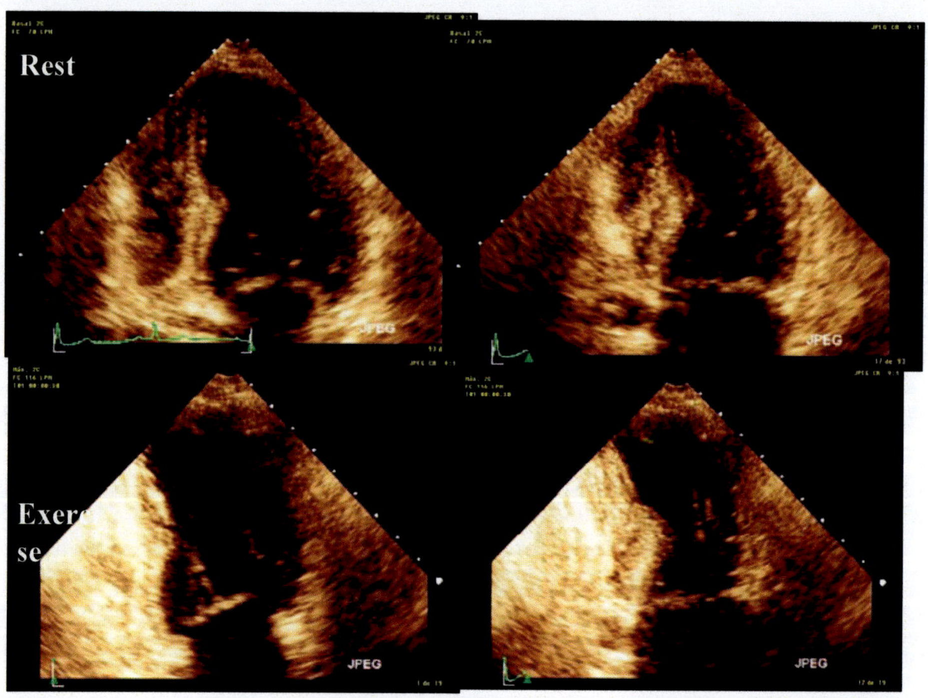

Figure 4. 2-Ch apical views at rest and peak exercise in the same patient as in Fig 3. There are hypokinesia in anteroapical and posteroapical segments during exercise.

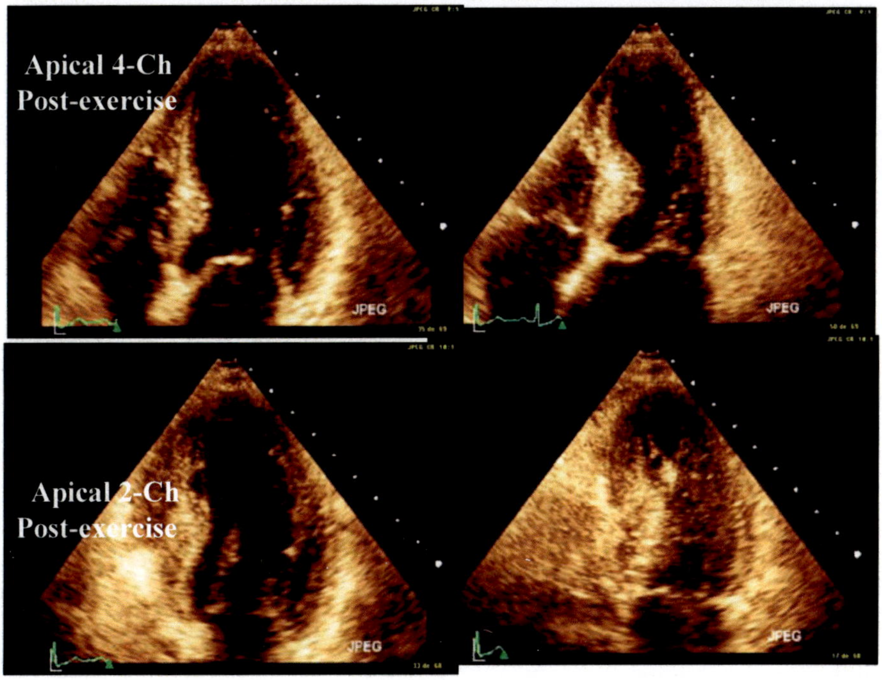

Figure 5. Post-exercise imaging in the same patient as in Figs 3 and 4, in the 4-Ch (top) and 2-Ch views (bottom). Although apical WMA are still evident, these WMA are less notorious than at peak exercise.

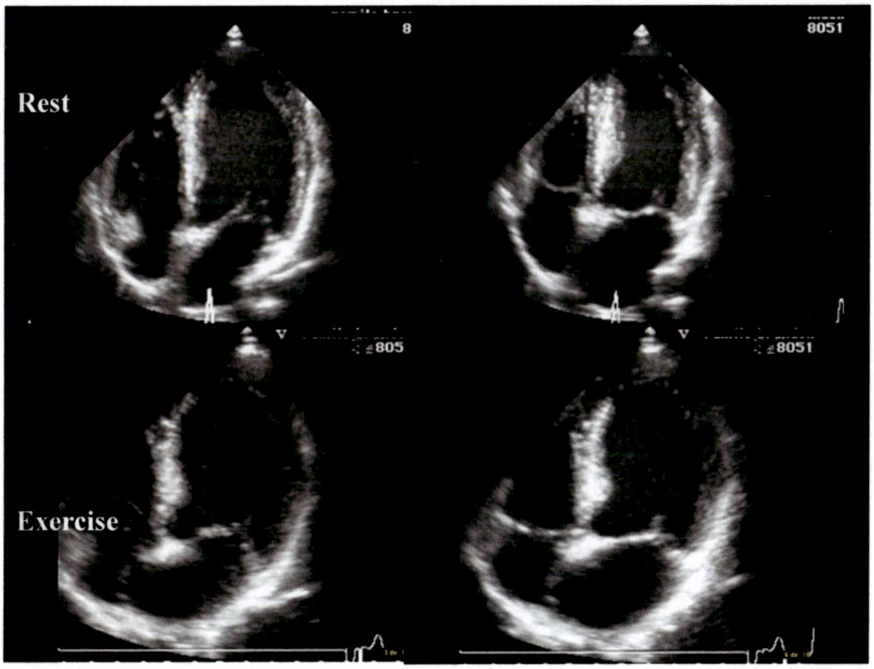

Figure 6. Resting echo (top) and peak exercise echo (bottom) in the 4-Ch apical view (diastolic frames on the left, systolic frames on the right) in a patient with multivessel CAD (95% stenoses in the left main, left anterior descending, and circumflex arteries, and 75% stenosis in the right coronary artery). At rest, wall motion is normal, whereas at exercise both global WMA and LV dilation are observed.

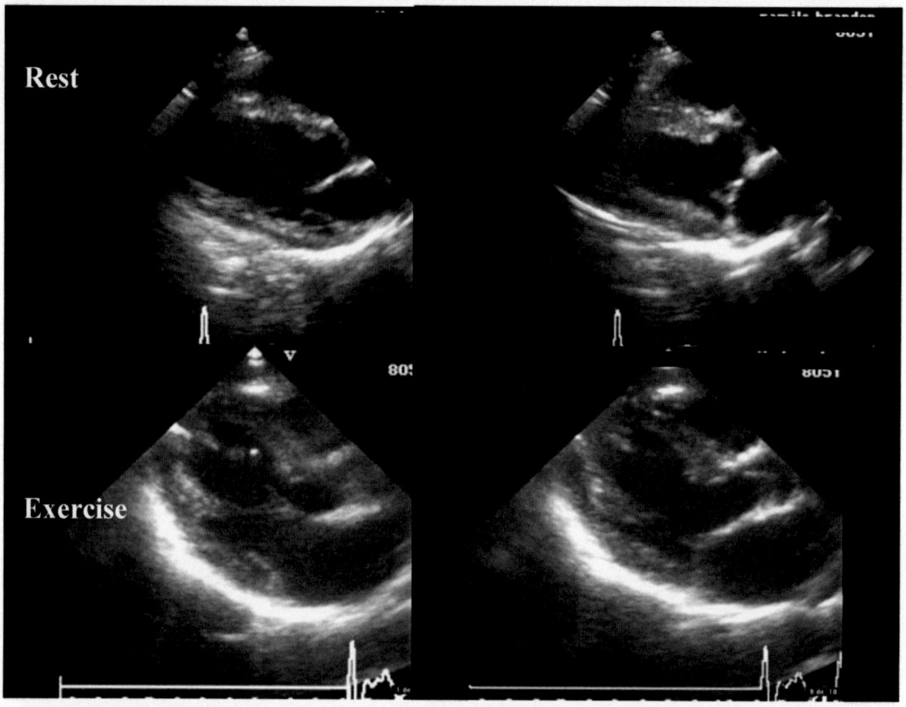

Figure 7. Parasternal short-axis views at rest and peak exercise in the same patient as in Fig 6.

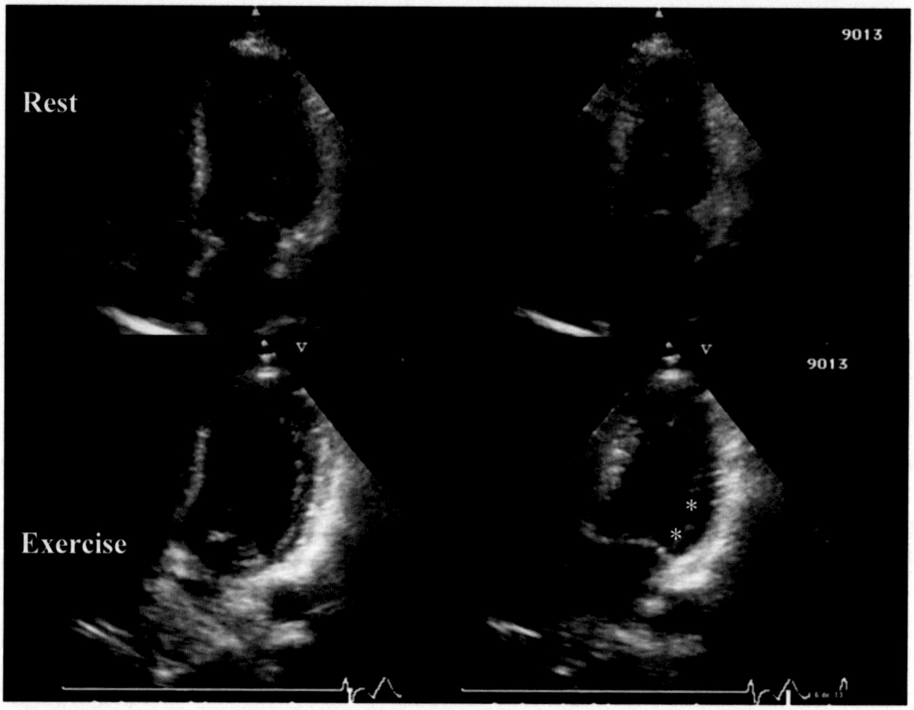

Figure 8. Resting echo (top) and peak exercise echo (bottom) in the 4-Ch apical view (diastolic frames on the left, systolic frames on the right) in a patient with a severe lesion in a marginal obtuse branch (99% stenosis). Wall motion is normal at rest, whereas lateral severe hypokinesia was seen at peak stress.

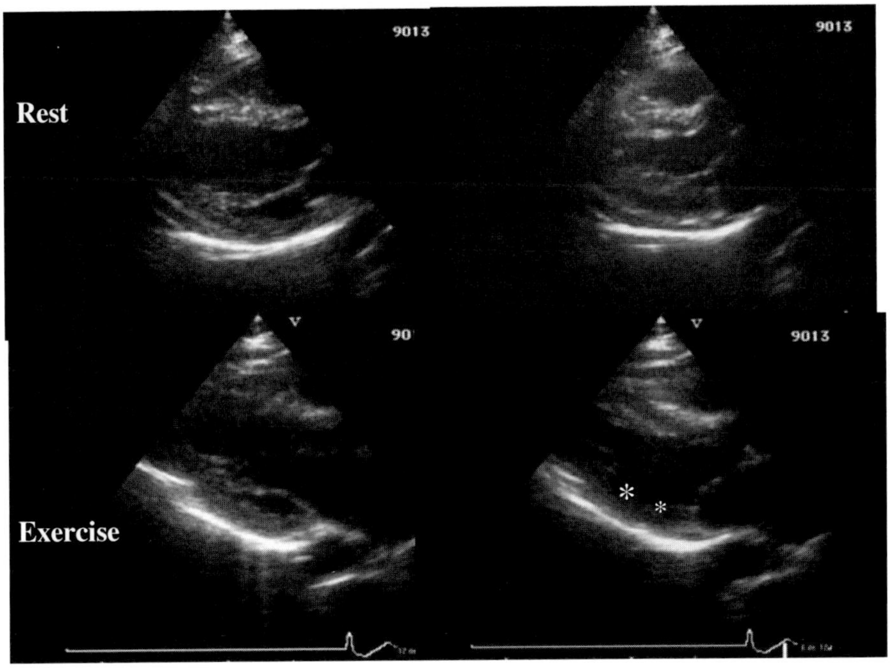

Figure 9. Resting echo (top) and peak exercise echo (bottom) in the parasternal long-axis view (diastolic frames on the left, systolic frames on the right) in the same patient as in Fig 8, showing inferior severe hypokinesia at peak exercise.

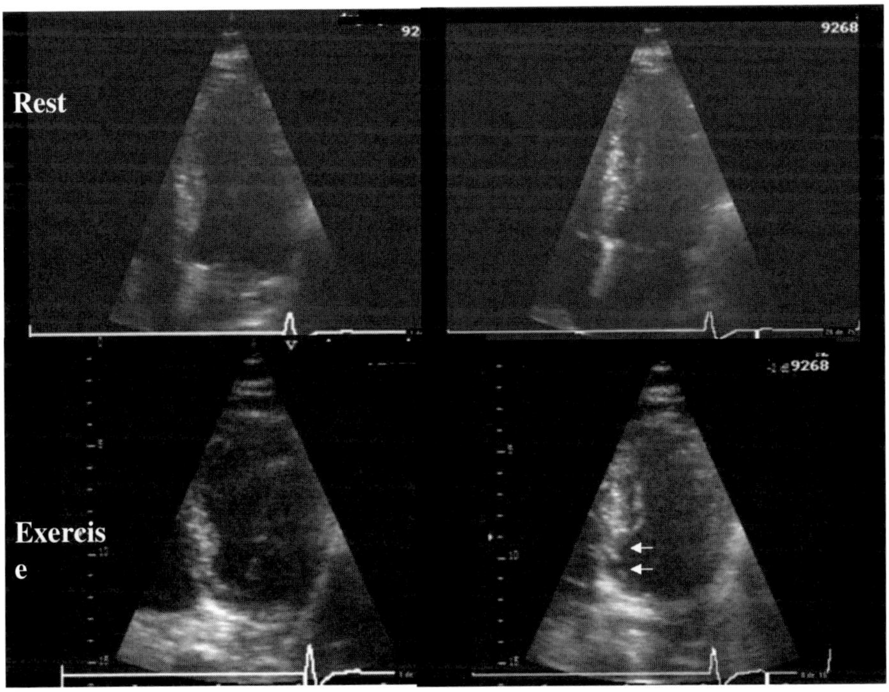

Figure 10. Resting echo (top) and peak exercise echo (bottom) in the 4-Ch apical view (diastolic frames on the left, systolic frames on the right) in a patient with a severe lesion in the right coronary artery (90% stenosis). Wall motion is normal at rest, whereas infero-septal akinesia was seen at peak stress.

Exercise Echo Limitations

The main limitation is the existence of a % of patients with bad acoustic window. This % has obviously diminished in recent years with the introduction of harmonic imaging, available in all the modern equipments. In the remaining 5-10% of cases with bad acoustic window contrast agents can be used to increase border detection. However, the need for an "excellent" vision is more a need for pharmacological stress echo, where all the diagnostic power is limited to the imaging, than for exercise echo where other important diagnostic and prognostic information based on symptoms, ECG, and functional capacity is provided.

Secondly, the nature of the test makes imaging acquisition more difficult than during pharmacological stress, due to the higher increase in both heart and respiratory rates with the former. It has been said that pharmacological stress echo represents the elementary and secondary school whereas exercise echo the University (18).

Thirdly, imaging interpretation by stress echo is made by a semi-quantitative approach, which has led to only moderate agreement between observers in different studies (19-20). However, this agreement is higher when either significant WMA or extensive CAD as defined by angiography are present.

Finally, some patients may have limited capacity for exercising and, as 85% of the theoretically maximal heart-rate is not achieved in up to 25-30% of the patients, these tests are often considered as non-conclusive. This % can be reduced by using atropine at sub-maximal or maximal effort, therefore reducing the need for pharmacological stressors (21).

Role of the New Technology

Exercise echo, as an echocardiographic technique, may be implemented with the new technology. As referred above, contrast agents for better border detection can be used in cases of suboptimal acoustic window in order to improve diagnostic accuracy (22), improve the accuracy of novel observers, and reduce the need for other explorations in case of non-conclusive tests. However, its use in a routine basis is not cost-effective (23). Contrast agents can also be used to look for myocardial perfusion defects during stress. As the defects of perfusion precede wall motion abnormalities, this technique has been used successfully, particularly during pharmacological stress (24), showing higher sensitivity than WMA although with lower specificity in some of these studies. However, the assessment of myocardial perfusion during exercise echo has several technical limitations.

Tissue Doppler imaging and speckle imaging can assess myocardial velocities and strain in different samples of the myocardium, increase the agreement between observers, and also the accuracy of non-trainers observers, but do not increase the accuracy of the visual assessment when this assessment is performed by trained observers (25-26). Speckle imaging can be effectively used to assess the torsional movement of the myocardium, which is diminished during ischemic conditions (27). However, no studies have evaluated this method during stress echo.

Finally, 3-dimensional echocardiography (3-DE) is able to acquire a full-volume of the myocardium in only 4-5 cardiac cycles. Then, any crops we want can be done at rest and stress to compare the different views in the 2 conditions (28-30). Although the imaging acquisition is therefore very quick, relatively much time is required to crop the needed views.

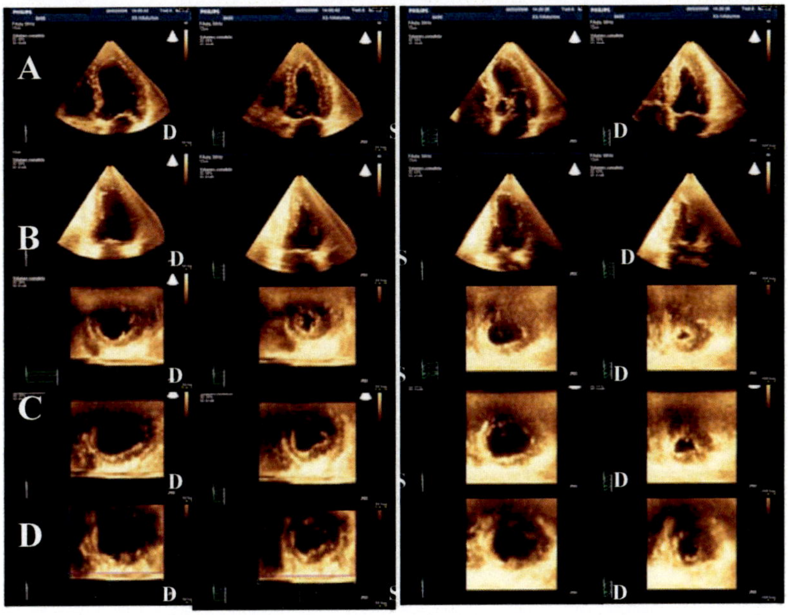

Figure 11. Cropped views obtained from a LV full-volume during 3-dimensional exercise echocardiography in resting conditions (left panel) and during peak exercise (right panel) in a normal subject. A: 4-Ch view; B: 2-Ch view; C: short-axis view at the apical level; D: short-axis view at the level of the papillary muscles; E: short-axis view at the basal level. Note the increase in thickness and displacement of all the LV segments from rest to exercise, and also the reduction in the LV cavity size.

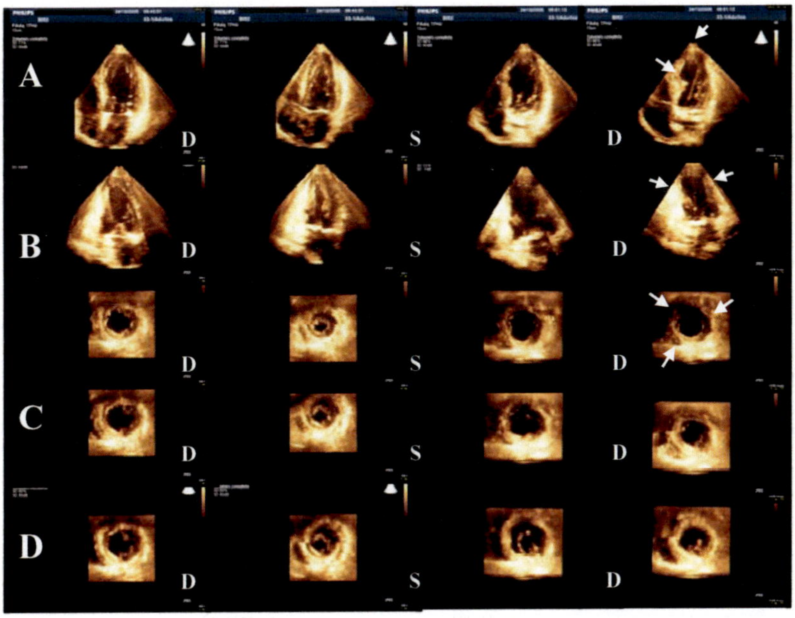

Figure 12. Cropped views obtained from a LV full-volume during 3-dimensional exercise echocardiography in resting conditions (left panel) and during peak exercise (right panel) in a patient with severe 3-vessels disease. During exercise, septoapical akinesia in the 4-Ch apical view (8-shaped LV), anterior and posterior hypokinesia in the 2-Ch apical view, akinesia and dilation in the short-axis apical view, and hypokinesia in the short-axis view at the papillary muscles view develop.

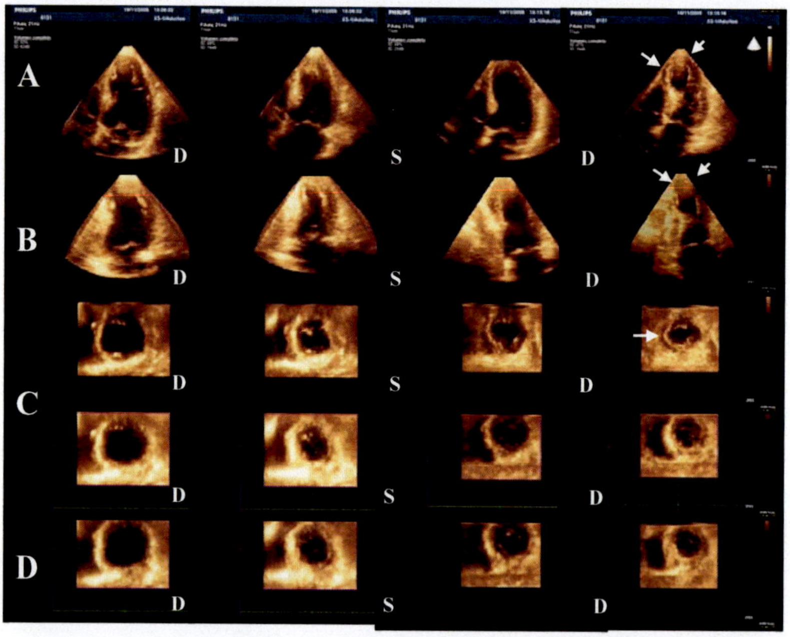

Figure 13. Cropped views obtained from a LV full-volume during 3-dimensional exercise echocardiography in resting conditions (left panel) and during peak exercise (right panel) in a patient with severe stenosis in the left anterior descending coronary artery. During exercise, septoapical akinesia in the 4-Ch apical view (8-shaped LV), apical akinesia in the 2-Ch apical view, and septal akinesia in the short-axis apical view develop.

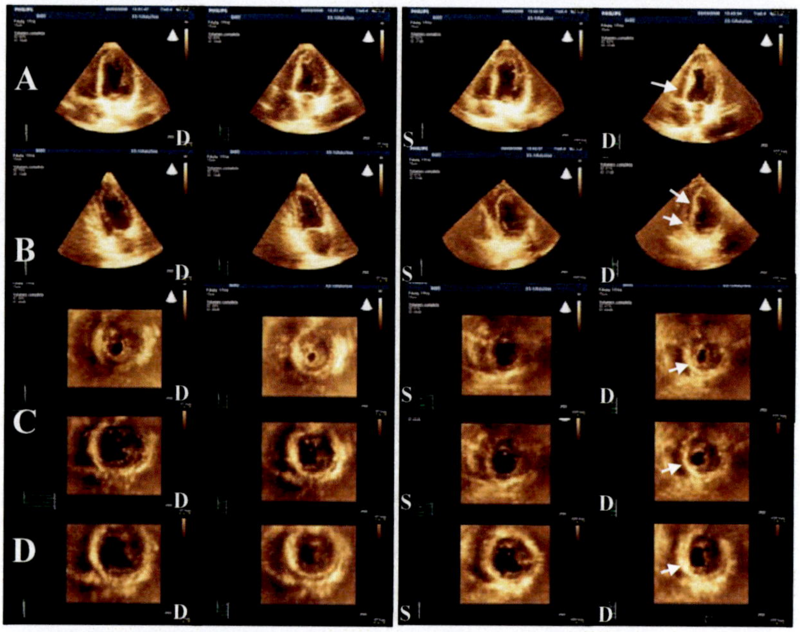

Figure 14. Cropped views obtained from a LV full-volume during 3-dimensional exercise echocardiography in resting conditions (left panel) and during peak exercise (right panel) in a patient with severe stenoses in both the left circumflex and right coronary arteries. Note the development during exercise of septobasal akinesia in the 4-Ch apical view, posterior akinesia in the 2-Ch apical view, and postero-septal akinesia in the short-axis views.

Diastolic Function Assessment

LV diastolic function impairment is associated to bad prognosis in patients with heart disease. Exercise echo can assess diastolic function during exercise. Among the numerous indexes of diastolic function, the ratio of early transmitral flow assessed by pulsed Doppler (E) to early diastolic annulus velocity assessed by tissue Doppler (e′) is closely related to LV end-diastolic pressures and can be easily measured. A high E/e′ index is associated to dyspnoea, bad functional capacity, exercise LV dysfunction and CAD (31-32). A change to a pseudonormalized LV inflow pattern is also associated to the same adverse variables (32). These measurements may help to clarify causes of dyspnoea in patients with different cardiac/noncardiac conditions.

Prognostic Value

Even before the development of stress echo, it was known that resting LV function and ischemia were important prognostic markers. These indicators can now be evaluated altogether. With each stress echo modality it has been demonstrated the independent prognostic value of the stress induced WMA, and also the excellent outcome of patients with a negative stress echo (<1% events/year) (33). Exercise echo is particularly useful for prognostic assessment because information on functional capacity parameters (Mets, heart rate x blood pressure product, % of age-predicted maximal achieved heart rate) is available.

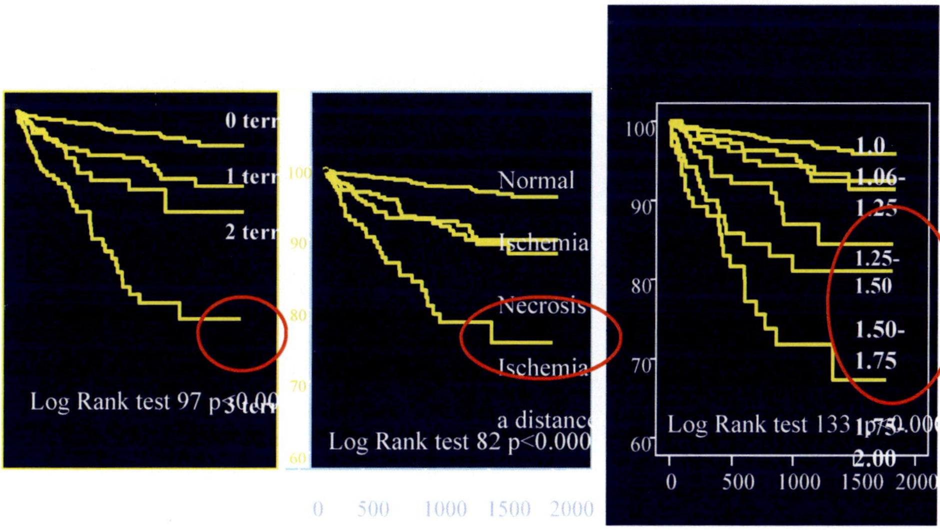

Figure 15. Kaplan-Meier survival curves of patients classified according to the number of involved territories, the exercise echo diagnosis category (normal, ischemia, necrosis, ischemia at a distance), and the peak WMA score index.

Exercise echo has its maximal cost-effectiveness in the assessment of patients with intermediate pre-test risk (8, 34). We have seen that exercise echo categorizes effectively patients with intermediate Duke score risk in those with higher or lower risk, but also stratifies patients with low Duke score risk, helping in the decision about the convenience of angiography in them (8). Several studies, as those performed in our institution, have shown that gender, functional capacity in Mets, heart rate x blood pressure product, resting LV function, and ischemia are independently associated to hard cardiac events (8-9), and how the value of exercise echo has incremental predictive value in patients with different pre-test probabilities of CAD (9). Patients with WMA in the 3 coronary territories, patients with peak wall motion score index >1.5, and patients with ischemia at a distance are at higher risk for cardiac events (35) (Fig 15).

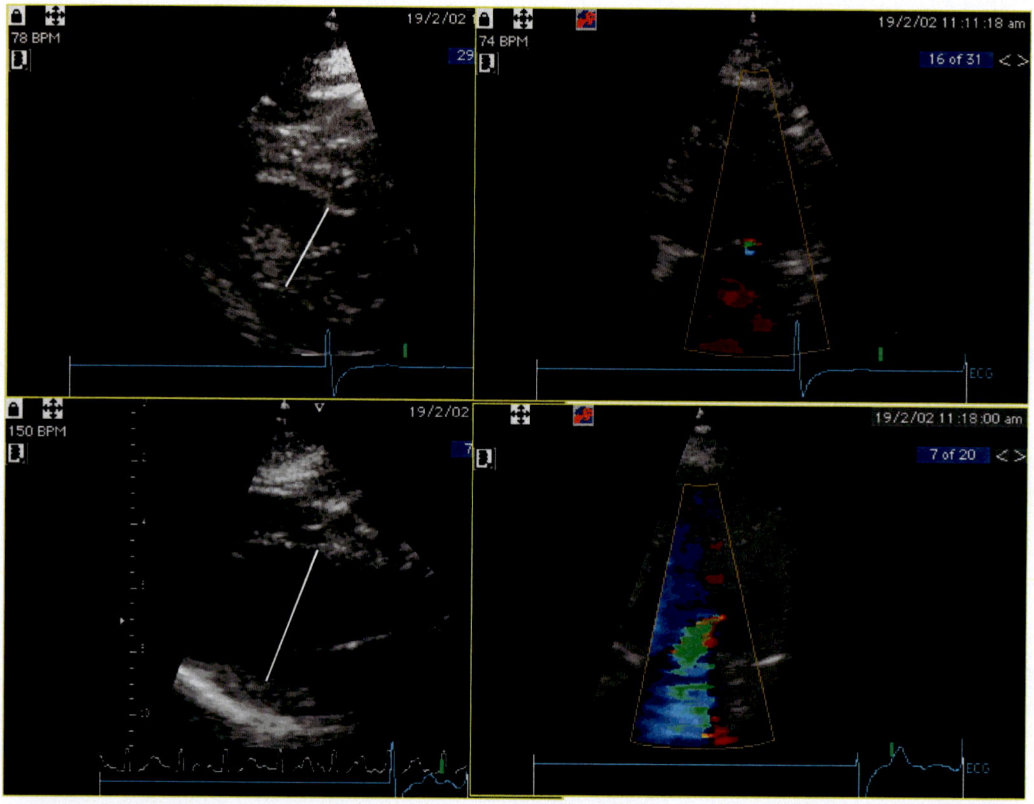

Figure 16. Example of a patient with exercise-induced LV dysfunction and mitral regurgitation (MR) worsening. Top: Resting parasternal long axis view at end-systole (left) and MR signal (right); Bottom: Peak exercise parasternal view at end-systole (left) and MR signal at post-exercise (right). Note the exercise-induce increase in LV dimension and the development of severe MR.

Moreover, exercise echo can also show increase or development of mitral regurgitation (MR) during exercise (36), which is due to LV functional remodelling related to LV dilation and impairment in LV function (Fig 16). However, this phenomenon is hardly seen with other kinds of stress, even in case of extensive CAD, because dobutamine and dipyridamole produce a significant preload reduction. Our group has demonstrated that MR increase or MR development during exercise echo is associated to poor outcome. In a recent study including almost 2000 patients, those with positive exercise echo and MR worsening had an event rate of 11% during a follow-up of 4 years, as compared to 6% in those with positive echo but without MR worsening (10) (Fig 17). MR worsening had independent value for the prediction of death, over WMA.

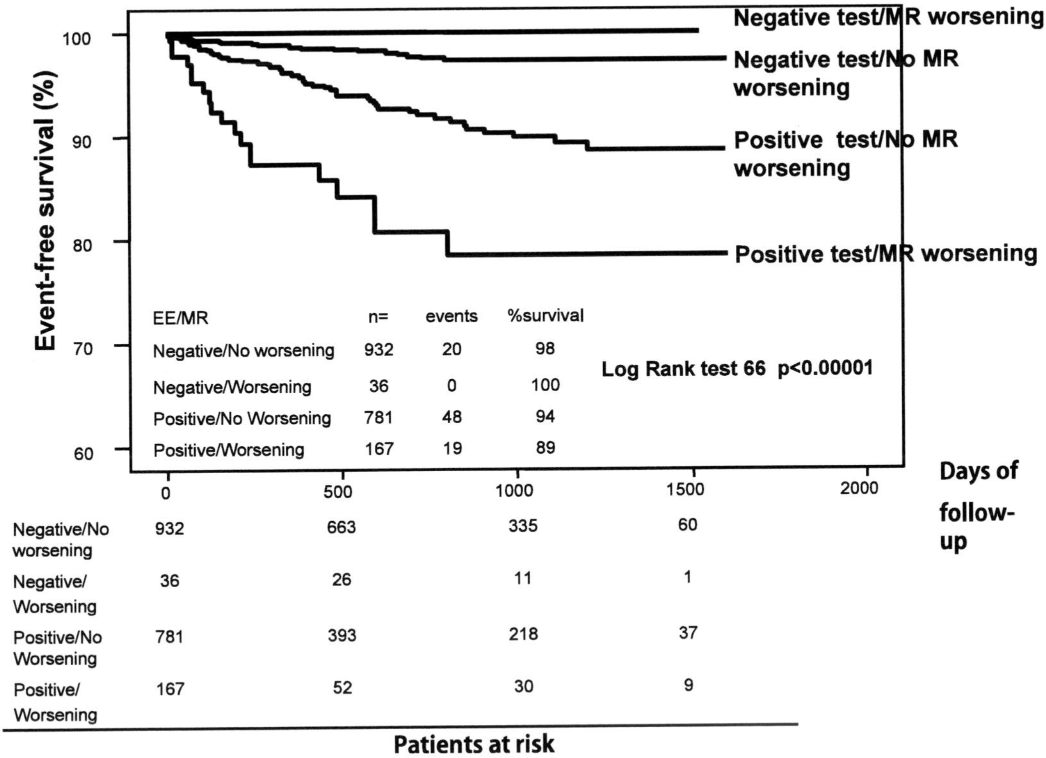

Figure 17. Kaplan-Meier survival curves of patients classified according to the exercise echo results and increase in mitral regurgitation from rest to post-exercise. Negative test/no MR worsening vs. negative test/MR worsening, p=NS; negative test/no MR worsening vs. positive test with or without MR worsening, p<0.0001; negative test/MR worsening vs. positive test with or without MR worsening, p<0.05; positive test/no MR worsening vs. positive test/MR worsening, p<0.001.

Conclusion

Due to its low cost, safety, diagnostic and prognostic capabilities, and absence of radiation, exercise echo should be considered as a first evaluation technique for patients with suspected or confirmed CAD. It represents a class I indication for patients with resting ECG abnormalities and for patients with non-conclusive or doubtful ECG exercise testing. Besides, exercise echo is an useful alternative to conventional exercise testing in centers with wide availability. The need for an exhaustive training seems not to be a serious limitation for a technique that, if implanted in environments where patients with CAD are seen, is cost-effective.

References

[1] Gohlke H, Samek L, Betz P, Roskamm H. Exercise testing provides additional prognostic information in angiographically defined subgroups of patients with coronary artery disease. *Circulation* 1983; 68: 979-985.

[2] Bonow RO, Kent KM, Rosing DR, Lan KK, Lakatos E, Borer JS, et al. Exercise-induced ischemia in mildly symptomatic patients with coronary artery disease and preserved left ventricular function: identification of subgroups at risk of death during medical therapy. *N Engl J Med* 1984; 311: 1339-1345.

[3] Iskandrian AS, Chae SC, Heo J, Stanberry CD, Wasserleben V, Cave V. Independent and incremental prognostic value of exercise single-photon emission computed tomography (SPECT) thallium imaging in coronary artery disease. *J Am Coll Cardiol* 1993; 22: 665-670.

[4] Gibbons RJ, Abrams J, Chatterjee K, Daley J, Deedwania PC, Douglas JS, et al. ACC/AHA 2002 guideline update for the management of patients with chronic stable angina--summary article: a report of the American College of Cardiology/American Heart Association Task Force on practice guidelines (Committee on the Management of Patients With Chronic Stable Angina). *J Am Coll Cardiol* 2003; 41: 159-68.

[5] Varga A, Garcia MA, Picano E. Safety of Stress Echocardiography (from the International Stress Echo Complication Registry). *Am J Cardiol* 2006; 98: 541-543.

[6] Picano E, Mathias W Jr, Pingitore A, Bigi R, Previtali M. Safety and tolerability of dobutamine-atropine stress echocardiography: a prospective, multicentre study. Echo Dobutamine International Cooperative Study Group. *Lancet* 1994; 344: 1190-2.

[7] Schinkel AF, Bax JJ, Geleijnse ML, Boersma E, Elhendy A, Roelandt JR, Poldermans D. Noninvasive evaluation of ischaemic heart disease: myocardial perfusion imaging or stress echocardiography? *Eur Heart J* 2003; 24: 789-800.

[8] Peteiro JC, Monserrat L, Pineiro M, Calvino R, Vazquez JM, Marinas J et al. Comparison of exercise echocardiography and the Duke treadmill score for risk stratification in patients with known or suspected coronary artery disease and normal resting electrocardiogram. *Am Heart J* 2006;151:1324.e1-e10

[9] Peteiro JC, Monserrat L, Bouzas A, Pinon P, Marinas J, Bouzas B et al. Risk stratification by treadmill exercise echocardiography. *J Am Soc Echocardiogr* 2006; 19: 894-901.

[10] Peteiro JC, Monserrat L, Bouzas A, Piñon P, Mariñas J, Piñeiro M et al. Prognostic value of mitral regurgitation assessment during exercise echocardiography in patients with known or suspected coronary artery disease. *J Am Soc Echocardiogr* 2006; 19: 1229-1237.

[11] Einstein AJ, Moser KW, Thompson RC, Cerqueira MD, Henzlova MJ. Radiation dose to patients from cardiac diagnostic imaging. *Circulation* 2007; 116: 1290-1305.

[12] Beleslin BD, Ostojic M, Stepanovic J, Djordjevic-Dikic A, Stojkovic S, Nedeljkovic M, et al. Stress echocardiography in the detection of myocardial ischemia. Head-to-head comparison of exercise, dobutamine and dipyridamole test. *Circulation* 1994; 90:1168-1176

[13] Fox K, Garcia MA, Ardissino D, Buszman P, Camici PG, Crea F et al. ESC Guidelines on the management of stable angina pectoris: executive summary: the Task Force on the

Management of Stable Angina Pectoris of the European Society of Cardiology. *Eur Heart J* 2006; 27: 1341-81.

[14] Peteiro J, Fabregas R, Monserrat L, Álvarez N, Castro-Beiras A. Comparison of treadmill exercise echocardiography before and after exercise in the evaluation of patients with known or suspected coronary artery disease. *J Am Soc Echocardiogr* 1999; 12: 1073-1079.

[15] Peteiro J, Garrido I, Monserrat L, Aldama G, Calvino R, Castro-Beiras A. Comparison of peak and postexercise treadmill echocardiography with the use of continuous harmonic imaging acquisition. *J Am Soc Echocardiogr* 2004; 17: 1044-1049.

[16] Park TH, Tayan N, Takeda K, Jeon HK, Quinones MA, Zoghbi WA. Supine bicycle echocardiography improved diagnostic accuracy and physiologic assessment of coronary artery disease with the incorporation of intermediate stages of exercise. *J Am Coll Cardiol* 2007; 50: 1857-1863.

[17] Bourdillon PD, Broderick TM, Sawada SG, Armstrong WF, Ryan T, Dillon JC, et al. Regional wall motion index for infarct and noninfarct regions after reperfusion in acute myocardial infarction: comparison with global wall motion index. *J Am Soc Echocardiogr.* 1989; 2: 398-407.

[18] Picano E, ed. *Stress echocardiography* (4ª ed). Springer-Verlag, Berlin, 2003.

[19] Hoffmann R, Marwick TH, Poldermans D, Lethen H, Ciani R, van der Meer P et al. Refinements in stress echocardiographic techniques improve interinstitutional agreement in interpretation of dobutamine stress echocardiograms. *Eur Heart J* 2002; 23: 821-829

[20] Peteiro, AM Alonso, R Florenciano, C Gzalez-Juanatey, G de la Morena, M Moreno, MA Rodríguez. Intercenters concordance in the interpretation of exercise echocardiography. *Rev Esp Cardiol* 2006; 59: 33-40.

[21] Peteiro J, Garrido I, Monserrat L, Aldama G, Salgado J, Castro-Beiras A. Exercise echocardiography with addition of atropine. *Am J Cardiol* 2004; 94: 346-348.

[22] Dolan MS, Riad K, El-Shafei A, Puri S, Tamirisa K, Bierig M, et al. Effect of intravenous contrast for left ventricular opacification and border definition on sensitivity and specificity of dobutamine stress echocardiography compared with coronary angiography in technically difficult patients. *Am Heart J* 2001; 142: 908-915.

[23] Moir S, Shaw L, Haluska B, Jenkins C, Marwick TH. Left ventricular opacification for the diagnosis of coronary artery disease with stress echocardiography: an angiographic study of incremental benefit and cost-effectiveness. *Am Heart J* 2007; 154: 510-8

[24] Rakhit DJ, Becher H, Monaghan M, Nihoyannopoulos P, Senior R. The clinical applications of myocardial contrast echocardiography. *Eur J Echocardiogr* 2007; 8: S24-9

[25] Cain P, Baglin T, Case P, Spicer D, Short L, Marwick TH. Application of tissue Doppler to interpretation of dobutamine echocardiography and comparison with quantitative coronary angiography. *Am J Cardiol* 2001; 87: 525-531.

[26] Hanekom L, Cho GY, Leano R, Jeffriess L, Marwick TH. Comparison of two-dimensional speckle and tissue Doppler strain measurement during dobutamine stress echocardiography: an angiographic correlation. *Eur Heart J* 2007; 28: 1765-72.

[27] Helle-Valle T, Crosby J, Edvardsen T, Lyseggen E, Amundsen BH, Smith HJ et al. New noninvasive method for assessment of left ventricular rotation: speckle tracking echocardiography. *Circulation* 2005; 112: 3149-1356.

[28] Ahmad M, Xie T, McCulloch M, Abreo G, Runge M. Real-time three-dimensional dobutamine stress echocardiography in assessment of ischemia: comparison with two-dimensional dobutamine stress echocardiography. *J Am Coll Cardiol* 2001; 37: 1303-1309.

[29] Matsumura Y, Hozumi T, Arai K, Sugioka K, Ujino K, Takemoto Y, et al. Non-invasive assessment of myocardial ischaemia using new real-time three-dimensional dobutamine stress echocardiography: comparison with conventional two-dimensional methods. *Eur Heart J* 2005; 26:1625-1632.

[30] Peteiro J, Perez R, Perez D, Estevez R, Barge E et al. Comparison of 2 and 3-dimensional exercise echocardiography for the detection of coronary artery disease. *J Am Soc Echocardiogr* 2007; 20: 959-67.

[31] Burgess MI, Jenkins C, Sharman JE, Marwick TH. Diastolic stress echocardiography: hemodynamic validation and clinical significance of estimation of ventricular filling pressure with exercise. *J Am Coll Cardiol* 2006; 47: 1891-900.

[32] Peteiro J, Pazos P, Bouzas A, Piñon P, Estevez R, Castro-Beiras A. Assessment of diastolic function during exercise echocardiography: annulus mitral velocity or transmitral flow pattern*? J Am Soc Echocardiogr* 2008; 21: 178-84

[33] Metz LD, Beattie M, Hom R, Redberg RF, Grady D, Fleischmann KE. The prognostic value of normal exercise myocardial perfusion imaging and exercise echocardiography: a meta-analysis. *J Am Coll Cardiol* 2007; 49: 227-37.

[34] Marwick TH, Shaw L, Case C, Vasey C, Thomas JD. Clinical and economic impact of exercise electrocardiography and exercise echocardiography in clinical practice. *Eur Heart J* 2003; 24: 1153-1163.

[35] Prognostic value of treadmill exercise echocardiography. Peteiro-Vazquez J, Monserrat L, Mariñas J, Garrido IP, Bouzas M, et al. *Rev Esp Cardiol.* 2005; 58: 924-933

[36] Peteiro J, Freire E, Montserrat L, Castro-Beiras A. The effect of exercise on ischemic mitral regurgitation. *Chest* 1998; 114: 1075-82.

In: Heart Disease in Men
Editors: A.B. Todd and M.H. Mosley, pp. 365-380
ISBN: 978-1-60692-297-2

Chapter 18

CHANGES IN RESEARCH FOCUS WITH TIME. THE OSLO-STUDY OF 1972/73 AND UNTIL TODAY

Lise Lund Håheim[1]
Norwegian Knowledge Centre for the Health Services, Oslo, Norway

Abstract

Heart disease has been the focus for researchers for many years. The focus has changed and new factors are being investigated. This is illustrated following the Oslo-Study of 1972/73 until today. New knowledge was needed to curb the increasing incidence and mortality from heart disease in Norway. The Oslo-study was conducted on men only who were at higher risk than women at the time. Traditional risk factors as total serum cholesterol, triglycerides, serum glucose, blood pressure, BMI and smoking were at center of the investigation both for intervention and for long term follow-up analyses. Later focus has been on the vascular inflammation that is a central effect mechanism linked to arteriosclerosis looking into markers of endothelial function, C-reactive protein, antigens of oral bacteria, and environmental factors. With the general increase in BMI and hence Type 2 diabetes related factors on BMI increase as metabolic syndrome, physical activity at leisure, repeated weight reduction are receiving important attention. Continued research into the disease mechanism in heart disease has brought forward a lot of knowledge for primary and secondary heart disease prevention.

Introduction

Historic Changes in Cardiovascular Disease in Norway

The CVD occurrence in the Norwegian population has varied in different periods of time. In Norway there have been distinct changes in rates of coronary heart disease (CHD) during the last 80 years. Men have been at greater risk than women as in many other countries. These observations have given rise to a persistent focus and a concentrated effort to unravel the disease etiology and prevalence in the Norwegian population.

[1] E-mail address: lise.lund.haheim@nokc.no. Tel no.: +47 90 11 33 98 Fax: +47 23 25 50 10. Contact information: Norwegian Knowledge Centre for the Health Services, POBox 7004 St.Olavs plass, N-0130 Oslo Norway

Part of the explanation and understanding can be sought in the past history. Norway experienced a period of deprivation during the second World War 1940-45. The shortage of many food items and other commodities led to rationing in the war period [1]. During the war was observed a subsequent reduction in CHD mortality rates. The knowledge from this forced situation is useful in studying etiologic and developmental aspects of heart disease.

The nutrition was poor and insufficient for many people as the war progressed [1]. Sugar and meat became scarce commodities as well as cigarettes and liquor. Production decreased for milk with 35%, grain 15%, meat and bacon 50%, fish catch 30%, potatoes and fruit decreased somewhat. Production of vegetables increased considerably. Physical activity was possibly higher than during later times. The changes in nutrition in terms of sugar shortage were also observed in reduced dental caries rates among school children [2]. The lower rate of CHD mortality during the war years was not likely to have been due to improved treatment. Mortality rates of CHD are in general terms influenced by factors affecting disease incidence and subsequent treatment or lifestyle factors. Nutrition status, low rate of smoking, and higher level of physical activity are factors that lends themselves to explain the lower rate of mortality in this period. Nor was the stress and strain experienced in this period a seriously contributing factor.

Norwegian mortality data registered by Statistics Norway goes back to 1856 [3]. The general mortality increased during the war, but the mortality of CHD and diabetes were reduced and there was a reduction in hypertension [1]. During the subsequent slowly rising post war affluence the rates of CHD increased and continued rising into the 50'ies and 60'ies and were reaching serious concern. Myocardial infarction (MI) increased at a higher rate than stroke. The increase was more pronounced among men over 40 years than for women [3].

On this background, studies to further the knowledge and understanding of this increase in CHD led to the start of a series of research projects [4, 5]. As men suffered more often than women from CHD the research focused on men initially. With the positive results of the intervention study on cholesterol lowering diet Leren initiated the Oslo-study in 1972/73 [6]. This was the first population based study in Norway and only men were invited to participate. It was soon to be followed by the Tromsø study in 1974 and later the County studies both on men and women [7, 8]. The latter studies were extended to all counties and involved a health screening of 40-42 year old men and women. Later, new studies developed in different parts of Norway. This research effort reflected the great concern for the increasing disease burden in CVD which was developing in Norway these years.

In the period 1962 to 1974 50 % of all deaths were due to CVD. The prevalence of CVD has sunk since the seventies. In 2004 this proportion was reduced to 38% [3]. National and international research had given knowledge as basis for the increased efforts in prevention of risk through drugs, lifestyle changes, smoking cessation and information campaigns on dietary measures and a call for increased physical activity. As research has progressed knowledge on risk factors have been consolidated. However, these factors did not explain all the variation in the pattern of CHD worldwide. This has spurred new analyses and new studies seeking to understand more fully the development from the intermediate stages to the presenting heart disease on members of the Oslo cohort.

This presentation will follow the development of the Oslo-Study focusing on the intervention studies, the epidemiologic risk factor analysis, long term follow-up on incidence and mortality of MI, and comparison with stroke. In the Oslo-study men only were invited as they experienced by far the largest incidence and mortality of CHD at the time. The study concentrated on young and middle aged men as this was believed to be the age-groups with the largest potential for prevention of CHD. Further, the two intervention studies will be reported together with the follow-up study of the diet and smoking cessation study 20 years later. The cohort was invited for a second screening in 2000 to the Oslo II study.

The Oslo Study 1972/73

In 1972/73 this health survey for CVD was carried out in Oslo, Norway, with the aim of studying risk factors, risk factor intervention, and epidemiology of cardiovascular disease [6]. With the years it has been well described in many publications and PhD dissertations some of which are presented here [9-13]. In short, all men living in the city of Oslo aged 40-49 were invited and a 7% sample of men aged 20-39. They answered a questionnaire, had a blood sample taken and height and weight measured. The blood sample taken in the non fasting state was analyzed for total serum cholesterol, triglycerides and glucose. The questionnaire included questions on the CVD history and diabetes, symptoms of CVD, smoking habits, mental stress and strain, physical activity at leisure and at work. Two intervention studies of five years duration were carried out and the men of lowest cardiovascular risk were examined [10, 12, 13]. The research has focused on traditional risk factors and confirming their importance also in this cohort. The two intervention studies were a cholesterol reducing diet and smoking cessation intervention and a drug trial on hypertension reduction. Further, long term follow-up with regard to incidence and mortality of cardiovascular diseases and total mortality have been carried out at 4 2/3, 7 1/2, 12, 18, 21, and 27 years [12, 14-25]. In 2000 the men living in Oslo were invited to a new health examination and survey [26, 43].

Traditional Risk Factors

Previous knowledge on possible risk factors determined which factors to be examined in 1972/73 screening as more information on these factors were called for. From the blood samples were recorded the level s of total serum cholesterol, triglycerides, and glucose, all in a non-fasting state. The questionnaire they filled in gave information on smoking pattern, physical activity at leisure and at work, mental stress and strain (four questions), medical history on CVD and diabetes and symptoms of CVD according to Rose questionnaire.

From this screening were selected persons with increased risk of heart disease to two intervention studies. The surviving men of the diet and smoking cessation study were invited to take part in a new diet intervention study named DOIT in 1977 [42]. Follow-up on incidence and mortality of CVD events were done several times since the screening. No repeat survey was carried out until year 2000 in the study named Oslo II, and it will be reported below [26].

Men of this cohort also took part in other intervention studies together with other persons recruited to these studies: HYRIM [27], and LIFE [28]. The 1972/73 cohort data with follow-up data on CVD events is also included in a major meta-analysis of one million adults in the Prospective Studies Collaboration [29-31]. Results will not be reported here.

1. Intervention Studies

In order to study the effect of reducing risk factors for CHD and stroke and thus reducing the event rate of CVD and stroke two randomized controlled trials of five years duration were carried out starting in 1974:

1) Lifestyle intervention by cholesterol lowering diet and smoking cessation [32]

The intervention was cholesterol reducing diet and smoking cessation versus no intervention in the trial of 1,232 men (born 1923-1932) of high risk of CVD [9]. The inclusion criteria were serum cholesterol concentrations of 6.9–9.0 mmol/L and systolic blood pressure <150 mm Hg. The five-year results showed that mean serum cholesterol concentrations were approximately 13% lower in the intervention group than in the control group and the mean fasting serum triglycerides fell by 20% in the intervention group compared with controls. 80% of the men in both groups smoked tobacco daily at the start of the study. The mean tobacco consumption fell by 45% more in the intervention group than in the control group. Smoking cessation was reported by 25% of the smokers in the intervention group compared to 17% in the control group. After 5 years the incidence of myocardial infarction (fatal and non-fatal) and sudden death was 47% lower in the intervention group than in the controls ($p = 0.028$, two-tailed log rank test). Adding stroke events did not alter the group difference. The trial was successful in showing the preventive effect of cholesterol lowering diet combined with smoking cessation on MI. Analyses 16 years after trial closure showed a sustained long term effect among the participants [41].

2) Drug treatment in mild hypertension [33].

The drug trial enrolled 406 actively treated men and 379 controls. Drug treatment started with hydrochlorothiazide. If systolic blood pressure remained above 140 mm Hg and/or diastolic blood pressure above 90 mm Hg, alphamethyldopa was added. If there were side effects, methyldopa was replaced with propranolol. The control group was not given a placebo. After five years the results showed that cerebrovascular events occurred only in the control group, 7 versus 0. There was no effect on major cardiovascular morbidity comparing groups as established by randomization, with 18 events in the treatment group and 20 events in the control group. There was no difference between the groups in total mortality and mortality from cardiovascular events.

The screening data and these two studies resulted in a number of papers focusing on associations observed by single factors or associations between factors explaining effects and prediction of events. Some of these results were:

Serum triglycerides and serum uric acid in thiazide treated and untreated patients in mild hypertension were compared [34]. Overall there was no change in triglycerides or cholesterol after three years of study. It was observed that some patients receiving treatment experienced increased values of triglycerides and uric acid. The treatment increased the pretreatment positive correlation between uric acid and triglycerides.

The antihypertensive treatment and effect on serum glucose level was analyzed. It was observed that moderate thiazide doses did not have significant effects on serum glucose levels. Propranolol in combination with thiazide seemed to increase the level of serum glucose [35].

A positive correlation was found between blood pressure and serum cholesterol among "healthy" men aged 20-49 of the screened population [36]. Body mass index and serum triglycerides significantly influence the relationship but not other factors measured.

The intercorrelation of serum cholesterol, cigarette smoking and body weight [37] was found to be stronger than in other studies on analyses of the screening data of the "healthy" men aged 20-49 years.

Mental stress as measured by four questions on trait and stage of mental stress to indicate a Type A personality was not found to predict heart disease in early or late follow-up analyses [22, 38]. One of these questions on stress was found to be a consistent trait into later life as observed in the Oslo II study [39].

Socioeconomic status measured by a combination of income and education was confirmed as an independent related predictor of CHD mortality after adjusting for serum cholesterol, systolic blood pressure, and cigarette smoking [40]. The lowest CHD mortality was found in social status Group III (middle class).

2. Longterm Follow-Up on Incidence and Mortality

The trend in incidence of MI and stroke was sparse when the Oslo-study started. At that time no local or national CVD registry had been established. Long term follow-up on incidence was therefore important to study. For the period 1972-93 hospital journals were searched to obtain the date of the first occurrence of MI and stroke. Mortality data were made available by Statistics Norway. These data allowed the study of incidence per se and associated risk factor analyses. Trend analyses were done at several points in time after 4 3/4, 7 1/2, 12, 18, 21, 27 years. The figures 1 and 2 show the development with regard to fatal and non-fatal MI and stroke after 21 years of follow-up. The decrease in incidence was more pronounced and started earlier for MI than stroke. The results indicated that both primary and secondary prevention had been successful in this period. The mortality rate was lower for the persons taking part in the Oslo- study than in the general Norwegian population [21]. The different stroke diagnoses of cerebral infarction, cerebral hemorrhage, subarachnoid hemorrhage, and unspecified stroke showed different trends related to their etiology [23].

Risk factor analyses of MI at 12 years follow-up confirmed previous analyses and other studies in that increasing age, total serum cholesterol, systolic and diastolic blood pressure, triglycerides, BMI, height (inversely), daily smoking, and physical exercise at leisure (inversely) predicted MI incidence and mortality [15]. The same factors predicted total mortality except BMI did not, but serum glucose did. Risk factors of stroke at 12 years follow-up ere as increased diastolic blood pressure, age, daily cigarette smoking and physical activity at leisure (inversely). Analyses at 21 years follow-up were done per specific stroke diagnosis and showed how they varied according to these diagnoses indicating the differences in etiology [16]. Cerebral infarction had similar risk factor pattern to MI. Increased blood pressure was the overall important predictor of any kind of stroke diagnoses. The long term follow-up also showed that the different risk factors imposed their effect differently. Whereas age, smoking, systolic blood pressure, and increased blood pressure gave a rather immediate increased risk of MI, BMI had a latency period of about 10 years (Table 1) [22]. Dose response with increasing amount of smoking in terms of number of cigarettes, pipe and cigars were shown for stroke [19]. We failed to find mental stress and strain (based on four questions) to predict CVD events [22]. Glucose alone did not predict MI but in interaction with BMI [17]. Men taking anti hypertensive drugs at study start had increased risk of stroke [18]. The men with the lowest levels of risk factors were examined in 1974. The analyses after 16 years showed that even small changes in ECG predicted later Mi events [13].

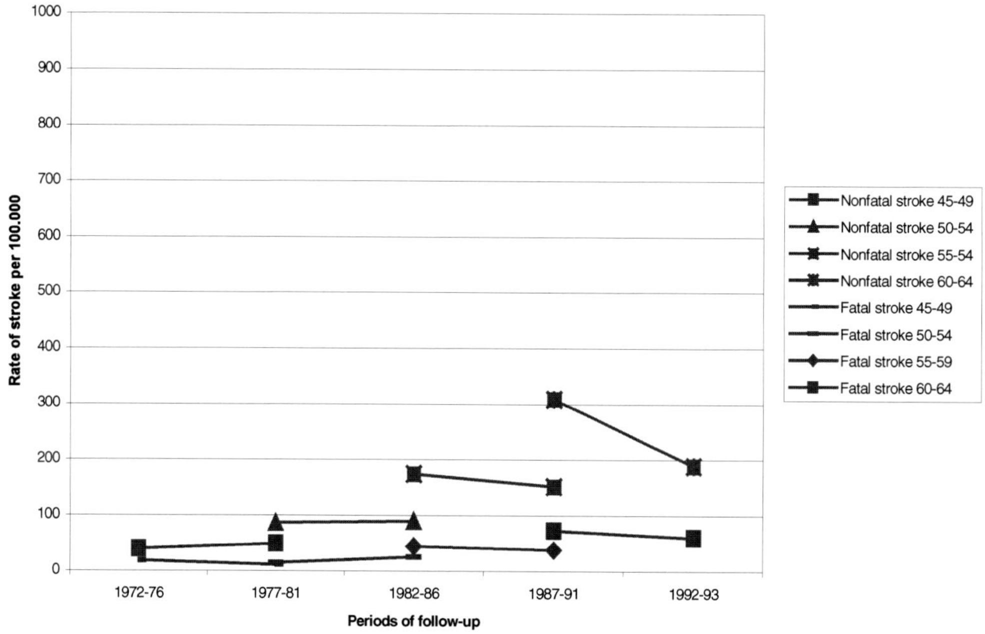

Figure 1.

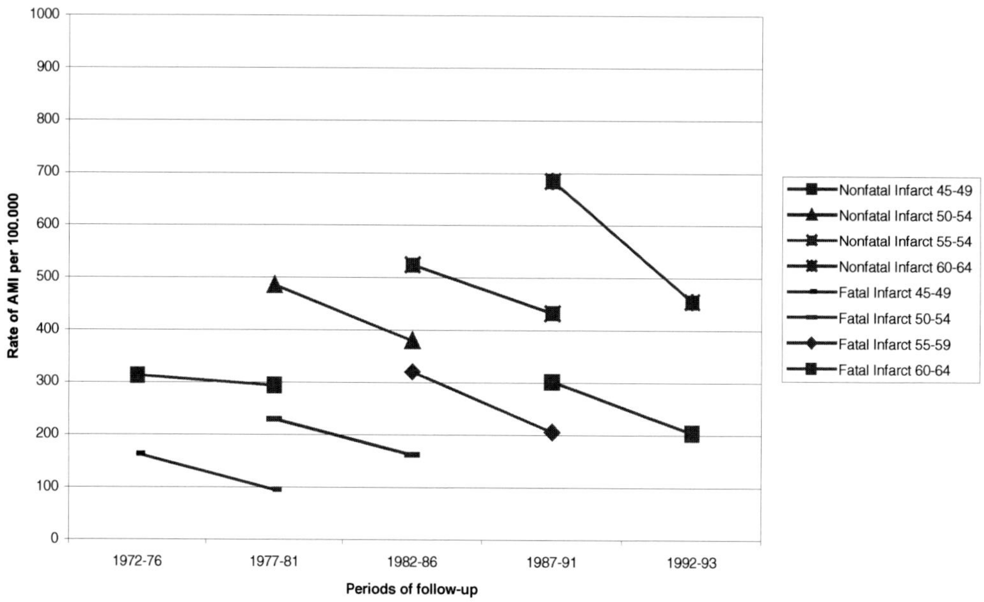

Figure 2.

Table 1. Relative risks (RR) with 95% CI and trends for risk factor's predictivity for fatal CHD (Cox proportional hazards regression analyses. Men who had died previous to the current 5-y period were excluded. Person-y were calculated from the start of each 5-y period of follow-up

Risk factor	1-5 y RR (95% CI) N=71	6-10 y RR (95% CI) N=106	11-15 y RR (95% CI) N=145	16-21 y RR (95% CI) N=163	Trend (P value)
Age (y)	1.15 (1.06-1.26)	1.13 (1.05-1.21)	1.07 (1.01-1.14)	1.11 (1.05-1.17)	0.30
Total cholesterol (mmol/l)	1.22 (1.06-1.40)	1.30 (1.18-1.44)	1.39 (1.27-1.52)	1.24 (1.08-1.42)	0.74
Systolic BP (mmHg)	1.02 (1.01-1.04)	1.02 (1.01-1.03)	1.02 (1.01-1.03)	1.02 (1.01-1.03)	0.59
Smoker (yes=1, no=0)	3.84 (2.00-7.34)	3.09 (1.89-5.06)	2.32 (1.58-3.42)	1.96 (1.40-2.74)	0.01
BMI (kg/m2)	0.96 (0.89-1.04)	0.99 (0.93-1.06)	1.03 (0.98-1.08)	1.06 (1.01-1.10)	0.002
Triglycerides (mmol/l)	1.02 (0.95-1.09)	0.98 (0.91-1.06)	1.00 (0.94-1.06)	1.02 (0.96-1.08)	0.87
Glucose (mmol/l)	1.05 (0.86-1.28)	0.92 (0.74-1.14)	1.06 (0.92-1.22)	1.03 (0.89-1.18)	0.89
Physical activity Sedentary	1.0	1.0	1.0	1.0	
Moderate	0.60 (0.36-1.01)	0.60 (0.39-0.93)	0.88 (0.59-1.31)	1.08 (0.73-1.60)	0.05
Intermediate/vigorous	0.42 (0.18-0.94)	0.57 (0.31-1.06)	0.75 (0.43-1.32)	1.21 (0.73-1.99)	0.04
Mental stress					
Chooses high activity rather than a peaceful life	1.62 (0.97-2.68)	1.26 (0.83-1.92)	0.89 (0.62-1.28)	0.82 (0.59-1.14)	0.03
Increased psychic tension or irritation during the last y	0.62 (0.33-1.14)	1.21 (0.78-1.86)	1.05 (0.71-1.54)	1.32 (0.93-1.87)	0.19
Increased pressure due to deadlines at work	0.60 (0.36-1.00)	0.93 (0.61-1.42)	1.08 (0.75-1.56)	0.95 (0.68-1.33)	0.25

Novel Risk Factors

Much research has been and is being done in the field of CVD. Several aspects in CVD remain unresolved and needed to be examined further in a Norwegian cohort. The Oslo cohort had not been reexamined at regular intervals, but it was of great interest to make follow-up studies of these men. A follow-up intervention study, DOIT, was done using the well known diet and smoking study participants. Several aspects were addressed as diet intervention, measure change in risk factors from the first trial, and address an investigation into markers of epithelial activation. The other study, Oslo II, was a new survey of the formerly invited men to the Oslo-study in 1972/73. The aim was to observe the changes in risk factors over 28 years, register a new set of risk factors to address a wider range of health issues, and to be the basis for sub-studies to test new research hypotheses.

1. The Doit Study

The men taking part in the intervention study of diet and smoking were invited to a new 3 year intervention study in 1997 [42]. The 910 survivors were contacted to participate in the Diet and Omega-3 Intervention Trial (DOIT). The aim was to study markers of epithelial activation in a randomized controlled study of 2x2 factorial design. The serum factors studied were sE-selectin, intercellular adhesion molecule 1 (ICAM-1), vascular cell adhesion molecule 1 (VCAM-1), thrombomodulin (TM), von Willebrand factor (vWF), and tissue-type plasminogen activator antigen (tPAag), and in addition were levels of total cholesterol, HDL cholesterol, triglycerols, glucose, and fatty acids measured. The interventions were *1*) control (no dietary counseling and placebo capsules), *2*) dietary counseling (and placebo capsules), *3*) n–3 PUFA capsules (and no dietary counseling), and *4*) dietary counseling and n–3 PUFA capsules combined. The study results indicated the mode of action in this dietary intervention. Each intervention (dietary counseling or n–3 PUFA supplements) reduced sTM and sICAM-1 concentrations and indicated decreased endothelial activation. tPAag was reduced by dietary counseling and not with n–3 PUFA supplements.

2. Oslo II Study

The Oslo II study has brought forward analyses on novel risk factors with respect to heart disease as oral infections, insulin resistance/ metabolic syndrome, mental stress, and weight loss periods [26, 43]. All invited men in 1972/73 habiting in Oslo (n=12,764) were invited for a second health screening named Oslo II in 2000. In all 5,323 men attended both health screenings. A total of 1,207 attended the first only or attended the Oslo II only. Not invited were men taking part in other intervention studies, but had taken part in the first screening (n=1,834). Baseline data for these men were later added to the data file of Oslo II (n=7,157). The second round of the Oslo-study included a health examination where a non-fasting blood sample was taken to estimate total serum cholesterol, triglycerides and glucose as in the first survey and HDL as a novel factor. Anthropometric measures as height, and weight were taken as well as waist and hip measurements as new variables. The participants filled in two questionnaires according to their age. The main questionnaire was more extensive than that in

1972/73 including new areas of research such as more health information, diet, alcohol consumption, mental health, social factors, and drug use. The second form included variables to complement the information with that received in the first survey. In addition were information on dental status and history, history of physical activity at leisure, weight loss, and grade of well being.

The main research focus was on the change in risk factors among the men over this 28 year period [43]. The dominant result was the significant increase in BMI of all age groups and, in particular, it was largest in the young men (figure 3). This coincided with a reduced level of physical activity at leisure, increasing levels of systolic blood pressure, total serum cholesterol and triglycerides. Diastolic blood pressure did not change most likely due to treatment of antihypertensiva. Height was reduced on average 2 cm. Medication by anti hypertensive and cholesterol reducing drugs were increased compared to the first screening. The most encouraging observation was the reduction to 17% daily smokers. A number of factors were found that could explain this increase namely increasing triglycerides, systolic blood pressure, age, non fasting glucose, physical activity (inversely) and smoking (inversely). Having stopped smoking was related to an increased BMI. Daily smoking in both 1972/73 and 2000 and daily smoking in 2000 but not in 1972/73 were inversely related [26].

Stored serum samples were analyzed for C-reactive protein (CRP) and antibodies for four common commencals of periodontal disease, *Porphyromonas gingivalis, Tannerella forsythia, Treponema denticola,* and *Aggregatibacter actinomycetemcomitans,* with the aim of mapping their association with myocardial infarction [45].

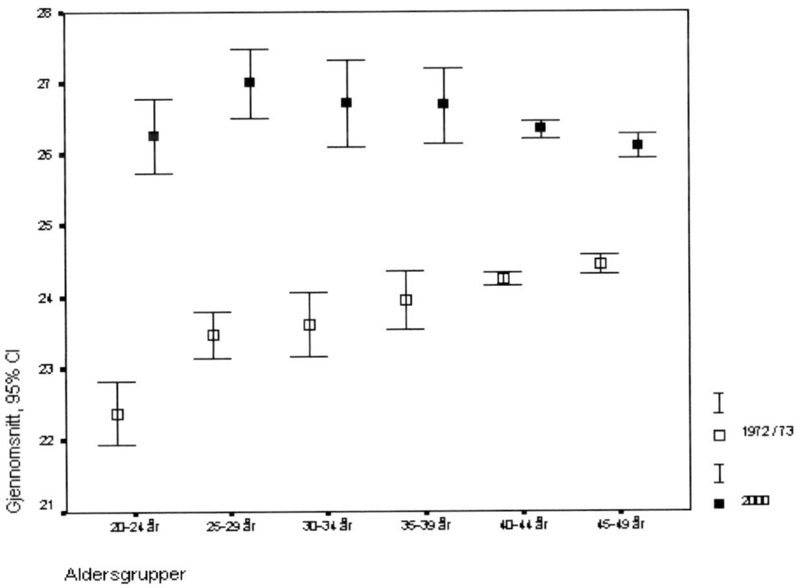

Figure 3. 28-years change in mean BMI from 1972/73 to 2000. The Oslo II study 2000.

Table 2. Logistic regression analyses for relative risk of myocardial infarction by combinations of antibodies of bacteria which cause marginal periodontitits.

Analytic models: upper quartile level of antibodies (OD reading) versus lower* or CRP	Univariate (crude) analysis			Adjusted analysis I †			Adjusted analysis II ‡		
	Odds Ratio	95%CI	P-value	Odds Ratio	95% CI	P-value	Odds Ratio	95% CI	P-value
Model 1									
One of any four bacteria PG, TF, TD, AA	1.30	1.02-1.65	0.032	1.29	1.02-1.65	0.037	1.31	1.01-1.69	0.039
Model 2									
One of any three bacteria PG, TD, AA not TF	1.29	1.02-1.62	0.036	1.29	1.02-1.64	0.033	1.29	1.01-1.66	0.042
Model 3									
One of any three bacteria TF, TD, AA not PG	1.19	0.94-1.50	0.148	1.18	0.93-1.49	0.164	1.19	0.93-1.52	0.175
Model 4									
One of any three bacteria PG, TF, AA not TD	1.28	1.01-1.62	0.040	1.26	0.997-1.60	0.053	1.23	0.96-1.58	0.101
Model 5									
One of any three bacteria PG, TF, TD not AA	1.13	0.90-1.43	0.304	1.13	0.89-1.42	0.322	1.12	0.88-1.43	0.361

Table 2. Continued

Analytic models: upper quartile level of antibodies (OD reading) versus lower* or CRP	Univariate (crude) analysis			Adjusted analysis I †			Adjusted analysis II ‡		
	Odds Ratio	95%CI	P-value	Odds Ratio	95% CI	P-value	Odds Ratio	95% CI	P-value
Model 6									
CRP – Trend			0.018	-	-	-			0.68
Quartile 1	1.00						1.00		
Quartile 2 vs 1	1.31	0.92-1.85	0.131				1.12	0.78-1.63	0.54
Quartile 3 vs 1	1.38	0.99-1.94	0.059				1.08	0.75-1.55	0.70
Quartile 4 vs 1	1.73	1.24-2.42	0.001				1.24	0.86-1.79	0.24
One of any four bacteria PG, TF, TD, AA	1.33	1.04-1.68	0.021				1.30	1.01-1.68	0.041

Bold type indicates that 95% CI does not include 1.0.

* Analytic model of number of bacteria (and CRP in last model) with upper quartile antibody level versus lower value. The 75 percentile of OD values of antibodies were: PG=212, TF=103, TD= 73, AA=111, and CRP=3.9 mg/l.

† Analyses adjusted for C-reactive protein (CRP) in 2000 (quartile values).

‡ Analyses adjusted for known risk factors for acute myocardial infarction; CRP in 2000 and daily smoking, total serum cholesterol, systolic blood pressure, Body Mass Index, triglycerides and non-fasting glucose adjusted for time since last meal measured in 1972/73. In the last model, the combined variable of CRP and any one of four bacteria was used.

PG = *Porphyromonas gingivalis.*

TF = *Tannerella forsythia.*

TD = *Treponema denticola.*

AA = *Aggregatibacter actinomycetemcomitans.*

All men reporting a history of MI (n=548) were compared with controls (n=625) in a case-control study design. The results showed a 30% significant increased risk of MI with antibody levels in the upper quartile range for at least one of four bacteria. This indicates that that the combined effect of several bacteria rather than a single one is causal to the occurrence of MI (Table 2). Time since infarct was not of influence. CRP was found to be associated with increased risk of MI in univariate analysis, but not when antibody levels were included in the multivariate model. Analyses on extraction history have been undertaken showing increased risk by extractions due to oral infections versus other causes [46].

Cardiovascular disease has been associated with several environmental exposures. A study has been carried out to understand the patophysiological mechanism whereby temperature, ambient air pollution and tobacco smoke exposure affect lung tissue and hence may influence the immune system and thereby initiate a systemic inflammatory response [47, 48]. With Oslo II data has been shown that short-term variations in both ambient air pollution and temperature were significantly associated with increases in serum concentrations of lung Clara cell protein 16 kD, a biomarker that has recently been used to assess altered lung epithelial permeability. Earlier analyses testing the association of the mean of first 5-year level of air pollution after screening at the home address of the participants of the Oslo I study did not find a significant association with CVD, but lung cancer after 27 years follow-up [27].

The Oslo II data has also been analyzed by making composite risk factors. This method was done to find out whether factors defining a healthy lifestyle predicted just that [44]. Metabolic syndrome is a generally well known composite risk factor and has been used to study metabolic syndrome versus diabetes (ref). A factor as repeated slimming periods and its effect on BMI has also been studied [50].

Conclusion

The main focus in the Oslo-study research has been on risk of heart disease, myocardial infarction. Both intervention studies and long term follow-up has been done. Results of risk factor analyses on predictors of incidence and mortality of heart disease and stroke have been published as well as risk factor associations and intermediary end points. This research shows that heart disease is a complex disease of a multifactor origin and development. To this date the full list of causal items for CVD events is still not clear. Novel risk factors as oral infections, CRP, and air pollution as well as in depth analyses of traditional factors as physical activity and composite factors as metabolic syndrome help our understanding of heart disease and make us better equipped to advice on heart disease prevention and its squeals.

References

[1] Toverud G. The influence of war and postwar conditions on the teeth of Norwegian school children. III Discussion of food supply and dental condition in Norway and other European countries. *Milbank Mem Fund Q* 1957;35:373-459

[2] Toverud G. Dental caries in Norwegian children during and after the last World War. A Preliminary Report. *Proc R Soc Med* 1949;42:249-58.

[3] Statistics Norway. Chapter: Pedersen AG. Mortality trend in change: From infections to life style. In: Causes of Mortality 1850–2004. Historic Health Statistics. In Norwegian. Oslo; Statistics Norway; 2007.http://www.ssb.no/emner/03/00/sa94/del-ii-1b.pdf
[4] Leren P. The effect of plasma cholesterol lowering diet in male survivors of myocardial infarction. Thesis. Oslo, Norway. Universitetsforlaget 1966.
[5] Natvig H, Borchrevink CF, Dedichen J, Owren PA, Schiøtz EH, Westlund K. A controlled trial of the effect of linoleic acid on incidence of coronary heart disease. The Norwegian vegetable oil experiment 1965-66. *Scand J Clin Lab Invest* 1968;22:Suppl 105.
[6] Leren P, Askevold EM, Foss OP, Froili A, Grymyr D, Helgeland A, Hjermann I, Holme I, Lund-Larsen PG, Norum KR. The Oslo study. Cardiovascular disease in middle-aged and young Oslo men. *Acta Med Scand Suppl.* 1975;588:1-38. No abstract available.
[7] Thelle DS, Førde OH, Try K, Lehmann E. The Tromsø Heart Study. Methods and Main Results of the Cross-sectional Study. *Acta Med Scand* 1976;200:107-118.
[8] Bjartveit K. The cardiovascular disease study in Norwegian counties. Background, organization, results from first screening. *Acta Med Scand* 1983;Suppl 675:1-184.
[9] Håheim L Lund. Epidemiology of stroke in middle-aged men. *The Oslo Study*. Thesis. Oslo, University of Oslo, 1998.
[10] Hjermann I. *Coronary Heart Disease Prevention*. Thesis. Oslo, Norway: University of Oslo 1980.
[11] Helgeland A. Medikamentell behandling av mild hypertensjon av middelaldrende men. Thesis. Oslo, Norway: University of Oslo 1981.
[12] Holme I. Coronary risk factors and their possible causal role in the development of coronary heart disease. Thesis. *The Oslo Study*. Oslo, Norway: Ullevål Hospital 1982.
[13] Lund-Larsen PG. ECG in health and disease. Thesis. University of Tromsø, 1994.
[14] Holme I, Helgeland A, Hjermann I, Leren P, Lund-Larsen PG. Four and two-thirds years incidence of coronary heart disease in middle-aged men: the Oslo study. *Am J Epidemiol.* 1980 Jul;112(1):149-60.
[15] Håheim LL, Holme I, Hjermann I, Leren P. The predictability of risk factors with respect to incidence and mortality of myocardial infarction and total mortality. A 12-year follow-up of the Oslo Study, Norway. *J Intern Med.* 1993 Jul;234(1):17-24.
[16] Håheim LL, Holme I, Hjermann I, Leren P. Risk factors of stroke incidence and mortality. A 12-year follow-up of the Oslo Study. *Stroke*. 1993 Oct;24(10):1484-9.
[17] Håheim LL, Holme I, Hjermann I, Leren P. Nonfasting serum glucose and the risk of fatal stroke in diabetic and nondiabetic subjects. 18-year follow-up of the Oslo Study. Stroke. 1995 May;26(5):774-7. Erratum in: *Stroke* 1997 May;28(5):1092.
[18] Håheim LL, Holme I, Hjermann I, Leren P. Risk of fatal stroke according to blood pressure level: an 18-year follow-up of the Oslo Study. *J Hypertens.* 1995 Aug;13(8):909-13.
[19] Håheim LL, Holme I, Hjermann I, Leren P. Smoking habits and risk of fatal stroke: 18 years follow up of the Oslo Study. *J Epidemiol Community* Health. 1996 Dec;50(6):621-4.
[20] Holme I, Håheim LL, Hjermann I. [Predictors for 21-year incidence of myocardial infarction in the Oslo study 1972/73]. *Tidsskr Nor Laegeforen.* 2003 Apr 10;123(8):1050-3. Norwegian. No abstract available.

[21] Håheim LL, Holme I, Hjermann I, Leren P, Tonstad S. Trends in the incidence of acute myocardial infarction and stroke: a 21-year follow-up of the Oslo study. *Scand Cardiovasc J.* 2004 Aug;38(4):216-21.

[22] L Lund Håheim, S Tonstad, I Hjermann, P Leren, I Holme. Predictivity of body mass index and other risk factors for fatal coronary heart disease: a 21-year prospective cohort study. *Scand J Public Health.* 2007;35:4-10.

[23] Lund Håheim L, Holme I, Hjermann I, Leren P, Tonstad S. Comparative analyses of risk factor profile for the incidence of subarachnoid and intracerebral haemorrhage, cerebral infarction and unspecified stroke during 21-years' follow-up in men. *Scand J Public Health.* 2006;34:589-97.

[24] Nafstad P, Lund Håheim L, Ofstad B, Gram F, Holme I, Hjermann I, Leren P. Urban air pollution and mortality in a cohort of Norwegian men. *Environmental Health Perspectives* 2004;112:610-5.

[25] Nafstad P, Lund Håheim L, Ofstad B, Gram F, Holme I, Hjermann I, Leren P. Lung cancer and air pollution. A 27 year follow up of 16 209 Norwegian men. Thorax 2003;58:1071-1076.

[26] Lund Haheim L, Lund Larsen PG, Sogaard AJ, Holme I. Risk factors associated with body mass index increase in men at 28 years follow-up. *QJM. 2006* Oct;99(10):665-71. Epub 2006 Sep 17.

[27] Anderssen SA, Hjelstuen AK, Hjermann I, Bjerkan K, Holme I. Fluvastatin and lifestyle modification for reduction of carotid intima-media thickness and left ventricular mass progression in drug-treated hypertensives. *Atherosclerosis.* 2005 Feb;178(2):387-97.

[28] Dahløf B, Devereux RB, Kjeldsen SE, Julius S, Beevers G, de Faire U, Fyhrquist F, Ibsen H, Kristiansson K, Lederballe-Pedersen O, Lindholm LH, Nieminen MS, Omvik P, Oparil S. Cardiovascular morbidity and mortality in the Losartan Intervention For Endpoint reduction in hypertension study(LIFE): a randomized trial against atenolol. *Lancet* 2002; 359: 995-1003.

[29] Prospective Studies Collaboration. Cholesterol, diastolic blood pressure, and stroke: 13,000 strokes in 450,000 people in 45 prospective cohorts. *Lancet* 1995;346:1647-1653.

[30] Prospective Studies Collaboration. Collaborative overview ('meta-analysis') of prospective observational studies of the associations of usual blood pressure and usual cholesterol levels with common causes of death: protocol for the second cycle of the Prospective Studies Collaboration. *J Cardiovasc Risk* 1999;6:315-320.

[31] Prospective Studies Collaboration. Age-specific relevance of usual blood pressure to vascular mortality: one million adults in 61 prospective cohorts. *Lancet* 2002;360:1903-1913.

[32] Hjermann I, Velve KB, Holme I, Leren P. Effect of diet and smoking intervention on the incidence of coronary heart disease. A randomized trial in healthy men. The Oslo Study. *Lancet* 1981;ii:1303-1310.

[33] Helgeland A. Treatment of mild hypertension: A five year controlled drug trial. The Oslo Study. *Am J Med* 1980;69:725-732.

[34] Helgeland A, Hjermann I, Holme I, Leren P. Serum triglycerides and serum uric acid in untreated and thiazide-treated patients with mild hypertension. The Oslo study. *Am J Med.* 1978 Jan;64(1):34-8.

[35] Helgeland A, Leren P, Foss OP, Hjermann I, Holme I, Lund-Larsen PG. Serum glucose levels during long-term observation of treated and untreated men with mild hypertension. The Oslo study. *Am J Med.* 1984 May;76(5):802-5.

[36] Hjermann I, Helgeland A, Holme I, Lund-Larsen PG, Leren P. The association between blood pressure and serum cholesterol in healthy men: the Oslo study. *J Epidemiol Community Health.* 1978 Jun;32(2):117-23.

[37] Hjermann I, Helgeland A, Holme I, Lung-Larsen G, Leren P. The intercorrelation of serum cholesterol, cigarette smoking and body weight. The Oslo Study. *Acta Med Scand.* 1976;200(6):479-85.

[38] Holme I, Froili A, Leren P. Mental "stress" and coronary risk factors. The Oslo study. *J Oslo City Hosp.* 1977 Jan;27(1):3-7. No abstract available.

[39] Søgaard AJ, Dalgard OS, Holme I, Røysamb E, Håheim LL. Associations between type A behaviour pattern and psychological distress: 28 years of follow-up of the Oslo Study 1972/1973.Soc Psychiatry *Psychiatr Epidemiol.* 2008 Mar;43(3):216-23. Epub 2007 Dec 14.

[40] Holme I, Helgeland A, Hjermann I, Leren P. Socio-economic status as a coronary risk factor: the Oslo study. *Acta Med Scand Suppl.* 1982;660:147-51.

[41] I Holme, LL Haaheim, S Tonstad, I Hjermann. Effect of dietary and antismoking advice on the incidence of myocardial infarction: A 16-year follow-up of the Oslo Diet and Antismoking Study after its close. *Nutrition, Metabolism and Cardiovascular Diseases* 2006;16:330-338.

[42] Hjerkinn EM, Seljeflot I, Ellingsen I, Berstad P, Hjermann I, Sandvik L, Arnesen H. Influence of long-term intervention with dietary counselling, long-chain n-3 fatty acid supplements, or both on circulating markers of endothelial activation in men with long-standing hyperlipidemia. *Am J Clin nutr.* 2005 Mar;81(3):583-9.

[43] Håheim LL, Holme I, Søgaard AJ, Lund-Larsen PG. [Changes in cardiovascular risk factors among men in Oslo during 28 years]. *Tidsskr Nor Laegeforen.* 2006 Sep 7;126(17):2240-5. Norwegian.

[44] Holme I, Søgaard AJ, Lund Larsen PG, Tonstad S, Lund Håheim L. Lønner det seg å leve sunt? Resultater fra Oslo-undersøkelser blant de samme menn i 1972/3 og i år 2000. [Is a healthy lifestyle worthwhile?]. *Tidsskr Nor Laegeforen.* 2006 Sep 7;126(17):2246-9. Norwegian.

[45] Lise Lund Håheim, Ingar Olsen, Per Nafstad, Per Schwarze, Kjersti S. Rønningen. Antibody Levels to Single Bacteria or in Combination Evaluated against Myocardial Infarction. In Press. *Journal of Clinical Periodontology.*

[46] Ingar Olsen, Per Nafstad, Per Schwarze, Kjersti Skjold Rønningen, Lise Lund Håheim. Tooth Extractions, *Bacterial Antibodies*, C-reactive Protein and Myocardial Infarction. Poster presentation. IADR conference 2007. New Orleans.

[47] Madsen C, Nafstad P, Eikvar L, Schwarze PE, Ronningen KS, Haaheim LL. Association between tobacco smoke exposure and levels of C-reactive protein in the Oslo II Study. *Eur J Epidemiol.* 2007;22(5):311-7. Epub 2007 May 5.

[48] Christian Madsen, Kevin L. Durand, Per Nafstad, Per E. Schwarze, Kjersti S. Rønningen, Lise L. Haheim. Associations between environmental exposures and serum concentrations of Clara cell protein among elderly men in Oslo, Norway. Submitted.

[49] Holme I, Tonstad S, Sogaard AJ, Larsen PG, Haheim LL. Leisure time physical activity in middle age predicts the metabolic syndrome in old age: results of a 28-year follow-up of men in the Oslo study. *BMC Public Health.* 2007 Jul 12;7(147):154.

[50] Holme I, Sogaard AJ, Haheim LL, Larsen PG, Tonstad S. Repeated Weight Loss is Associated with the Metabolic Syndrome and Diabetes: Results of a 28 Year Re-screening of Men in the Oslo Study.*Metab Syndr Relat Disord.* 2007 Jun;5(2):127-35.

In: Heart Disease in Men
Editors: A.B. Todd and M.H. Mosley, pp. 381-390
ISBN: 978-1-60692-297-2

Chapter 19

Diabetic Nephropathy - A Ticking Cardiovascular Bomb

Ole Torffvit*

Internal Medicine, Endocrinology and Nephrology,
Renal laboratory, Biomedical Centrum, Lund, Institution of Clinical Sciences,
Department of Nephrology, University hospital Lund, Sweden

Abstract

Diabetic nephropathy with the early sign called microalbuminuria is associated with silent myocardial ischemia. It has a poor prognosis with more than seven times higher mortality than in diabetic patients without albuminuria. A multifactorial approach is necessary in order to reach full effect of treatment. With such the risk for cardiovascular disease and mortality may decrease by 50%.

The Definition of Microalbuminuria?

The definition is "a urine albumin concentration above normal not detected by the dipstick" or more exact:

U-albumin: 21-200 mg/l or 31-300 mg/day or 20-200 μg/min or

ACI = U-albumin/U-creatinine = Albumin creatinine index 3-20 mg/mmol

Levels above these are referred to as albuminuria = macroalbuminuria = diabetic nephropathy.

---

* E-mail address: Ole.Torffvit@med.lu.se. Ole Torffvit, Associate professor, has done research on diabetic nephropathy and other diabetic complications since 1983 and was the secretary of the European diabetic nephropathy study group (EDNSG) 2000-2003. Postmailadress: Vårdcentralen Höör, Storgatan 2, 243 30 Höör, Sweden

The Characteristics of the Diabetic Heart

Several studies have shown the diabetic heart is characterized by increased sympatic activity with increased heart rate (*Nielsen. Diabetic Med 1999;16:555-562; Valensi P. Diabetes Care 2001;24:339-343)* and asymptomatic myocardial ischemia in as much as 26% of the patients (*Janand-Delenne B. Diabetes Care 1999;22:1396-1400; Bacci S. Eur J Endocrinol 2002;147:649-654; de Lorenzo A. Am J Cardiol 2002;90:827-83).* Left ventricle hypertrophy with systolic myocardial dysfunction may exist independent of the existence of ischemic heart disease *(Bouchard A. Am J Med 1989;87:160-66 ; Strong Heart study. Circulation 2000;101:2271-2276).*

Microalbuminuria in Non-diabetic Patients

Microalbuminuria may be found even in apparently healthy subjects without diabetes and is often associated with hypertension, increased triglycerides and decreased HDL. These patients have increased risk of developing diabetes within three years (*Haffner SM. Arteriosclerosis 1990;10:727-31; Mykkänen L. Diabetes 1994;43:552-557*). Furthermore, the degree of albuminuria is associated with the number of stenotic coronary arteries (*Geluk CA. Netherlands Heart J 2007;15(4):133-41*).

Microalbuminuria in Diabetic Patients

As for the non-diabetic subjects these patients have hypertension, increased triglycerides, apolipoprotein B, LDL and decreased HDL. Fibrinogen and homocystein levels and QT time on ECG may be increased (*Jones SL. BMJ 1989;298:487-90; Niskanen L. Diabetologia 1990;33:237-243; Chici A. Diabetologia 1998;41:684-93; Earle KA. J Diab Compl 2000;14:277-80*). Left ventricular systolic and diastolic dysfunction is frequent in both type 1 (insulin-dependent) and 2 (non-insulin-dependent) diabetic patients (*Guglielmi MD. Diabetes Care 1995; 18:353-60; Strong Heart study. JACC 2003;41:2922-8*).

Micro-Macroalbuminuria in Diabetic Patients

A third of diabetic patients may have silent myocardial ischemia and half of these patients have albuminuria (*Wackers FJT. Diabetes Care 2004;27:1954-61; Valensi P. Diabetes Care 2005; 28:2722-27*). A fourth of type 1 diabetic patients with microalbuminuria have silent myocardial ischemia (*Earle KA. Diabetologia 1996;39:854-56*) while half of type 2 diabetic patients with microalbuminuria have silent ischemia (*Rutter MK. JACC 2002;40:56-61; Wackers FJT. Diabetes Care 2004;27:1954-61*). When the patients have reached the level macroalbuminuria, i.e. diabetic nephropathy, they have left ventricular hypertrophy (*Kimball TR. Circulation 1994;90:357-61; Sato A. Diabetologia 1999;42:76-80*), diffuse myocardial fibrosis, increased thickness of the walls of the arterioles and subendothelial and subintimal deposits of acid mucopolysacharides as well as hypertrophy of the medial layer (*Rubler S. Am J Card 1972;30:595-602; Genda A. Clin Cardiol 1986;9:375-82*).

At the time for renal transplantation a third of the type 1 diabetic patients have more than 50% stenosis of the coronary arteries and one fifth have a stenosis of more than 75% of the vessel lumen (*Manske CL. Lancet 1992;340:998-1002; Weinrauch L. Circulation 1978;58:1184-90*). These patients have often had myocardial infarction before the invasive diagnostic procedure (*Thomas GN. Diabetologia 2004;47:1528-1534*).

In our study of type 2 diabetic patients with micro-macroalbuminuria which were examined with renal biopsy on this indication, all had diabetic nephropathy in combination with nephrosclerosis. All 40 patients participating performed an exercise provocation test for diagnosis of myocardial ischemia or a scintiography (n=17). 19 patients had a pathologic test and eight had stenosis of several arteries or the left main artery and thus were treated with PTCA/CABG (*Torffvit O. Diabetes Metab 2003;29:4S297, 2473*). Thus, half of the patients without symptoms were diagnosed as having major artery stenosis. The eight patients who performed an invasive treatment had, however, one symptom in common, dyspnoea at physical exercise misinterpreted as poor physical condition.

Prognosis for Non-diabetic Patients with Microalbuminuria

Apparently healthy non-diabetic subjects with microalbuminuria have a poor prognosis. They also have an increased development and growth of artery plaques (*Jörgensen L. Eur Heart J 2007; 28:363-369*). One fifths of the patients with both hypertension and microalbuminuria died within six years (*Agewall S. Am J Card 1997;80:164-69*). The mortality after myocardial infarction was 74% in non-diabetic patients with microalbuminuria compared with 12% in those without microalbuminuria (3 years of follow-up)(*Berton G. Diabetologia 2004;47:1511-1518*). In a large population study (n = 22368) the mortality increased with the degree of albuminuria for both non-diabetic and diabetic patients *(EPIC-Norfolk Study, United Kingdom, Yuyun MF. Am J Epidemiology 2004;159:284-93).*

Prognosis for Diabetic Patients with Microalbuminuria

Diabetic patients have a worse prognosis than non-diabetic patients. After PCI (percutaneous cardiac intervention) the mortality is higher in the diabetic patients (*Marso SP. 1999;33:1269-77*). After myocardial infarction the mortality was 68% in those with microalbuminuria compared to the patients without (34%) (three years observations time)(*Berton G. Diabetologia 2004;47:1511-1518*). Both type 1 and type 2 diabetic patients with microalbuminuria had seven times higher risk for dying in heart disease than patients without microalbuminuria (*Schmitz A. Diabet Med 1988;5:126-34; Messent JWC. Kidney Int 1992;41:836-839; Stephenson JM. Diabet Med 1995;12:149-55; Mattock MB. Diabetes 1998;47:1786-192; Valmadrid CT. Arch Intern Med 2000;160:1093-1100; Riu FR. J Diab Compl 2003;17:235-242*).

Prognosis for Patients with Albuminuria with or without Diabetes

Cardiac death in a study of 2253 patients was clearly increased in patients with proteinuria with or without diabetes but the prognosis was poorer in diabetic patients (*Natali A.*

Diabetologia 2000;43:632-641). As many as 69% of diabetic patients with albuminuria may die within 10 years (*Damsgaard EM. Diabetologia 1993;36:1030-36; Tuomilehto J. Diabetologia 1998;41:784-90; Mühlhauser I. Diabet Med 2000;17:727-34*).

The cardiovascular mortality in type 1 diabetic patients with albuminuria may be 18 times increased and in microalbuminuric diabetic patients five times increased compared with those with normal urinary albumin excretion (table 1).

Table 1. 12 years of relative risk for death, cardiovascular death, in diabetic patients with macro- and microalbuminuria (type 1 diabetes).

			MACRO albuminuria vs. normoalbuminuria		**MICRO albuminuria vs. normoalbuminuria**	
	Dead (N)	**Survivors (N)**	**RR adjusted for age, gender**	**RR adjusted for age gender +confounders[1]**	**RR adjusted for age, gender**	**RR adjusted for age, gender + confounders[1]**
Dead	56	406	9.0 (4.5-18.1)***	4.9 (2.3-10.6)***	1.1 (1.04-1.1)***	NS
CVD death[2]	25	437	18.3 (5.2-64.1)***	8.2 (2.1-31.7)**	4.9 (1.2-19.8)*	NS

[1]confounders = mean systolic and diastolic blood pressure, HbA_{1c} levels and treatment for hypertension
[2]CVD death = cardiovascular death (heart, stroke or other vascular death)
RR = relative risk and 95% CI = confidence interval. = p<0.05, ** = p<0.01, *** = p<0.001 vs. Normoalbuminuria. (*Torffvit O. Diabet Med 2005;22:723-729*).

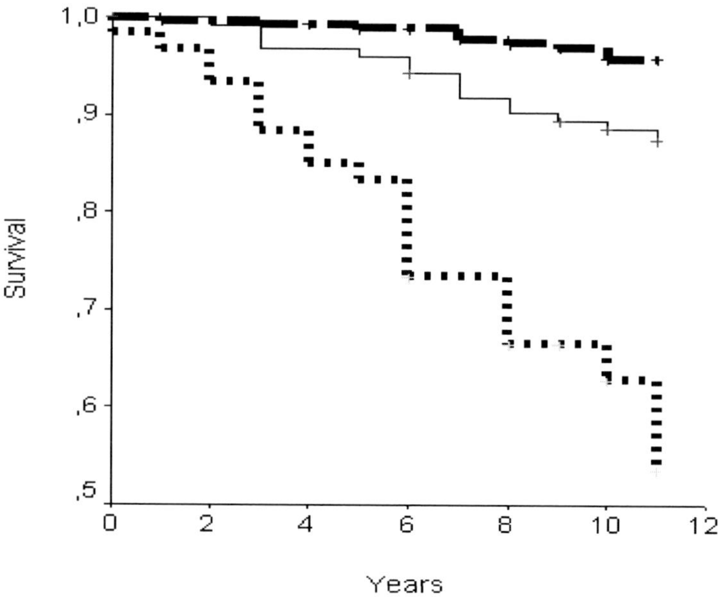

Figure 1. Type 1 diabetes. survival curves for patients with normo-, micro- and macro-albuminuria. (*Torffvit O. Diabet Med 2005;22:723-729*).

As shown in Fig 1 only 50% of type 1 diabetic patients with albuminuria (the stippled line) survived 10 years, while less, 20%, of the type 2 diabetic patients survived (fat line Fig 2). An association was found between the degree of albuminuria and mean systolic blood pressure during 24 hours (Fig 3). Furthermore, an increased blood pressure during the night was associated with decreased glomerular function (Fig 4).

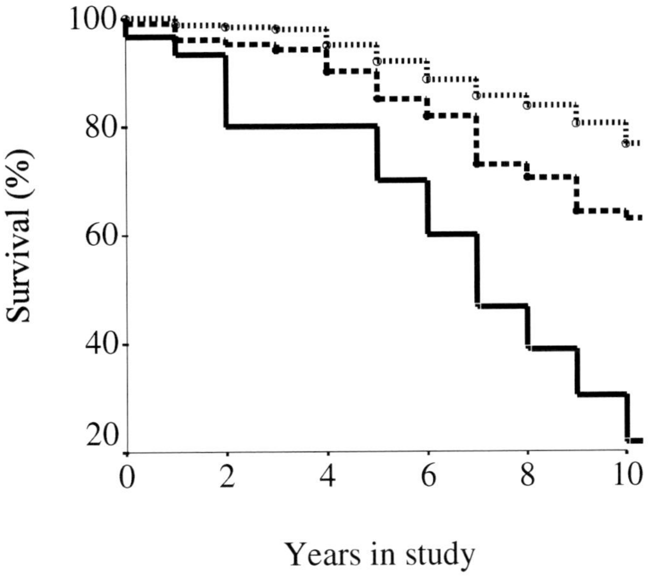

Figure 2. Type 2 diabetes: survival curves for patients with normo, micro- and macroalbuminuria (*Torffvit O. J Diab Compl 2001;15:307-313*).

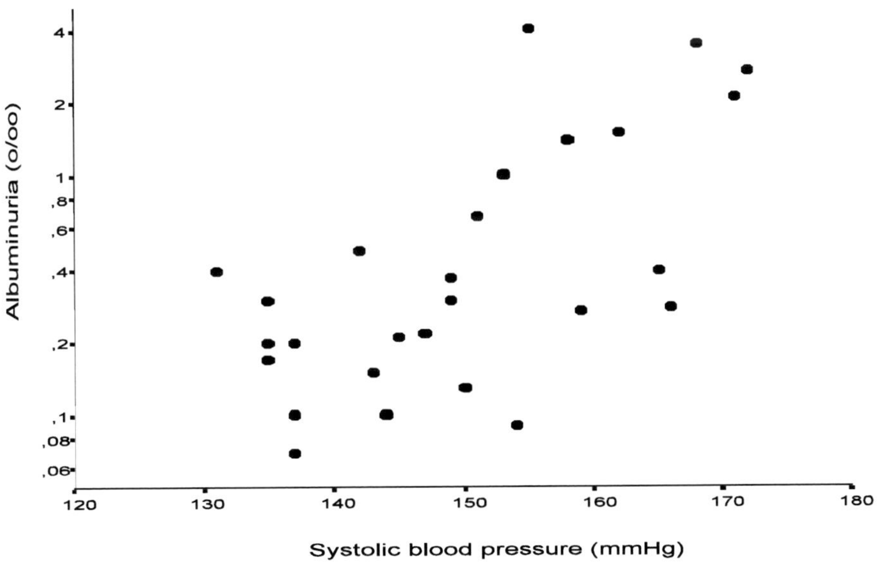

Figure 3. Type 2 diabetes: 24 hours blood pressure and albuminuria.

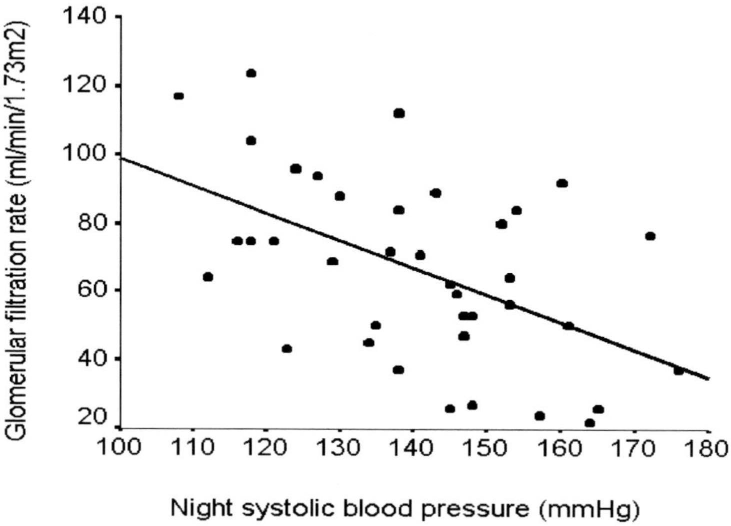

Figure 4. Type 2 diabetes: night blood pressure and glomerular function.

Treatment

Treatment may be expected to be equally effective for both heart and kidney disease (*HOPE study. Lancet 2000;355:253-59*). However, a multifactorial approach is necessary in order to reach the full effect (*Gäde P. New Eng J Med 2008; 358 (6): 580-592*). When patients with asymptomatic myocardial ischemia were treated 79% improved on treatment with statins, ASA and ACE inhibitors (*Wackers FJTh. Diabetes Care 2007;30(11): 2892-2898*).

Treat Microalbuminuria!

Today it is recommended to treat microalbuminuria even when the blood pressure apparently is normal. If the degree of albuminuria increases it has been found to be associated with a doubling of the risk for death in heart disease (*Spoelstra-DE Man AME. Diabetes Care 2001;24:2097-2101*). In contrast, a decrease in the degree of albuminuria leads to a lesser risk for death in heart disease (*Zandbergen AAM. Diabetes Care 2007;30:3119-3121*).

It is important to perform randomised prospective double blind studies on selected patients but equally important is epidemiological observation studies of patients treated in daily clinical practice. In our prospective observation study we found the risk for developing myocardial infarction to be decreased three times if the patients were on ACE inhibition compared with Ca- or Beta blockers (Fig 5).

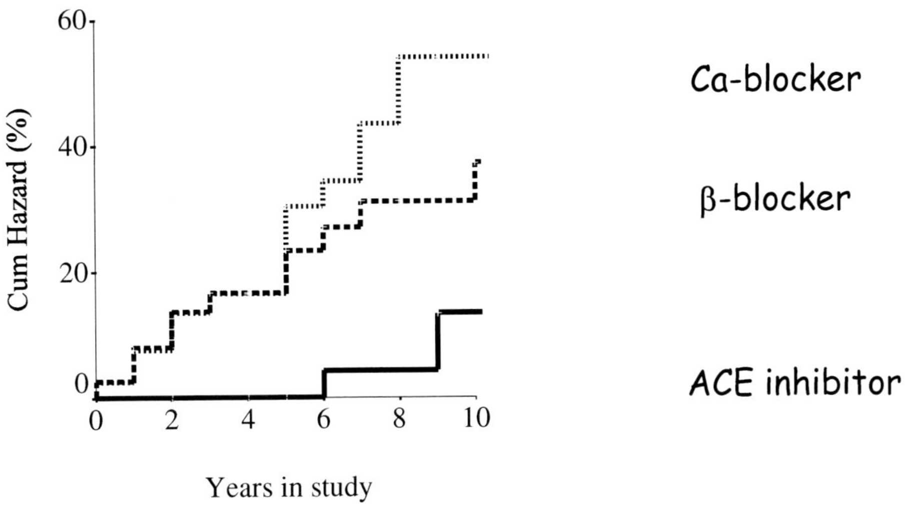

Figure 5. Development of myocardial infarction in Type 2 diabetic patients in 10 years, effect of treatment with Ca-, Beta-blockers and ACE inhibitors (*Torffvit, J Diabetes Compl 2001;15:307-13*).

Multifactorial Treatment

The most important study of multifactorial treatment was done in the Steno Memorial Hospital in Copenhagen and showed a 50% decrease in the risk for cardiovascular disease in type 2 diabetic patients during eight years (*Gäde P. NEJM 2003;348:383-393;Gäde P. NEJM 2008;358(6):580-592*). We found that cardiovascular disease and mortality decreased with mulfactorial treatment, which included invasive procedures such as CABG/PCI (Table 2). These procedures has been shown to decrease mortality by 57% during one years treatment of type 1 diabetic patients with kidney disease (*Manske CL. Lancet 1992;340:998-1002*).

Table 2. Four year observations study of Type 2 diabetic patients treated in our specialised policlinic for diabetic nephropathy (DNM) compared to previous observations (historical). The years in the headline refers to start of observation:

	DNM (1998-99) n=69	Historical (1985-88) N=37	P-value
Death	11 (16%)	10 (27%)	NS
Myocardial infarction (MI)	5 (7%)	7 (19%)	NS
Heart failure (HF)	2 (3%)	5 (14%)	P<0,05
Stroke	3 (4%)	4 (11%)	NS
Death/MI/HF/stroke	16 (23%)	17 (46%)	P<0,05

Postprandial p-glucose Treatment

Treatment aiming only for a normal fasting glucose has never been proven to have any effect on development of complications (*Bonora E. Diabetologia 2001;44:2107-2114*). In contrast, aiming for normal postprandial glucose (= mealcontrol) decreases the risk for myocardial infarction and death (*Hanefeld M. Diabetologia 1996;39:1577-83; Shichiri M. Diabetes Care 2000; 23 (S2):B21-29* (*The Kumamoto study*); *The DECODE study. Arch Int Med 2001; 161:397-404*).

Finally Some Short Consideration of Treatment

Sulfonylurea (SU)

SU have effect on the heart: They inhibit ATP sensitive potassium channels. Glibenclamide may worsen myocardial ischemia while glimepiride may improve ischemia (*Meier JJ. Review in Heart 2004;90:9-12*).

Sulfonylurea and Metformine

Patients with renal failure or even better patients with increased levels of serum creatinine should not be treated with SU or metformine. Even so patients with liver failure or high age should not be treated! Insulin treatment in such cases is preferred. Repaglinide or nateglinide have short halftime in serum and may be given. Glimepiride have lesser risk for hypoglycaemia than the other SU and even have an antiaggregatory effect on trombocytes which in vitro is better than ASA (*Siluk D. Diabetologia 2002;45:1034-1037*).

Glitazones = Tiazolidiniones

These should not be given to patients with renal-, heart- or liver failure. They may induce oedema and anaemia.

Effect of Insulin on the Heart

Insulin has several positive effects on the heart especially vasodilatation (*Sundell J. Diabetologia 2002;45:775-782*), anti-inflammatory and anti-atherogenic effect (*Dandona P. Diabetologia 2002;45:924-930*). Insulin prevent ischemia in ischemic heart disease in contrast to glibenclamide (*Scognamiglio R. Diabetes 2002;51:808-812*).

Recommendations for Treatment of Diabetic Patients with Diabetic Nephropathy

Direct acting per oral drug or insulin analogue for the meal
Postprandial p-glucose < 9 mmol/l
ACE inhibitor or AII blockers
daytime systolic blood pressure < 140 mmHg
night time systolic blood pressure < 130 mmHg

References

Agewall S. *Am J Card* 1997;80:164-69
Bacci S. *Eur J Endocrinol* 2002;147:649-654
Berton G. *Diabetologia* 2004;47:1511-1518
Bonora E. *Diabetologia* 2001;44:2107-2114
Bouchard A. *Am J Med* 1989;87:160-66
Chici A. *Diabetologia* 1998;41:684-93
Damsgaard EM. *Diabetologia* 1993;36:1030-36
Dandona P. *Diabetologia* 2002;45:924-930
The DECODE study. *Arch Int* Med 2001; 161:397-404
de Lorenzo A. *Am J Cardiol* 2002;90:827-83
Earle KA. *Diabetologia* 1996;39:854-56
Earle KA. *J Diab Compl* 2000;14:277-80
EPIC-Norfolk Study, UK, Yuyun MF. *Am J Epidemiology* 2004;159:284-93
Geluk CA. *Netherlands Heart J* 2007;15(4):133-41
Genda A. *Clin Cardiol* 1986;9:375-82
Guglielmi MD. *Diabetes Care* 1995; 18:353-60
Gäde P. *NEJM* 2003;348:383-393
Gäde P. *New Eng J Med* 2008; 358 (6): 580-592
Haffner SM. *Arteriosclerosis* 1990;10:727-31
Hanefeld M. *Diabetologia* 1996;39:1577-83
HOPE study. *Lancet* 2000;355:253-59
Janand-Delenne B. *Diabetes Care* 1999;22:1396-1400
Jones SL. *BMJ* 1989;298:487-90
Jörgensen L. *Eur Heart J* 2007; 28:363-369
Kimball TR. *Circulation* 1994;90:357-61
Manske CL. *Lancet* 1992;340:998-1002
Marso SP. 1999;33:1269-77
Mattock MB. *Diabetes* 1998;47:1786-192
Meier JJ. *Review in Heart* 2004;90:9-12
Messent JWC. *Kidney Int* 1992;41:836-839
Mühlhauser I. *Diabet Med* 2000;17:727-34
Mykkänen L. *Diabetes* 1994;43:552-557
Natali A. *Diabetologia* 2000;43:632-641
Nielsen. *Diabetic Med* 1999;16:555-562
Niskanen L. *Diabetologia* 1990;33:237-243
Riu FR. *J Diab Compl* 2003;17:235-242
Rubler S. *Am J Card* 1972;30:595-602
Rutter MK. *JACC* 2002;40:56-61
Sato A. *Diabetologia* 1999;42:76-80
Schmitz A. *Diabet Med* 1988;5:126-34
Scognamiglio R. *Diabetes* 2002;51:808-812
Shichiri M. *Diabetes Care* 2000; 23 (S2):B21-29 (The Kumamoto study)
Siluk D. *Diabetologia* 2002;45:1034-1037

Spoelstra-DE Man AME. *Diabetes Care* 2001;24:2097-2101
Strong Heart study. *Circulation* 2000;101:2271-2276
Strong Heart study. *JACC* 2003;41:2922-8
Stephenson JM. *Diabet Med* 1995;12:149-55
Sundell J. *Diabetologia* 2002;45:775-782
Thomas GN. *Diabetologia* 2004;47:1528-1534
Torffvit O. *J Diab Compl* 2001;15:307-313
Torffvit O. *Diabetes Metab* 2003;29:4S297, 2473
Torffvit O. *Diabet Med* 2005;22:723-729
Tuomilehto J. *Diabetologia* 1998;41:784-90
Valensi P. *Diabetes Care* 2001;24:339-343
Valensi P. *Diabetes Care* 2005; 28:2722-27
Valmadrid CT. *Arch Intern Med* 2000;160:1093-1100
Wackers FJT. *Diabetes Care* 2004;27:1954-61
Wackers FJTh. *Diabetes Care* 2007;30(11): 2892-2898
Weinrauch L. *Circulation* 1978;58:1184-90
Zandbergen AAM. *Diabetes Care* 2007;30:3119-3121

INDEX

A

abdomen, 65, 251, 256
abnormalities, 23, 61, 62, 63, 92, 105, 245, 248, 250, 252, 253, 254, 255, 257, 258, 265, 294, 307, 348, 349, 350, 351, 356, 361
absolute zero, 175
absorption, 54, 224, 297
abstinence, 255
ACC, 71, 180, 289, 316, 332, 362
access, 28, 83, 203, 263, 278, 279, 283, 284, 287, 288, 290, 291, 324, 328
accessory pathway, 53, 60, 63, 324
accidents, 151
accounting, 11, 26, 108, 335
accuracy, viii, ix, xv, 75, 76, 77, 78, 93, 96, 134, 136, 137, 182, 227, 267, 270, 347, 348, 356, 363
ACE inhibitors, 386, 387
ACE-inhibitor, 303
acetate, 66
achievement, 107, 296, 327
ACI, 381
acid, 17, 25, 27, 66, 115, 172, 175, 176, 260, 294, 323, 326, 330, 368, 377, 378, 379, 382
acidosis, 174, 180
acoustic, 7, 12, 356
actin, 176
action potential (AP), 4, 5, 10, 11, 13, 21
activation, 4, 5, 13, 21, 26, 48, 52, 62, 64, 105, 106, 108, 260, 372, 379
activators, 296
acute, xi, xii, xiv, 53, 68, 69, 96, 99, 106, 109, 118, 119, 120, 122, 128, 133, 167, 168, 172, 174, 177, 178, 179, 180, 181, 182, 195, 197, 199, 201, 205, 208, 221, 233, 236, 239, 240, 245, 246, 247, 248, 253, 255, 256, 257, 259, 260, 261, 262, 263, 264, 265, 266, 267, 269, 270, 271, 272, 273, 294, 302, 304, 308, 310, 311, 313, 325, 327, 344, 363, 375, 378
acute coronary syndrome, xi, 96, 167, 168, 172, 173, 174, 178, 179, 180, 181, 199, 205, 208, 233, 236, 240, 260, 262, 263, 269, 270, 271, 344
acute lymphoblastic leukemia, 239
acute stress, 327
Adams, 121, 258
adaptability, x, 101, 106
adaptation, 164
additives, 266
adenosine, 79, 81, 92, 94, 296
adherens junction, 3
adhesion, 194, 335, 372
adipose, 220, 224, 225, 226, 230, 239, 249, 251
adipose tissue, 220, 224, 225, 226, 230, 239, 249, 251
adjustment, xiii, xiv, 103, 130, 146, 158, 207, 219, 223, 230, 234, 239, 275, 276, 279, 284, 286, 287, 288, 298, 307, 339
administration, 24, 52, 66, 110, 111, 163, 185, 198, 251, 302, 303, 304
administrative, 291
adolescence, 274, 327
adolescents, 103, 108, 109, 117, 120, 164, 165, 166, 238, 272
adult, xiv, xv, 11, 23, 146, 147, 150, 151, 153, 156, 157, 159, 160, 161, 162, 163, 164, 165, 166, 193, 248, 268, 277, 289, 317, 318, 319, 324, 328, 329, 330, 331, 332
adult population, 23
adulthood, xv, 146, 158, 161, 164, 166, 238, 249, 317, 318, 319, 321, 324
adults, x, xiii, xiv, 17, 108, 109, 113, 116, 145, 146, 147, 148, 150, 151, 152, 153, 154, 156, 157, 158, 159, 160, 161, 162, 163, 164, 165, 166, 170, 219, 220, 221, 238, 270, 271, 272, 277, 317, 318, 328, 329, 331, 332, 367, 378
adverse event, 110, 211, 212, 222, 233, 234, 235, 237, 286
aerobic, 326
aetiology, 184
aetiopathogenesis, xi, 183
affective disorder, 102, 110, 114, 115, 121, 122
Africa, 321
African American, 17, 37
African Americans, 17, 37
age, xi, xii, xiv, 15, 16, 18, 25, 36, 46, 81, 135, 141, 151, 152, 154, 160, 166, 167, 169, 177, 183, 185,

188, 189, 193, 194, 220, 221, 223, 226, 227, 238, 250, 253, 254, 255, 259, 263, 268, 270, 272, 273, 276, 278, 279, 281, 283, 284, 286, 287, 288, 291, 293, 298, 307, 308, 318, 319, 323, 324, 330, 334, 335, 336, 337, 340, 341, 342, 369, 372, 373, 380, 384, 388
agent, 18, 21, 211, 296, 310
agents, 47, 49, 51, 73, 93, 94, 110, 111, 223, 224, 226, 245, 246, 255, 295, 297, 298, 300, 301, 305, 306, 309, 310, 327, 356
aggregation, 108, 171
aggression, 111, 114, 115, 152
aggressive behavior, 116, 148, 150, 151
aggressive therapy, 211
aggressiveness, 107, 157
aging, 40
agonist, 66
aid, xi, xiii, 167, 202, 212, 219
AIDS, 246, 314
air, 327, 376, 378
air embolism, 327
air pollution, 376, 378
akathisia, 109, 110
akinesia, 51, 351, 355, 357, 358
albumin, xi, 167, 174, 180, 381, 384
albuminuria, xvi, 381, 382, 383, 384, 385, 386
alcohol, 51, 65, 107, 133, 137, 142, 170, 254, 373
alcohol abuse, 254
alcohol consumption, 65, 170, 254
alcohol dependence, 254
alcohol use, 254
alcoholic cardiomyopathy, 254
alcoholics, 251, 254, 255
aldosterone, 261, 262
algorithm, 277, 324, 339
alkaline, 187, 188
alkaline phosphatase, 187, 188
alkaloids, 68
allele, 9, 12, 17, 29
alleles, 17
allergy, 199
allograft, 273
alpha, 106, 173, 250, 265
alternative, 21, 26, 49, 212, 226, 227, 236, 291, 323, 325, 348, 349, 361
alternatives, 309
alveolar macrophage, 194, 200
alveolar macrophages, 194, 200
ambient air, 376
American Heart Association, 71, 76, 97, 117, 180, 221, 289, 309
amine, 41, 251, 362
amino, 17, 25, 66, 172, 260, 270, 294
amino acid, 17, 25, 66, 172, 260, 294
amino acids, 260
aminoglycosides, 224, 239
Amiodarone, 323
amniocentesis, 323
amplitude, 15, 22, 61, 109
amputation, 102
Amsterdam, 3, 125, 333
amyloid, 172, 252
amyloidosis, 51, 252, 258, 272
anaemia, 66, 260, 388
anastomosis, 129, 338
anatomy, xi, 127, 128, 133, 135, 136, 139, 141, 167, 275, 276, 319, 320, 324, 338, 348
androgen, 335
androgens, 225, 334, 335
anemia, 73, 251, 322, 326, 333
anesthesiologist, xv, 317, 320, 322, 327, 329, 331
anesthesiologists, 328
aneurysm, 216, 248, 249, 253, 320, 327, 328
angina, x, 78, 96, 99, 101, 108, 178, 181, 194, 208, 260, 265, 272, 275, 296, 309, 336, 338, 342, 345, 346, 349
angiogenesis, 214
angiogram, 86, 95, 194
angiography, viii, ix, 58, 63, 76, 83, 86, 88, 90, 95, 96, 97, 131, 133, 186, 206, 208, 277, 295, 348, 349, 356, 360, 363
angioplasty, ix, 76, 94, 133, 135, 214, 342
Angiotensin, 323
angiotensin II, 173, 323
angiotensin receptor antagonist, 262
angiotensin-converting enzyme (ACE), 262, 313, 386, 387, 388
angulation, 127, 128, 130, 133, 136, 137, 138, 141
animal models, 334
animals, 30
annealing, 30
anomalous, 322
anorexia, 251
ANOVA, 186, 188, 189, 190, 191, 192
ANP, 260, 262, 266, 267, 268
antacids, 297, 298
antagonist, 306, 314
antagonists, 262, 306, 323
antiarrhythmic, 16, 107, 110, 255, 325
anti-atherogenic, 388
antibiotic, 185, 321
antibiotics, 247, 322
Antibodies, 187, 189, 190, 196, 198, 200, 379
antibody, xii, 176, 184, 185, 187, 194, 200, 214, 246, 375, 376
anticoagulant, 266
anticoagulants, 323, 326
anticoagulation, 327
anticonvulsants, 111
antidepressant, 103, 107, 108, 109, 110, 112, 113, 114, 117, 120, 122
antidepressant medication, 103, 109, 112, 120, 122
antidepressants, 22, 23, 50, 107, 108, 109, 110, 113, 116, 120, 122, 255
antigen, 197, 199, 372
antihistamines, 22, 23
antihypertensive agents, 110, 305
antihypertensive drugs, 304

antioxidant, 170, 213
antiphospholipid syndrome, 252
anti-platelet, 214, 222
antipsychotic, 110, 116
antipsychotics, 110, 114
antitoxin, 247
ants, 34, 79
anxiety, 46, 52, 103, 105, 109, 110, 116, 118, 119, 123, 148, 149, 150, 151, 152, 163, 166
anxiety disorder, 149, 151
aorta, 248, 320, 322, 327, 328
aortic aneurysm, 249
aortic dilatation, 328
aortic regurgitation, 248
aortic stenosis, 53, 163, 309, 322, 326
aortic valve, 318, 322, 324, 328
apathy, 251
Apo E, 343
appetite, 105
application, 71, 131, 214, 239
Arabia, 11
arginine, 294
arrest, 20, 23, 234, 306
arrhythmia, 4, 5, 6, 7, 8, 11, 12, 13, 15, 16, 17, 18, 26, 28, 29, 30, 31, 33, 34, 35, 39, 40, 43, 44, 247, 324, 340
arrhythmias, vii, viii, x, 4, 5, 11, 17, 18, 22, 23, 24, 26, 28, 29, 30, 31, 36, 39, 41, 42, 43, 45, 46, 47, 52, 53, 59, 60, 61, 62, 63, 68, 101, 110, 111, 244, 245, 248, 249, 252, 253, 254, 321, 322, 324, 326, 327, 329, 331
arrhythmogenesis, 5, 26, 30, 38
arterial hypertension, 313, 314
arteries, ix, xiv, 59, 76, 84, 85, 86, 93, 94, 95, 170, 171, 179, 213, 214, 259, 264, 271, 294, 295, 308, 326, 327, 331, 353, 383
arteriography, 93, 97
arterioles, 54, 382
arteriosclerosis, xvi, 365
artery, vii, viii, ix, xii, xiv, xv, 30, 45, 47, 53, 58, 63, 69, 70, 75, 76, 77, 78, 79, 83, 84, 86, 89, 93, 94, 95, 96, 97, 98, 100, 104, 105, 108, 114, 115, 117, 119, 133, 141, 143, 170, 171, 179, 181, 195, 196, 198, 200, 201, 205, 208, 212, 213, 214, 215, 216, 240, 248, 249, 250, 252, 255, 257, 260, 265, 271, 272, 275, 276, 277, 278, 279, 280, 281, 282, 283, 285, 286, 287, 288, 289, 290, 291, 293, 294, 295, 302, 303, 307, 309, 310, 311, 313, 316, 319, 320, 322, 325, 326, 331, 333, 334, 335, 338, 339, 340, 341, 342, 343, 344, 345, 346, 347, 349, 352, 353, 355, 358, 362, 363, 364, 383
arthritis, 221, 248, 279
artificial heart valve, 260
ascites, 251, 254, 258
ASD, 318, 319, 320, 322, 325, 326, 327, 328
Asia, 21, 321
aspartate, 174
aspiration, 252, 296
aspirin, 121, 173, 211, 222, 309
assessment, viii, xi, xv, 37, 45, 62, 68, 81, 82, 87, 93, 94, 95, 96, 97, 103, 104, 146, 147, 153, 164, 167, 170, 182, 257, 265, 270, 315, 319, 320, 323, 339, 347, 348, 349, 356, 359, 362, 363, 364
assessment procedures, 147
asymptomatic, 23, 40, 41, 49, 61, 181, 211, 215, 245, 248, 250, 252, 253, 265, 311, 318, 382, 386
asystole, 60, 61, 62, 72
ataxia, 51, 245, 254, 258
atherogenesis, 169, 185, 200, 335
atherosclerosis, 170, 171, 179, 184, 185, 194, 195, 196, 197, 198, 199, 200, 211, 252, 293, 294, 295, 308, 309, 310, 311, 334, 335, 343
atherosclerotic plaque, 106, 169, 179, 260, 293, 295, 335
atherothrombotic, 172
athletes, 53, 54, 59, 68, 69
Atlas, 179
ATP, 388
atresia, 319
atria, vii, 3, 4, 5, 6, 26, 260, 262
atrial fibrillation, 6, 12, 18, 20, 23, 24, 26, 27, 38, 42, 43, 53, 221, 254, 258, 325
atrial flutter, 254, 327
atrial myxoma, 53
atrial natriuretic peptide, 262, 264, 269, 272
atrial septal defect, 165, 318
atrio-ventricular, 328
atrioventricular block, 32, 33, 70, 107
atrioventricular node, 27
atrium, vii, 3
atrophy, 50, 51, 52, 57, 66, 67, 73, 251, 254, 312
atropine, 60, 356, 363
attachment, 185, 186, 189, 213
attacks, viii, 11, 12, 45, 47, 109
attention problems, 148, 152, 158
attitudes, 163
atypical, 58, 110, 257, 349
auditory stimuli, 34
auscultation, 60
Australia, 117, 219, 220, 233, 238
autism, 8, 12, 34
autoantibodies, 185, 195, 199
autoantibody, 28
autoimmune, 6, 51, 73, 185, 195, 200
autoimmune disease, 185
autoimmunity, 184, 197
automaticity, 5
autonomic activity, 49
Autonomic Nervous System, viii, 45, 47, 49, 67
autonomic neuropathy, 52, 73, 249
autonomy, 161
autopsy, xi, 167, 206, 256, 257
autosomal dominant, 9, 24, 25, 43, 253
autosomal recessive, 41, 254
availability, 23, 227, 288, 319, 320, 321, 348, 361
averaging, 58, 61
avoidance, 130, 326
awareness, 318, 319

axon, 68

B

B cell, 194
back pain, 299
background noise, 175
bacteremia, 196, 246
bacteria, xvi, 184, 197, 198, 365, 374, 375, 376
bacterial, xi, 183, 184, 196, 197, 198, 199, 246
bacterial infection, 196
balloon angioplasty, 202, 203
Baroreflex, 68
Baroreflex function, 68
barrier, 323
barriers, 146
Bax, 362
B-cell, 196, 198
behavior, x, 101, 106, 108, 109, 113, 114, 115, 116, 118, 119, 121, 148, 150, 151, 152, 156, 158, 159, 160, 165
behavioral problems, 147, 148, 149, 150, 152, 158
behaviours, 108, 165
beliefs, 103, 112
bell, 7, 12, 16
beneficial effect, 109, 208, 213, 214, 303, 304, 306
benefits, xiii, 125, 131, 132, 219, 276, 302, 305, 335, 349
benign, 217, 252
benzodiazepines, 225
beriberi, 251, 254
beta blocker, 50
beta-blockers, 34, 305, 309
bias, 266, 276, 288, 336
bicuspid, 318, 322, 327, 328
bifurcation, xii, 132, 133, 141, 142, 201, 205
binding, 13, 21, 174, 175, 176, 180, 214, 298
binge drinking, 254
bioavailability, 297, 301
biocompatible, xii, 201
biodegradable, xii, 202, 213
biological activity, 261
biological processes, xii, 201
biological psychiatry, 119
biomarker, xi, 167, 168, 172, 177, 376
biomarkers, xi, xiv, 167, 168, 169, 174, 177, 178, 179, 180, 259, 264, 265, 273
biopsy, 244, 246, 250, 252, 253, 383
bipolar, 103, 109, 112, 117
bipolar disorder, 103, 112, 117
birth, 8, 11, 12, 160, 162, 169, 260, 274, 318
birth control, 160, 162
births, 318
black-box, 108, 110
bladder, 254
bleeding, 224, 234, 235, 236, 326
blocks, 340
blood, vii, viii, ix, xii, xvi, 3, 4, 45, 46, 47, 49, 51, 53, 54, 55, 56, 57, 59, 60, 61, 62, 64, 65, 66, 68, 69, 70, 77, 78, 79, 94, 97, 100, 105, 106, 108, 117, 122, 126, 170, 174, 177, 183, 186, 187, 199, 206, 212, 221, 223, 224, 225, 247, 260, 262, 263, 265, 266, 268, 269, 270, 276, 295, 296, 301, 303, 304, 307, 309, 314, 320, 322, 338, 342, 349, 350, 359, 360, 365, 367, 368, 369, 372, 373, 375, 377, 378, 379, 384, 385, 386, 388
blood flow, vii, ix, 45, 46, 53, 54, 56, 57, 69, 70, 77, 78, 97, 100, 224, 295, 296, 303, 320
blood pressure, viii, xvi, 45, 47, 49, 51, 54, 55, 56, 57, 59, 60, 61, 64, 65, 66, 68, 79, 105, 106, 108, 117, 122, 221, 223, 224, 262, 296, 301, 304, 309, 314, 349, 350, 359, 360, 365, 369, 373, 378, 379, 385, 386
Blood pressure, 314
blood sampling, 223
blood transfusion, 247, 338, 342
blood vessels, vii, 65, 126, 276
bloodstream, 248
BMI, xvi, 220, 221, 225, 226, 227, 228, 229, 232, 233, 235, 237, 365, 369, 370, 371, 373, 376
body composition, xiii, 219, 220, 221, 225, 227, 228, 231, 232, 237
body fat, 221, 251
body fluid, 246
body image, 146, 159, 162, 163
body mass index, xiii, 219, 225, 339, 378
body size, xiii, 219, 221, 225, 226, 227, 228, 229, 230, 231, 236, 237, 276, 290, 336, 338, 345
body weight, xiii, 219, 222, 225, 226, 232, 239, 241, 369, 379
bolus, 17, 98, 236
bone resorption, 184
borderline, 24, 109, 149
Boston, 68, 101, 163
bowel, 50
boys, 220, 253
bradyarrhythmia, 24
bradycardia, vii, 5, 7, 12, 20, 23, 24, 32, 40, 41, 45, 47, 48, 56, 61, 62, 63, 72, 325, 328
brain, xiv, 46, 47, 48, 55, 118, 259, 262, 263, 264, 269, 270, 271, 272, 273, 274
brain natriuretic peptide (BNP), xiv, 259, 262, 263, 269, 271, 272, 273, 274
brainstem, 47, 48, 49, 56, 62
branching, 142
breakdown, 299
British Columbia, 275, 277, 278, 279, 280, 286, 291
bronchitis, 248
Brugada syndrome, 6, 20, 21, 22, 33, 39, 40, 43, 53, 60
buffer, 187, 188
bundle branch block, 19, 22, 107
bupropion, 108, 121
burning, 250
bypass, xiv, xv, 94, 105, 117, 185, 275, 276, 277, 280, 281, 282, 283, 285, 287, 288, 289, 290, 291,

294, 297, 320, 333, 334, 338, 339, 340, 341, 342, 343, 344, 345, 346
bypass graft, 275, 280, 289, 290, 340, 342

C

C. diphtheriae, 247
Ca^{2+}, 5, 7, 12, 13, 16, 20, 26
cachexia, 251
calcification, 130
calcium, x, 5, 8, 9, 12, 13, 14, 21, 26, 34, 39, 42, 49, 101, 106, 111, 116, 119, 138, 223, 249, 255, 314
calcium channel blocker, x, 49, 101, 106, 111, 116
calibration, 15, 25
calorimetry, 239
calreticulin, 41
cAMP, 296
campaigns, 366
Canada, vii, 102, 186, 187, 275, 277, 289, 291, 330
cancer, 50, 116, 168, 169, 251, 279, 280, 282, 285, 287, 378
Candida, 247
capacitance, 54
capacity, 225, 264, 276, 302, 303, 306, 309, 313, 314, 321, 326, 331, 356, 359, 360
capillary, 255, 302
capsule, 256
carbohydrates, 65
carbon, 212
carbon dioxide, 212
cardiac arrest, 9, 12, 18, 106, 113, 116
cardiac arrhythmia, 26, 28, 30, 31, 33, 34, 35, 39, 40, 47, 52, 249, 326, 329
cardiac catheterization, viii, 75, 76, 78, 83, 86, 89, 96, 97, 276, 288, 290, 320
cardiac function, xiii, 5, 37, 177, 243, 250, 258, 262, 274, 301, 309, 336
cardiac involvement, 246, 247, 248, 252
cardiac muscle, 248
cardiac myocytes, 260, 301
cardiac operations, 336
cardiac output, viii, 45, 47, 49, 52, 53, 54, 62, 63, 72, 224, 249, 251, 262, 302, 303, 322, 325, 327
cardiac pacemaker, 40
cardiac risk, 107, 312
cardiac surgery, 23, 110, 164, 165, 253, 270, 289, 291, 321, 325, 328, 330, 334, 346
cardiac tamponade, 252
cardiologist, xv, 61, 317, 319, 320, 322, 323, 324, 326, 327, 328, 329
cardiology, xii, xiii, xv, 79, 95, 97, 113, 114, 115, 119, 120, 126, 168, 174, 196, 200, 201, 208, 219, 223, 233, 236, 317, 327, 328, 348
cardiomyocytes, 3, 12, 21, 33, 35, 262
cardiomyopathy, vii, ix, xiii, xiv, 26, 27, 30, 41, 43, 53, 54, 61, 76, 96, 99, 111, 142, 243, 244, 245, 246, 247, 249, 252, 253, 254, 255, 256, 257, 258, 266, 309
cardiopulmonary, 245, 302, 329, 338
cardiopulmonary bypass, 338
cardiovascular disease, vii, xi, xiii, xvi, 6, 102, 104, 105, 106, 107, 108, 112, 115, 120, 121, 122, 170, 179, 189, 195, 196, 197, 219, 220, 221, 238, 259, 270, 271, 301, 310, 311, 312, 316, 319, 336, 367, 377, 381, 387
Cardiovascular disease (CVD), 167, 168, 179, 184, 376, 377
cardiovascular function, 111, 221
cardiovascular morbidity, 26, 122, 249, 304, 368
cardiovascular physiology, 261
cardiovascular risk, 105, 106, 111, 116, 165, 196, 221, 310, 367, 379
cardiovascular system, 106, 213, 249
carotid sinus, vii, 45, 48, 49, 57, 59, 60, 63, 67, 70
carotid sinus syncope, 59
carrier, 11, 15, 17, 23, 28, 204, 212, 213
CAT, 348
cataplexy, 47
cataracts, 253
catechol, 297
catecholamine, 24, 41, 52
catecholamines, 105, 118
category a, 47
catheter, 79, 126, 127, 136, 214, 318, 324, 325, 331
catheterization, viii, xiv, 75, 76, 77, 78, 83, 84, 85, 86, 89, 93, 96, 97, 201, 275, 276, 277, 278, 281, 283, 284, 286, 287, 288, 290, 320
catheters, 126, 133
cattle, 247
Caucasian, 185, 221
causation, 334
cell, 4, 5, 6, 21, 66, 106, 132, 136, 143, 170, 171, 172, 174, 175, 176, 178, 179, 194, 198, 199, 213, 214, 248, 261, 335, 372, 376, 379
cell adhesion, 372
cell line, 198
cell lines, 198
cell membranes, 6
cell surface, 21
Centers for Disease Control, 237
central nervous system, 66, 248, 254, 260
ceramic, 213
cerebral blood flow, 54, 55, 56, 59, 69, 70
cerebral hemorrhage, 369
cerebral hypoperfusion, viii, 45, 47, 56, 57, 59, 69, 70
cerebrospinal fluid, 54
cerebrovascular, 55, 56, 57, 69, 70, 279, 280, 282, 285, 287, 304, 336, 368
cerebrovascular disease, 57, 279, 280, 282, 285, 287, 336
cerebrovascular diseases, 57
cervical cancer, 169
Chagas disease, 247, 256
channel blocker, 22, 50, 119
channelopathy, 42

channels, 3, 4, 5, 6, 11, 12, 13, 21, 30, 33, 34, 39, 132, 388
chaperones, 196
chemokines, 122, 171
chemosis, 248
chemotherapeutic agent, 224, 226
chemotherapy, 98, 239, 252
childhood, 9, 15, 26, 36, 164, 166, 239, 319, 321, 326
children, x, xi, 9, 16, 22, 40, 108, 117, 120, 145, 146, 160, 162, 167, 170, 179, 220, 222, 238, 249, 253, 256, 269, 272, 274, 299, 301, 318, 325, 366, 376
China, 123
Chi-square, 83, 280
chloroquine, 255
cholesterol, xvi, 169, 170, 172, 173, 211, 221, 293, 310, 334, 335, 365, 366, 367, 368, 369, 371, 372, 373, 375, 377, 378, 379
cholinergic, 110
chorionic villus sampling, 323
chromosome, 23, 25, 26, 33, 42, 260
chronic disease, 102, 116, 162
chronic diseases, 102, 116
chronic fatigue syndrome, 68
chronic illness, 165
chronic obstructive pulmonary disease, 279, 285, 315, 339, 340
chronically ill, 160, 165
cigarette smoking, 293, 369, 379
cigarettes, 366, 369
cimetidine, 299
circulation, 48, 49, 54, 56, 57, 61, 65, 69, 175, 270, 271, 296, 313
cirrhosis, 254
classes, 141, 246
classical, 169, 173, 174, 251
classification, 47, 67, 221, 262, 342
cleavage, 266
cleft palate, 8, 12
clinical diagnosis, 178, 307
clinical examination, xiv, 170, 243, 244
clinical presentation, 47, 50, 174, 243, 253
clinical psychology, 120, 121
clinical symptoms, 28
clinical syndrome, 21
clinical trial, xii, 23, 38, 109, 168, 169, 178, 201, 204, 205, 207, 208, 211, 217, 233, 237, 264, 297, 300, 301, 308, 309, 312, 313
clinical trials, xii, 23, 109, 201, 204, 205, 207, 211, 217, 233, 237, 264, 297, 300, 301, 309
clinically significant, 111, 252, 305
clinician, xiii, 94, 107, 208, 219, 222, 225, 226
clinics, xv, 317, 318, 319, 321, 329
clonidine, 64
cloning, 31, 34
clopidogrel, 211, 214, 216, 222
closure, 162, 318, 320, 368
clozapine, 110, 111, 120, 123, 255
CME, 97
CNV, 28
Co, 30
CO2, 54, 55, 56, 69, 188
coagulation, 173, 303, 327, 335
coagulation factor, 327
coagulation factors, 327
coarctation, 320, 322, 327, 328
cobalt, 174
cocaine, 22, 255
cocaine abuse, 255
coding, 6, 9, 32, 52
codon, 17
codons, 29
coenzyme, 251
cognitive, 105, 115, 155, 157, 163, 321
cognitive function, 157
cohort, 37, 113, 116, 119, 150, 157, 160, 166, 182, 198, 270, 277, 286, 305, 310, 311, 344, 366, 367, 372, 378
coil, 320
Collaboration, 71, 289, 320, 330, 367, 378
collagen, 170, 171, 172, 203, 249
collateral, xi, 167, 300, 320
Columbia, 333
Columbia University, 333
combined effect, 376
combined oral contraceptives, 323
communication, 5, 100, 112, 161
communities, 120
community, 46, 102, 162, 182, 210, 269, 270, 274, 318, 319, 321, 326, 328
co-morbidities, 336, 337, 339
comorbidity, 103, 112, 269, 278, 279, 284, 291
compensatory effect, 262
competence, 329
competitive sport, 326
competitiveness, 107
complement, 210, 373
complexity, xv, 128, 133, 136, 141, 333
compliance, 54, 173, 323
complications, 141, 216, 244, 248, 252, 253, 255, 265, 308, 324, 338, 340, 381, 388
components, 3, 5, 106, 107, 111, 172
composition, xiii, 30, 147, 171, 219, 227
compounds, ix, 18, 76, 78, 213, 296
comprehension, xii, 202, 208
Compton effect, 100
computation, 226, 228
computed tomography, 77, 319
computer software, 83
concentration, 26, 54, 169, 172, 175, 184, 186, 187, 197, 212, 222, 223, 224, 234, 238, 239, 262, 263, 266, 268, 273, 297, 301, 305, 381
conception, 323
concordance, 363
concrete, 56, 150
conduction, vii, 3, 4, 6, 19, 20, 22, 23, 27, 28, 30, 32, 33, 39, 40, 43, 52, 53, 61, 63, 107, 110, 247, 250, 252, 253, 254, 255, 258, 324, 327, 328, 331

confidence, 77, 84, 103, 211, 231, 283, 285, 287, 337, 384
confidence interval, 77, 84, 103, 211, 283, 285, 287, 337, 384
confidence intervals, 77, 84, 103, 211, 337
configuration, 5, 141, 212
conflict, 330
conflict of interest, 330
confounders, 184, 279
confounding variables, 307
congenital heart disease, x, xi, xiv, 145, 146, 158, 163, 164, 165, 166, 264, 267, 317, 318, 330, 331, 332
congestive heart failure (CHF), ix, xiv, 76, 78, 95, 96, 98, 100, 103, 118, 121, 236, 244, 245, 247, 253, 255, 256, 269, 279, 313, 317, 322, 326, 327, 336, 339, 340, 341, 342
Congress, 97
conjunctiva, 247
connective tissue, 170, 184, 227, 245, 305
connective tissue diseases, 305
consciousness, 47, 51, 56, 59
consensus, 39, 66, 175, 180, 202, 269, 312, 316
consent, 79, 186
constipation, 247
constraints, 288
constrictive pericarditis, 252
consulting, 120, 121, 328
consumers, 251
consumption, 49, 65, 170, 254, 258, 297, 299, 313, 323, 349, 368, 373
contraceptives, 323, 326
contractions, 254
contracts, vii, 3
contrast agent, 356
control, x, xii, 44, 54, 57, 62, 67, 68, 69, 98, 102, 105, 107, 123, 125, 126, 127, 128, 135, 140, 141, 154, 155, 156, 157, 162, 168, 175, 183, 185, 186, 187, 188, 189, 190, 192, 193, 194, 204, 238, 258, 279, 289, 294, 307, 308, 314, 315, 330, 368, 372
control group, xii, 135, 154, 155, 156, 157, 168, 183, 186, 188, 189, 190, 192, 193, 204, 294, 368
controlled trials, 64, 66, 215, 216, 308, 368
conversion, 6, 22
convulsion, 59
COPD, 306, 337, 342
Copenhagen, 198, 258, 387
Coping, 160
coronary angioplasty, 180
coronary arteries, xi, 54, 83, 91, 94, 97, 128, 167, 168, 205, 215, 248, 252, 255, 276, 294, 295, 320, 335, 338, 358, 382, 383
coronary artery bypass graft, xiv, xv, 105, 275, 281, 282, 283, 287, 289, 290, 291, 333, 339, 341, 343, 344, 345, 346
coronary artery disease, vii, viii, xii, xiv, xv, 30, 53, 63, 75, 77, 78, 86, 87, 79, 93, 94, 96, 98, 104, 105, 114, 119, 170, 181, 196, 198, 200, 208, 216, 240, 249, 250, 252, 255, 260, 265, 271, 277, 279, 281, 286, 291, 293, 294, 295, 307, 308, 309, 310, 311, 316, 320, 333, 334, 335, 343, 347, 348, 349, 351, 353, 356, 359, 360, 361, 362, 363, 364
coronary bypass surgery, 290, 291, 334, 342, 345
coronary heart disease, x, 101, 106, 114, 115, 116, 117, 119, 120, 122, 123, 169, 184, 194, 195, 196, 197, 198, 199, 221, 310, 311, 365, 377, 378
correlation, viii, xii, 15, 31, 37, 70, 76, 84, 88, 89, 95, 98, 183, 188, 190, 194, 195, 266, 308, 363
correlation coefficient, 188, 190
correlations, 39, 87, 95, 331
cortex, 47
corticosteroids, 247, 253
corticotropin, 114
cortisol, 105, 114, 122
Corynebacterium, 246
Corynebacterium diphtheriae, 246
cosmetics, 159
cost-effective, 356
costs, 77, 94, 102, 112, 131, 222, 263, 349
cotinine, 194
cough, 59, 64, 256
coughing, 47
counseling, 162, 323, 327, 372
covariate, 157, 222, 223, 227, 229
C-reactive protein, xii, xvi, 172, 182, 183, 195, 196, 197, 200, 264, 365, 373, 375, 379
creatine, 174, 175, 180, 181
creatine kinase, 174, 175, 180, 181
creatinine, 229, 234, 239, 297, 326, 336, 381, 388
credit, 95, 97
criticism, 93
crops, 356
cross-sectional, x, 101, 163, 184, 330
cross-sectional study, 163
crosstalk, 29, 30
CRP, xii, 172, 173, 177, 178, 183, 184, 185, 188, 190, 191, 192, 194, 195, 373, 374, 375, 376
CRT, 324
crying, 105, 121
CSF, 114, 120
CT scan, 128
C-terminal, 25, 33, 44, 266
C-terminus, 27
culture, 188, 193, 247
curing, 312
CVD, xi, xiv, 167, 168, 169, 170, 172, 173, 178, 259, 293, 294, 295, 302, 308, 309, 365, 366, 367, 368, 369, 370, 372, 376, 384
cyanosis, 159, 322, 323, 326
cyanotic, 151, 156, 264, 322
cycles, xv, 347, 350, 351, 356
cyclohexanol, 120
cyclophosphamide, 255
cystine, 172
cysts, 247, 248, 250
cytochrome, 111, 301
cytokine, 105, 194
cytokines, 106, 122, 171, 179

cytomegalovirus, 195, 246
cytoplasm, 175, 176
cytosol, 5
cytosolic, 20, 26, 174, 175
cytotoxicity, 185, 198
Czech Republic, 259

D

DAD, 5, 26
daily living, 342
Danon disease, 249
data set, 116, 286, 288
database, 179, 276, 277, 291, 307, 342
de novo, 13, 205, 215
deafness, 11
death, vii, viii, x, xi, xiv, 5, 6, 9, 12, 16, 17, 18, 21, 23, 24, 33, 36, 37, 38, 39, 41, 45, 59, 63, 101, 102, 104, 105, 112, 113, 118, 121, 167, 169, 178, 184, 207, 208, 209, 210, 211, 222, 240, 245, 247, 248, 249, 252, 255, 257, 263, 264, 265, 275, 276, 278, 283, 284, 285, 286, 287, 288, 309, 316, 317, 323, 324, 326, 328, 346, 361, 362, 368, 378, 383, 384, 386, 388
death rate, 18
deaths, 21, 108, 169, 178, 213, 221, 236, 259, 277, 283, 366
decay, ix, 11, 29, 32, 76, 78, 83, 87, 93, 94
decision making, xv, 77, 169, 269, 347
decisions, ix, 76, 348
defecation, 59, 64
defects, 5, 12, 27, 40, 52, 162, 163, 165, 250, 253, 319, 322, 326, 330, 356
defibrillator, viii, 18, 23, 26, 45, 318, 331
deficiency, 21, 43, 50, 68, 245, 251, 294, 299, 326
deficit, xiii, 219
deficits, 251
definition, 66, 67, 94, 115, 208, 210, 221, 363, 381
deformation, xv, 127, 347
degenerate, 6
degradation, 11, 29, 30, 180, 212, 266, 294, 296
degrading, 179
dehydration, 49, 54
dehydrogenase, 19, 37, 39, 174, 176
delinquent behavior, 152
delivery, 30, 79, 96, 126, 128, 133, 136, 137, 212, 213, 214, 217, 255, 318, 323, 329
demand, xi, 94, 167, 174, 304, 321
dementia, 221, 251, 279, 280, 282, 285, 287
demographic characteristics, 222
demographics, 223, 226
denervation, 38, 42, 49, 52
denial, 150
densitometry, 227
density, 172, 173, 179, 187, 293
dental caries, 366
dental plaque, 184
depolarization, 4, 5, 9, 11, 39
deposition, 213, 250, 252, 257, 316
deposits, 184, 250, 382
depressed, x, 101, 103, 105, 106, 108, 109, 112, 113, 120, 121, 122, 148, 150, 161, 165
depression, x, 46, 101, 102, 103, 104, 105, 106, 107, 109, 110, 111, 112, 113, 114, 115, 116, 117, 118, 119, 120, 121, 122, 123, 148, 150, 151, 152, 166, 193, 221, 251, 293, 309
depressive disorder, 103, 105, 115, 117, 120, 121, 149
depressive symptoms, 105, 115, 118
deprivation, 366
destruction, 184, 194
desynchronization, 59
detection, viii, xi, 13, 45, 78, 86, 97, 98, 120, 167, 168, 174, 175, 177, 181, 187, 272, 273, 295, 347, 348, 356, 362, 364
developed countries, xiv, 169, 317, 318, 321
developed nations, 251, 322, 326
developing countries, xiv, 317, 318, 319, 320, 321, 322, 329
diabetes, xi, xii, xiv, xvi, 51, 52, 102, 113, 116, 119, 170, 173, 183, 185, 201, 212, 221, 238, 249, 250, 254, 259, 266, 270, 279, 280, 282, 285, 286, 287, 293, 294, 295, 298, 307, 308, 310, 315, 319, 336, 340, 365, 366, 367, 376, 382, 383, 384, 385, 386
diabetes mellitus, xiv, 173, 249, 254, 270, 280, 282, 285, 287, 293, 294, 295, 298, 307, 315, 319, 336, 340
diabetic nephropathy, xvi, 382, 383, 387
diabetic patients, xvi, 119, 212, 315, 381, 382, 383, 384, 385, 387
diagnostic criteria, 105, 147, 149
diagnostic markers, 269
dialysis, 339, 340
Diamond, 216
diaphragm, 254
diarrhea, 248, 300
diastole, 4, 129
diastolic blood pressure, 49, 368, 369, 378, 384
Diastolic dysfunction, 258
diastolic pressure, 60, 304, 359
diet, 155, 157, 335, 366, 367, 368, 372, 373, 377, 378
dietary, 251, 366, 372, 379
dietary intake, 251
diets, 334, 335
dilated cardiomyopathy, 95, 245, 247, 250, 256, 258, 273
dilation, 203, 250, 353, 357, 360
diluent, 187, 188
diphtheria, 246
direction control, 128, 130, 138, 141
directionality, 211
disability, 102, 112, 169, 321, 327
discomfort, 92, 159, 256, 262, 319
disease progression, 178, 254, 262

diseases, vii, xiv, 27, 28, 46, 50, 53, 55, 57, 63, 102, 112, 168, 193, 221, 223, 236, 244, 245, 248, 257, 259, 262, 264, 267, 269, 295, 319, 367
disorder, 12, 17, 23, 24, 26, 34, 39, 43, 103, 105, 106, 115, 116, 121, 249, 250, 254, 257, 311, 322, 326
dispersion, 38
displacement, 357
disposition, xiii, 219, 239, 350
disseminate, 248
distress, 155, 157, 158, 160, 161, 162, 266
distribution, 18, 62, 179, 217, 224, 232, 250, 279, 281, 286, 296, 330
diuretic, 258
diuretics, 49, 111, 305
diving, 7, 9
dizziness, 18, 23, 49, 51, 169, 300
DNA, 17, 184
Dobutamine, 79, 100, 362
dominance, 95
donor, 213, 326
donors, 268, 270
dopamine, 106, 108, 118, 223
Doppler, xv, 56, 70, 97, 271, 315, 347, 356, 359, 363
dosage, 112, 239, 298
dose-response relationship, 306
dosing, xiii, 212, 220, 222, 223, 224, 225, 226, 227, 228, 231, 233, 234, 235, 236, 237, 240, 241, 297, 301, 304
double-blind trial, 215
Down syndrome, 326
DPQ, 149, 150
drainage, 322, 325
drinking, 71, 254
drug delivery, 212, 213, 215
drug exposure, xiii, 219, 223, 224, 236, 237
drug interaction, 297, 302, 314
drug manufacturers, 108
drug therapy, 72, 239, 310
drug treatment, 6, 108
drug use, 114, 122, 373
drug-induced, 13, 35
drugs, x, xii, xiii, 14, 16, 17, 49, 50, 53, 59, 64, 65, 66, 101, 106, 109, 111, 113, 117, 120, 122, 165, 201, 204, 212, 219, 220, 222, 223, 224, 225, 226, 228, 229, 230, 231, 236, 237, 255, 265, 295, 297, 301, 302, 305, 307, 309, 312, 314, 323, 325, 326, 327, 366, 370, 373
DSM, 149
DSM-IV, 151
dual chamber pacing, 65
duration, 5, 10, 11, 13, 21, 43, 108, 238, 300, 307, 308, 309, 310, 324, 328, 367, 368
dysarthria, 51
dyskinesia, 351
dyslipidemia, 103, 105, 221, 293, 307, 311
dyspepsia, 299
dysphagia, 247, 254
dysphoria, 112
dysplasia, 30
dyspnea, 182, 256, 262, 272
dysregulation, 302
dystrophin, 253

E

ears, 8, 12
eating, 65, 247
echocardiogram, 92, 252, 267
echoing, 133
eclampsia, 255
ecological, x, 101, 109, 119
edema, 247, 248, 251
Eden, 199
Education, 165, 317, 328
EEG, 58
effusion, 252
egg, 204
elderly, 23, 47, 49, 50, 59, 67, 70, 72, 102, 103, 106, 112, 114, 115, 118, 120, 121, 122, 230, 251, 267, 269, 270, 279, 288, 289, 379
elderly population, 114
electrical cardioversion, 325
electrical properties, 29
electricity, vii, 3
electrocardiogram (ECG), 5, 13, 39, 92, 295, 362
electrodes, 62
electrolyte, 17, 34, 249, 254
electrolyte imbalance, 34, 249
electrolytes, 16, 251, 296
electrophysiological properties, 63
electrophysiological study, 22, 58, 63, 328
electrophysiologists, 325
electrophysiology, 21, 43
ELISA, xii, 172, 183, 187, 188, 267
emboli, 256, 320
embolism, 168, 323
embolization, 320
embolus, 53
emission, 362
emotion, 47
emotional, 9, 24, 102, 109, 146, 147, 148, 149, 150, 151, 152, 153, 154, 156, 157, 158, 159, 161
emotional disorder, 102
emotions, 47
employment, xii, 146, 165, 201, 321
encapsulated, 169
encapsulation, 212
encephalitis, 248
encoding, 5, 13, 27
encyst, 248
endocarditis, xiv, 246, 252, 317, 318, 321, 324, 326, 328, 330, 340
endocardium, 3
endorphins, 47
endothelial cell, xii, 170, 172, 179, 194, 199, 201, 213, 214, 261, 296

endothelial cells, xii, 172, 194, 201, 214, 296
endothelial dysfunction, 195, 293, 294, 302, 303, 305, 307, 310, 311
endothelial progenitor cells, 214
endothelin-1, 270
endothelium, 171, 172, 213, 294, 302
endurance, 54, 59, 68, 69
energy, 80, 109, 176, 251
England, vii, 108, 120
enlargement, 176, 244
enteritis, 251, 256
environment, 28, 29
environmental factors, xvi, 15, 27, 223
enzymatic, 296
enzyme inhibitors, 50, 323
enzymes, 171, 173, 174, 245, 248, 260, 296, 297, 300
eosinophilia, 248
epicardium, 3
epidemic, 220
epidemiology, 114, 119, 120, 197, 293, 346, 367
epilepsy, viii, 33, 45, 47, 59, 115
epinephrine, 16, 17, 37
epithelial cell, 250
epithelial cells, 250
epitope, 198
epitopes, 194, 196, 198, 266
Epstein-Barr virus, 246
equipment, viii, 75, 127, 128, 132, 140, 227, 320
erectile dysfunction, 293, 310, 311, 312, 314, 315, 316
ergonomics, 137
erosion, xi, 167, 260
erythematous, 248
erythrocytosis, 327
erythropoietin, 52, 68, 73
Escherichia coli, 198
EST, 78, 79, 94
esters, 169
estimating, 229
estradiol, 335
Estrogen, 218, 323, 334, 335, 343
estrogen receptors, 334
estrogens, 225
ethnicity, 268
etiology, xiv, xv, 52, 64, 71, 259, 260, 269, 295, 307, 310, 323, 333, 365, 369
eukaryotic cell, 29
Europe, 168, 222, 234
Europeans, 5
evening, 64
evolution, x, 47, 125, 258, 264
examinations, xiv, 16, 243, 244, 247
excitation, vii, 3, 4
exclusion, xiii, 177, 219, 318
excretion, 118, 225, 251, 260, 384
exercise, viii, xv, 7, 8, 9, 11, 14, 17, 25, 53, 54, 59, 60, 63, 65, 76, 78, 79, 80, 92, 98, 99, 174, 253, 264, 295, 302, 303, 306, 309, 312, 313, 314, 316, 317, 326, 331, 347, 348, 349, 350, 351, 352, 353, 354, 355, 356, 357, 358, 359, 360, 361, 362, 363, 364, 383
exertion, 9, 309
exons, 9, 17
expenditures, 318
experimental condition, 61
expert, 257, 310, 316, 320
expertise, xv, 227, 317, 318, 320, 321, 326, 328, 329
exposure, xiii, 194, 219, 223, 224, 236, 237, 248, 255, 306, 320, 335, 376, 379
externalizing, 150, 152, 158
externalizing problems, 152
extracellular matrix, 172
extraction, 268, 325, 376
extrapolation, 227, 237
extrasystoles, 7, 15, 25
eyelid, 247

F

Fabry disease, 250
facial expression, 51
facial nerve, 248
factor analysis, 366
factor VII, 173
factor Xa, 233
factorial, 372
failure, vii, viii, xi, xiii, 45, 47, 50, 51, 52, 56, 66, 67, 69, 70, 72, 73, 99, 105, 114, 119, 134, 135, 167, 168, 177, 219, 231, 236, 247, 249, 250, 251, 255, 257, 259, 260, 262, 263, 265, 266, 267, 269, 271, 272, 323, 340, 387
fainting, 66
false negative, 54, 86, 95
false positive, 54, 62, 86
familial, xiii, 5, 24, 28, 29, 40, 41, 42, 43, 59, 243, 244
family, 11, 12, 16, 18, 21, 22, 23, 24, 26, 27, 28, 33, 63, 103, 113, 160, 199, 212, 254, 296, 321
family history, 18, 21, 63, 254
family life, 160
family members, 16, 22, 23, 27, 28
family physician, 103
family planning, 321
fasting, 79, 83, 367, 368, 373, 388
fasting glucose, 373, 388
fat, 220, 221, 224, 225, 226, 227, 228, 232, 250, 252, 385
fatal arrhythmia, 29
fatigue, 23, 51, 68, 118, 169, 256, 262
fatty acid, 174, 175, 372, 379
fatty acids, 174, 372
fax, 101
FDG, 96
fear, 47, 66
February, 345
feces, 247

feedback, 105
feelings, x, 102, 106, 109, 146, 149, 153, 157, 159, 161
feet, 65, 127
females, xi, 9, 15, 146, 152, 153, 157, 158, 159, 160, 161, 162, 169, 175, 183, 225, 226, 229, 257, 329, 340
ferritin, 250
fertility, 160, 162
fetal, 16, 32, 36, 322, 323, 326
fetus, 23, 323
fetuses, 260
fever, 22, 23, 247, 248
fibers, 47, 48, 298
fibrillation, 5, 6, 23, 26, 28, 42, 43, 52, 54, 61, 254, 327
fibrin, 214
fibrinogen, 111, 195
fibrinolysis, 240, 303, 335
fibronectin, 214
fibrosis, 23, 27, 43, 170, 171, 244, 249, 252, 253, 255, 265, 324, 382
fibrous cap, 171
film, 93
films, 131
filtration, 62, 229, 230
Finland, 165
Finns, 32
first generation, 134, 213
first-time, 286
fish, 366
fitness, 326
fixed rate, 137
flexibility, 137, 141, 235
flow, vii, ix, 3, 45, 46, 53, 54, 55, 56, 57, 59, 69, 70, 76, 77, 78, 94, 97, 100, 133, 170, 173, 203, 206, 214, 224, 294, 295, 296, 303, 309, 320, 359, 364
fluctuant, 305
fluctuations, 57
fluid, 54, 62, 65, 137, 296
fluoroscopy, 93, 127, 128, 130, 131, 132, 134, 135, 136
fluoxetine, 119
flushing, 299, 300
focusing, 29, 366, 368
folic acid, 323, 330
food, 251, 297, 298, 366, 376
Food and Drug Administration (FDA), 108, 110, 122, 174, 306
Ford, 181, 184, 185, 196, 197, 272
Fox, 30, 35, 98, 117, 182, 309, 316, 362
fracture, 138, 325
frameshift mutation, 9, 24, 44
Framingham study, 46, 66
France, 257, 297
free radical, 174, 180
free radicals, 174, 180
freedom, 121
Freedom of Information Act (FOIA), 79
friction, 130, 131, 246
functional aspects, 226
funds, 288
fungal, 247
fungal infection, 247
fungi, 322

G

gait, 51, 253, 254
ganglion, 18, 51
gastric, 297
gastrointestinal, 49, 252, 340
gastrointestinal tract, 49, 252
gender, x, xi, xv, 9, 13, 15, 27, 36, 135, 145, 146, 152, 153, 157, 158, 161, 162, 163, 169, 175, 177, 189, 250, 268, 272, 273, 276, 289, 290, 333, 334, 335, 336, 337, 338, 339, 340, 341, 342, 343, 344, 345, 346, 360, 384
gender differences, 146, 152, 153, 157, 158, 161, 169, 333, 342, 346
gender effects, 146, 152
gender role, 339
gene, 7, 8, 9, 11, 12, 13, 16, 17, 19, 20, 21, 23, 24, 25, 26, 27, 28, 29, 30, 31, 32, 33, 34, 37, 38, 39, 40, 41, 42, 43, 44, 52, 68, 214, 250, 253, 260, 273
gene expression, 30
general anesthesia, 327
General Health Questionnaire, 149, 150, 152, 150, 164
general practitioner, 103, 263
general practitioners, 103, 263
generation, 5, 6, 135, 174, 216, 319
generators, 325
genes, 5, 6, 7, 9, 10, 13, 15, 16, 19, 21, 26, 28, 29, 30, 31, 44, 335
genetic mutations, 5
genetic testing, 36, 254
genetics, 223
Geneva, 179
genome, 17, 246
genotype, 14, 15, 16, 17, 21, 36
genotypes, 14, 21, 35
gentamicin, 239
geriatric, 114, 120, 121, 122
germline mutations, 28
Gestalt, 96
gestation, 255
Gibbs, 100, 238
gingival, 185, 193, 199
gingivitis, xii, 183, 185, 193, 199
girls, 220
glaucoma, 103
global networks, 321
glossitis, 251
glossopharyngeal nerve, 47
glucose, xvi, 334, 365, 367, 368, 369, 372, 373, 375, 377, 379, 388

glycation, 316
glycogen, 249
glycoprotein, 249
glycosylation, 308
goals, 234, 327
gold, xi, 167, 177, 226
gold standard, xi, 167, 177, 226
gout, 103
government, 78, 220
grafting, xiv, 275, 280, 281, 282, 283, 285, 287, 289, 290, 291, 339, 340, 341, 345, 346
grafts, 128, 205, 333, 340, 342
grain, 366
Gram-negative, 184
Gram-positive, 184
granulomas, 245, 253
gravity, 52
GroEL, 185, 196
groups, xii, xiv, 52, 65, 135, 139, 150, 151, 152, 170, 173, 178, 183, 184, 185, 186, 188, 189, 190, 191, 192, 194, 195, 204, 208, 210, 211, 231, 246, 268, 275, 277, 279, 281, 286, 288, 323, 334, 336, 368, 373
growth, xiii, 199, 207, 214, 219, 234, 303, 323, 325, 383
growth factor, 199, 214
guidance, 142
guidelines, xiii, 180, 181, 219, 221, 231, 233, 235, 279, 289, 290, 312, 314, 348, 362
Guillain-Barré syndrome, 50
guilt, 109
gynecologist, 323

H

H_2, 241
HADS, 149, 150
haematocrit, 66
half-life, 65, 93, 172, 177, 260, 266, 297, 300, 301, 309
hallucinations, 148
haloperidol, 118
handling, 26
hands, 132
haplotype, 43
happiness, 157
harm, 117, 211
harmful effects, 160
Harvard, 101
hazards, 371
HBV, 246
HDL, 170, 335, 372, 382
headache, 59, 65, 300
healing, 206, 207, 212, 213
health, xv, 77, 103, 112, 118, 120, 146, 153, 154, 156, 157, 158, 160, 161, 162, 164, 165, 166, 168, 169, 193, 220, 226, 230, 263, 291, 317, 318, 319, 321, 329, 330, 333, 366, 367, 372, 373, 377
health care, 77, 103, 263, 319, 321
health care costs, 77, 263
health information, 373
health problems, 154
health services, 118, 165, 291
health status, 146, 153, 154, 156, 157, 158, 160, 161, 162, 164, 165, 220
healthcare, 117
hearing, 11, 32, 300, 312
hearing loss, 300, 312
heart, vii, viii, ix, x, xi, xiv, xv, xvi, 3, 4, 5, 6, 9, 13, 16, 17, 18, 23, 24, 26, 29, 30, 31, 32, 33, 34, 36, 37, 38, 39, 41, 42, 44, 45, 46, 47, 48, 49, 51, 52, 53, 54, 55, 56, 58, 60, 61, 62, 63, 67, 68, 69, 70, 71, 75, 76, 78, 79, 80, 81, 82, 83, 87, 91, 92, 94, 95, 96, 97, 98, 99, 100, 101, 102, 103, 104, 105, 106, 107, 108, 109, 110, 111, 112, 113, 114, 115, 116, 117, 118, 119, 120, 121, 122, 123, 125, 126, 143, 145, 146, 147, 149, 151, 153, 155, 157, 158, 159, 161, 162, 163, 164, 165, 166, 167, 169, 171, 173, 175, 177, 178, 179, 180, 181, 182, 183, 184, 185, 194, 195, 196, 197, 198, 199, 201, 203, 216, 217, 219, 221, 222, 223, 224, 236, 238, 243, 244, 245, 246, 247, 248, 249, 250, 251, 252, 253, 254, 255, 256, 257, 258, 259, 260, 261, 262, 263, 264, 265, 266, 267, 269, 270, 271, 272, 273, 274, 275, 276, 279, 280, 282, 285, 287, 288, 289, 293, 294, 295, 302, 303, 304, 309, 310, 311, 312, 313, 314, 316, 317, 318, 319, 320, 321, 322, 323, 324, 325, 326, 327, 329, 330, 331, 332, 333, 336, 339, 340, 341, 342, 344, 345, 346, 347, 349, 356, 359, 360, 362, 363, 364, 365, 366, 367, 369, 372, 376, 377, 378, 381, 382, 383, 384, 386, 387, 388, 389, 390
heart block, 110, 111, 248, 257, 327
heart disease, vii, viii, ix, x, xi, xiv, xvi, 23, 26, 36, 42, 45, 46, 47, 52, 53, 55, 60, 63, 99, 101, 102, 106, 107, 113, 114, 115, 119, 121, 145, 146, 149, 155, 158, 163, 164, 165, 166, 169, 183, 184, 194, 195, 196, 197, 199, 211, 221, 245, 247, 251, 256, 259, 260, 262, 264, 267, 269, 272, 310, 311, 316, 317, 318, 320, 322, 323, 330, 331, 336, 344, 359, 365, 366, 367, 369, 376, 377, 383, 386, 388
heart failure, xiv, 98, 104, 112, 118, 119, 120, 121, 177, 178, 182, 221, 222, 238, 249, 251, 252, 253, 254, 255, 256, 257, 258, 259, 260, 261, 262, 263, 264, 265, 266, 267, 269, 270, 271, 272, 273, 274, 280, 282, 285, 287, 294, 295, 302, 303, 304, 310, 313, 317, 318, 321, 322, 342, 346
heart rate, 5, 6, 9, 17, 18, 24, 44, 49, 51, 52, 54, 61, 62, 68, 79, 105, 107, 115, 116, 117, 121, 122, 223, 224, 251, 302, 304, 309, 314, 320, 359, 360, 382
heartbeat, 176
heartburn, 300
heat, xi, 51, 183, 196, 197, 198, 199, 200
heat shock protein, xi, 183, 196, 197, 198, 199, 200
height, 220, 226, 227, 228, 229, 232, 239, 367, 369, 372
Helicobacter pylori, 196
hematological, 247

hemiplegia, 279, 280, 282, 285, 287
hemochromatosis, 245, 250, 257
hemodialysis, 269
hemodynamic, 78, 98, 255, 262, 302, 305, 306, 309, 314, 319, 320, 322, 324, 327, 337, 364
hemodynamic effect, 302
hemodynamics, 70, 266, 303, 313, 319, 324
hemoptysis, 256
hemorrhage, 49, 248
hemorrhages, 248
hemostasis, 302
Heparin, 238
hepatitis, 246, 256
hepatitis B, 246
hepatomegaly, 251
hepatosplenomegaly, 247
hERG, 32
heritability, 162
herpes, 246
herpes simplex, 246
herpes virus, 246
herpes zoster, 246
heterogeneity, 210
heterogeneous, 9, 21, 147, 260
high density lipoprotein, 310
high fat, 297
high risk, 18, 23, 38, 108, 110, 112, 173, 177, 182, 195, 240, 267, 270, 276, 277, 279, 281, 288, 293, 309, 319, 322, 323, 324, 342, 368
high-density lipoprotein, 211
high-fat, 298
hip, 113, 372
hips, 250
histamine, 110
histological, 249, 252
HIV, 102, 246, 256, 306
HIV/AIDS, 102
homeostasis, 54, 105, 296
homocysteine, 170, 172
homology, 172, 184
Honda, 200
Hong Kong, 196
hopelessness, x, 102, 107, 109, 113
hormone, 102, 114, 177, 260
hormones, 270
horse, 247, 257
hospital, x, 46, 61, 82, 83, 101, 103, 106, 112, 116, 117, 118, 120, 122, 126, 131, 166, 178, 264, 269, 270, 276, 277, 278, 283, 284, 285, 288, 289, 290, 318, 319, 327, 338, 339, 343, 345, 369, 381
hospital anxiety and depression scale, 166
hospital stays, 289, 345
hospitalization, x, 57, 63, 101, 106, 116, 121, 222, 238, 264
hospitalizations, 151, 303
hospitalized, 119, 264, 344
hospitals, 231, 277
host, 185, 248
hostility, 107, 148, 149, 150, 151
House, 113, 116
HRS, 71
HSP, xi, xii, 183, 185, 186, 187, 190, 191, 193, 194, 195, 196
HSP60, xi, xii, 183, 184, 185, 186, 187, 189, 190, 191, 192, 193, 194, 195
human, xi, xii, 32, 34, 35, 40, 41, 42, 43, 44, 66, 68, 97, 179, 180, 183, 184, 186, 187, 191, 194, 195, 196, 197, 198, 199, 200, 246, 257, 271, 273, 295, 305, 313, 316
human brain, 273
human immunodeficiency virus, 246
human subjects, 199
humans, 39, 69, 126, 203, 239
hybrid, 320
hydration, 326, 327
hydro, 224, 233
hydrolysis, 173
hydrophilic, 224, 233
hydroxide, 188
hygiene, 184, 321
hyperacidity, 103
hyperactivity, 105
hypercholesteremia, 336
hypercoagulable, 256
hyperemia, 97, 303
hyperglycemia, 333
hyperkeratosis, 251
hyperlipidemia, 310, 379
hyperplasia, 204, 208
hypersensitive, 66
hypersensitivity, vii, 45, 48, 49, 52, 57, 60, 63, 67, 70, 301
hypertension, x, xiv, 51, 57, 65, 66, 67, 72, 101, 105, 121, 170, 221, 222, 249, 252, 255, 259, 270, 274, 286, 293, 294, 295, 302, 304, 305, 310, 313, 314, 315, 319, 320, 322, 326, 327, 331, 336, 366, 367, 368, 378, 379, 382, 383, 384
hypertensive, xiii, 51, 243, 252, 304, 305, 310, 370, 373
hypertrophic cardiomyopathy, 246, 249, 257
hypertrophy, 244, 249, 250, 254, 257, 267, 274, 307, 336, 339, 382
hyperventilation, 55, 56, 57
hypocapnia, 47, 55, 56, 57
hypokalemia, 13, 65, 254
hypokinesia, 351, 352, 354, 355, 357
hypomagnesemia, 254
hypoperfusion, 54, 56
hypotension, vii, viii, 45, 46, 47, 48, 49, 51, 56, 57, 65, 66, 67, 70, 72, 108, 110, 111, 296, 299, 301, 327
hypotensive, 49, 72, 301
hypotensive drugs, 49
hypothalamic, 49
hypothalamus, 47
hypothermia, 251
hypothesis, xiii, 52, 66, 69, 119, 184, 194, 208, 219, 231, 233, 264

hypothyroidism, 16, 103
hypoventilation, 56, 253
hypoventilation syndrome, 253
hypovolemic shock, 69
hypoxemia, 271, 315, 322, 326
hypoxia, 47, 69, 168, 265, 314

I

iatrogenic, 208
ideal body weight, 225, 239
identification, 17, 25, 29, 32, 52, 60, 62, 68, 135, 136, 168, 177, 198, 289, 362
identity, 235
idiopathic, xiii, 24, 26, 27, 64, 243, 244, 257, 258, 263, 270, 305, 314, 326
idiopathic pulmonary hypertension, 314
IFN, 171, 173
IgG, xii, 14, 183, 184, 185, 187, 188, 189, 190, 192, 193, 194, 195
IKr, 5, 7, 11, 12, 19, 31, 34, 44
IKs, 5, 7, 8, 9, 11, 12, 13, 19, 20, 31, 34, 42
IL-1, 173
IL-6, 172, 173
ileostomy, 102
Illinois, 212
IMA, xi, 167, 174, 180
images, viii, ix, xv, 76, 78, 79, 80, 81, 82, 83, 86, 87, 92, 93, 94, 96, 98, 99, 127, 128, 129, 134, 137, 141, 142, 347, 349, 350, 351
imaging, viii, ix, xiv, xv, 75, 76, 77, 78, 79, 80, 82, 87, 88, 93, 95, 96, 97, 98, 100, 134, 142, 177, 243, 250, 253, 255, 264, 303, 319, 320, 347, 349, 350, 353, 356, 362, 363, 364
imaging modalities, 319, 320
imaging techniques, 264, 349
imbalances, 17
immersion, 227
immune reaction, 198
immune response, xii, 106, 119, 183, 193, 194, 197, 199
immune system, 106, 119, 376
immunity, 118, 198
immunoassays, 266
immunoglobulin, 198, 258
immunoglobulin G, 198
immunohistochemical, 173
immunology, 195, 196, 199
immunomodulatory, 204
immunoreactivity, 120
immunosuppression, 106
immunosuppressive, 252
implantable cardioverter defibrillators (ICD), 3, 18, 21, 26, 253, 318, 324, 325
implants, 320
impotence, 50, 250, 310, 311, 316
impulsive, 115
impulsiveness, 107, 111
in situ, 260
in utero, 38
in vitro, 17, 118, 174, 214, 266, 388
in vivo, 97, 117, 142, 260, 266
inactivation, 5, 11, 27, 38
inactive, 260, 266
incentive, 226
incidence, ix, xvi, 12, 21, 60, 63, 76, 86, 98, 102, 111, 116, 168, 207, 208, 210, 238, 247, 252, 253, 255, 258, 264, 300, 309, 318, 323, 325, 326, 335, 365, 366, 367, 368, 369, 376, 377, 378, 379
inclusion, 104, 208, 246, 277, 318, 368
inclusion bodies, 246
income, 369
incubation, 247, 248
incubation period, 247, 248
independent variable, xv
India, 330
Indian, 330
indication, viii, 45, 63, 132, 207, 301, 306, 325, 361, 383
indicators, 289, 346, 359
indices, 108, 191
individualization, xiii, 219, 222, 223, 226, 227, 231, 236
inducer, 301, 306
induction, 22, 48, 54, 63, 296, 306
industrialized countries, 104
industry, 222, 226
inertia, 138
infants, 16, 17, 18, 249, 319
infarction, xi, 81, 82, 86, 91, 92, 116, 167, 175, 178, 180, 182, 240, 255, 261, 262, 267, 269, 273, 311, 340, 366, 368, 369, 376, 377, 378, 383, 387, 388
infection, xv, 172, 184, 194, 196, 197, 198, 246, 247, 248, 251, 256, 317, 322, 324, 340
infections, 51, 194, 196, 197, 246, 247, 248, 256, 372, 376, 377
infectious, xiii, 243, 245, 248
infertility, 253
inflammation, xi, xii, xvi, 98, 172, 183, 184, 185, 194, 195, 197, 198, 199, 252, 253, 260, 365
inflammatory, xi, xiii, 64, 77, 78, 94, 120, 168, 169, 171, 172, 183, 184, 194, 195, 197, 203, 206, 213, 243, 248, 376
inflammatory cells, 171
inflammatory disease, 77, 184
inflammatory mediators, 172
inflammatory response, 169, 203, 206, 213, 376
inflammatory responses, 213
inflation, 203
influenza, 246
informed consent, 79
infrastructure, 321
ingestion, 71, 248
inheritance, 23, 26, 253, 323
inherited, 4, 5, 6, 24, 25, 28, 30, 31, 36, 39
inherited disorder, 6

inhibition, 30, 137, 233, 299, 300, 301, 303, 313, 314, 386
inhibitor, 39, 66, 72, 179, 213, 247, 261, 296, 297, 299, 301, 302, 304, 305, 309, 312, 316, 387, 388
inhibitors, xiv, 50, 108, 121, 173, 262, 294, 295, 296, 297, 299, 300, 301, 303, 309, 311, 312, 314, 323
inhibitory, 297
inhibitory effect, 297
initiation, xi, 5, 110, 167, 172
injection, 79, 93, 98, 132, 136, 143, 214
injections, 129, 323
injuries, 107
injury, viii, ix, 23, 76, 77, 78, 81, 82, 86, 90, 102, 172, 180, 199, 203, 213, 214, 255, 259, 264, 334, 335
innate immunity, 195
inner ear, 11
innervation, 51, 52, 55, 57, 68
iNOS, 316
insertion, 27, 85, 127, 213, 260
insight, ix, 67, 76
insomnia, 109
instability, 51, 174, 337
institutions, 135, 139, 279, 283
instruction, 126, 321
instruments, 113, 146, 147, 150, 152, 156, 157, 163, 168, 187, 188, 266
insulin, 173, 249, 253, 372, 388
insulin resistance, 173, 253, 372
insurance, 226, 318, 321
integration, 128, 130, 131, 140, 327
integrity, xii, 201
intensity, 250
intensive care unit, 66, 320, 338
interaction, 13, 28, 29, 33, 69, 70, 111, 306, 316, 318, 370
interactions, 4, 111, 212, 297, 299, 302
intercellular adhesion molecule, 372
interface, 126
interference, 29, 157
interferon, 106, 171
interferon gamma, 171
interleukin-1, 106, 115, 118
internal environment, 171
internalizing, 150
internet, 97
internist, xv, 317, 329
interpersonal relations, x, 101, 106, 161
interpersonal relationships, x, 101, 106, 161
interpretation, 86, 92, 95, 96, 97, 230, 319, 320, 350, 356, 363
interstitial, 62, 173, 249, 251, 253, 255, 296, 306
interstitial lung disease, 306
interval, 8, 10, 15, 18, 24, 60, 61, 108, 224, 264, 270, 299, 304, 305
intervention, ix, xv, xvi, 6, 23, 29, 76, 77, 93, 96, 121, 128, 141, 142, 143, 170, 173, 175, 177, 178, 195, 202, 210, 211, 215, 238, 239, 276, 288, 295, 317, 319, 320, 321, 322, 327, 328, 333, 334, 365, 366, 367, 368, 372, 376, 378, 379, 383
interview, 113, 151
interviews, 147
intestine, 102
intimacy, 161
intracellular signaling, 296
intracerebral, 378
intracranial, 54, 69
intramuscular, 65
intramyocardial, 136
intraocular, 59
intraocular pressure, 59
intraoperative, 338, 339
intrauterine growth retardation, 323
intravascular, 65, 77, 206, 335
intravenous, 79, 110, 118, 240, 327, 340, 363
intrinsic, xii, 54, 201, 336
introns, 17
invasive, 47, 62, 63, 65, 174, 175, 177, 240, 320, 329, 383, 387
inversion, 53, 111
Investigations, 93, 245, 247, 249, 251, 253, 255, 257
investment, 139
ion channels, 3, 5, 6
ionic, 6, 26, 33
ions, 4, 5, 174, 274, 290
iris, 51
iron, 180, 250, 257, 326
iron deficiency, 326
irradiation, 128, 131, 135, 141, 214, 255, 258
irritability, 106, 111
irritation, 371
ischaemia, 23, 174, 175, 180, 349, 364
ischaemic heart disease, 362
ischemia, viii, ix, xi, 53, 76, 77, 78, 81, 82, 86, 87, 90, 92, 93, 94, 95, 96, 97, 99, 167, 168, 174, 180, 259, 307, 309, 347, 348, 351, 359, 360, 362, 364, 382, 388
ischemic, viii, xiii, xv, 45, 47, 86, 96, 99, 108, 113, 196, 205, 211, 243, 261, 265, 267, 300, 304, 308, 309, 316, 326, 347, 356, 364, 382, 388
ischemic heart disease, 99, 113, 211, 316, 388
isoforms, 175, 295
isolation, 246
isotope, 78, 79, 80, 81, 82, 83, 85, 86, 89, 91, 92, 93, 94, 96
Isotope, 91, 92
isotopes, viii, 75, 78, 93, 95
isozyme, 300
isozymes, 297, 302
Israel, 41, 129
Italy, 45, 101, 114, 201
iteration, 132

J

JAMA, 66, 71, 72, 73, 216, 238, 240, 311, 313, 315, 316
January, 103, 112, 277, 338, 344, 345
Japan, 12, 31, 106, 118, 243
Japanese, 246, 272, 330
Jefferson, 216
Jordan, 67, 68, 70, 71, 73
judge, 127
Jun, 257, 258, 379, 380
Jung, 123
jury, 81, 82
justification, 239

K

K^+, 5, 9, 12, 16, 26, 36, 39, 44
kidney, 252, 262, 269, 386, 387
kidneys, 52, 252
killing, vii
kinase, 176, 181
Kinase, 181, 218
kinetics, 21, 98, 99
King, 183, 185, 217, 276, 290
knockout, 32

L

labeling, 301, 306
labor, 322
laboratory studies, 244
lactate dehydrogenase, 174, 176
lactic acid, 251
lamellar, 250
lamina, 170, 171
laminar, 170
language, 162
larvae, 248
latency, 369
later life, 115, 369
Latin-American countries, 247
LDL, 170, 171, 172, 173, 185, 335, 382
lead, viii, x, 13, 15, 16, 21, 22, 25, 26, 29, 30, 45, 47, 52, 76, 93, 95, 106, 111, 112, 125, 131, 136, 138, 146, 151, 194, 208, 228, 229, 231, 246, 248, 250, 251, 253, 255, 266, 318, 325, 328, 334
lean body mass, 251
learning, 135, 137, 139
left atrium, vii, 3
left ventricle, vii, 3, 67, 252, 261
left ventricular, ix, xiv, 48, 66, 76, 79, 86, 90, 91, 92, 98, 122, 143, 177, 181, 182, 244, 248, 249, 250, 251, 253, 254, 256, 257, 259, 260, 263, 264, 265, 267, 270, 271, 272, 273, 274, 278, 289, 302, 303, 309, 313, 322, 324, 336, 339, 341, 342, 347, 362, 363, 382
leisure, xvi, 365, 367, 369, 373
lesions, ix, 76, 78, 86, 128, 132, 133, 134, 135, 136, 138, 140, 141, 143, 168, 170, 185, 203, 205, 215, 216, 247, 248, 250, 252, 295, 320, 322, 326, 334, 335, 349
leukemia, 239
leukocyte, 195
LIFE, 367, 378
life expectancy, 169, 222, 238
lifestyle, 46, 169, 170, 366, 376, 377, 378, 379
lifestyle changes, 169, 366
life-threatening, 31, 62, 63, 248
lifetime, 6, 163
likelihood, 11, 246, 265, 284
limbic system, 47
limitation, xii, 93, 201, 262, 320, 356, 361
limitations, ix, 28, 76, 82, 96, 132, 153, 154, 155, 156, 157, 159, 162, 220, 225, 228, 263, 320, 356
linear, 136, 225, 231, 233, 284
links, 311
linoleic acid, 377
lipid, 169, 170, 171, 172, 179, 224, 250
lipids, 249
lipophilic, 224, 228, 298
lipoprotein, 172, 173, 179, 211, 293, 310, 335, 344
lipoproteins, 172, 179
liquor, 366
lithium, 111, 114, 117, 122, 255
liver, 102, 250, 251, 252, 254, 256, 279, 280, 282, 285, 287, 297, 388
liver disease, 250, 254, 280, 282, 285, 287, 297
liver failure, 388
localization, 7, 12, 34, 99, 349
location, 27, 32, 175, 212, 334, 335
locus, 11, 16, 23, 25, 26, 27
London, 37, 39, 41, 167, 183, 187, 239
longitudinal studies, 291
long-term, x, 46, 104, 111, 112, 114, 115, 118, 123, 145, 147, 153, 162, 195, 200, 205, 207, 211, 213, 254, 255, 258, 263, 264, 266, 272, 276, 295, 303, 314, 333, 337, 338, 339, 340, 342, 345, 346, 379
lordosis, 253
loss of consciousness, vii, viii, 45, 46, 47, 48, 52, 54, 56, 59, 61, 62, 70
loss of libido, 50
low molecular weight, 240
low risk, 64, 277, 281
low-density, 198, 211
low-density lipoprotein, 198, 211
low-density lipoprotein receptor, 198
LPO, 80
lumbar, 253, 323
lumen, 78, 83, 93, 171, 202, 203, 206, 207, 212, 214, 383
luminal, 173, 206, 338
lung, ix, xv, 76, 79, 80, 81, 87, 91, 95, 98, 103, 272, 297, 305, 306, 307, 317, 320, 323, 326, 327, 376

lung cancer, 376
lung disease, 103, 272, 306, 307
lungs, vii, 3, 252
lupus, 245, 252, 258
lupus erythematosus, 102, 245, 252
lymph, 247
lymphadenopathy, 247
lymphocyte, 246, 252
lysine, 27, 180
lysis, 185, 194

M

macrophage, 170, 171, 173, 179, 185, 194
macrophages, 171, 173
magnet, 126, 130, 137, 138
magnetic, x, 125, 126, 127, 128, 130, 131, 132, 133, 134, 135, 136, 137, 138, 141, 142, 143, 177, 250, 257, 319, 320, 348
magnetic field, x, 125, 126, 128, 130, 133, 137, 138, 141
magnetic resonance, 177, 250, 257, 319, 348
magnetic resonance imaging, 177, 250, 319
magnets, x, 125, 126, 137, 138
maintenance, xiii, 49, 54, 82, 131, 219, 225, 236, 237, 303, 329
major depression, 102, 103, 104, 105, 107, 112, 114, 115, 118, 119, 123, 163
major depressive disorder, 117, 120, 149
males, xi, 9, 15, 50, 145, 146, 152, 153, 157, 158, 159, 160, 161, 162, 169, 175, 183, 225, 226, 228, 229, 232, 250, 300, 301, 315, 336, 340
malignancy, 247
malignant, 39, 41, 102, 340
malnutrition, 251, 254, 258
management, xv, 23, 29, 30, 35, 38, 63, 65, 66, 68, 71, 79, 92, 94, 96, 112, 117, 168, 169, 178, 180, 181, 182, 198, 216, 240, 256, 257, 279, 280, 282, 283, 284, 285, 287, 290, 295, 306, 313, 314, 317, 318, 319, 322, 323, 324, 326, 327, 328, 329, 333, 348, 349, 362
mania, 109, 112
manipulation, 127, 130
manpower, xv, 317, 318, 319, 321, 329
manufacturer, 80, 176
MAO, 50
mapping, 130, 136, 143, 373
Marfan syndrome, 322
marital status, 160, 165
market, xii, 139, 201, 295
market penetration, 139
marketing, 226, 234
Massachusetts, 293, 307, 310
maternal, 36, 255, 322, 323, 326
matrix, 80, 171, 172, 173, 179
matrix metalloproteinase, 173
maturation, 323
meals, 49, 64, 65, 297
measurement, 60, 115, 134, 137, 147, 172, 174, 175, 176, 177, 178, 227, 250, 269, 270, 272, 274, 306, 363
measures, 64, 153, 156, 157, 226, 227, 305, 326, 330, 366, 372
meat, 247, 248, 257, 366
mechanical properties, 54
media, 203
median, 186, 188, 189, 190, 191, 192, 193
mediators, 55, 172
medical care, 321
medication, 23, 108, 110, 111, 113, 237, 260, 276, 300, 314
medications, 23, 108, 109, 111, 116, 122, 255, 300, 301, 302, 304, 305, 321
medicine, x, xii, xiii, 78, 87, 93, 95, 97, 102, 107, 114, 115, 116, 118, 119, 120, 121, 122, 123, 174, 196, 201, 202, 208, 219, 222, 224, 256, 291, 312, 332, 348
medulla, 118
membranes, 173
men, vii, x, xiv, xv, xvi, 21, 46, 68, 102, 103, 116, 121, 122, 160, 169, 197, 199, 220, 221, 226, 254, 257, 258, 275, 276, 277, 278, 279, 280, 281, 283, 284, 286, 288, 290, 293, 294, 295, 297, 298, 300, 304, 305, 307, 308, 309, 310, 311, 314, 315, 316, 333, 334, 335, 336, 337, 338, 339, 340, 341, 342, 343, 345, 346, 365, 366, 367, 368, 369, 370, 372, 373, 376, 377, 378, 379, 380
meningitis, 248
meningoencephalitis, 247, 248
mental health, 110, 113, 156, 157, 373
mental health professionals, 113
mental illness, 112
mental retardation, 8, 12, 249
meta-analysis, 113, 114, 120, 122, 123, 207, 208, 210, 211, 216, 228, 308, 315, 364, 367, 378
metabolic, xiii, xvi, 17, 54, 59, 173, 219, 221, 225, 227, 233, 243, 249, 303, 306, 334, 335, 365, 372, 376, 380
metabolic syndrome, xvi, 173, 221, 365, 372, 376, 380
metabolism, 54, 69, 99, 106, 115, 118, 225, 230, 297, 301
metabolite, 260, 297
metalloproteinase, 179
metals, 174
metastases, 246
metastatic, 246
methionine, 172
metric, xiii, 219, 221, 226, 227, 228, 237
Mg^{2+}, 16
mice, 27, 43, 184, 185, 198, 334, 335
microbial, xi, xii, 183, 184, 185, 186, 187, 189, 190, 194, 197, 198, 199
microbiota, 196
microscopy, 250
microvascular, 249, 307
middle class, 369

middle-aged, 118, 377
migraine, 52
migration, 213, 214, 261
milk, 366
miniaturization, 203
Minnesota, 303
minority, 111
miRNAs, 30
misconception, 93
misconceptions, 78, 162
mitochondria, 176
mitochondrial, 98, 99, 197, 249
mitral, 244, 246, 250, 252, 253, 260, 264, 265, 273, 320, 322, 360, 361, 362, 364
mitral regurgitation, 246, 253, 360, 361, 362, 364
mitral stenosis, 264, 273, 322
mitral valve, 244, 250, 252, 260, 320, 322
MMP-2, 173
MMP-3, 173
MMP-9, 173
MMPs, 173
modalities, 29, 169, 246, 319, 320, 348, 349
modality, 276, 310, 359
modeling, 224, 235, 237, 240
models, 38, 137, 141, 142, 184, 213, 223, 224, 239, 279, 284, 285, 287, 334, 335, 374, 375
modifier gene, 15
modulation, 49, 54, 55
molecular mechanisms, 26, 33
molecular mimicry, 185
molecular weight, 240
molecules, 3, 29, 31, 233
monoclonal, 173
monoclonal antibodies, 173
monocyte, 199
monocytes, 194
monomeric, 260
mononuclear cell, xii, 172, 183, 187, 199
mononuclear cells, xii, 172, 183, 187, 199
monotherapy, 304, 314
mood, x, 102, 103, 104, 109, 111, 112, 117
mood disorder, x, 102, 103, 104, 112
morbidity, ix, xiii, 26, 93, 94, 101, 103, 104, 107, 112, 114, 115, 120, 122, 153, 219, 221, 249, 259, 276, 304, 313, 319, 322, 324, 325, 345, 368, 378
morning, 51, 65, 304, 305
morphology, 22, 24, 136
mortality, viii, ix, xii, xiii, xiv, xv, xvi, 25, 45, 46, 63, 93, 94, 101, 102, 104, 107, 112, 113, 114, 115, 116, 118, 119, 122, 123, 153, 164, 168, 169, 177, 178, 181, 195, 196, 201, 207, 209, 210, 211, 215, 219, 220, 221, 226, 235, 238, 249, 259, 263, 264, 265, 269, 270, 271, 275, 276, 277, 279, 286, 288, 289, 290, 304, 309, 310, 313, 319, 320, 322, 324, 333, 334, 335, 336, 337, 338, 339, 340, 341, 342, 343, 345, 365, 366, 367, 368, 369, 376, 377, 378, 381, 383, 384, 387
mortality rate, 104, 112, 178, 210, 211, 215, 276, 277, 337, 341, 366, 369
mortality risk, 114, 226
MOS, 166
motion, 92, 95, 244, 309, 348, 350, 351, 352, 353, 354, 355, 356, 360, 363
motivation, 109
motor function, 157
mountains, 94
mouse, 30, 34, 335
mouse model, 335
movement, 126, 129, 132, 136, 138, 203, 356
MPI, viii, 75, 76, 77, 78, 79, 82, 84, 86, 92, 93, 94, 95, 96
MRI, 16, 58, 319, 320
mRNA, 11, 29, 30, 32, 177
mucosa, 248, 252
multidimensional, 153, 315
multidisciplinary, 57, 327
multiple myeloma, 51, 98
multiple sclerosis, 102
multivariate, 278, 279, 284, 288, 376
murmur, 246
muscle, 8, 12, 26, 27, 49, 55, 68, 106, 169, 170, 171, 172, 174, 175, 176, 180, 203, 213, 214, 220, 226, 227, 230, 244, 248, 249, 251, 253, 254, 261, 294, 296, 297, 300, 302, 303, 316
muscle atrophy, 251
muscle cells, 55, 170, 171, 203, 296, 303
muscle contraction, 26, 175
muscle mass, 227
muscle tissue, 226
muscle weakness, 253
muscles, 65, 253, 357
muscular dystrophy, 43, 253, 258
musculoskeletal, 252
mutant, 9, 11, 29, 32, 35, 39
mutation, 6, 9, 10, 11, 12, 13, 15, 16, 17, 18, 19, 20, 21, 22, 24, 25, 26, 27, 28, 29, 31, 32, 33, 34, 35, 37, 38, 39, 40, 41, 42, 43, 44, 249
mutations, 5, 6, 8, 9, 10, 11, 12, 13, 16, 18, 21, 22, 23, 24, 25, 26, 27, 28, 29, 30, 31, 32, 33, 34, 37, 38, 39, 40, 41, 42, 44, 68, 250, 253
myalgia, 247, 299
Mycobacterium, 186
myeloma, 50, 51, 98
myocardial infarction, vii, viii, x, xi, xii, xiv, 30, 53, 61, 76, 77, 78, 86, 90, 96, 99, 101, 104, 112, 116, 118, 119, 121, 122, 123, 167, 168, 169, 174, 176, 180, 185, 195, 197, 199, 201, 205, 209, 238, 240, 245, 249, 257, 259, 261, 263, 264, 269, 271, 272, 273, 294, 311, 316, 336, 338, 363, 373, 374, 375, 377, 378, 379, 383, 386, 387
myocardial ischemia, ix, xvi, 60, 63, 76, 77, 180, 208, 252, 315, 347, 348, 362, 381, 382, 383, 386, 388
myocardial necrosis, xi, 167, 175, 246, 263
myocarditis, 111, 123, 244, 245, 246, 247, 248, 252, 255, 256, 257, 258
myocardium, viii, ix, xi, xiii, xv, 3, 13, 54, 63, 76, 78, 81, 83, 86, 88, 89, 90, 93, 94, 95, 96, 97, 99,

167, 177, 243, 246, 249, 250, 252, 253, 255, 301, 303, 347, 356
myocyte, 4, 89, 99, 174, 177
myocytes, 3, 4, 5, 26, 177
myofibril, 176
myofibrillar, 251
myoglobin, 174, 175, 176, 180
myopathy, 174, 249
myosin, 176
myositis, 248, 258
myotonic dystrophy, 245, 253, 254, 258

N

Na^+, 4, 7, 11, 12, 21, 27, 33, 39
Nash, 316
national, xii, 114, 117, 182, 201, 307, 315, 330, 369
National Institutes of Health, 237
natural, 32, 163, 179, 208, 211, 323
nausea, 51, 59, 169, 248
navigation system, 126, 142, 143
neck, 49, 102, 169
necrosis, xi, 106, 115, 167, 168, 173, 174, 175, 178, 199, 200, 246, 263, 264, 270, 348, 351, 359
negative attitudes, 161
negative emotions, 161
negative life events, 161
negative outcomes, 147
nematode, 247
neonatal, 32, 230, 271, 323
neonates, 11, 32, 260
neoplasms, 102
neoplastic, 64, 246
nephropathy, 135, 381
nerve, 68, 106, 298, 312
nerve fibers, 298
nerves, 47, 55, 254
nervous system, 47
Netherlands, 3, 129, 145, 186, 258, 382, 389
network, 29, 217, 332
neuralgia, 46, 64
neurodegeneration, 50
neurogenic, 46, 54, 55, 66, 71, 73, 308, 316
neurohormonal, 105, 260, 262, 273
neuroleptic, 110
neurological disease, 54, 59, 60, 62
neurologist, 60
neuromuscular diseases, 23
neuronal survival, 118
neurons, 65
neuropathy, 250, 307, 308
neurosyphilis, 248
neuroticism, 149, 150, 152
neurotransmitters, 106
New England, 256, 276, 290, 342, 343
New Jersey, 101
New Orleans, 379
New York, 97, 100, 114, 116, 118, 120, 240, 302, 312, 333, 336
next generation, 214
NHS, 167
Ni, 316
Nielsen, 33, 34, 120, 263, 272, 382, 389
nifedipine, 223
nitrate, 61, 98, 314
nitrates, 296, 299, 301, 309, 316
nitric oxide, 47, 294, 296, 299, 302, 303, 305, 308, 311, 313
Nitric oxide (NO), 213, 294, 296, 297, 299, 300
nitric oxide synthase, 294, 294, 311
nocturnal polyuria, 73
noise, 7, 11, 12, 16, 175
non-invasive, viii, 56, 75, 77, 130, 319, 320, 329, 348
non-linear, 233
non-smokers, xii, 183, 188, 189, 191, 194
norepinephrine, 50, 51, 52, 65, 66, 68, 73, 106, 108, 115, 118, 264
normal, 6, 9, 11, 12, 13, 14, 15, 16, 21, 24, 29, 51, 56, 60, 67, 68, 69, 81, 84, 92, 97, 98, 111, 154, 156, 157, 159, 160, 172, 175, 194, 196, 203, 222, 224, 225, 226, 227, 230, 231, 232, 233, 234, 237, 251, 254, 256, 260, 263, 265, 266, 269, 278, 294, 296, 313, 351, 352, 353, 354, 355, 357, 359, 362, 364, 381, 384, 386, 388
North America, 72, 256, 321, 346
Northeast, 248
Northern Ireland, 178
Norway, xvi, 365, 366, 367, 369, 376, 377, 379
novel biomarkers, 168
NPR, 261
NS, ix, 30, 76, 85, 88, 89, 91, 143, 361, 384, 387
N-terminal, xi, 25, 167, 180, 182, 266, 269, 270, 271, 272, 273, 274
nuclear, 78, 79, 83, 87, 95, 97, 348
nuclear medicine physician, 78
nucleotides, 296
nucleus, 61, 62, 115
nurse, 248
nurses, 328
nursing, 123, 327
nutrition, 366

O

obese, xiii, 219, 220, 221, 222, 224, 225, 226, 227, 228, 230, 231, 232, 233, 234, 235, 236, 237, 239, 240, 241, 249
obese patients, 230, 234, 236, 237
obesity, xiii, 168, 173, 219, 220, 221, 222, 224, 230, 234, 235, 237, 238, 239, 249, 259, 293, 319
observations, 70, 206, 365, 383, 387
obstetricians, 328
obstruction, viii, 45, 47, 260, 309
obstructive sleep apnea, 306

occlusion, 53, 130, 205, 303, 325
odds ratio, 284, 285, 287, 307
odynophagia, 247
Odyssey, 141
oedema, 260, 388
oil, 377
old age, xi, 167, 380
Omega-3, 372
oncological, 28
oncology, 226
online, 237, 238, 240, 241, 312
opacification, 363
open heart surgery, 151, 288
operator, 130, 131, 288, 320
optical, 186, 188, 190
Optical Coherence Tomography, 142
optical density, 188, 190
oral, xvi, 71, 184, 213, 297, 312, 313, 314, 323, 326, 331, 365, 372, 376, 388
oral hygiene, 184
organ, vii, xi, 3, 27, 67, 106, 167, 244, 247, 326
organic, 109, 295, 298, 300, 301, 314
organism, 247, 322
organization, 377
orientation, x, 125, 127, 128, 131, 138, 141
orthopnea, 256
orthostatic hypotension, vii, 45, 47, 50, 51, 52, 54, 56, 60, 65, 66, 67, 68, 70, 72, 73, 107, 108, 110, 252, 301
orthostatic intolerance, 57, 67, 69, 70
ostium, ix, 76, 84, 93
out-of-hospital, 116
outpatient, 328
outpatients, 164, 310
overload, 12, 14, 249, 257, 260, 262
overweight, xiii, 219, 220, 228, 237, 238
oxidation, 179, 335
oxidative, 213
oxidative stress, 213
oxide, 47, 294, 296, 299, 302, 303, 305, 308, 311, 313
oxygen, xi, 46, 167, 174, 303, 304, 313, 349
oxygen consumption, 313, 349
oxygenation, 69, 306, 314

P

PACE, 71, 72
pacemaker, 23, 24, 40, 63, 64, 72, 324, 325, 327
pacemakers, 29, 137, 253
Pacific, 248
pacing, viii, 18, 23, 38, 45, 64, 65, 72, 137, 320, 325, 329, 331
paclitaxel, 212, 213
pain, 47, 59, 78, 103, 154, 156, 157, 169, 172, 174, 182, 196, 245, 248, 253, 256, 299, 308, 311, 348, 349
palliative, 66, 318, 319, 320, 321, 322, 326
palpitations, 16, 18, 49, 51
pancreas, 254
panic attack, 109
panic disorder, 149
Pap, 271
paper, 103, 220, 239
parabolic, ix, 77, 97
paracrine, 265
paradoxical, 48, 56, 323, 327
paralysis, 8, 12, 247
parameter, 188, 224, 225, 230, 231, 239, 304
parasitic infection, 247
parasympathetic, 55
parenthood, 165
parents, 160, 323
Parkinson, 50, 51, 102, 103
paroxetine, 64, 72
paroxysmal nocturnal dyspnea, 256
particles, 171, 335
passive, 56, 62, 65, 95, 161
patent ductus arteriosus, 318
pathogenesis, 4, 28, 29, 49, 52, 56, 67, 121, 195, 199, 245, 256, 294
pathogenic, 16, 17, 27, 28, 184
pathogens, 184, 196, 197, 198
pathology, 6, 28, 199
pathophysiological, vii, 39, 47, 45, 54, 63, 67, 105, 120, 174, 177
pathophysiological mechanisms, vii, 45, 105, 120, 174
pathophysiology, 5, 21, 27, 28, 47, 67, 243, 247
pathways, viii, 29, 45, 48, 54, 60, 61, 63, 224, 296, 297, 302, 324, 325, 334
patient care, ix, 18, 76, 78, 92
patient management, 178, 329
patients, viii, ix, x, xi, xii, xiii, xiv, xv, xvi, 6, 9, 11, 12, 13, 14, 15, 16, 17, 18, 21, 22, 23, 24, 25, 26, 27, 28, 29, 30, 32, 36, 37, 38, 40, 41, 42, 43, 45, 46, 47, 50, 51, 52, 53, 56, 57, 58, 59, 60, 61, 62, 63, 64, 65, 66, 67, 69, 70, 71, 72, 73, 78, 86, 93, 96, 98, 99, 100, 101, 102, 103, 104, 105, 106, 107, 108, 109, 110, 111, 112, 113, 114, 115, 116, 117, 118, 119, 120, 121, 122, 123, 134, 135, 143, 145, 146, 147, 148, 149, 150, 151, 152, 153, 154, 155, 156, 157, 158, 159, 160, 161, 162, 163, 164, 165, 168, 169, 172, 173, 174, 175, 176, 177, 178, 179, 180, 181, 182, 183, 184, 185, 186, 187, 188, 189, 190, 192, 193, 194, 195, 196, 197, 198, 199, 201, 202, 205, 207, 208, 210, 211, 212, 215, 216, 222, 231, 234, 235, 236, 237, 240, 243, 245, 246, 247, 248, 249, 250, 251, 252, 253, 254, 255, 256, 258, 259, 261, 262, 263, 264, 265, 266, 267, 269, 270, 271, 272, 273, 274, 275, 276, 277, 278, 279, 280, 281, 282, 283, 284, 285, 286, 287, 288, 289, 290, 291, 294, 295, 297, 298, 300, 301, 302, 303, 304, 305, 306, 307, 308, 309, 310, 311, 312, 313, 314, 315, 316, 317, 318, 319, 320, 321, 322, 323, 324, 325, 326, 327, 328, 329, 330, 331, 333, 334, 335, 336, 337, 339, 340, 342, 344, 345, 347, 348, 349,

356, 359, 360, 361, 362, 363, 368, 378, 381, 382, 383, 384, 385, 386, 387, 388
Paxil, 72
PBMC, 187, 194
PCR, 246, 256
peak concentration, 263
pearls, 296
pediatric, xiv, xv, 164, 165, 317, 318, 319, 328, 329, 331
pediatric patients, xiv, 164, 317
pediatrician, xv, 317, 329
peer, 275
peer review, 275
peers, x, 145, 146, 147, 152, 155, 158, 160, 161
penetrance, 15, 24, 27
penis, 296, 316
peptic ulcer, 102, 279, 280, 285
peptic ulcer disease, 279, 285
peptide, 12, 172, 177, 182, 194, 214, 218, 260, 261, 263, 264, 265, 266, 267, 269, 270, 271, 272, 273, 274, 313
peptides, xi, xiv, 167, 168, 178, 182, 198, 259, 260, 261, 262, 263, 264, 265, 266, 267, 268, 269, 270, 271, 272, 274
percentile, 175, 375
perception, 153, 156, 159
perceptions, 154, 156
performance, 54, 114, 134, 135, 157, 159, 174, 214, 239, 286, 289, 325, 341, 348
perfusion, vii, viii, 45, 46, 53, 54, 55, 56, 57, 75, 78, 97, 98, 255, 262, 356, 362, 364
pericardial, 53, 246, 252, 255
pericardial effusion, 246
pericardial tamponade, 53
pericarditis, 246, 252
pericardium, 255
periodic, 8, 12, 319
periodontal, xi, 183, 184, 186, 189, 193, 195, 197, 198, 200, 373
periodontal disease, xi, 183, 184, 193, 195, 197, 198, 373
periodontitis, xi, 183, 184, 185, 189, 192, 193, 194, 195, 196, 197, 198, 199
periodontium, 184
Peripheral, xii, 183, 187, 282, 285, 287
peripheral blood, 199
peripheral blood mononuclear cell, 199
peripheral nerve, 254
peripheral nervous system, 252
peripheral neuropathy, 251
peripheral vascular disease, 279, 295, 311, 336, 339, 340, 341, 342
permeability, 5, 303, 376
permeation, 11
permit, 3
personal, 94, 153, 157, 160, 161, 208, 293
personal autonomy, 161
personality, 107, 109, 114, 115, 121, 147, 150, 151, 152, 153, 369
personality disorder, 107, 109
personality traits, 107, 147, 150, 151, 152, 153
PET, 96
P-glycoprotein, 99
pH, 187
pharmaceutical, 108, 211, 295
pharmaceutical companies, 108
pharmacokinetic, 223, 239, 306
pharmacokinetics, 73, 239, 297, 300, 310
pharmacological, 22, 39, 72, 115, 174, 203, 212, 237, 348, 349, 356
pharmacology, xiv, 120, 240, 294
pharmacotherapy, xiii, 220
pharyngitis, 246, 247
phenothiazines, 255
phenotype, 9, 11, 13, 17, 24, 27, 28, 29, 33, 35, 40, 43
phenotypes, 9, 11, 12, 27, 28, 29, 33, 34, 35
phenotypic, 21, 327
Philadelphia, 30, 67, 69, 179, 330
philosophy, xii, 201
phlebotomy, 250
phobic anxiety, 148, 152
phone, 61
phosphate, 187
phosphodiesterase, xiv, 294, 295, 311, 312, 313, 314
Phosphodiesterase inhibitors, 312
phospholipids, 173
photoreceptor, 297
photoreceptor cells, 297
phototransduction, 296
phylogeny, 184
physical activity, xvi, 24, 65, 251, 262, 365, 366, 367, 373, 376, 380
physical aggression, 107
physical exercise, xi, 24, 59, 167, 369, 383
physical health, 154, 156, 157
physicians, xiii, 71, 103, 104, 113, 122, 126, 169, 234, 240, 243, 291, 321, 328, 333
physics, 93
physiological, xiii, 49, 64, 107, 219, 268, 296, 305, 322, 348
physiology, 118, 199
pig, 213, 247
pigs, 134, 213
pilot study, 37, 163, 270, 297
pituitary, 297, 301
pituitary gland, 297, 301
placebo, 64, 65, 66, 71, 72, 73, 300, 303, 304, 306, 307, 308, 309, 312, 313, 316, 331, 368, 372
planning, 321
plaque, xi, 167, 168, 170, 171, 172, 173, 178, 179, 184, 193, 199, 204, 208, 260, 295, 335
plaques, 170, 173, 179, 184, 197, 203, 293, 383
plasma, 49, 50, 52, 105, 107, 115, 172, 173, 174, 182, 214, 224, 225, 250, 251, 262, 263, 266, 268, 269, 270, 271, 272, 273, 299, 301, 305, 377
plasma levels, 270, 273, 299, 301
plasminogen, 172, 372

platelet, 108, 111, 171, 172, 213, 296, 327
platelet aggregation, 213
platelet count, 111
platelet-activating factor, 179
platelets, 106, 296
platforms, 176, 177, 213
play, ix, xiv, xv, 28, 55, 101, 114, 131, 184, 213, 246, 259, 261, 262, 265, 296, 333, 334, 335
pleasure, 113
pneumonia, 248, 251
poisoning, 108
pollution, 376, 378
polycythemia, 327
polymer, 204, 212, 213, 214
polymer-based, 215, 216
polymers, xii, 201, 213
polymorphism, 17, 35, 37
polymorphisms, 13, 42
polypeptide, 172
polysaccharide, 214
polystyrene, 187
polyuria, 73
poor, xv, xvi, 104, 107, 137, 157, 160, 177, 179, 237, 252, 290, 307, 308, 318, 322, 323, 325, 326, 327, 336, 337, 341, 342, 345, 347, 360, 366, 381, 383
population, x, xi, xiii, 5, 17, 22, 23, 46, 54, 72, 103, 105, 109, 111, 114, 116, 119, 136, 145, 146, 147, 148, 151, 152, 153, 154, 155, 156, 158, 160, 162, 163, 164, 168, 172, 175, 177, 178, 181, 182, 197, 205, 206, 207, 210, 219, 220, 222, 223, 224, 226, 227, 228, 230, 231, 232, 233, 234, 236, 237, 239, 264, 265, 267, 272, 275, 294, 300, 304, 308, 318, 321, 324, 328, 329, 330, 365, 366, 369, 383
pore, 9, 11, 32, 40
pork, 248
portability, 319
positive correlation, 368, 369
postmortem, 247
postoperative, xiv, 275, 276, 278, 284, 286, 288, 289, 319, 338, 339, 340, 345
postoperative outcome, 289, 345
postpartum, 16, 18
postpartum period, 16, 18
post-translational, 7, 12
posture, 64, 65
potassium, 12, 13, 18, 21, 31, 32, 33, 34, 35, 388
potassium channels, 12, 13, 21, 34, 388
potatoes, 366
poverty, 318
power, 173, 210, 215, 356
preclinical, 213, 294
predictability, 377
prediction, 100, 173, 174, 175, 271, 337, 339, 340, 361, 368
predictive model, 107
predictors, xiv, xv, 103, 105, 107, 114, 115, 119, 162, 166, 208, 217, 259, 264, 273, 302, 310, 333, 334, 336, 337, 339, 340, 341, 342, 345, 376
preeclampsia, 255
pre-eclampsia, 322
pre-existing, 173, 295
preference, 96, 161
pregnancy, xv, 16, 36, 146, 160, 162, 255, 256, 317, 321, 322, 323, 324, 326, 327, 330
pregnant, 255, 322, 329
pregnant women, 255
premature contraction, 254
prematurity, 323
premium, 127
president, 100
pressure, viii, xvi, 45, 47, 49, 51, 54, 55, 56, 57, 59, 60, 61, 62, 64, 65, 66, 68, 69, 70, 79, 105, 106, 108, 117, 122, 221, 223, 224, 249, 251, 254, 260, 261, 262, 296, 301, 302, 304, 305, 306, 309, 313, 314, 349, 350, 359, 360, 364, 365, 368, 369, 371, 373, 375, 377, 378, 379, 384, 385, 386, 388
prevention, xii, xvi, 71, 72, 113, 120, 123, 173, 201, 221, 222, 311, 324, 325, 330, 345, 365, 366, 367, 369, 376
preventive, 64, 173, 255, 368
priapism, 299
primary amyloidosis, 252
primary care, 79, 110, 112, 113, 118, 177, 182, 238, 263, 270
proarrhythmia, 35
probability, 223, 235, 237, 264, 278, 349
proband, 16
probe, 127, 185, 350
problem solving, 160
procoagulant, 322
production, 54, 128, 129, 142, 171, 172, 177, 194, 213, 294, 297, 299, 300, 308
productivity, 318
progesterone, 323
prognosis, viii, xi, xiii, xvi, 40, 45, 63, 66, 167, 168, 178, 182, 243, 247, 252, 256, 271, 272, 273, 274, 291, 302, 307, 359, 381, 383
prognostic factors, xiv, 259, 263, 269
prognostic marker, 359
prognostic value, 181, 182, 264, 269, 271, 295, 359, 362
program, 226, 328, 329
proinflammatory, 105, 106, 122
prokaryotic, 184
prokaryotic cell, 184
prolapse, vii, 128, 133
proliferation, 171, 172, 191, 194, 213, 214, 261
promote, 213, 214, 335
promoter, 28, 43
promoter region, 28
propagation, 5, 6
property, 21
prophylactic, 18, 122
prophylaxis, 71, 321, 326, 327
propofol, 255
propranolol, 368
prosthesis, 203, 323
protection, 121, 265

protein, 4, 5, 6, 7, 8, 11, 12, 19, 20, 26, 28, 29, 30, 32, 35, 172, 174, 175, 176, 179, 187, 192, 195, 196, 197, 198, 199, 200, 214, 246, 247, 249, 251, 264, 298, 376, 379
protein binding, 174, 298
protein synthesis, 247
proteins, xi, 3, 4, 33, 167, 174, 175, 176, 183, 184, 195, 196, 197, 198, 200, 250, 334, 335
proteinuria, 250, 383
proteolytic enzyme, 173, 260
prothrombin, 111, 173
protocol, 61, 79, 83, 98, 222, 324, 349, 378
protocols, viii, 18, 61, 75, 76, 79, 98, 267, 348
prototype, 298
protozoa, 247
provocation, 383
proximal, viii, 45, 47, 53, 84, 85, 93, 276, 278, 280, 282
proxy, 288
psychiatric disorder, viii, 45, 47, 63, 68, 106, 120
psychiatric disorders, viii, 45, 47, 63, 68, 106, 120
psychiatric illness, 151, 164
psychiatric morbidity, 103, 120
psychiatric patients, x, 101
psychiatrist, xv, 317, 323, 329
psychological distress, 379
psychological health, 154
psychological problems, 151, 327
psychological stress, 120, 122
psychological well-being, 166
psychologist, 331
psychology, 117, 120, 327
psychopathology, 107, 147, 150, 151, 159, 163, 164, 166
psychopharmacology, 117, 120, 122
psychoses, 103
psychosocial functioning, x, xi, 145, 146, 158, 159, 161, 162
Psychosomatic, 114, 115, 116, 118, 119, 120, 121, 122, 123, 163, 166
psychotic, 151
psychoticism, 148, 152
psychotropic drug, 111, 117, 118
psychotropic drugs, 111, 117, 118
PsycINFO, 104
public, xv, 122, 321, 333
public health, 122
Public Health Service, 122
public interest, xv, 333
PUFA, 372
pulmonary artery pressure, 302, 313
pulmonary circulation, 305
pulmonary embolism, xi, 53, 167, 240
pulmonary hypertension, xiv, xv, 53, 252, 253, 294, 295, 297, 302, 305, 312, 313, 314, 315, 317, 323, 327
pulmonary vascular resistance, 302, 305, 327
pulmonic stenosis, 320
pulmonic valve, 322
pulmonologist, 273
pulse, 111, 251, 304
pumping, vii, 3
pupil, 59
Purkinje, vii, 3
P-value, 374, 375, 387
pyramidal, 254
pyrene, 199
pyrophosphate, 251

Q

QRS complex, 61
QT interval, 6, 9, 11, 12, 13, 14, 15, 16, 17, 19, 21, 28, 30, 42, 108, 110, 111, 251
QT prolongation, 12, 301
quality of life, viii, ix, 46, 63, 101, 104, 146, 153, 154, 155, 156, 157, 158, 160, 161, 162, 163, 164, 165, 209, 303, 342, 347
quartile, 178, 188, 374, 375, 376
questionnaire, 150, 151, 156, 293, 295, 307, 367, 372
questionnaires, 116, 147, 150, 156, 372
quinidine, 301
Quinones, 363

R

race, 308, 340
radiation, 132, 245, 255, 320, 361, 362
radical, 174, 298, 312
radiofrequency, 324, 331
radiotherapy, 255, 258, 298
range, xi, xiii, 21, 49, 54, 127, 135, 137, 138, 148, 149, 150, 152, 154, 155, 159, 167, 172, 176, 177, 178, 185, 186, 188, 189, 190, 191, 192, 193, 219, 221, 222, 223, 224, 225, 226, 227, 228, 229, 230, 231, 235, 237, 245, 282, 308, 329, 372, 376
raphe, 115
rat, 99, 115, 118, 334
ratings, 147, 151
RDP, 132
reactants, 172
reactive oxygen, 213, 249
reactive oxygen species, 213, 249
reactivity, 69, 70, 105, 109, 117, 194
reading, viii, 76, 86, 374, 375
reality, 95
recall, 296
receptors, 5, 41, 47, 49, 52, 61, 65, 66, 110, 260, 261, 297, 300, 334, 335
recession, 185, 186
recognition, 104, 112, 256, 308
reconstruction, 80, 129, 130, 133, 134, 136, 141, 143, 320
recovery, 11, 59, 60, 79, 80, 99, 105, 119, 120, 245
recurrence, 17, 234, 322, 323, 325
redistribution, 99

reduction, vii, viii, xvi, 11, 27, 45, 46, 47, 48, 49, 52, 53, 54, 55, 56, 57, 60, 61, 62, 63, 64, 78, 86, 95, 103, 109, 110, 132, 135, 168, 173, 174, 178, 211, 212, 213, 214, 234, 249, 264, 276, 298, 303, 304, 305, 306, 343, 357, 360, 365, 366, 367, 373, 378
refining, 202
refractory, 4, 18, 21, 53, 65, 72, 73, 256
regeneration, 213
regional, ix, xii, 17, 76, 78, 92, 97, 99, 114, 201
registries, xii, 201, 205, 207, 208, 211, 214
Registry, 36, 43, 135, 216, 217, 218, 277, 362
regression, 230, 231, 278, 285, 287, 371, 374
regression analysis, 230
regressions, 288
regular, 15, 65, 212, 314, 319, 327, 372
regulation, 13, 44, 66, 105, 118, 184, 262, 265, 303
rehabilitation, 326
rejection, 159, 161, 266, 273
relapse, 114
relationship, ix, 11, 40, 76, 79, 88, 89, 90, 91, 95, 98, 113, 115, 119, 120, 174, 190, 195, 196, 206, 220, 223, 224, 228, 231, 233, 234, 237, 239, 263, 264, 300, 306, 308, 340, 369
relationships, x, 43, 98, 101, 106, 118, 159, 161, 162, 195, 234, 239
relatives, 18, 37
relaxation, 55, 253, 294, 296, 300, 308, 316
relevance, 42, 270, 271, 311, 378
reliability, 87, 182, 270
remodeling, 30, 261, 264
remodelling, xi, 167, 213, 260, 263, 360
renal, xi, 51, 62, 83, 102, 141, 167, 178, 223, 229, 230, 235, 237, 239, 240, 250, 260, 262, 263, 266, 273, 279, 280, 282, 285, 286, 287, 297, 298, 326, 337, 339, 340, 383, 388
renal disease, 102, 279, 280, 282, 285, 286, 287, 297
renal dysfunction, 141
renal failure, 51, 178, 266, 337, 339, 340, 388
renal function, 83, 223, 230, 235, 237, 239
renin, 249, 260
repair, 166, 214, 260, 326, 327, 328, 331
reperfusion, 99, 363
replication, xii, 25, 28, 201
repolarization, 5, 12, 13, 21, 30, 35, 37, 38, 39, 111
reproduction, 160
research, vii, xi, xv, xvi, 18, 30, 111, 114, 116, 117, 118, 119, 122, 140, 153, 162, 167, 168, 169, 196, 198, 199, 213, 224, 228, 237, 291, 296, 302, 313, 327, 329, 333, 337, 342, 365, 366, 367, 372, 373, 376, 381
research and development, 296
researchers, x, xii, xv, 101, 201, 365
resection, 325
reservoirs, 213
resistance, 54, 55, 56, 57, 69, 128, 173, 251, 253, 262, 302, 305, 320, 322, 327, 372
resolution, 58, 59, 61, 107, 121, 300
resources, 131, 179, 238, 288, 318, 319, 321, 329, 349
respiratory, 99, 174, 246, 248, 266, 340, 356
respiratory failure, 340
respiratory rate, 356
response time, 138
responsiveness, 161, 249
restenosis, 202, 203, 204, 205, 206, 208, 211, 213, 214, 216, 217
restrictive cardiomyopathy, 252, 253
resuscitation, 329
retention, 50, 96, 97, 99, 212, 262
reticular activating system, vii, 45, 46
reticulum, 5, 26
retina, 59, 296, 297
retrograde amnesia, 59
returns, 256
revascularization, xiv, 202, 204, 205, 206, 208, 210, 211, 215, 275, 276, 277, 279, 286, 288, 290, 291, 333, 345, 348, 349
revolutionary, 204
rheumatic, 264, 318, 322, 330
rheumatic heart disease, 318, 322
rheumatoid arthritis, 279, 280, 282, 285, 287
rhinitis, 299
rhythm, 5, 6, 15, 24, 26, 64, 110, 258, 314, 349
rice, 251
right ventricle, vii, 3, 271, 313, 327
rigidity, 51
rings, 246
risk, ix, x, xi, xiv, xv, xvi, 4, 9, 11, 12, 15, 16, 17, 18, 21, 23, 31, 32, 35, 37, 44, 62, 65, 76, 89, 93, 94, 96, 98, 101, 102, 103, 104, 105, 106, 107, 108, 109, 110, 111, 112, 113, 114, 115, 116, 117, 118, 119, 120, 122, 133, 135, 138, 151, 160, 161, 167, 168, 170, 172, 173, 176, 178, 181, 182, 183, 184, 185, 194, 195, 196, 197, 200, 207, 209, 211, 212, 221, 226, 233, 234, 236, 237, 238, 254, 255, 257, 258, 259, 263, 264, 265, 267, 270, 271, 272, 275, 276, 277, 278, 279, 280, 281, 282, 283, 284, 285, 286, 287, 288, 289, 293, 294, 295, 301, 307, 309, 310, 311, 312, 313, 315, 316, 319, 321, 322, 323, 324, 325, 326, 327, 328, 330, 333, 334, 335, 336, 337, 338, 339, 340, 342, 343, 346, 359, 360, 361, 362, 365, 366, 367, 368, 369, 370, 371, 372, 373, 374, 375, 376, 377, 378, 379, 381, 382, 383, 384, 386, 387, 388
risk assessment, xi, 112, 167, 168, 272, 327, 342
risk factors, xi, xiv, xv, xvi, 98, 105, 111, 115, 118, 165, 168, 170, 183, 184, 221, 238, 255, 259, 263, 275, 277, 288, 293, 295, 307, 310, 311, 321, 322, 323, 330, 333, 334, 335, 336, 337, 339, 340, 365, 366, 367, 368, 369, 370, 372, 373, 375, 376, 377, 378, 379
risk profile, 334, 335, 336
risks, 110, 113, 160, 162, 276, 279, 346, 349, 371
RNA, 44
roadmap, 130
robotic, 320
ROI, 78, 80, 82, 83, 88, 94, 95
Rome, 101

room temperature, 187, 188
Rouleau, 115, 272
rural, 288
Russia, 321

S

SA node, 328
sadness, 109
safety, xii, xiv, 107, 108, 120, 143, 201, 202, 207, 210, 213, 215, 294, 303, 309, 315, 316, 348, 361
saline, 79, 187
Salmonella, 256
salt, 64, 65, 251
sample, x, 102, 103, 147, 148, 149, 150, 151, 152, 154, 155, 156, 157, 182, 187, 269, 367, 372
sampling, 223, 231, 323
sand, 236
sarcoidosis, 253, 258
satisfaction, 163
saturation, 250, 327
Saudi Arabia, 11
scaffold, 203
scalar, 227, 228
scaling, 227
Scandinavia, 166
scar tissue, 138
scarcity, 231
SCD, 5, 16, 18, 324
scheduling, 278
schizophrenia, 110, 114
schizophrenic patients, 110
Schmid, 269
school, 166, 220, 356, 366, 376
scintigraphy, 98, 100
scores, 105, 136, 148, 149, 308, 337
search, 68, 104, 209, 213
search terms, 104
searches, 104
second generation, 215
secrete, 171
secretion, 54, 199, 265, 300
sedative, 108
sedatives, 50
sedentary, 68
seeding, 214
seizure, 103
seizures, 24
selecting, 111, 237
selective serotonin reuptake inhibitor, 72, 108
selectivity, 296, 297, 306
self-care, 305
self-confidence, 159
self-esteem, x, 102, 106, 149, 152, 159
self-report, 113, 150, 156
self-reports, 150, 152, 158
self-worth, x, 102, 106
senescence, 37
senile, 252
sensitivity, viii, xi, xiv, xv, 9, 31, 52, 65, 75, 77, 86, 93, 148, 152, 167, 174, 175, 177, 259, 262, 296, 347, 348, 350, 356, 363
sepsis, 51, 251, 340
septum, 244, 246
sequelae, 151, 245, 319, 321, 327, 328
series, 135, 176, 187, 245, 366
serology, 246
serotonergic, 108, 110
serotonin, 47, 66, 72, 106, 108, 115, 118, 121
serum, xii, xiv, xvi, 34, 52, 105, 170, 172, 180, 181, 183, 184, 185, 186, 187, 188, 189, 190, 192, 193, 194, 195, 197, 198, 199, 200, 239, 245, 248, 250, 259, 263, 264, 266, 274, 293, 297, 326, 334, 335, 365, 367, 368, 369, 372, 373, 375, 376, 377, 378, 379, 388
serum albumin, 180
services, 103, 104, 118, 169, 291, 321, 328
severity, xiv, 12, 29, 51, 78, 94, 96, 97, 109, 122, 180, 200, 211, 259, 260, 262, 264, 277, 278, 289, 293, 307, 308, 327, 334, 335
sex, 152, 155, 157, 158, 160, 226, 227, 239, 263, 270, 276, 278, 279, 280, 281, 283, 286, 289, 339, 345
sex steroid, 239
sexual activity, 157, 293, 305, 307
sexual behavior, 160
sexual health, 165
sexual intercourse, 298
shape, 130
shares, xi, 172, 183
sheep, 188, 213
shock, xi, 69, 137, 183, 195, 196, 197, 198, 199, 200, 337
shocks, 325
shoot, 79, 80
shortage, 366
shortness of breath, 169, 177, 262, 271
short-term, 104, 112, 286, 338, 348, 376
shoulder, 171, 173
shunt surgery, 325
shunts, 320, 322, 325
sibling, 323
siblings, 323
sick sinus syndrome, 24, 40, 250
side effects, 60, 65, 110, 111, 213, 296, 297, 300, 321
SIDS, 16, 17, 25, 36, 41
Siemens, 129
sign, xvi, 39, 59, 108, 247, 251, 253, 263, 311, 381
signaling, 296, 303, 335
signaling pathway, 296
signalling, 29
signals, 5, 47, 48, 56, 61, 169
significance level, 84, 188
signs, 43, 50, 59, 111, 159, 247, 251, 252, 253, 265

sildenafil, 295, 296, 297, 298, 300, 301, 302, 303, 304, 305, 306, 307, 308, 309, 312, 313, 314, 315, 316, 331
simulation, 240
sine, 16
Singapore, 315
sinoatrial node, 27
sinus, 6, 12, 15, 20, 23, 24, 25, 27, 32, 40, 46, 47, 49, 52, 58, 64, 111, 122, 250, 273, 320, 324, 325, 327, 328
sinus rhythm, 64, 273
sites, 21, 59, 126, 174, 185, 187, 212, 214, 252, 264, 276, 335
Sjogren, 52
skeletal muscle, 8, 12, 174, 175, 176, 180, 248, 249, 253, 254, 303
skills, 112, 328, 329
skin, 159, 247, 248, 250, 251, 252
SLE, 252
sleep, 7, 9, 11, 51, 103, 105, 109, 155, 306
sleep disorders, 103, 109
small intestine, 297
smoke, 199
smokers, xii, 183, 185, 186, 188, 189, 191, 194, 198, 200, 341, 368, 373
smoking, xi, xii, xvi, 168, 183, 184, 188, 189, 194, 221, 293, 310, 336, 365, 366, 367, 368, 369, 372, 373, 375, 378, 379
smoking cessation, 366, 367, 368
smooth muscle, 55, 169, 170, 171, 172, 203, 213, 214, 261, 294, 296, 297, 302, 303, 316
smooth muscle cells, 55, 170, 171, 203, 296, 303
SND, 24, 27
SNP, 13, 14, 17, 27, 28
SNPs, 17, 27, 28, 29
SNS, 13
social activities, 154, 156, 157
social adjustment, 321
social factors, 373
social integration, 327
social policy, 114
social psychology, 114, 115, 121
social relations, 113
social status, 369
social support, 161, 166
social work, 317, 329
sodium, 4, 5, 7, 8, 11, 13, 19, 20, 21, 22, 23, 27, 30, 33, 34, 35, 37, 40, 42, 43, 111, 188, 213, 260
sodium hydroxide, 188
software, 80, 82, 84, 126, 129, 132, 134, 135, 137, 140, 188
solutions, xii, xiii, 201, 202
somatic complaints, 148, 152
somatic mutations, 28
somatization, 148, 152
somatostatin, 114
South America, 247, 321
South Asia, 28
Southeast Asia, 21
Spain, 347
spastic, 99
spatial, 350
species, xi, 17, 183, 184, 185, 198, 213, 248, 249, 294
specificity, viii, xi, xiv, xv, 75, 77, 93, 167, 174, 175, 177, 259, 347, 348, 356, 363
SPECT, 80, 98, 99, 100, 362
spectrum, xi, xiii, 35, 40, 167, 193, 219, 237, 326
speculation, 305
speech, 51
speed, 28, 132, 349
sphincter, 300
spillovers, 51
spinal cord, 102, 254
sporadic, 24, 28
sports, 146, 326
spouse, 150
SSS, 23, 24
stability, 7, 12, 33, 173, 180, 214
stabilization, 131
stabilizers, 111
stable angina, 197, 211, 215, 278, 288, 309, 316, 342, 349, 362
stages, xi, 105, 109, 110, 113, 134, 167, 168, 264, 363, 366
standard deviation, 282
standard model, 4
standardization, 230
Staphylococcus, 322
statin, 173, 195
statins, 173, 311, 386
statistical analysis, 231
statistics, 178, 237, 238, 291
steady state, 17, 225
steel, 127, 212
Stem cell, 136
stem cells, 137
STEMI, 178
stenosis, vii, viii, xii, 76, 78, 83, 87, 88, 90, 91, 97, 163, 201, 215, 257, 276, 278, 281, 295, 319, 320, 322, 328, 348, 353, 354, 355, 358, 383
stenotic lesions, 86, 326
stent, ix, xii, 76, 85, 133, 134, 135, 136, 138, 141, 142, 201, 202, 203, 204, 206, 207, 208, 209, 210, 211, 212, 213, 214, 215, 216, 217, 218
sterilisation, 214
sternocleidomastoid, 49
sternum, 79
steroid, 239
steroid hormone, 239
steroid hormones, 239
steroids, 252
stiffness, 51, 253, 304
stimulus, 7, 12, 48
STO, 271
stock, 65
stomach, 297
stomatitis, 185

storage, 62, 173, 245, 249, 257
storms, 18
strain, 356, 363, 366, 367, 369
strategies, xiii, 24, 30, 64, 114, 131, 133, 139, 219, 220, 222, 233, 235, 236, 237
stratification, 33, 62, 181, 182, 264, 269, 270, 313, 324, 348, 362
strength, 151, 295
stress, viii, ix, xv, 7, 9, 16, 24, 25, 37, 58, 60, 70, 75, 76, 78, 79, 80, 81, 82, 85, 86, 89, 92, 93, 94, 95, 96, 98, 99, 100, 105, 114, 117, 120, 122, 198, 199, 213, 260, 261, 294, 295, 309, 311, 321, 322, 324, 327, 347, 348, 349, 351, 354, 355, 356, 359, 360, 362, 363, 364, 366, 367, 369, 371, 372, 379
stress echocardiogram, 363
stressors, 17, 105, 356
stretching, 260, 262
stroke, 26, 221, 264, 309, 336, 339, 340, 366, 368, 369, 370, 376, 377, 378, 384, 387
strokes, 168, 378
structural defect, 318, 325
students, 107
subacute, 207
subarachnoid hemorrhage, 369
subcutaneous tissue, 220
subgroups, 204, 205, 211, 215, 362
subjective, 146, 153, 154, 156, 157, 158, 161, 162, 166
substance abuse, 112
substances, 13, 54, 213, 214
substrates, vii, xii, 45, 201, 301
success rate, 132, 134, 135, 324
sudden infant death syndrome, 34, 36, 37, 38, 39, 41
suffering, xiv, 62, 63, 106, 193, 306, 317
sugar, 307, 366
suicidal, x, 101, 102, 103, 104, 106, 107, 108, 109, 110, 111, 113, 118, 119, 122
suicidal behavior, x, 101, 102, 106, 108, 109, 113, 118, 119
suicidal ideation, 107, 108, 110, 113
suicide, x, 101, 102, 103, 104, 106, 107, 108, 109, 110, 111, 112, 113, 114, 115, 116, 117, 118, 119, 120, 121, 122
suicide attempters, 103, 112, 122
suicide attempts, 114, 116
suicide rate, 109, 114
sulphur, 172
summer, 248
Sun, 33, 42, 266, 273, 307, 315, 343
superiority, 134, 135, 174, 213
supplements, 372, 379
supply, xi, 46, 141, 167, 174, 308, 321, 376
suppression, 12, 24, 199, 204, 251
supraventricular arrhythmia, 6
supraventricular tachycardia, 327
surface area, 225, 239, 335, 338
surface modification, 213
Surgeon General, 112, 122
surgeons, 71, 202, 276, 277, 288, 289, 320, 321, 328, 329, 333, 343, 344
surgeries, 318, 321, 327, 329
surgery, xiv, xv, 23, 51, 71, 94, 102, 105, 110, 117, 142, 151, 162, 163, 164, 165, 202, 247, 253, 265, 270, 275, 276, 277, 278, 279, 280, 281, 283, 284, 286, 287, 288, 289, 290, 291, 294, 317, 319, 320, 321, 324, 325, 326, 327, 328, 330, 331, 333, 334, 335, 336, 337, 339, 340, 341, 342, 343, 344, 345, 346
surgical, xiv, xv, 146, 159, 161, 162, 164, 166, 178, 202, 275, 276, 277, 286, 288, 289, 317, 318, 319, 320, 321, 324, 325, 326, 329, 333, 334, 335, 336, 337, 340, 346
surgical intervention, 178, 317, 319
surgical resection, 325
survival, x, xi, 114, 116, 118, 119, 145, 146, 167, 177, 178, 224, 240, 252, 264, 272, 273, 276, 277, 288, 289, 326, 336, 339, 340, 341, 342, 346, 359, 361, 384, 385
survival rate, x, 145, 177, 264
surviving, 165, 367
survivors, 164, 245, 258, 372, 377
susceptibility, 17, 27, 198
swallowing, 47
Sweden, 216, 290, 381
swelling, 247, 248
switching, 109
sympathetic, vii, 9, 13, 31, 38, 42, 45, 47, 48, 49, 51, 52, 55, 57, 62, 65, 66, 68, 69, 105, 106, 108, 118, 260, 262
sympathetic denervation, 38, 42
sympathetic fibers, 47
sympathetic nervous system, 13, 68, 105, 262
symptom, vii, 18, 25, 45, 46, 57, 59, 63, 148, 178, 208, 302, 307, 383
symptoms, 12, 16, 18, 21, 23, 24, 26, 28, 49, 50, 51, 57, 58, 59, 60, 61, 62, 64, 66, 67, 70, 105, 109, 111, 113, 114, 115, 118, 121, 122, 123, 147, 148, 150, 151, 152, 153, 155, 157, 159, 163, 164, 169, 177, 194, 211, 215, 248, 252, 253, 254, 255, 256, 260, 265, 275, 294, 295, 300, 310, 336, 341, 342, 346, 348, 350, 356, 367, 383
syndrome, xi, xv, 4, 6, 9, 10, 12, 14, 15, 17, 18, 20, 21, 22, 23, 30, 31, 32, 33, 34, 35, 36, 37, 38, 39, 40, 42, 43, 44, 47, 50, 51, 52, 53, 57, 67, 68, 70, 96, 150, 167, 168, 172, 179, 240, 246, 253, 254, 260, 262, 265, 266, 271, 310, 317, 322, 323, 324, 326, 327, 331, 338, 376
synergistic, 296, 301
synthesis, 11, 40, 172, 214, 247, 296
syphilis, 248, 249
systemic circulation, 296
systemic lupus erythematosus, 102, 252
systemic sclerosis, 102
systems, 52, 61, 126, 129, 134, 137, 143, 244
systolic blood pressure, 49, 60, 368, 369, 373, 375, 388
systolic pressure, 251, 305

T

T cell, 171, 184, 194, 195, 198
T cells, 171
tachycardia, 5, 6, 7, 12, 16, 20, 23, 24, 25, 26, 41, 42, 51, 52, 54, 61, 62, 68, 70, 111, 251, 253, 260, 324, 325, 327, 331
tachycardia-bradycardia syndrome, 23
task force, 66, 180, 314, 326
TdP, 6, 14, 15
Tea, 67
teachers, 329
team members, 327
technetium, 78
technician, 87
technicians, 87
technology, x, xv, 93, 125, 131, 132, 134, 135, 137, 139, 140, 141, 142, 176, 177, 202, 213, 320, 321, 347, 348, 356
teenagers, 78
teens, 318
teeth, xi, 8, 12, 183, 185, 186, 376
telephone, 11, 110, 113
temperature, 187, 376
tendons, 227
Tennessee, 257
tension, 371
termination codon, 29
territory, 351
test statistic, 281, 283
testes, 297, 301
testosterone, 334
tetralogy, 163, 165, 331
Tetralogy of Fallot, 156, 318, 319
TGF, 265
thallium, 99, 362
theory, 49, 52, 207, 230, 239
therapeutic approaches, 29, 120
therapeutic interventions, 72
therapeutics, 121
therapy, 13, 15, 17, 18, 21, 23, 24, 29, 36, 63, 64, 71, 72, 73, 102, 110, 113, 121, 173, 185, 195, 207, 210, 211, 213, 214, 215, 217, 222, 223, 231, 234, 237, 239, 241, 247, 249, 250, 252, 255, 257, 258, 264, 265, 271, 274, 296, 304, 305, 306, 307, 309, 310, 312, 314, 320, 324, 325, 331, 362
Thiamine, 245, 251
thiazide, 368
thoracic, 159, 341
thoracotomy, 163, 325
thorax, 62
thought problems, 148
threat, 169
threatened, 107, 161
threatening, 57, 62
three-dimensional, 228, 364
threshold, 288, 309
thrombin, 213, 214
thromboembolic, 222, 233, 236, 240, 314, 315
thromboembolism, 221, 240, 247, 306
thrombolytic therapy, 238
thrombomodulin, 372
thrombosis, xii, 106, 168, 171, 172, 195, 197, 198, 201, 206, 207, 208, 211, 214, 215, 216, 217, 218, 248, 252, 255, 260, 319, 323, 325, 328
thrombotic, 320, 326
thrombus, 128, 171, 203, 206, 208, 260, 325
thyrotoxicosis, 322
time, xii, xiii, xiv, xvi, 4, 21, 25, 27, 29, 49, 64, 77, 78, 82, 83, 89, 94, 95, 96, 102, 104, 105, 107, 109, 111, 112, 119, 125, 130, 131, 132, 134, 135, 136, 137, 139, 141, 173, 180, 192, 194, 201, 202, 203, 209, 210, 212, 214, 219, 221, 224, 225, 226, 264, 275, 276, 277, 278, 279, 281, 283, 284, 286, 287, 288, 290, 291, 295, 297, 300, 301, 306, 307, 309, 311, 320, 322, 326, 334, 336, 348, 349, 350, 356, 365, 366, 369, 375, 380, 382, 383, 388
time consuming, 137
timing, 265, 269, 276, 288, 319
tin, 176
tinnitus, 300
tissue, xi, xiii, xv, 130, 138, 167, 168, 170, 174, 175, 180, 184, 194, 202, 203, 219, 220, 224, 225, 226, 227, 230, 245, 249, 250, 251, 260, 296, 297, 303, 305, 316, 347, 359, 363, 376
Titan, 127
titration, 236
TLR, 210
TMP, 13
TNF, 265
tobacco, 194, 198, 199, 342, 368, 376, 379
tobacco smoke, 194, 198, 199, 376, 379
Tokyo, 243
tolerance, 55, 64, 65, 69, 71, 302, 307, 316, 326
tonsillitis, 246
tort, 141
total cholesterol, 172, 335, 372
toxic, xiii, 51, 212, 243, 245, 294
toxicity, 111, 120, 123, 180, 223, 234, 247, 301
toxin, 178, 247
toxoplasmosis, 246
trace elements, 251
tracers, ix, 77, 78, 97
tracking, 363
trade, 209, 295
tradition, 202
traffic, 151
trainees, 327, 328
training, xv, 97, 112, 127, 157, 181, 317, 321, 326, 328, 329, 332, 350, 361
traits, x, 102, 107, 109, 147, 149
trajectory, 130, 133
trans, 329
transcatheter, 142
transcription, 177
transcripts, 32
transducer, 350

transduction, 300
transferrin, 250
transforming growth factor, 199
transfusion, 338
transfusions, 338
transgenic, 27
transgenic mice, 27
transient ischemic attack, viii, 45, 47
transition, 105, 172, 174, 321, 327
transition metal, 174
transition period, 327
transition rate, 105
transitional countries, 169
transitions, 115
translation, 30, 177
translational, 174
translocation, 5
transmembrane, 9
transmission, 17, 160, 247, 250
transplant, 266, 272, 329
transplantation, xv, 252, 253, 266, 270, 273, 317, 320, 326, 383
transport, 99, 217, 335
trastuzumab, 255, 265
trauma, xi, 51, 167, 175, 325
traumatic events, 151
travel, 248
treatable, 151, 246
tremor, 51
trend, 117, 136, 168, 303, 304, 324, 369, 377
Treponema denticola, 373, 375
trial, xv, 27, 38, 65, 71, 72, 122, 127, 168, 169, 177, 178, 195, 207, 208, 215, 216, 230, 240, 303, 304, 306, 307, 308, 312, 313, 314, 315, 316, 317, 367, 368, 372, 377, 378
trial and error, 127
tricuspid valve, 260, 324
tricyclic antidepressant, 107, 255
tricyclic antidepressants, 107, 255
trigeminal, 47
triggers, vii, 31, 45, 59, 64
triglyceride, 334
triglycerides, xvi, 365, 367, 368, 369, 372, 373, 375, 378, 382
Triglycerides, 371
trust, 208
tubular, 250
tumor, 106, 115, 199, 200, 264
tumor necrosis factor, 106, 115, 199, 200, 264
tumour, 173, 270
two-dimensional, 142, 364
two-way, 304
type 1 diabetes, 308, 384
type 2 diabetes, 116, 221, 238, 293, 307, 308, 315
type 2 diabetes mellitus, 293, 315

U

ubiquitous, 199, 296
ulcer, 282, 287
ulcerative colitis, 102
ultrasonography, 315
ultrasound, 77, 97, 303, 335
uncertainty, 64, 109, 300
underlying mechanisms, 49, 64
uniform, 15, 212, 213
United Kingdom, 167, 168, 169, 220, 307, 383
United States, vii, xiii, 162, 169, 219, 220, 234, 318
univariate, 336, 341, 376
university students, 107
unmasking, 16, 17, 94
unstable angina, 168, 176, 177, 180, 181, 240, 336
upper respiratory tract, 246
urbanization, 169
uric acid, 326, 368, 378
urinary, 50, 51, 59, 103, 118, 251, 384
urinary retention, 50
urine, 250, 381
urology, 73

V

vagus, 48
vagus nerve, 48
validation, 162, 164, 289, 291, 364
validity, viii, 75, 77, 78, 86
values, xiv, 9, 51, 56, 57, 172, 181, 188, 207, 228, 229, 230, 231, 235, 259, 263, 264, 265, 268, 271, 368, 375
valvular heart disease, xiv, 255, 259, 267, 274, 309, 320
variability, 28, 43, 105, 107, 108, 115, 116, 117, 121, 122, 123, 212, 223, 227, 231, 239
variable, xv, 6, 18, 109, 194, 231, 237, 249, 279, 284, 286, 288, 308, 333, 334, 375
variables, x, 98, 113, 145, 146, 263, 279, 324, 359, 372, 373
variation, xv, 17, 21, 27, 29, 44, 54, 68, 187, 276, 279, 333, 366
vascular disease, 279, 280, 282, 285, 287, 294, 295, 308, 311, 319, 331, 336, 339, 340, 341, 342
vascular inflammation, xvi
vascular prostheses, 214
vascular system, 170
vasculature, 56, 66, 213, 214, 294
vasculitis, 252
vasoconstriction, 48, 54, 55, 56, 57, 62, 65, 69, 70, 108, 260, 262, 303
vasoconstrictor, 334
vasodilatation, 48, 54, 55, 260, 388
vasodilation, 48, 49, 55, 62, 65, 97, 294, 296, 299, 303, 304, 306, 311, 313
vasodilator, 296, 304, 305, 313, 320

vasomotor, 251, 294
vasopressin, 47, 66
vasospasm, 96
vasovagal syncope, 49, 51, 57, 59, 61, 64, 65, 67, 69, 70, 71, 72
vector, 126, 247
vegetable oil, 377
vegetables, 366
VEGF, 214
vein, viii, 45, 47, 52, 128, 129, 133, 205
velocity, 57, 69, 70, 271, 304, 359, 364
venlafaxine, 108, 117, 122
venous pressure, 254
ventilation, 303, 327
ventricle, 319, 325, 326, 382
ventricles, vii, 3, 4, 5, 6, 260
ventricular arrhythmia, xiv, 5, 11, 12, 21, 23, 24, 41, 105, 106, 254, 317, 324, 340, 348
ventricular arrhythmias, xiv, 5, 11, 12, 21, 23, 24, 41, 105, 106, 254, 317, 324, 348
Ventricular fibrillation (VF), 5, 18, 21, 24, 106
ventricular septal defect, xiv, 157, 163, 259, 264, 318
ventricular septum, 254
ventricular systolic dysfunction, xv, 260, 320, 324
ventricular tachycardia, 5, 6, 12, 16, 20, 23, 26, 41, 42, 52, 54, 61, 111, 253, 324, 331
venue, 305
verapamil, 71, 223
Vermont, 162
versatility, 128
vertebral artery, viii, 45, 47, 53, 58
vertebrobasilar, viii, 45
vertigo, 300
vessels, xi, xii, 55, 56, 57, 95, 128, 129, 130, 132, 136, 141, 142, 167, 172, 177, 201, 276, 296, 308, 338, 341, 345, 348
Victoria, 186, 187
violent, 112
viral infection, 246
viral myocarditis, 245, 246
virus, 246, 256
virus infection, 256
viruses, 245, 246
viscera, 220
visible, 61, 130, 133, 159
vision, 49, 59, 248, 299, 300, 356
visualization, 320
vitamins, 251
VLDL, 170
vomiting, 59, 248
VSD, 318, 320, 322, 326, 328
vulnerability, 28

W

waiting times, 281, 282, 283
waking, 73
Wales, vii, 120
walking, 306, 349
war, 366, 376
war years, 366
warfarin, xiii, 220, 222
water, 212, 251, 260, 262
wavelengths, 93
weakness, 248, 253
wear, 203
weight gain, 111
weight loss, 373
weight reduction, 365
Weinberg, 257, 289, 345
wellbeing, 102, 146, 153, 162, 166
wells, 188
wheelchair, 51
wild type, 9
wires, 127, 132, 133, 134, 135, 137, 138, 142
witnesses, 59
women, x, xiv, xv, xvi, 18, 46, 102, 103, 107, 118, 122, 160, 169, 177, 197, 220, 221, 226, 250, 255, 258, 275, 276, 277, 278, 279, 280, 281, 283, 284, 286, 288, 289, 290, 323, 324, 330, 333, 334, 335, 336, 337, 338, 339, 340, 341, 342, 343, 344, 345, 346, 349, 365, 366
work activity, 46
workforce, 332
workload, 222
workstation, 129
World Health Organization, 155, 156, 164, 165, 176, 178, 179, 220, 221, 237, 256, 306
World War, 366, 376
worms, 248
worry, 165
wound infection, 340
writing, 295

X

X-linked, 250, 253

Y

yield, ix, 28, 61, 77, 94, 121, 193, 319
young adults, 108, 163, 164, 165, 166, 170, 272
young men, 21, 373
young women, 163, 336

Z

zinc, 174
zoonosis, 256